Hacker & Moore's

E S S E N T I A L S   O F

OBSTETRICS & GYNECOLOGY

03/01/20

Hacker & Moore's

ESSENTIALS OF
OBSTETRICS & GYNECOLOGY

Neville F. Hacker, MD

Professor of Gynaecologic Oncology
Conjoint, University of New South Wales
Director, Gynaecological Cancer Centre
Royal Hospital for Women
Sydney, Australia

Joseph C. Gambone, DO, MPH, Executive Editor

Professor Emeritus of Obstetrics and Gynecology
David Geffen School of Medicine at UCLA
Attending Physician, Ronald Reagan UCLA Medical Center
Clinical Professor of Obstetrics and Gynecology
Western University of Health Sciences
College of Osteopathic Medicine of the Pacific
Private Infertility and Reproductive Endocrinology Practice, Durango, Colorado

Calvin J. Hobel, MD

Miriam Jacobs Chair in Maternal-Fetal Medicine
Cedars-Sinai Medical Center
Professor of Obstetrics and Gynecology
Professor of Pediatrics
David Geffen School of Medicine at UCLA
Los Angeles, California

Sixth Edition

ELSEVIER

ELSEVIER

1600 John F. Kennedy Blvd.
Ste 1800
Philadelphia, PA 19103-2899

HACKER & MOORE'S ESSENTIALS OF OBSTETRICS & GYNECOLOGY, SIXTH EDITION
INTERNATIONAL EDITION

ISBN: 978-1-4557-7558-3

ISBN: 978-0-323-34053-3

Notices

Knowledge and best practice in this field are constantly changing. As new research and experience broaden our understanding, changes in research methods, professional practices, or medical treatment may become necessary.

Practitioners and researchers must always rely on their own experience and knowledge in evaluating and using any information, methods, compounds, or experiments described herein. In using such information or methods they should be mindful of their own safety and the safety of others, including parties for whom they have a professional responsibility.

With respect to any drug or pharmaceutical products identified, readers are advised to check the most current information provided (i) on procedures featured or (ii) by the manufacturer of each product to be administered, to verify the recommended dose or formula, the method and duration of administration, and contraindications. It is the responsibility of practitioners, relying on their own experience and knowledge of their patients, to make diagnoses, to determine dosages and the best treatment for each individual patient, and to take all appropriate safety precautions.

To the fullest extent of the law, neither the Publisher nor the authors, contributors, or editors, assume any liability for any injury and/or damage to persons or property as a matter of products liability, negligence or otherwise, or from any use or operation of any methods, products, instructions, or ideas contained in the material herein.

Previous editions copyrighted 2010, 2004, 1998, 1992, and 1986.

Library of Congress Cataloging-in-Publication Data

Hacker & Moore's essentials of obstetrics & gynecology / [edited by] Neville F. Hacker, Joseph C. Gambone, Calvin J. Hobel.—6th edition.
     p. ; cm.
   Hacker and Moore's essentials of obstetrics and gynecology
   Essentials of obstetrics and gynecology
   Preceded by Hacker and Moore's essentials of obstetrics and gynecology / [edited by] Neville F. Hacker, Joseph C. Gambone, Calvin J. Hobel.
   Includes bibliographical references and index.
   ISBN 978-1-4557-7558-3 (pbk. : alk. paper)–ISBN 978-0-323-34053-3 (international edition)
   I. Hacker, Neville F., editor. II. Gambone, Joseph C., editor. III. Hobel, Calvin J., editor. IV. Title: Hacker and Moore's essentials of obstetrics and gynecology. V. Title: Essentials of obstetrics and gynecology.
   [DNLM: 1. Obstetrics–methods. 2. Genital Diseases, Female. 3. Pregnancy Complications. WQ 100]
   RG101
   618—dc23

2015035364

Acquisitions Editor: James Merritt
Developmental Editor: Julia Rose Roberts
Publishing Services Manager: Catherine Jackson
Project Manager: Rhoda Howell
Design Manager: Renee Duenow
Illustrations Manager: Nichole Beard
Marketing Manager: Melissa Darling

Working together
to grow libraries in
developing countries

www.elsevier.com • www.bookaid.org

Printed in Canada

Last digit is the print number: 9 8 7 6 5 4 3 2

This edition is dedicated to our wives,
Estelle Hacker, Marge (Morris) Gambone, and Marsha Lynn Hobel.

Their understanding and support for the time and effort required
to complete this project was *essential*.

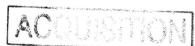

Contributors

Carolyn J. Alexander, MD
Southern California Reproductive Center
Beverly Hills, California;
Clinical Associate Professor
David Geffen School of Medicine at UCLA
University of California, Los Angeles
Los Angeles, California

Jonathan S. Berek, MD, MMS
Laurie Kraus Lacob Professor
Chair, Department of Obstetrics and Gynecology
Stanford University School of Medicine
Director, Stanford Women's Cancer Center
Director, Stanford Health Care Communication
    Program
Stanford, California

Lony C. Castro, MD, FACOG
Professor of Obstetrics & Gynecology
Specialist Maternal-Fetal Medicine
College Mentor, Dept. of Medical Education
California University of Science and Medicine,
    College of Medicine (CalMed-COM)
Colton, CA

Sara Churchill, MD
Resident Physician
Department of Obstetrics and Gynecology
Cedars Sinai Medical Center
Los Angeles, California

Daniel A. Dumesic, MD
Professor, Department of Obstetrics and Gynecology
Division Chief, Reproductive Endocrinology and
    Infertility
David Geffen School of Medicine at UCLA
University of California, Los Angeles
Los Angeles, California

Michael L. Friedlander, PhD, FRACP
Conjoint Professor of Medicine
Prince of Wales Clinical School
University of New South Wales
Sydney, Australia

Brian J. Koos, MD, DPhil
Professor, Department of Obstetrics and Gynecology
David Geffen School of Medicine at UCLA
University of California, Los Angeles
Los Angeles, California

Amy R. Lamb, PhD, CNM
Nurse-Midwife and Researcher
Obstetrics and Gynecology
Cedars-Sinai Medical Center
Los Angeles, California

Anita L. Nelson, MD
Professor, Department of Obstetrics and Gynecology
David Geffen School of Medicine at UCLA
University of California, Los Angeles
Los Angeles, California;
Medical Director, Research Division
California Family Health Council
Los Angeles, California

William H. Parker, MD
Health Sciences Clinical Professor
Department of Obstetrics and Gynecology
UCLA School of Medicine
Santa Monica, California

Andrea J. Rapkin, MD
Professor of Obstetrics and Gynecology
David Geffen School of Medicine at UCLA
University of California, Los Angeles
Los Angeles, California

Bassam H. Rimawi, MD, FACOG
Department of Gynecology and Obstetrics
Division of Reproductive Infectious Diseases and
    Maternal Fetal Medicine
Emory University School of Medicine
Atlanta, Georgia

Ingrid A. Rodi, MD
Health Sciences Clinical Professor
Director, Fertility Services
UCLA Medical Center
Santa Monica, California

Amy E. Rosenman, MD, FACOG, FPMRS
Health Sciences Clinical Professor of Obstetrics and
   Gynecology
David Geffen School of Medicine at UCLA
University of California, Los Angeles
Los Angeles, California

David E. Soper, MD
J. Marion Sims Professor
Department of Obstetrics and Gynecology
Medical University of South Carolina
Charleston, South Carolina

John Williams III, MD
Clinical Professor
Department of Obstetrics and Gynecology
David Geffen School of Medicine at UCLA
University of California, Los Angeles
Director of Reproductive Genetics
Department of Obstetrics and Gynecology
Cedars-Sinai Medical Center
Los Angeles, California

Mark Zakowski, MD
Associate Professor of Anesthesiology
Adjunct, Charles Drew University of Medicine and
   Science
Chief, Obstetric Anesthesiology, Cedars-Sinai Medical
   Center
Los Angeles, California

Preface

It has been thirty years since the first edition of *Essentials of Obstetrics and Gynecology* was published. As stated in the Preface to the First Edition, there was then, and continues to be today, a need for a textbook that covers the *essential* aspects of the specialty of Obstetrics and Gynecology, which is written primarily for the student and resident physician training in the field. The text has become known as "Hacker and Moore" over the years, as a tribute to the pioneering work of the original editors. The late J. George "Jerry" Moore was the Professor and Chairman of Obstetrics and Gynecology at the University of California at Los Angeles (UCLA), and the concept for the book was his. Neville Hacker was then an Assistant Professor in the Department and was in charge of the Student Clerkship. He was co-opted by Jerry to co-edit the book, after the entire UCLA faculty had agreed to participate in its writing.

The first edition of any textbook contains the vision and forms the foundation of the intent of the work, as outlined in the original preface. The editors have always felt that a new edition should be published only when there was significant new clinical information to report. Based on that standard, we believe it is now time for the sixth and latest edition of "Hacker and Moore" to be published.

Medical education is continuously evolving, and has changed significantly since the first edition of this textbook was published in 1986. The internet with its world-wide web and other technologies have made information instantly available to students and residents on a mobile phone or tablet during a clinical meeting. They are being taught to be life-long learners and information seekers. The classroom dynamics have been flipped in the past decade, in the sense that information transfer and gathering occurs before a seminar, with classroom time now increasingly devoted to discussions and problem solving by teams of students supported by diverse faculty mentors. This is appropriate, because health care is increasingly being delivered by multidisciplinary teams of professionals rather than by individual practitioners. With the ever-increasing complexity of medical and surgical care, this trend is expected to continue.

Textbooks have the recognized disadvantage of not always containing the latest information on a topic and of having a limited "shelf life." But just as newspapers and periodicals (printed or electronic) provide a "first and early draft" of human history and require frequent correction over time, medical texts should contain and document the time-tested facts of a discipline, along with newer information viewed through the prism of evidence-based and safe practice. It is our belief that textbooks will continue to provide the *reliable essentials* of all clinical practice, including the practice of obstetrics and gynecology.

All of the 42 chapters in this edition have been updated. Some chapters have been completely rewritten. Others have been modified due to changes in clinical practice. As was the case in previous editions of this text, we have worked to include only the "essentials" of obstetrics and gynecology, making difficult choices about the breadth and depth of the material presented. Every attempt has been made to include material consistent with the learning objectives and goals proposed by the Association of Professors in Gynecology and Obstetrics (APGO), available on their website at www. apgo.org.

In addition to the authors and editors of this current edition, we wish to acknowledge and thank those who have contributed to all previous editions.* Their knowledge and wisdom contained in their words, some of

Contributors from all previous editions: Juan J. Arce, Carol L. Archie, Ricardo Azziz, Martha J. Baird, Richard A. Bashore, A. David Barnes, Michael J. Bennett, Narender N. Bhatia, Jennifer Blake, Clifford Bochner, J. Robert Bragonier, Charles R. Brinkman III, Michael S. Broder, Philip G. Brooks, John E. Buster, Maria Bustillo, Richard P. Buyalos, Mary E. Carsten (deceased), Anita Bachus Chang, R. Jeffrey Chang, George Chapman, Ramen H. Chmait, Gautam Chaudhuri, Kenneth A. Conklin, Irvin M. Cushner (deceased), Alan H. DeCherney, Catherine Marin DeUgarte, William J. Dignam (deceased), John A. Eden, Bruce B. Ettinger, Ozlem Equils, Robin Farias-Eisner, Larry C. Ford (deceased), Michelle Fox, Janice I. French, Ann Garber, Anne D.M. Graham, Paul A. Gluck, William A. Growdon, John Gunning (deceased), Lewis A. Hamilton, Hunter A. Hammill, George S. Harris, Robert H. Hayashi, James M. Heaps, Howard L. Judd (deceased),
Continued

which remain in this edition, form the foundation of this work and will continue to enlighten future students of obstetrics and gynecology.

We greatly appreciate, and wish to acknowledge, the support and professionalism of James Merritt and his excellent production staff, particularly Rhoda Howell, Rachel McMullen, Amy Meros, and Julia Roberts at Elsevier. We hope that the knowledge acquired from this book will encourage many to pursue a more in depth study of the specialty.

Joseph C. Gambone (Executive Editor)
Neville F. Hacker
Calvin J. Hobel

Daniel A. Kahn, Samir Khalife, Ali Khraibi, Matthew Kim, Oscar A. Kletzky (deceased), Grace Elizabeth Kong, Larry R. Laufer, Thomas B. Lebherz (deceased), Joel B. Lench, Ronald S. Leuchter, John K.H. Lu, Michael C. Lu, Donald E. Marsden, John Marshall, Ruchi Mathur, James A. McGregor, Arnold L. Medearis deceased) David R. Meldrum, Robert Monoson, J. George Moore (deceased), Thomas R. Moore, John Morris (deceased), Suha H.N. Murad, Sathima Natarajan, Lauren Nathan, John Newnham, Tuan Nguyen, Bahij S. Nuwayhid, Gary Oakes, Dotun Ogunyemi, Aldo Palmieri, Groesbeck P. Parham, Ketan S. Patel, Margareta D. Pisarska, Gladys A. Ramos, Anthony E. Reading, Robert C. Reiter, Jean M. Ricci (Goodman), Michael G. Ross, Edward W. Savage, William D. Schlaff, Mousa Shamonki, James R. Shields, Klaus J. Staisch (deceased), Eric Surrey, Khalil Tabsh, Christopher M. Tarnay, Maryam Tarsa, Nancy Theroux, Paul J. Toot, Maclyn E. Wade (deceased), Nathan Wasserstrum, Barry G. Wren, and Linda Yielding.

Contents

Hacker & Moore's

ESSENTIALS OF
OBSTETRICS &
GYNECOLOGY

Introduction

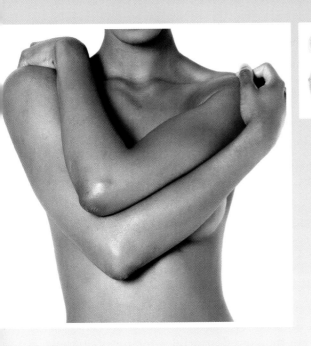
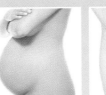
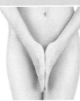
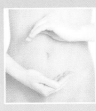
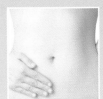

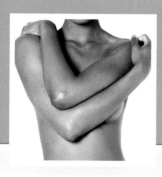

CHAPTER 1

A Life-Course Perspective for Women's Health Care
Safe, Ethical, Value-Based Practice with a Focus on Prevention

CALVIN J. HOBEL • JOSEPH C. GAMBONE

CLINICAL KEYS FOR THIS CHAPTER

- Clinical practice in obstetrics and gynecology, based upon the principles of safe, ethical and value-based care, is facilitated by viewing wellness and sickness in the context of a **life-course perspective.** Effective clinical care of mother and child must begin early, even before conception, and continue throughout life.
- Adaptive developmental plasticity and epigenetic modification of genes during and after pregnancy can have a significant impact on chronic diseases later in life.
- Clinicians should incorporate the major ethical principles of nonmaleficence, beneficence, autonomy, and justice into their practices, along with the duties

and ideals of confidentiality and multidisciplinary collaboration.
- Regulatory, economic, and public pressure make assessment and improvement of safety and value essential in the delivery of women's health care. Optimal health outcomes can only be achieved when principles from continuous quality assessment and high reliability organizations are combined with the systematic approach of safety science and evidence-based medicine.
- The promising area of clinical preventive services in obstetrics and gynecology, as in all heath care, is transforming the practice of medicine in a very positive way.

This chapter of *Essentials of Obstetrics and Gynecology* is being revised at a time when the health and wellness of the population of the United States and some other developed countries of the world are being evaluated and questioned. A recent study by the Harvard Business School conducted by Professor Michael Porter and his team ranked the United States only 70th in the world in terms of overall health and wellness. **Despite the fact that the United States spends far more on health care** (nearly 18% of gross domestic product or GDP) **than any other nation, it continues to be ranked only about 37th out of 191 nations for health status and health system performance.** Further, the United States is ranked only 46th for average life-expectancy and 42nd for infant mortality by the World Health Organization (WHO). Clearly, the United States must strive to improve its standing on these and other measures of performance. This is especially important at a time when the health care delivery system enters the era of the Affordable Care Act (ACA), and efforts to provide care to all citizens at a reasonable cost are underway.

Obstetrics and gynecology is one of the most exciting and challenging areas of health care, with a number of significant opportunities for improvement such as infant and maternal mortality. The specialty provides students and young physicians in training with the knowledge and skills necessary to improve the health of women and their children very early in their lives. In this first chapter of the book, some basic principles and guidelines for improving health care are provided, and several important factors that are influencing the health of women and their children are suggested.

Principles of Practice

There are four basic principles for practicing and improving health care. First, the safety of our patients must always be paramount. In recent years we have made major improvements in patient safety, in large part by emphasizing teamwork and implementing practices proven to be effective in the airline industry. **Second, we must be true to our personal pledge made when taking the Hippocratic Oath—to adhere to ethical practices. Third, we must transform to a value-based system of health care delivery.** Because medicine has become very complex, we must be open to a more cost-effective multidisciplinary approach to both diagnostic and therapeutic practice. Performance improvement efforts, practice management skills, and effective communication are all necessary to efficiently optimize clinical outcomes and value. **Fourth,** and perhaps most importantly, **we must focus on the prevention and early mitigation of disease,** in addition to our continued focus on its treatment. This should occur in a patient-centered manner, meeting their needs and expectations.

For this reason, we emphasize an approach called a *life-course perspective for clinical practice,* beginning with preconception health, continuing throughout pregnancy, the postpartum period (interconception health), and then giving children and their mothers a **health perspective** for adopting and maintaining healthy living.

Before delving more deeply into these principles of practice (safety, ethics, value, and prevention), some newer concepts about the origins of disease are important to mention.

LIFE-COURSE PERSPECTIVE

When does disease begin and lead to pathology and illness during the course of life?

First, although genetics is beginning to provide a much better understanding of the etiology of poor health, it probably accounts for only about one-third of the direct causes. Imprinted genes from both the mother and the father play an important role in passing on characteristics to the offspring. This imprinting process maintains the phenotype of the family in subsequent generations. However, some imprinted and nonimprinted genes can be upregulated or downregulated by subsequent epigenetic modifications, due to environmental influences. For example, person X with gene A has a disease but person Y with the same gene does not. Clearly there is more to human development and disease risk than genetic makeup. Currently it is thought that factors such as poverty or abnormal health behaviors (poor nutrition and smoking) and/or environmental conditions can influence the expression of gene A without actually changing its genomic makeup. This may occur directly or these factors may activate another gene, A-2 downstream, which may then affect gene A. This process whereby human cells can have the same genomic makeup but different characteristics is referred to as **epigenetics (literally meaning "on top of genetics"), an exciting new frontier.**

The developmental origins of adult disease hypothesis (Barker hypothesis) postulates that perturbations in the gestational environment may influence the development of adult diseases such as cardiovascular disease, obesity, diabetes, and stroke. Current evidence suggests that this occurs through the reprogramming of gene expression via epigenetic changes in chromatin structure. Epigenetic changes in chromatin structure include altered DNA methylation by both histone acetylation and methylation.

Since the last edition of this text, investigators have determined that alterations in the in utero environment during pregnancy may result in modifications to the chromatin structure. These modifications may lead to persistent changes in postnatal gene expression which may render the child more susceptible to early onset adult disease. **The conditions during pregnancy that account for these epigenetic changes are preeclampsia, preterm birth, intrauterine growth restriction (IUGR), obesity, diabetes, poor nutrition, smoking, and some cancers.** Even the mothers with these pregnancy conditions are themselves at greater risk for cardiovascular disease, hypertension, and diabetes later in life. The onset for these conditions occurs earlier in life compared to those women who have normal pregnancies. Thus **having a normal pregnancy may be protective of disease later in life.**

It is now thought that the effect of harmful behaviors and our environment on the expression of our genes may account for up to 40% of all premature deaths in the United States. Two of the top behavioral factors related to this premature death rate are obesity (and its usual physical inactivity) and smoking. Environmental exposures to metals, solvents, pesticides, endocrine disruptors, and other reproductive toxicants are also major concerns.

Second, in human biology, a phenomenon called *adaptive developmental plasticity* **plays a very important role in helping to adjust behavior to meet any environmental challenge.** In order to understand human development over time *(a life-course perspective),* one must first understand what is normal and what adverse circumstances may challenge and then change normal development of the fetus. **These protective modifications of growth and development which are programmed in utero to prevent fetal death, may become permanent.** The price the fetus may pay for short-term survival is later vulnerability to conditions such as obesity, hypertension, insulin resistance, atherosclerosis, and even diabetes.

In relation to individual X and individual Y with the same genomic makeup but different in utero environmental influences, metabolic changes that may be initiated in utero in response to inadequate nutritional supplies (Figure 1-1) can lead to insulin resistance and eventually the development of type 2 diabetes. These adaptive changes can even result in a reduced number of nephrons in the kidneys as a stressed fetus conserves limited nutritional resources for more important organ systems in utero. This can then lead to a greater risk of hypertension later in life.

This series of initially protective but eventually harmful developmental changes was first described in humans by David Barker, a British epidemiologist, who carefully assessed birth records of individuals

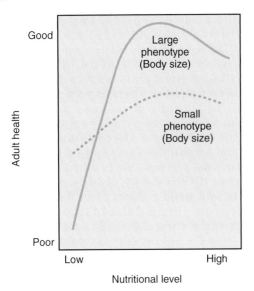

FIGURE 1-1 The potential effects of intrauterine nutrition on subsequent adult health. There are genetic, nutritional, and environmental causes of poor fetal growth leading to a small phenotype. Having a large phenotype at birth has advantages. These data form the basis of the "developmental origins of adult disease" hypothesis (Barker hypothesis). Having a low birth weight increases the risk for diseases and conditions such as hypertension, atherosclerosis, stroke, and diabetes later in life. For example, a nutritionally deprived fetus in utero may develop insulin resistance as an adaptation to preserve glucose supply to the brain rather than releasing it from the circulation to other less important tissues. Later in life, the insulin resistance that was protective in utero could increase the risk of diabetes as an adult. (From Bateson P, Barker D, Clutton-Brock T, et al: Developmental plasticity and human health. *Nature* 430:419-421, 2004. Adapted by permission from Macmillan Publishers Ltd.)

and linked low birth weight (<2500 grams) to the development of hypertension, diabetes, atherosclerosis, and stroke later in life. The association between poor fetal growth during intrauterine life, insulin resistance, and cardiovascular disease is known as the *Barker hypothesis.* The process whereby a stimulus or insult, at a sensitive or critical period of fetal development, induces permanent alterations in the structure and functions of the baby's vital organs is now commonly referred to as *developmental programming.*

Third, another important concept in the life-course perspective is allostasis, which describes the body's ability to maintain stability during physiologic change. A good example of allostasis is found in the body's stress response. When the body is under stress (biological or psychological), it activates a stress response. The sympathetic system kicks in and adrenalin flows to make the heart pump faster and harder (with the end result of delivering more blood and oxygen to vital organs including the brain). The hypothalamic-pituitary-adrenal (HPA) axis is also activated to produce more cortisol, which has many actions to prepare the body for fight or flight.

Normally, as soon as the fight or flight is over, the stress response is turned off. The body's sympathetic response is counteracted by a parasympathetic response, which fires a signal via the vagal nerve to slow down the heart, and the HPA axis is shut off by cortisol via negative feedback mechanisms. Negative feedback mechanisms are common to many biological systems and work very much like a thermostat. When the room temperature falls below a preset point, the thermostat turns on the heat. Once the preset temperature is reached, the heat turns off the thermostat. Stress turns on the HPA axis to produce cortisol. Cortisol, in turn, turns off the HPA axis to keep the stress response in check.

This stress response works well for acute stress but it tends to break down under chronic stress. In the face of chronic and repeated stress, the body's stress response is always turned on, and over time will wear out. The body goes from being "stressed" to being "stressed out"—from a state of allostasis to **allostatic overload.** This describes the cumulative wear and tear on the body's adaptive systems from chronic stress. Helpful physiologic mechanisms that initially protect may eventually be harmful.

The life-course perspective synthesizes both the developmental programming mechanisms of early life events and allostatic overload mechanisms of chronic life stress into a longitudinal model of health development. It is a way of looking at life not as disconnected stages, but as an integrated continuum. Thus to promote a healthy first pregnancy, preconception health should be a priority. To promote preconception health, adolescent health must be provided to young girls so that as women having children, they are free of diseases such as diabetes, hypertension, and obesity and have been encouraged to eat a healthy diet and to abstain from using tobacco products. Rather than episodic care that many women now receive, as a specialty we must strive toward disease prevention and health promotion over the continuum of a woman's life.

IMPACT ON PUBLIC HEALTH

The public health implications of the Barker hypothesis and other life-course events are significant. This is the beginning of an exciting era in medicine where young physicians and other health care professionals can begin to take charge of these events and change our health care delivery system in a very positive way. Patients should be encouraged to take responsibility for improving their own health, particularly by practicing healthy behaviors early in life. They should also be encouraged to improve and maintain a healthy "green" environment. Currently there are only a few environmental and behavioral factors that have been clearly identified as part of the Barker hypothesis. Many others are yet to be discovered.

Adaptive developmental plasticity will take place secondary to changes in genes as a result of environmental and behavioral practices. Even the controversial concept of climate change may play a role in this phenomenon. Biological processes are very powerful and frequently unpredictable. Physicians must increasingly strive for a safe, ethical, and value-based practice.

In order to facilitate the improvement of the health and wellness of women and children, four basic principles of practice should guide our strategy: **patient safety, ethical practice, value,** and the need for a **patient-centered focus on prevention,** as follows.

Patient Safety—The First Principle of Practice

Safety in health care is not a new concept. Facilities have had safety programs in place since the early 1900s, but these programs have traditionally focused on emergency preparedness, environmental safety, security, and infection control. The term *patient safety,* meaning avoidance of medical error, was first coined by the American Society of Anesthesiologists in 1984, when they inaugurated the Anesthesia Patient Safety Foundation to give assurance that the effects of anesthesia would not harm patients.

Medical errors now rank as the fifth leading cause of death in the United States. The Institute of Medicine (IOM) published an alarming report in 1999 called *To Err Is Human: Building a Safer Health System.* This report estimated that between 44,000 and 98,000 Americans die each year as a result of medical errors. **Error is defined as failure of a planned action to be completed as intended (e.g., failing to operate when obvious signs of appendicitis are present) or the use of a wrong plan to achieve an aim (e.g., wrong diagnosis, wrong medication administered).** Medication errors alone, occurring either in or out of the hospital, are estimated to account for over 7,000 deaths annually. According to the National Council on Patient Information and Education, "more than 2/3 of all physician visits end with a prescription." An estimated 39-49% of all medication errors occur at the stage of drug ordering. **Patient noncompliance also contributes to medical errors.**

The U.S. Pharmacopoeia (USP) MedMARx error tracking service estimates that as many as 100,000 medication errors occur annually. Because reporting is voluntary and does not include all medical facilities in the United States, the scope of the problem is likely to be much larger. A preventable adverse drug event (ADE) is one type of medication error. Administering the incorrect drug, an incorrect dose, wrong frequency, or incorrect route may cause an ADE.

A drug that cures one patient's condition may be the one that causes another patient's injury or death due to an adverse drug reaction (ADR). The latter may account for 1 out of 5 injuries or deaths for hospitalized patients. ADRs commonly occur from an overdose, a side effect, or an interaction among several concomitantly administered drugs. **In order to minimize ADRs, health care providers should avoid the following actions:**

1. **Prescribing unnecessary medications**
2. **Treating mild side effects of one drug with a second, more toxic drug**
3. **Misinterpreting a drug's side effect for a new medical problem** and prescribing another medication
4. **Prescribing a medication when there is any uncertainty about dosing**

In the absence of automated systems, providers should strive to write legibly and use only approved abbreviations and dose expressions. Most health care facilities publish and circulate an acceptable list of appropriate abbreviations, as a means of reducing medication errors.

MEDICAL ERROR REPORTING

According to the U.S. Agency for Healthcare Research & Quality (AHRQ), "Reporting is an important component of systems to improve patient safety." Incident reporting is an important and inexpensive method to detect medical error and prevent future adverse events. Unfortunately, this method may fail to impact clinical outcomes effectively, because most hospital reporting systems do not capture the majority of errors. **Reporting should be considered a quality improvement process (focused on system failures) rather than a performance evaluation method (blaming individual providers).**

As a founding member of the National Patient Safety Foundation and the National Patient Safety Partnership, the Joint Commission on the Accreditation of Healthcare Organizations (JCAHO), now more commonly known as The Joint Commission (TJC), has formed a coalition with the U.S. Pharmacopoeia (USP), the American Medical Association (AMA), and the American Hospital Association (AHA) to create patient safety reporting principles. Recognizing that fear of liability discourages error reporting, TJC has advised the U.S. Congress that federal statutory protection must be afforded to those who report medical error. **An anonymous nonpunitive environment will encourage reporting.** Many states have implemented mandatory reporting systems for selected medical errors to improve patient safety and reduce errors. Others consider incident reporting and analysis as peer review activities immune from liability. **The IOM report recommends that health care providers be required to report errors that result in serious harm. Information collected should be made available to the public.** AHRQ publishes case summaries of reported medical errors and near misses on their website.

DISCLOSURE OF MEDICAL ERROR

The National Patient Safety Foundation (NPSF) was one of the first organizations to address the issue of disclosure. Their position, finalized in November 2000, states, **"When a health care injury occurs, the patient and the family or representatives are entitled to a prompt explanation of how the injury occurred and its short- and long-term effects.** When an error contributed to the injury, the patient and the family or representatives should receive a truthful and compassionate explanation about the error and the remedies available to the patient. They should be informed that the factors involved in the injury will be investigated so that steps can be taken to reduce the likelihood of similar injury to other patients."

The Joint Commission now requires hospitals to disclose any serious harm caused by medical errors to the harmed parties. Disclosing an error can be very difficult for physicians because they may struggle with intense feelings of incompetence, betrayal of the patient, and fear of litigation. **Studies suggest that physicians with good relationship skills are less likely to get sued. Furthermore, suits are settled more rapidly and for less money if errors are disclosed early. Simple rules for disclosing errors include: admit the mistake, acknowledge the listener's anger, speak slowly, and stop frequently to allow the listener to talk.** Usually, the attending physician is the one who should make the disclosure and offer an apology.

Ethical Practice— The Second Principle

Obstetrics and gynecology encompasses many high-profile areas of ethical concern such as in vitro fertilization (IVF) and other assisted reproductive technologies (ART), abortion, the use of aborted tissue for research or treatment, surrogacy, contraception for minors, and sterilization of persons with a mental illness. Nevertheless, most ethical problems in the practice of medicine arise in cases in which the medical condition or desired procedure itself presents no moral problem. **In the past, the main areas of ethical concern have related to the competence and beneficence of the physician. Current areas of ethical concern should include the goals, values, individual and appropriate cultural preferences of the patient, as well as those of the community at large.** Consideration of such issues enriches the study of obstetrics and gynecology by emphasizing that scientific knowledge and technical skills are most meaningful in a social and moral context.

During the day-to-day consideration of ethical dilemmas in health care, a number of principles or ideals and the concepts derived from them are commonly accepted and taken into account. Four such principles or ideals are **nonmaleficence, beneficence, autonomy, and justice; these are generally accepted as the major ethical concepts that apply to health care.**

NONMALEFICENCE

The principle of *primum non nocere* or "first, do no harm" originates from the Hippocratic school, and although few would dispute the basic concept, in day-to-day medical practice, physicians and their patients may need to accept some harm from treatment (such as necessary surgical trauma) in order to achieve a desired outcome. However, there is an ethical obligation to be certain that recommended medical treatment, surgery, or diagnostic testing is not likely to cause *more harm* than benefit.

BENEFICENCE

The duty of beneficence, or the promotion of the welfare of patients, is an important part of the Hippocratic Oath. Most would see its strict application as an ideal rather than a duty, however. One could save many suffering people in a Third World country by practicing there or by giving a large portion of one's income in aid, but few would consider it a moral duty to do so. On the other hand, **when the concept of beneficence involves a specific patient encounter, the duty applies.** A physician prevented by conscience from participating in the performance of an abortion, for example, would generally be expected to provide lifesaving care for a woman suffering complications after such a procedure—putting her welfare first.

AUTONOMY

The right of self-determination is a basic concept of biomedical ethics. **To exercise autonomy, an individual must be capable of effective deliberation and be neither coerced into a particular course of action nor limited in her or his choices by external constraints.** Being capable of effective deliberation implies a level of intellectual capacity and the ability to exercise that capacity. There are a number of situations in which it may be reasonable to limit autonomy: (1) to prevent harm to others, (2) to prevent self-harm, (3) to prevent immoral acts, or (4) to benefit many others.

The concept of **informed consent** is derived directly from the principle of autonomy, and from a desire to protect patients and research subjects from harm. **There is general agreement that consent must be genuinely voluntary and made after adequate disclosure of information.** As a minimum, when a patient consents to a procedure in health care, the patient should be informed about the expectation of benefit as well as the other reasonable alternatives and possible risks that are known. Table 1-1 provides a useful checklist

TABLE 1-1

THE *PREPARED* SYSTEM: A CHECKLIST TO GUIDE PATIENT AND PROVIDER IN THE PROCESS OF INFORMED CONSENT

P	lan	The course of action being considered
R	eason	The indication or rationale
E	xpectation	The chances of benefit and failure
P	references	Patient-centered priorities (utilities) and cultural preferences affecting choice
A	lternatives	All other reasonable options
R	isks	The potential for harm from treatment
E	xpenses	All direct and indirect costs
D	ecision	Fully informed collaborative choice and consent

Modified from Reiter RC, Lench JB, Gambone JC: Consumer advocacy, elective surgery, and the "golden era of medicine." *Obstet Gynecol* 74:815–817, 1989.

(PREPARED) that expands on the minimum information required.

The exercise of autonomy may put considerable stress and conflict on those providing health care, as in the case of a woman with a ruptured ectopic pregnancy who refuses a lifesaving blood transfusion for religious reasons and dies despite the best efforts of the medical team. More complex questions may be raised by court-ordered cesarean deliveries for the benefit of the fetus.

JUSTICE

Justice relates to the way in which the benefits and burdens of society are distributed. The general principle that equals should be treated equally was espoused by Aristotle and is widely accepted today, but it does require that one be able to define the relevant differences between individuals and groups. Some believe all rational persons to have equal rights; others emphasize need, effort, contribution, and merit; still others seek criteria that maximize both individual and social utility. **In most Western societies, race, sex, and religion are not considered morally legitimate criteria for the distribution of benefits, although they too may be taken into account in order to right what are perceived to be historic wrongs, in programs of affirmative action.** When resources are scarce, issues of justice become even more problematic. There are often competing claims from parties who appear equal by all relevant criteria, and the selection criteria themselves become a moral issue. Most modern societies find the *rational* rationing of health care resources to be appropriate and acceptable (Figure 1-2).

OTHER DUTIES OF ETHICAL PRACTICE

Confidentiality is a cornerstone of the relationship between physician and patient. This duty arises from

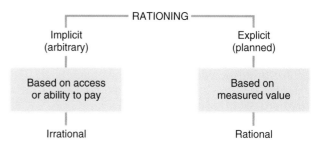

FIGURE 1-2 Representation of arbitrary rationing commonly based on access or ability to pay versus planned clinical resource management based on measured value. *Explicit* rationing is objectionable to many despite the fact that *implicit* rationing still occurs.

considerations of autonomy but also helps promote beneficence, as is the case with honesty. In obstetrics and gynecology, conflicts can arise as in the case of a woman with a sexually transmitted infection who refuses to have a sexual partner informed, or a school-aged child seeking contraceptive advice or an abortion.

There are many other situations in which conflicting responsibilities make confidentiality a difficult issue. The U.S. Health Insurance Portability and Accountability Act (HIPAA) mandates strict rules that physician practices and health care facilities must adhere to regarding the confidentiality and security of patient health care records. Some are concerned that these regulations could restrict the flow of information about patient care and may hinder efforts to improve overall performance.

Caring for a pregnant woman creates a unique **maternal-fetal relationship** because the management of the mother inevitably affects her baby. Until recently, the only way by which an obstetrician could produce a healthy baby was by maintaining optimal maternal health, but as the fetus becomes more accessible to diagnostic and therapeutic interventions, new problems emerge. **Procedures performed on behalf of the fetus may violate the personal integrity and autonomy of the mother.** The obstetrician with a dual responsibility to mother and fetus faces a potential conflict of interest. **Most conflicts will be resolved due to the willingness of most women to undergo considerable self-sacrifice to benefit their fetus.** When a woman refuses consent for a procedure that presents her with significant risk, her autonomy will generally be respected. However, there may be cases in which an intervention that is likely to be efficacious carries little risk to the mother and can reasonably be expected to prevent substantial harm to the fetus. These have occasionally ended in a court-ordered intervention.

Health care is a multidisciplinary activity and respectful and collegial relationships with other health professionals are very important. Although the physician has traditionally been the only decision maker, this situation has often caused concern among other health care professionals. **There is increasing**

recognition that other clinicians involved in health care have a right to participate in any decision making. Physicians have not been as aware of the sensitivities of the nursing profession and other allied health professionals as they should have been. For example, the decision to either operate or not on a newborn with severe spina bifida inevitably leaves nurses with responsibilities to the infant, the parents, and the doctor that may be in direct conflict with their personal values. They may rightly request to be party to the decision-making process, and although the exact models whereby such a goal may be achieved are debatable, physicians must be aware of the legitimate moral concerns of nurses and others involved.

Health care delivery takes place in a very complex environment and **relationships with other interested parties is becoming increasingly important. Hospitals, health insurance companies, and governments all claim an interest in what services are made available or paid for,** and this may prevent individual patients from receiving what their physician may consider optimal care. This poses moral problems not only for physicians on a case-by-case basis but also for insurance companies and society as a whole. **An atmosphere of mutual *trust* should be sought, earned, and practiced in these relationships.**

Finally, and very importantly, all physicians and other health care providers should be mindful of a potential **conflict of interest** that may occur during practice or during performance of committee work at the local or national level. Even the *appearance* of a conflict between a personal interest and the duty to put patient care interest first can undermine the confidence that patients and the public have in them.

MALPRACTICE AND MALOCCURRENCE

Medical malpractice refers to care that is negligent and below the accepted standard. **When an undesired outcome occurs irrespective of the care that is given, it is referred to properly as medical maloccurrence.** The system of tort law that currently applies to medical malpractice in the United States *distorts* the difference between these two events in many cases. Clearly there is preventable medical error resulting from negligent care, but many of these events are not properly addressed in our system. **Too often medical maloccurrence is judged to be malpractice.**

The interface of medicine and the law raises major ethical issues because legality and morality are not always synonymous. Professional liability insurance premiums for obstetricians are testimony to the relevance of legal issues to obstetric practice. Professional liability is affecting every major decision that is made by the practicing obstetrician and gynecologist, and under these conditions, the "tunnel vision" that ensues may obscure the ability to see clear answers to ethical questions.

Value—The Third Principle of Practice

The mandate from payers (government and employers) and the public to measure and improve the effectiveness and efficiency (value) of health care services is clear. Unfortunately, change based on adoption of national standards derived from evidence-based practice and randomized controlled trials (RCTs) alone may be too expensive and slow to meet this mandate. Furthermore, the results from RCTs may not always establish how diagnostic and therapeutic procedures actually work in clinical practice. **For these reasons, health care organizations, including schools of public health and physician groups, must develop the tools to identify and adopt best practices and improve clinical outcomes locally.**

Value in health care is defined as "clinical outcomes considering the resources used," or results divided by the costs of care. Figure 1-3 illustrates a collaborative process that may be used to involve the patient in the determination of *value* when decisions about treatments are being made. The past 40 years that have been devoted to the measurement and pursuit of quality improvement have not been successful in terms

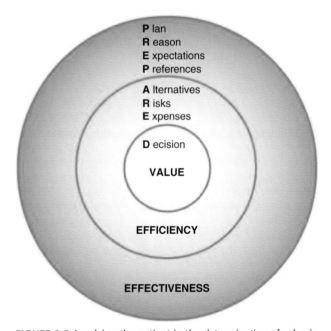

FIGURE 1-3 Involving the patient in the determination of value in decision making. Defining the Plan or Procedure along with its Reason or indication, its evidence-based Expectations, and the patient-centered Preferences for it helps to determine its effectiveness. Further defining of all other Alternatives, the associated Risks and complications along with all Expenses (Costs) determines its efficiency. Making a collaborative Decision based on this process helps to determine the Value of the treatment. (Modified from Gambone JC, Reiter RC, Hagey S: Clinical outcomes in gynecology: hysterectomy. *Curr Probl Obstet Gynecol Fertil* 16(4), 1993.)

SURGICAL SAFETY CHECKLIST

Before induction of anaesthesia →	Before skin incision →	Before patient leaves operating room
(with at least nurse and anaesthetist)	(with nurse, anaesthetist, and surgeon)	(with nurse, anaesthetist, and surgeon)

Before induction of anaesthesia
(with at least nurse and anaesthetist)

Has the patient confirmed his/her identity, site, procedure, and consent?
☐ Yes

Is the site marked?
☐ Yes
☐ Not applicable

Is the anaesthesia machine and medication check complete?
☐ Yes

Is the pulse oximeter on the patient and functioning?
☐ Yes

Does the patient have a:

Known allergy?
☐ No
☐ Yes

Difficult airway or aspiration risk?
☐ No
☐ Yes, and equipment/assistance available

Risk of >500 ml blood loss (7 ml/kg in children)?
☐ No
☐ Yes, and two IVs/central access and fluids planned

Before skin incision
(with nurse, anaesthetist, and surgeon)

☐ **Confirm all team members have introduced themselves by name and role.**

☐ **Confirm the patient's name, procedure, and where the incision will be made.**

Has antibiotic prophylaxis been given within the last 60 minutes?
☐ Yes
☐ Not applicable

Anticipated critical events

To surgeon:
☐ What are the critical or non-critical steps?
☐ How long will the case take?
☐ What is the anticipated blood loss?

To anaesthetist:
☐ Are there any patient-specific concerns?
☐ How long will the case take?

To nursing team:
☐ Has sterility (including indicator results) been confirmed?
☐ Are there equipment issues or concerns?

Is essential imaging displayed?
☐ Yes
☐ Not applicable

Before patient leaves operating room
(with nurse, anaesthetist, and surgeon)

Nurse verbally confirms:
☐ The name of the procedure
☐ Completion of instrument, sponge, and needle counts
☐ Specimen labeling (read specimen labels aloud, including patient name)
☐ Whether there are any equipment problems to be addressed

To surgeon, anaesthetist, and nurse:
☐ What are the key concerns for recovery and management of this patient?

This checklist is not intended to be comprehensive. Additions and modifications to fit local practice are encouraged.

FIGURE 1-4 Surgical safety checklist. (Based on the WHO Surgical Safety Checklist: Available at http://whqlibdoc.who.int/publications/2009/9789241598590_eng_Checklist.pdf, © World Health Organization 2009. All rights reserved.)

of reducing the high cost of care, particularly in the United States. Transforming health care organizations into high reliability organizations (HROs) that deliver patient-centered value has become the main focus of performance improvement today.

HIGH RELIABILITY IN HEALTH CARE

Recent progress in health care outcomes has been attained by introducing the concepts and tools of HROs into health care delivery facilities. The two industries that have led as HROs have been commercial aviation and nuclear power plants. **In aviation, the adoption of checklists and crew resource management (CRM) has improved commercial aviation safety significantly.** The concepts of CRM (called medical team management in health care) are now being adopted for high-risk procedures in trauma centers and operating rooms. The development of high reliability teams for decision-

making is replacing the older solo "captain of the ship" principle for high-risk, high-consequence health care activities. One checklist developed for health care for use in the operating room (Figure 1-4) was tested worldwide by the WHO and resulted in a 47% reduction in surgical mortality and a 36% reduction in inpatient complications. **The use of medical teams in health care has resulted in similar reductions in both mortality and morbidity.** Both of these interventions are relatively inexpensive when compared to the gains and both are highly effective.

Patient-Centered Prevention— The Fourth Principle of Practice

The prevention and mitigation of existing disease has become an extremely important and sometimes overlooked area of value-based practice. The famous American humorist, Will Rogers, said many years ago that people should only pay their doctors when they are well and not sick. This suggests a frustration that he was reflecting publicly that medical practice had neglected the promotion of wellness, resulting in a high cost of sickness. As health care treatment becomes more expensive and complex, there is a greater incentive for government, private industry, and individuals to invest in preventive services.

There are several good examples of effective preventive interventions that are now available in obstetric and gynecologic practice. **In obstetrics, the newer techniques for mitigating intrauterine fetal damage from chronic stress that may result in short- and long-term morbidity** (see Chapters 7 and 9) **are increasingly successful.** And **in gynecology, the vaccination against human papillomavirus (HPV) infection to prevent cervical cancer** (see Chapters 22 and 38) is a major advance. Box 1-1 contains a life-course perspective of other early, effective preventive opportunities.

BOX 1-1

LIFE-COURSE PERSPECTIVE OF EARLY PREVENTION OPPORTUNITIES

- Preconception counseling (see Chapter 7)
- Antepartum care and nutrition counseling (see Chapter 7)
- Intrapartum care and surveillance (see Chapters 9 and 10)
- Newborn screening (see Chapter 8 and pediatric care textbooks*)
- Well-baby visits, breastfeeding and nutrition counseling (see pediatric care textbooks*)
- Childhood and adolescent screening and Immunizations (see pediatric care textbooks*)
- Adult preventive health screening (see Table 1-2)

*For example, Kliegman R, Behrman R, Jenson H, et al: *Nelson's textbooks of pediatrics,* ed 18, Philadelphia, 2007, Saunders.

TABLE 1-2

RECOMMENDED PREVENTIVE HEALTH SCREENING FOR WOMEN

Intervention/Procedure	Risk(s)
Pap smear from age 21 irrespective of sexual activity: age 21-29, every 3 yr; age 30-65, every 3 yr with cytology only or every 5 yr with HPV testing added; age >65, only with history of significant CIN. After total hysterectomy (corpus and cervix) cytology not needed (see Chapter 38)	Cervical dysplasia/cancer
Annual breast exam ages >39 and every 1-3 yr age 20-39; high risk women should consider annual exam; screening mammography annually starting at age 40; USPSTF recommends starting at age 50; breast self-exam not universally recommended (see Chapter 29)	Breast cancer
Smoking cessation counseling, warning about second-hand smoke exposure	Lung cancer, heart disease, other health risks associated with smoking
Sigmoidoscopy or colonoscopy (preferred) every 3-5 yr after age 50	Colorectal cancer
Height and weight measurement for BMI calculation (see Box 2-2)	Overweight and obesity
Regular blood pressure screening (every 2 yr)	Hypertension and stroke
Cholesterol/lipid profile every 5 yr until age 65	Heart disease
Total skin inspection and selective biopsies	Skin cancer (sun exposure)
Diet and exercise counseling; BMD testing for all women > age 64, or younger if at least one risk factor for osteoporosis (see Chapter 35)	Osteoporosis, fracture, and deformity
Blood sugar study with family history, obesity, or history of gestational diabetes	Diabetes mellitus; other comorbidities associated with obesity
Cervical sampling for *Chlamydia, N. gonorrhoeae,* syphilis, and HIV based on history of high-risk behavior (see Chapter 26)	Sexually transmitted infections
TSH starting at age 50 (see Chapter 35)	Thyroid disease
PPD of tuberculin for high-risk women	Tuberculosis

BMD, Bone mineral density; *BMI,* body mass index; *CIN,* cervical intraepithelial neoplasia; *HIV,* human immunodeficiency virus; *HPV,* human papillomavirus; *Pap,* Papanicolaou test; *PPD,* purified protein derivative; *TSH,* thyroid-stimulating hormone; *USPSTF,* United States Preventive Services Task Force.

IMMUNIZATIONS AND PREVENTIVE HEALTH SCREENING

Because public health recommendations for immunizations may change, it is best to check a reliable source periodically (e.g., www.cdc.gov) for the latest information before counseling patients. General recommendations include the following for women aged 19 to 49: measles, mumps and rubella (MMR), hepatitis B, and varicella for women who are nonimmune. Additionally, vaccination against HPV is currently recommended for girls and women aged 11 to 26, and a single dose of tetanus-diphtheria-pertussis (Tdap) for adults 19 to 64 years of age is now recommended to replace the next booster dose of tetanus and diphtheria toxoids (Td) vaccine. **Influenza vaccine** annually is recommended for all women older than age 50 and women aged 19 to 49 who are health care workers, who have chronic illnesses such as heart disease or diabetes mellitus, or who are pregnant or planning to become pregnant during the flu season. **Pneumococcal vaccine** is recommended for all women aged 65 and older, and those with chronic illnesses, alcoholism, or who are immunosuppressed. Meningococcal and hepatitis A vaccines may be indicated in some women with risk factors. **MMR, varicella, and HPV vaccines are contraindicated during pregnancy.**

Table 1-2 contains preventive screening recommendations for women. **These recommendations can change or be modified from time to time.** The American College of Obstetricians and Gynecologists (ACOG) and the United States Preventive Services Task Force (USPSTF) have websites that keep the recommendations up to date. **The promising area of preventive services in obstetrics and gynecology, as in health care generally, is transforming the practice of medicine in a very positive way.**

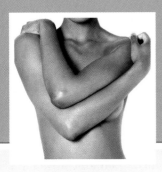

CHAPTER 2

Clinical Approach to the Patient

JOSEPH C. GAMBONE

CLINICAL KEYS FOR THIS CHAPTER

- The clinical approach to obstetric and gynecologic patients requires sensitivity and an understanding that medical issues related to birth and reproductive care require a trusting relationship between a woman and her obstetrician and gynecologist as well as all health care professionals that she may encounter.
- Recent changes in the acceptance of sexual roles in society mean that a nonjudgmental approach is needed. The physician should be careful not to assume that a casual and overly familiar approach is always acceptable to all patients, especially older ones.
- The obstetric history and physical examination should be complete and carefully performed with the goal of

providing care that results in the best clinical outcomes for the mother and her child.
- The gynecologic encounter may be for routine preventive care or may be to address a specific clinical problem that a woman may be having. Reproductive matters are of most interest during the early adult years. Concerns about chronic disorders typically arise later in life during the pre- and postmenopausal years.
- The physician and all health care professionals should be aware that certain groups of women, such as the pediatric, geriatric, and disabled, have special needs and concerns. Women who are in same-sex relationships and transgender women may also have special needs.

A careful history and physical examination should form the basis for patient evaluation and clinical management in obstetrics and gynecology, as in other clinical disciplines. This chapter outlines the essential details of the clinical approach to, and evaluation of, the obstetric and gynecologic patient. The clinical approach to female patients has evolved in recent years (see Chapter 28). It is important for the clinician who cares for women to refrain from making value judgments about sexual preferences and behavior, unless they are clearly unhealthy or dangerous. Some patients may have special needs in terms of their clinical care, and an accepting and understanding attitude is important. Pediatric and adolescent patients, the geriatric patient, as well as women with disabilities, also have unique gynecologic and reproductive needs and this chapter concludes with information about their evaluation and management.

Obstetric and Gynecologic Evaluation

In few areas of medicine is it necessary to be more sensitive to the emotional and psychological needs of the patient than in obstetrics and gynecology. By their very nature, the history and physical examination may cause embarrassment to some patients. The members of the medical care team are individually and collectively responsible for ensuring that each patient's privacy and modesty are respected while providing the highest level of medical care. Box 2-1 lists the appropriate steps for the clinical approach to the patient.

While a casual and familiar approach may be acceptable to many younger patients, it may offend others and be quite inappropriate for many older patients. Different circumstances with the same patient may dictate different levels of formality. Entrance to the

BOX 2-1

APPROACH TO THE PATIENT

The doctor should always:
- Knock before entering the patient's room.
- Identify himself/herself.
- Meet the patient initially when she is fully dressed, if possible.
- Address the patient courteously and respectfully.
- Respect the patient's privacy and modesty during the interview and examination.
- Ensure cleanliness, good grooming, and good manners in all patient encounters.
- Beware that a casual and familiar approach is not acceptable to all patients; it is generally best to avoid addressing an adult patient by her first name.
- Maintain the privacy of the patient's medical information and records.
- Be mindful and respectful of any cultural preferences.

patient's room should be announced by a knock and spoken identification. A personal introduction with the stated reason for the visit should occur before any questions are asked or an examination is begun. The placement of the examination table should always be in a position that maximizes privacy for the patient as other health care professionals enter the room. Any cultural beliefs and preferences for care and treatment should be recognized and respected.

Obstetric History

A complete history must be recorded at the time of the prepregnancy evaluation or at the initial antenatal visit. Several detailed standardized forms are available, but this should not negate the need for a detailed chronologic history taken personally by the physician who will be caring for the patient throughout her pregnancy. While taking the history, major opportunities will usually arise to provide counseling and explanations that serve to establish rapport and a supportive patient/physician encounter.

PREVIOUS PREGNANCIES

Each prior pregnancy should be reviewed in chronologic order and the following information recorded:
1. **Date of delivery** (or pregnancy termination).
2. **Location of delivery** (or pregnancy termination).
3. **Duration of gestation** (recorded in weeks). When correlated with birth weight, this information allows an assessment of fetal growth patterns. The gestational age of any spontaneous abortion is of importance in any subsequent pregnancy.
4. **Type of delivery** (or method of terminating pregnancy). This information is important for planning the method of delivery in the present pregnancy. A difficult forceps delivery or a cesarean delivery may require a personal review of the labor and delivery records.
5. **Duration of labor** (recorded in hours). This may alert the physician to the possibility of an unusually long or short labor.
6. **Type of anesthesia.** Any complications of anesthesia should be noted.
7. **Maternal complications.** Urinary tract infections, vaginal bleeding, hypertension, and postpartum complications may be repetitive; such knowledge is helpful in anticipating and preventing problems with the present pregnancy.
8. **Newborn weight** (in grams or pounds and ounces). This information may give indications of gestational diabetes, fetal growth problems, shoulder dystocia, or cephalopelvic disproportion.
9. **Newborn gender.** This may provide insight into patient and family expectations and may indicate certain genetic risk factors.
10. **Fetal and neonatal complications.** Certain questions should be asked to elicit any problems and to determine the need to obtain further information. Inquiry should be made as to whether the baby had any problems after it was born, whether the baby breathed and cried right away, and whether the baby left the hospital with the mother.

MENSTRUAL HISTORY

A good menstrual history is essential because it is the determinant for establishing the expected date of confinement (EDC). A modification of **Nägele rule** for establishing the EDC is to add 9 months and 7 days to the first day of the last normal menstrual period (LMP). For example:

LMP: July 20, 2015
EDC: April 27, 2016

This calculation assumes a normal 28-day cycle, and adjustments must be made for longer or shorter cycles. Any bleeding or spotting since the last normal menstrual period should be reviewed in detail and taken into account when calculating an EDC.

CONTRACEPTIVE HISTORY

This information is important for risk assessment. Hormonal contraceptives taken during early pregnancy have been associated with birth defects, and retained intrauterine devices (IUDs) can cause early pregnancy loss, infection, and premature delivery.

MEDICAL HISTORY

The importance of a good medical history cannot be overemphasized. In addition to common disorders, such as diabetes mellitus, hypertension, and renal disease, which are known to affect pregnancy outcome, all serious medical conditions should be recorded.

SURGICAL HISTORY

Each surgical procedure should be recorded chronologically, including date, hospital, surgeon, and complications. Trauma must also be listed (e.g., a fractured pelvis may result in diminished pelvic capacity).

SOCIAL HISTORY

Habits such as smoking, alcohol use, and other substance abuse are important factors that must be recorded and managed appropriately. The patient's contact or exposure to domesticated animals, particularly cats (which carry a risk of toxoplasmosis), is important.

The patient's type of work and lifestyle may affect the pregnancy. Exposure to solvents (carbon tetrachloride) or insulators (polychlorobromine compounds) in the workplace may lead to teratogenesis or hepatic toxicity.

Obstetric Physical Examination

GENERAL PHYSICAL EXAMINATION

This procedure must be systematic and thorough and performed as early as possible in the prenatal period. A complete physical examination provides an opportunity to detect previously unrecognized abnormalities. Normal baseline levels must also be established, particularly those of weight, blood pressure, funduscopic (retina) appearance, and cardiac status.

PELVIC EXAMINATION

The initial pelvic examination should be done early in the prenatal period and should include the following: (1) inspection of the external genitalia, vagina, and cervix; (2) collection of cytologic specimens from the exocervix (or ectocervix) and superficial endocervical canal; and (3) palpation of the cervix, uterus, and adnexa. The initial estimate of gestational age by uterine size becomes less accurate as pregnancy progresses. Rectal and rectovaginal examinations are also important aspects of this initial pelvic evaluation.

CLINICAL PELVIMETRY

This assessment, which is helpful for predicting potential problems during labor, should be carried out following the bimanual pelvic examination and before the rectal examination. It is important that clinical pelvimetry be carried out systematically. The details of clinical pelvimetry are described in Chapter 8.

Diagnosis of Pregnancy

The diagnosis of pregnancy and its location, based on physical signs and examination alone, may be quite challenging during the early weeks after a missed menses. Urine pregnancy tests in the office are reliable a few days after the first missed period, and office ultrasonography is used increasingly as a routine.

SYMPTOMS OF PREGNANCY

The most common symptoms in the early months of pregnancy are missed menses, urinary frequency, breast engorgement, nausea, tiredness, and easy fatigability. A missed or abnormal menses in a previously normally menstruating, sexually active woman should be considered to be caused by pregnancy until proven otherwise. Urinary frequency is most likely caused by the pressure of the enlarged uterus on the bladder.

SIGNS OF PREGNANCY

The signs of pregnancy may be divided into presumptive, probable, and positive.

Presumptive Signs

The presumptive signs are primarily those associated with skin and mucous membrane changes. Discoloration and cyanosis of the vulva, vagina, and cervix are related to the generalized engorgement of the pelvic organs and are, therefore, nonspecific. The dark discoloration of the vulva and vaginal walls is known as **Chadwick sign.** Pigmentation of the skin and abdominal striae are nonspecific and unreliable signs. The most common sites for pigmentation are the midline of the lower abdomen (linea nigra), over the bridge of the nose, and under the eyes. Pigmentation under the eyes is called chloasma or the mask of pregnancy. Chloasma is also an occasional side effect of hormonal contraceptives.

Probable Signs

The probable signs of pregnancy are those mainly related to the detectable physical changes in the uterus. During early pregnancy, the uterus changes in size, shape, and consistency. Early uterine enlargement tends to be in the anteroposterior diameter so that the uterus becomes globular. In addition, because of asymmetric implantation of the ovum, one cornu of the uterus may enlarge slightly (**Piskaçek sign).** Uterine consistency becomes softer, and it may be possible to palpate or to compress the connection between the cervix and fundus. This change is referred to as **Hegar sign.** The cervix also begins to soften early in pregnancy.

Positive Signs

The positive signs of pregnancy include the detection of a fetal heartbeat and the recognition of fetal movements. Endovaginal ultrasound is capable of detecting fetal cardiac activity as early as 6 weeks (from last menses) and fetal movement from about 7 to 8 weeks' gestation. Modern Doppler techniques for detecting the fetal heartbeat may be successful as early as 9 weeks and are nearly always positive by 12 weeks. Fetal heart tones can usually be detected with a stethoscope between 16 and 20 weeks. The multiparous woman generally recognizes fetal movements between 15 and 17 weeks, whereas the primigravida usually does not recognize fetal movements until 18 to 20 weeks.

LABORATORY TESTS FOR PREGNANCY

Pregnancy Tests

Tests to detect pregnancy have revolutionized early diagnosis. Although they are considered a probable sign of pregnancy, the accuracy of these tests is very good. All commonly used methods depend on the detection of human chorionic gonadotropin (hCG) or its β subunit in urine or serum. Depending on the specific sensitivity of the test, pregnancy may be suspected even prior to a missed menstrual period.

Diagnostic Ultrasonography

The imaging technique of ultrasonography has made a significant contribution to the diagnosis and evaluation of pregnancy. Using real-time ultrasonography, an intrauterine gestational sac can be identified at 5 menstrual weeks (21st postovulatory day) and a fetal image can be detected by 5 to 6 weeks. A beating heart is noted at 7 weeks or even sooner with the latest equipment.

Gynecologic History

Gynecologic history-taking must be systematic to avoid omissions, and it should be conducted with sensitivity and without haste.

PRESENT ILLNESS

The patient is asked to state her main complaint and to relate her present illness, sequentially, in her own words. Pertinent negative information should be recorded, and, as much as possible, questions should be reserved until after the patient has described the course of her illness. Generally, the history provides substantial clues to the diagnosis, so it is important to evaluate fully the more common symptoms encountered in gynecologic patients.

Abnormal Vaginal Bleeding

Vaginal bleeding before the age of 9 years and after the age of 52 years is cause for concern and requires investigation. These are the general limits of normal menstruation, and although the occasional woman may menstruate regularly and normally up to the age of 57 or 58 years, it is important to ensure that she is not bleeding from uterine cancer or from exogenous estrogens. Prolongation of menses beyond 7 days or bleeding between menses may connote abnormal ovarian function, uterine myomata, or endometriosis.

Abdominal Pain

Many gynecologic problems are associated with abdominal pain. The common gynecologic causes of acute lower abdominal pain are salpingo-oophoritis with peritoneal inflammation, torsion and infarction of an ovarian cyst, endometriosis, or rupture of an ectopic pregnancy. Patterns of pain radiation should be recorded and may provide an important diagnostic clue. Chronic lower abdominal pain is generally associated with endometriosis, chronic pelvic inflammatory disease, or large pelvic tumors. It may also be the first symptom of ovarian cancer.

Amenorrhea

The most common causes of amenorrhea are pregnancy and the normal menopause. It is abnormal for a young woman to reach the age of 16 without menstruating (primary amenorrhea). Pregnancy should be suspected in a woman between 15 and 45 years of age who fails to menstruate within 35 days from the first day of her last menstruation. In a patient with amenorrhea who is not pregnant, inquiry should be made about menopausal or climacteric symptoms such as hot flashes, vaginal dryness, or mild depression.

Other Symptoms

Other pertinent symptoms of concern include dysmenorrhea, premenstrual tension, fluid retention, leukorrhea, constipation, dyschezia, dyspareunia, and abdominal distention. Lower back and sacral pain may indicate uterine prolapse, enterocele, or rectocele.

MENSTRUAL HISTORY

The menstrual history should include the age at menarche (average is 12 to 13 years), interval between periods (21 to 35 days with a median of 28 days), duration of menses (average is 5 days), and character of the flow (scant, normal, heavy, usually without clots). Any intermenstrual bleeding (metrorrhagia) should be noted. The date of onset of the LMP and the date of the previous menstrual period should be recorded. Inquiry should be made regarding menstrual cramps (dysmenorrhea); if present, the age at onset, severity, and character of the cramps should be recorded, together with an estimate of the disability incurred. Midcycle pain *(mittelschmerz)* and a midcycle increase in vaginal secretions are usually indicative of ovulatory cycles.

CONTRACEPTIVE HISTORY

The type and duration of each contraceptive method must be recorded, along with any attendant complications. These may include amenorrhea or thromboembolic disease with hormonal contraceptives; dysmenorrhea, heavy bleeding (menorrhagia), or pelvic infection with the intrauterine device; or contraceptive failure with the diaphragm, or other barrier method.

OBSTETRIC HISTORY

Each pregnancy, delivery, and any associated complications should be listed sequentially with relevant details and dates.

SEXUAL HISTORY

The health of, and current relationship with, the husband or partner(s) may provide insight into the present complaints. Inquiry should be made regarding any pain (dyspareunia), bleeding, or dysuria associated with sexual intercourse. Sexual satisfaction should be discussed tactfully.

PAST HISTORY

As in the obstetric history, any significant past medical or surgical history should be recorded, as should the patient's family history. A list of current medications is important.

SYSTEMIC REVIEW

A review of all other organ systems should be undertaken. Habits (tobacco, alcohol, other substance abuse), medications, usual weight with recent changes, and loss of height (osteoporosis) are important parts of the systemic review.

Gynecologic Physical Examination

GENERAL PHYSICAL EXAMINATION

A complete physical examination should be performed on each new patient and repeated at least annually. The initial examination should include the patient's height, weight, and arm span (in adolescent patients or those with endocrine problems) and should be carried out with the patient completely disrobed but suitably draped. A body mass index (BMI) should be calculated (Box 2-2) and recorded. The examination should be systematic and should include the following points.

Vital Signs

Temperature, pulse rate, respiratory rate, and blood pressure should be recorded.

BOX 2-2

CALCULATIONS AND DESIGNATIONS* OF BODY MASS INDEX

Body mass index is calculated by dividing weight in kilograms (kg) by height in meters squared or weight in pounds by height in inches squared times 703.
- Less than 18.5 = underweight
- 18.5 to 25 = normal weight
- 25 to 29.9 = overweight
- 30 to 34.9 = class one obesity
- 35 to 39.9 = class two obesity
- 40 or greater = extreme obesity

*Data from the National Heart, Lung, and Blood Institute.

General Appearance

The patient's body build, posture, state of nutrition, demeanor, and state of well-being should be recorded.

Head and Neck

Evidence of supraclavicular lymphadenopathy, oral lesions, webbing of the neck, or goiter may be pertinent to the gynecologic assessment.

Breasts

The breast examination is particularly important in gynecologic patients (see Chapters 30 and 32).

Heart and Lungs

Examination of the heart and lungs is of importance, particularly in a patient who requires surgery. The presence of a pleural effusion may be indicative of a disseminated malignancy, particularly ovarian cancer.

Abdomen

Examination of the abdomen is critical in the evaluation of the gynecologic patient. The contour, whether flat, scaphoid, or protuberant, should be noted. The protuberant appearance may suggest ascites. The presence and distribution of hair, especially in the area of the escutcheon, should be recorded, as should the presence of striae or operative scars.

Abdominal tenderness must be determined by placing one hand flat against the abdomen in the nonpainful areas initially, then gently and gradually exerting pressure with the fingers of the other hand (Figure 2-1). Rebound tenderness (a sign of peritoneal irritation), muscle guarding, and abdominal rigidity should be gently elicited, again first in the nontender areas. A "doughy" abdomen, in which the guarding

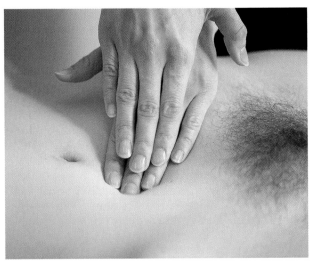

FIGURE 2-1 The abdomen is palpated by placing the left palm flat against the abdominal wall and then gently exerting pressure with the fingers of the right hand.

increases gradually as the pressure of palpation is increased, is often seen with a hemoperitoneum.

It is important to palpate any abdominal mass. The size should be specifically noted. Other characteristics may be even more important in suggesting the diagnosis, such as whether the mass is cystic or solid, smooth or nodular, fixed or mobile, and whether it is associated with ascites. In determining the reason for abdominal distention (tumor, ascites, or distended bowel), it is important to percuss carefully the areas of tympany (gaseous distention) and dullness. A large tumor is generally dull on top with loops of bowel displaced to the flanks. Dullness that shifts as the patient turns onto her side **(shifting dullness) is suggestive of ascites.**

Back

Abnormal curvature of the vertebral column (dorsal kyphosis or scoliosis) is an important observation in evaluating osteoporosis in a postmenopausal woman. Costovertebral angle tenderness suggests pyelonephritis, whereas psoas muscle spasm, which is associated with flexion of the hip, may occur with gynecologic infections, malignant infiltration, or acute appendicitis.

Extremities

The presence or absence of varicosities, edema, pedal pulsations, and cutaneous lesions may suggest pathologic conditions within the pelvis. The height of pitting edema should be noted (e.g., ankle, shin, to the knee, or above).

PELVIC EXAMINATION

The pelvic examination must be conducted systematically and with careful sensitivity. The procedure should be performed with smooth and gentle movements and accompanied by reasonable explanations.

Vulva

The character and distribution of hair, the degree of development or atrophy of the labia, and the character of the hymen (imperforate or cribriform) and introitus (virginal, nulliparous, or multiparous) should be noted. Any clitorimegaly should be noted, as should the presence of cysts, tumors, or inflammation of the **Bartholin gland.** The urethra and **Skene glands** should be inspected for any purulent exudates. The labia should be inspected for any inflammatory, dystrophic, or neoplastic lesions. Perineal relaxation and scarring should be noted because they may cause dyspareunia and defects in anal sphincter tone. The urethra should be "milked" for any inflammatory exudates, which if found should be cultured for pathologic organisms.

Speculum Examination

It is important to use an appropriately sized speculum (Figure 2-2), which should be warmed and lubri-

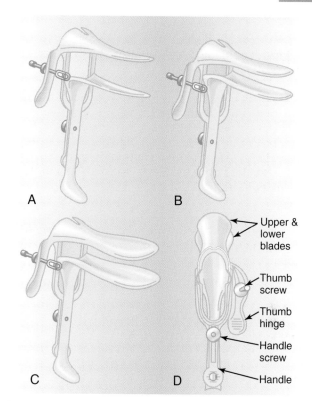

Upper & lower blades

Thumb screw

Thumb hinge

Handle screw

Handle

FIGURE 2-2 A, Pediatric speculum. **B,** Pederson speculum. **C,** Graves speculum. The Pederson speculum has narrower blades and is more appropriate for examining a nulliparous patient. **D,** Parts of a speculum.

cated with warm water only, so as not to interfere with the examination of cervical cytology or any vaginal exudate. After gently spreading the labia to expose the introitus, the speculum should be inserted with the blades entering the introitus transversely, then directed posteriorly in the axis of the vagina with pressure exerted against the relatively insensitive perineum to avoid contacting the sensitive urethra. As the anterior blade reaches the cervix, the speculum is opened to bring the cervix into view (Figure 2-3). As the vaginal epithelium is inspected, it is important to rotate the speculum through 90 degrees, so that lesions on the anterior or posterior walls of the vagina ordinarily covered by the blades of the speculum are not overlooked. Vaginal wall relaxation should be evaluated using either a Sims speculum or the posterior blade of a bivalve speculum. The patient is asked to bear down **(Valsalva maneuver)** or to cough to demonstrate any stress incontinence. If the patient's complaint involves urinary stress or urgency, this portion of the examination should be carried out before the bladder is emptied.

The cervix should be inspected to determine its size, shape, and color. The nulliparous patient generally has a conical, unscarred cervix with a circular, centrally placed os; the multiparous cervix is generally bulbous

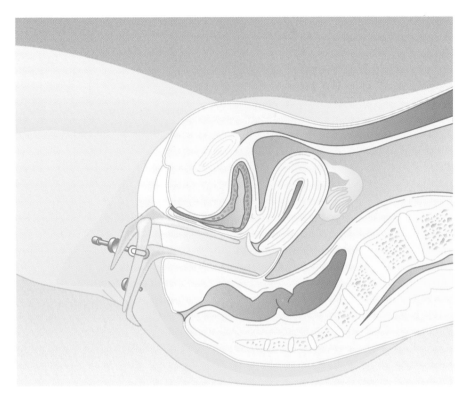

FIGURE 2-3 Proper insertion of the speculum so that the uterine cervix may be visualized.

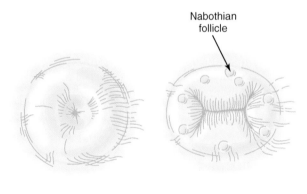

Nabothian follicle

A   NULLIPAROUS   B   MULTIPAROUS

FIGURE 2-4 Cervix of a nulliparous patient (A) and a multiparous patient (B). Note the circular os in the nulliparous cervix and the transverse os, resulting from lacerations at childbirth, in the multiparous cervix.

and the os has a transverse configuration (Figure 2-4). Any purulent cervical discharge should be cultured. Plugged, distended cervical glands (**nabothian follicles**) may be seen on the exocervix (or ectocervix). In premenopausal women, the squamocolumnar junction of the cervix is usually visible around the cervical os, particularly in patients of low parity. Postmenopausally, the junction is invariably retracted within the endocervical canal. A cervical cytologic smear (Papanicolaou, or Pap, smear), liquid-based sampling, or DNA probe for human papillomavirus (HPV) should be taken before the speculum is withdrawn. For the traditional Pap smear the exocervix (or ectocervix) is gently scraped with a wooden spatulum or plastic broom, and the endocervical tissue gently sampled with a cytobrush.

Bimanual Examination

The bimanual pelvic examination provides information about the uterus and adnexa (fallopian tubes and ovaries). During this portion of the examination, the urinary bladder should be empty; if it is not, the internal genitalia will be difficult to delineate, and the procedure is more apt to be uncomfortable for the patient. The labia are separated, and the gloved, lubricated index finger is inserted into the vagina, avoiding the sensitive urethral meatus. Pressure is exerted posteriorly against the perineum and puborectalis muscle, which causes the introitus to gape somewhat, thereby usually allowing the middle finger to be inserted as well. Intromission of the two fingers into the depth of the vagina may be facilitated by having the patient bear down slightly. **If insertion of two fingers causes undue patient discomfort, examination with the index finger alone may give more information.**

The cervix is palpated for consistency, contour, size, and tenderness to motion. **If the vaginal fornices are**

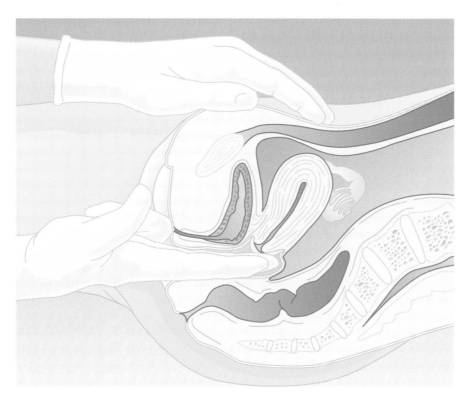

FIGURE 2-5 Bimanual evaluation of the uterus by exerting gentle pressure on the uterus with the vaginal fingers against the abdominal hand.

absent, as may occur in postmenopausal women, it is not possible to appreciate the size of the cervix on bimanual examination. This can be determined only on rectovaginal or rectal examination.

The uterus is evaluated by placing the abdominal hand flat on the abdomen with the fingers pressing gently just above the symphysis pubis. With the vaginal fingers supinated in either the anterior or the posterior vaginal fornix, the uterine corpus is pressed gently against the abdominal hand (Figure 2-5). As the uterus is felt between the examining fingers of both hands, the size, configuration, consistency, and mobility of the organ are appreciated. If the muscles of the abdominal wall are not compliant or if the uterus is retroverted, the outline, consistency, and mobility must be determined by ballottement with the vaginal fingers in the fornices; in these circumstances, however, it is impossible to discern uterine size accurately.

By shifting the abdominal hand to either side of the midline and gently elevating the lateral fornix up to the abdominal hand, it may be possible to outline a right adnexal mass (Figure 2-6). The left adnexa are best appreciated with the fingers of the left hand in the vagina (Figure 2-7). The examiner should stand sideways, facing the patient's left, with the left hip maintaining pressure against the left elbow, thereby

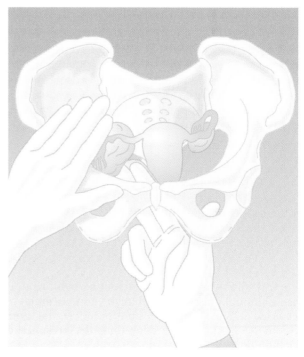

FIGURE 2-6 Bimanual examination of the right adnexa. Note that fingers of the right hand are in the vagina.

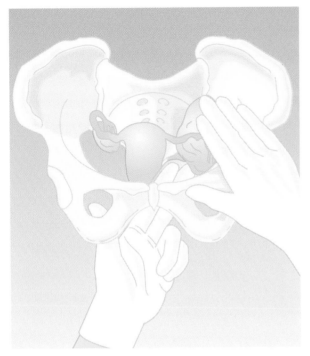

FIGURE 2-7 Bimanual examination of the left adnexa. Note that fingers of the left hand are in the vagina.

providing better tactile sensation because of the relaxed musculature in the forearm and examining hand. The **pouch of Douglas** is also carefully assessed for nodularity or tenderness, as may occur with endometriosis, pelvic inflammatory disease, or metastatic carcinoma.

It is usually impossible to feel the normal tube, and conditions must be optimal to appreciate the normal ovary. The normal ovary has the size and consistency of a shelled oyster and may be felt with the vaginal fingers as they are passed across the undersurface of the abdominal hand. The ovaries are very tender to compression, and the patient is uncomfortably aware of any ovarian compression or movement during the examination.

It may be impossible to differentiate between an ovarian or tubal mass or even a lateral uterine mass. Generally, left adnexal masses are more difficult to evaluate than those on the right because of the position of the sigmoid colon on the left side of the pelvis. An ultrasonic examination should be helpful for delineating these features.

RECTAL EXAMINATION

The anus should be inspected for lesions, hemorrhoids, or inflammation. Rectal sphincter tone should be recorded and any mucosal lesions noted. A guaiac test should be performed to determine the presence of occult blood.

A rectovaginal examination is helpful in evaluating masses in the cul-de-sac, the rectovaginal septum, or adnexa. It is essential in evaluating the parametrium in patients with cervical cancer. Rectal examination may also be essential in differentiating between a rectocele and an enterocele (Figure 2-8).

LABORATORY EVALUATION

Appropriate laboratory tests normally include a urinalysis, complete blood count, erythrocyte sedimentation rate, and blood chemistry analyses. Special tests, such as tumor marker and hormone assays, are performed when indicated.

ASSESSMENT

A reasonable differential diagnosis should be possible with the information gleaned from the history, physical examination, and laboratory tests. The plan of management should aim toward a chemical or histologic confirmation of the presumptive diagnosis, and the appropriate therapeutic options, along with the rationale for each option, should be recorded.

Patients with Special Needs

PEDIATRIC AND ADOLESCENT PATIENTS

Girls experience fewer gynecologic problems than do adult women, but their concerns need to be met effectively and skillfully in a way that will allay anxiety and create a positive attitude toward their gynecologic health. Unique complaints fall generally into a handful of categories: congenital anomalies, genital injuries, inflammation of the nonestrogenized genital tract, pubertal problems, and psychosexual concerns. Genital ambiguity, trauma, and vaginal bleeding in the prepubertal child are covered briefly in this chapter.

GENITAL AMBIGUITY

Dealing with genital ambiguity in the newborn requires a coordinated and timely response. **The family's psychological well-being must be addressed because they must feel confident in the gender identity of their child.** Ambiguity can result from masculinization of a female child due to exogenous hormone ingestion or maternal or fetal overproduction of androgen. It may also result from incomplete virilization of a male infant, hormonal insensitivity, gonadal dysgenesis, or chromosomal anomalies (see Chapters 18 and 20). **When assessing an infant with ambiguous genitalia, fluid and electrolyte balance should be monitored and blood drawn for 17-hydroxyprogesterone and cortisol to rule out 21-hydroxylase deficiency.** Life-threatening illness may be missed in children with the salt-losing form of congenital adrenal hyperplasia (see Chapter 33).

TRAUMA

Straddle injuries are the most common cause of trauma to the genitalia of a young girl, and the injuries have a

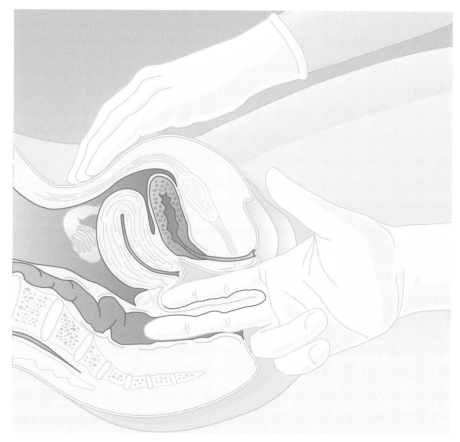

FIGURE 2-8 Rectovaginal bimanual examination. During the Valsalva maneuver, an enterocele will separate the two fingers.

seasonal peak when bicycles come out in the spring. The majority of these injuries are to the labia. Penetrating vaginal injuries can cause major intraabdominal damage with minimal external findings. **Sexual assault must always be considered.** After a life-threatening condition is ruled out, an ice pack, chilled bag of intravenous solution, or cool compress may be applied to the injured area and the child allowed to rest quietly for 20 minutes before being assessed further. Extensive injuries usually require examination under anesthesia and surgical repair.

In any case of trauma, concurrent damage to the rectum or urinary tract should be considered. **If there is any reason to suspect sexual or physical abuse, the child protection authorities must be notified, and the examination should include the collection of medicolegal evidence.**

VAGINAL BLEEDING IN THE PREPUBERTAL CHILD

Vaginal bleeding is a frequent and distressing complaint in childhood. Although it will most often be of benign etiology, more serious pathology must always be ruled out. Vaginal bleeding in the newborn is most often physiologic as a result of maternal estrogen withdrawal. In such cases, there should be supportive evidence of a hormonal effect, such as the presence of breast tissue and pale, engorged vaginal epithelium. Bleeding disorders are uncommon in this age group but should be considered. Vitamin K is routinely given to the newborn, but some parents may refuse the medication.

Precocious puberty (see Chapter 32) may present with vaginal bleeding, although most commonly other evidence of maturation will have preceded the bleeding and will be evident on examination. At the very least, a pale, estrogenized vaginal epithelium will be seen, and cytology from the vagina will confirm the hormonal effect. Transient precocious puberty may occur in response to a **functional ovarian cyst,** and vaginal bleeding may be triggered by the spontaneous resolution of the cyst. **Exogenous hormonal exposure** should be considered, because children have been known to ingest birth control pills. **Ovarian tumors** resulting in pseudoprecocious puberty should be ruled out.

Vulvovaginitis is common but is a diagnosis of exclusion. When bleeding is present, it is necessary to assess the vagina and to rule out a foreign body or vaginal tumor.

Vaginal tumors are the most serious possibility to be considered. **Sarcoma botryoides** classically presents with vaginal bleeding and grapelike vesicles. Fortunately, this is a rare tumor.

Geriatric Patients

The gynecologic assessment of the elderly woman may present a special challenge. Many older patients tend to underreport their symptoms, possibly because of a belief that any new physical problems are due to the normal aging process. Also, a fear of loss of their independence may contribute to this denial and this may lead to a delay of diagnosis and perhaps a worse prognosis. In addition to the routine gynecologic history and physical examination, these patients should be evaluated for any sensory impairments, such as visual or hearing loss, any impaired mobility, malnutrition, urinary incontinence, or confusion, which may be due to polypharmacy. Appropriate referral, when improvement can be reasonably expected, should be considered for these problems once identified.

Gynecologic conditions such as atrophic vaginitis, uterine and vaginal prolapse, and genital tract malignancies are among the more common problems encountered in the geriatric patient.

Patients with Disabilities

Women with developmental or acquired disabilities should receive the same high quality obstetric and gynecologic care as anyone else, with a goal of sustaining their best level of functioning. Assisting families of mentally or physically disabled individuals with obstetric or gynecologic problems or attending for them in special institutions can be quite challenging. The woman with a disability is a person with special and unique needs, and communicating to her a sense of caring and respect is paramount.

Lesbian, Gay, Bisexual, and Transgender Patients

This group of patients is composed of **l**esbian, **g**ay, **b**isexual, and **t**ransgender women and men and is known as **LGBT**. There is now recognition that women who are in a same-sex intimate relationship, as well as those who are transgender, need special consideration and understanding for the health issues that they may encounter. The U.S. Office of Prevention and Health Promotion points out that LGBT individuals, possibly because of the discrimination that they encounter, have higher rates of psychiatric disorders, substance abuse, and suicide. The obstetrician and gynecologist should be particularly sensitive to the needs that these women may have regarding their reproductive health. More information about the health disparities that the LGBT community may have can be found at www.healthypeople.gov/LGBT. For more detailed information about the specific needs that lesbian and transgender women may have, the American College of Obstetricians and Gynecologists Committee Opinion Number 525, dated May 2012 and reaffirmed in 2014, can be consulted at www.ACOG.org.

Female Reproductive Anatomy and Embryology

JOSEPH C. GAMBONE

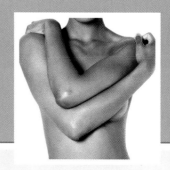

CLINICAL KEYS FOR THIS CHAPTER

- The upper vagina, cervix, uterus, and fallopian tubes are formed from the paramesonephric (müllerian) ducts. The absence of the Y chromosome leads to the development of the müllerian (female) system with virtual total regression of the mesonephric (wolffian) or male system. With the Y chromosome present, a testis is formed and müllerian-inhibiting substance is produced, creating the reverse situation.

- The vagina is a flattened tube extending from the hymenal ring at the vaginal introitus up to the fornices that surround the uterine cervix. The vaginal epithelium, which is stratified squamous in type, and not mucosal, is nonkeratinized and devoid of mucous glands and hair follicles.

- The blood supply to the ovaries is provided by the ovarian arteries, which arise from the abdominal aorta immediately below the renal arteries. The venous drainage of each ovary differs in that the right ovary drains directly into the inferior vena cava whereas the left ovary drains into the left renal vein.

- At the time of pelvic examination when a woman is in the dorsal-lithotomy position, the uterus may be palpated to be tilted forward in an anterior or anteverted position, in a midline position, or tilted backward in a posterior or retroverted position. The top or corpus of the uterus may also be folded forward (anteflexed) or backward (retroflexed). Most of the time this represents normal anatomic variation.

- Gynecologic surgeons use several types of skin incisions for the performance of "open" surgical procedures. The most common is the low transverse or Pfannenstiel incision. When more exposure is needed than anticipated, the skin incision can be extended and the rectus abdominis muscles divided with diathermy. This is called a Maylard incision. For most open operations for cancer, vertical incisions are desirable, because they can be readily extended to allow access to the upper abdomen.

Other chapters in this book deal with the disruptive deviations from normal female anatomy and physiology, whether they be congenital, functional, traumatic, inflammatory, neoplastic, or even iatrogenic. As the etiology and pathogenesis of clinical problems are considered in these other chapters, each should be studied in the context of normal anatomy, development, and physiology. A physician cannot practice obstetrics and gynecology effectively without understanding the physiologic processes that transpire in a woman's life as she passes through infancy, adolescence, reproductive maturity, and the climacteric. As the various clinical problems are addressed, it is important to consider those anatomic, developmental, and physiologic changes that normally take place at key points in a woman's life cycle.

This chapter presents the normal anatomy of the female reproductive tract along with its embryologic development and the anatomy of some important surrounding structures. Applied anatomic issues, such as the normal variation in uterine position and the types of surgical incisions used by gynecologic surgeons, are also covered.

Development of the External Genitalia

Before the seventh week of development, the appearance of the external genital area is the same in males and females. Elongation of the genital tubercle into a phallus with a clearly defined terminal glans portion is noted in the 7th week, and gross inspection at this time may lead to faulty sexual identification. Ventrally and caudally, the urogenital membrane, made up of both endodermal and ectodermal cells, further differentiates into the genital folds laterally and the urogenital folds medially. **The lateral genital folds develop into the labia majora, whereas the urogenital folds develop subsequently into the labia minora and prepuce of the clitoris.**

The external genitalia of the fetus are readily distinguishable as female at approximately 12 weeks (Figure 3-1). In the male, the urethral ostium is located conspicuously on the elongated phallus by this time and is smaller, because of urogenital fold fusion dorsally, which produces a prominent raphe from the anus to the urethral ostium. In the female, the hymen is usually perforated by the time delivery occurs.

Anatomy of the External Genitalia

The perineum represents the inferior boundary of the pelvis. It is bounded superiorly by the levator ani muscles and inferiorly by the skin between the thighs (Figure 3-2). Anteriorly, the perineum extends to the symphysis pubis and the inferior borders of the pubic bones. Posteriorly, it is limited by the ischial tuberosities, the sacrotuberous ligaments, and the coccyx. **The superficial and deep transverse perineal muscles cross the pelvic outlet between the two ischial tuberosities and come together at the perineal body. They divide the space into the urogenital triangle anteriorly and the anal triangle posteriorly.**

The urogenital diaphragm is a fibromuscular sheet that stretches across the pubic arch. It is pierced by the vagina, the urethra, the artery of the bulb, the internal pudendal vessels, and the dorsal nerve of the clitoris. Its inferior surface is covered by the crura of the clitoris, the vestibular bulbs, the greater vestibular (Bartholin) glands, and the superficial perineal muscles. The Bartholin glands are situated just posterior to the vestibular bulbs, and their ducts empty into the introitus just below the labia minora. They are often the site of gonococcal infections and painful abscesses.

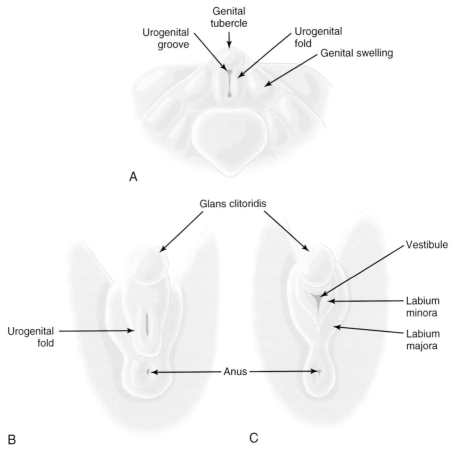

FIGURE 3-1 Development of the external female genitalia. **A,** Indifferent stage (approximately 7 weeks). **B,** Approximately 10 weeks. **C,** Approximately 12 weeks.

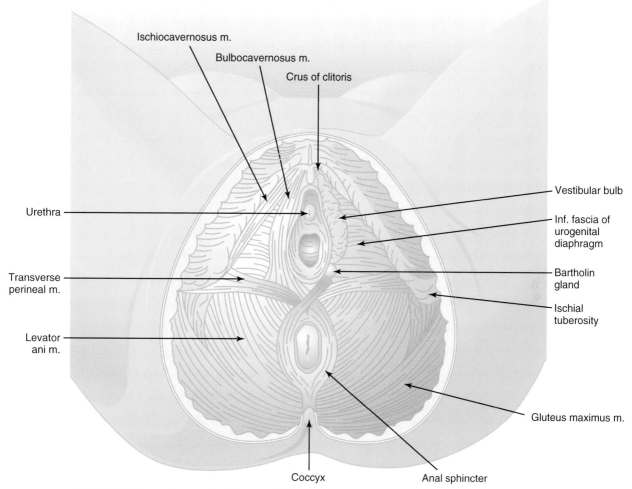

FIGURE 3-2 The perineum, showing superficial structures on the left and deeper structures on the right.

VULVA

The external genitalia are referred to collectively as the vulva. As shown in Figure 3-3, **the vulva includes the mons veneris, labia majora, labia minora, clitoris, vulvovaginal (Bartholin) glands, fourchette, and perineum.** The most prominent features of the vulva, the labia majora, are large, hair-covered folds of skin that contain sebaceous glands and subcutaneous fat and lie on either side of the introitus. The labia minora lie medially and contain no hair but have a rich supply of venous sinuses, sebaceous glands, and nerves. The labia minora may vary from scarcely noticeable structures to leaf-like flaps measuring up to 3 cm in length. Anteriorly, each splits into two folds. The posterior pair of folds attach to the inferior surface of the clitoris, at which point they unite to form the frenulum of the clitoris. The anterior pair are united in a hoodlike configuration over the clitoris, forming the prepuce. Posteriorly, the labia minora may extend almost to the fourchette.

The clitoris lies just in front of the urethra and consists of the glans, the body, and the crura. Only the glans clitoris is visible externally. The body, composed of a pair of corpora cavernosa, extends superiorly for a distance of several centimeters and divides into two crura, which are attached to the undersurface of either pubic ramus. Each crus is covered by the corresponding ischiocavernosus muscle. Each vestibular bulb (equivalent to the corpus spongiosum of the penis) extends posteriorly from the glans on either side of the lower vagina. Each bulb is attached to the inferior surface of the perineal membrane and covered by the bulbocavernosus muscle. These muscles aid in constricting the venous supply to the erectile vestibular bulbs and also act as the sphincter vaginae.

As the labia minora are spread, the vaginal introitus, guarded by the hymenal ring, is seen. Usually, the hymen is represented only by a circle of carunculae myrtiformes around the vaginal introitus. The hymen

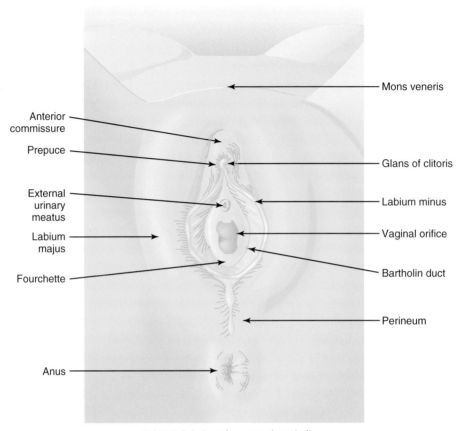

Anterior commissure
Prepuce
External urinary meatus
Labium majus
Fourchette
Anus

Mons veneris
Glans of clitoris
Labium minus
Vaginal orifice
Bartholin duct
Perineum

FIGURE 3-3 Female external genitalia.

may take many forms, however, such as a cribriform plate with many small openings or a completely imperforate diaphragm.

The vestibule of the vagina is that portion of the introitus extending inferiorly from the hymenal ring between the labia minora. The fourchette represents the posterior portion of the vestibule just above the perineal body. **Most of the vulva is innervated by the branches of the pudendal nerve. Anterior to the urethra, the vulva is innervated by the ilioinguinal and genitofemoral nerves.** This area is not anesthetized adequately by a pudendal block, and repair of paraurethral tears should be supplemented by additional subcutaneous anesthesia.

Internal Genital Development

The upper vagina, cervix, uterus, and fallopian tubes are formed from the paramesonephric (müllerian) ducts. Although human embryos, whether male or female, possess both paired paramesonephric and mesonephric (wolffian) ducts, **the absence of Y chromosomal influence leads to the development of the paramesonephric system** with virtual total regression

of the mesonephric system. With a Y chromosome present, a testis is formed and müllerian-inhibiting substance is produced, creating the reverse situation.

Mesonephric duct development occurs in each urogenital ridge between weeks 2 and 4 and is thought to influence the growth and development of the paramesonephric ducts. **The mesonephric ducts terminate caudally by opening into the urogenital sinus.** First evidence of each paramesonephric duct is seen at 6 weeks' gestation as a groove in the coelomic epithelium of the paired urogenital ridges, lateral to the cranial pole of the mesonephric duct. **Each paramesonephric duct opens into the coelomic cavity cranially** at a point destined to become a tubal ostium. Coursing caudally at first, parallel to the developing mesonephric duct, the blind distal end of each paramesonephric duct eventually crosses dorsal to the mesonephric duct, and the two ducts approximate in the midline. **The two paramesonephric ducts fuse terminally at the urogenital septum, forming the uterovaginal primordium.** The distal point of fusion is known as the **müllerian tubercle (Müller tubercle)** and can be seen protruding into the urogenital sinus dorsally in embryos at 9 to 10 weeks' gestation (Figure 3-4). **Later**

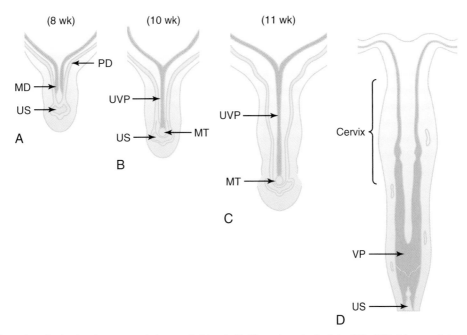

FIGURE 3-4 Early embryologic development of the genital tract **(A-C)** and vaginal plate **(D)**. *MD,* Mesonephric duct; *MT,* müllerian tubercle; *PD,* paramesonephric duct; *US,* urogenital sinus; *UVP,* uterovaginal primordium; *VP,* vaginal plate. (Redrawn from Didusch JF, Koff AK: Development of the vagina in the human fetus. *Contrib Embryol Carnegie Inst* 24:61, 1933.)

dissolution of the septum between the fused paramesonephric ducts leads to the development of a single uterine fundus, cervix, and, according to some investigators, the upper vagina.

Degeneration of the mesonephric ducts is progressive from 10 to 16 weeks in the female fetus, although vestigial remnants of the latter may be noted in the adult (Gartner duct cyst, paroöphoron, epoöphoron) (Figure 3-5). The myometrium and endometrial stroma are derived from adjacent mesenchyme; the glandular epithelium of the fallopian tubes, uterus, and cervix is derived from the paramesonephric duct.

Solid vaginal plate formation and lengthening occur from the 12th through the 20th weeks, followed by caudad to cephalad canalization, which is usually completed in utero. Controversy surrounds the relative contribution of the urogenital sinus and paramesonephric ducts to the development of the vagina, and it is uncertain whether the whole of the vaginal plate is formed secondary to growth of the endoderm of the urogenital sinus or whether the upper vagina is formed from the paramesonephric ducts.

VAGINA

The vagina is a flattened tube extending posterosuperiorly from the hymenal ring at the introitus up to the fornices that surround the cervix (Figure 3-6). **Its epithelium, which is stratified squamous in type, is normally devoid of mucous glands and hair follicles and is nonkeratinized.** Gestational exposure to diethylstilbestrol (taken by the mother) may result

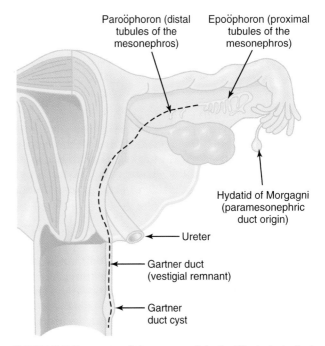

FIGURE 3-5 Remnants of the mesonephric (wolffian) ducts that may persist in the anterolateral vagina or adjacent to the uterus within the broad ligament or mesosalpinx.

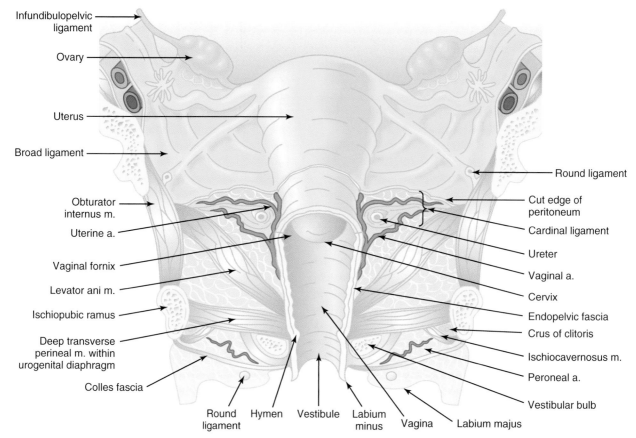

FIGURE 3-6 Coronal section of the pelvis at the level of the uterine isthmus and ischial spines, showing the ligaments supporting the uterus.

in columnar glands interspersed with the squamous epithelium of the upper two-thirds of the vagina (vaginal adenosis). Deep to the vaginal epithelium are the muscular coats of the vagina, which consist of an inner circular and an outer longitudinal smooth muscle layer. Remnants of the mesonephric ducts may sometimes be demonstrated along the vaginal wall in the subepithelial layers and may give rise to **Gartner duct cysts.** The adult vagina averages about 8 cm in length, although its size varies considerably with age, parity, and the status of ovarian function. An important anatomic feature is the immediate proximity of the posterior fornix of the vagina to the pouch of Douglas, which allows easy access to the peritoneal cavity from the vagina, by either culdocentesis or colpotomy.

UTERUS

The uterus consists of the cervix and the uterine corpus, which are joined by the isthmus. The uterine isthmus represents a transitional area wherein the endocervical epithelium gradually changes into the endometrial lining. In late pregnancy, this area elongates and is referred to as the lower uterine segment.

The cervix is generally 2 to 3 cm in length. In infants and children, the cervix is proportionately longer than the uterine corpus (Figure 3-7). The portion that protrudes into the vagina and is surrounded by the fornices is covered with a nonkeratinizing squamous epithelium. **At about the external cervical os, the squamous epithelium covering the exocervix (or ectocervix) changes to simple columnar epithelium, the site of transition being referred to as the squamocolumnar junction.** The cervical canal is lined by irregular, arborized, simple columnar epithelium, which extends into the stroma as cervical "glands" or crypts.

The uterine corpus is a thick, pear-shaped organ, somewhat flattened anteroposteriorly, that consists of largely interlacing smooth muscle fibers. The endometrial lining of the uterine corpus may vary from 2 to 10 mm in thickness (which may be measured by ultrasonic imaging), depending on the stage of the menstrual cycle. Most of the surface of the uterus is covered by the peritoneal mesothelium.

Four paired sets of ligaments are attached to the uterus (Figure 3-8). Each round ligament inserts on the anterior surface of the uterus just in front of the

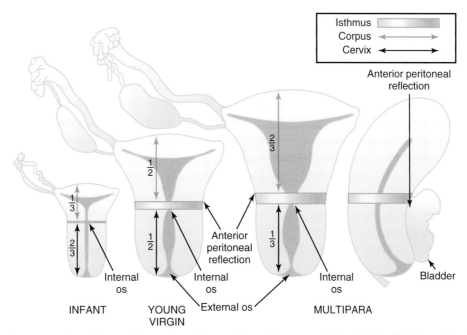

FIGURE 3-7 Changing proportion of the uterine cervix and corpus from infancy to adulthood. (Modified from Cunningham FG, Mac-Donald PC, Gant NF, et al, editors: *Williams obstetrics,* ed 20, East Norwalk, Conn, 1997, Appleton & Lange.)

fallopian tube, passes to the pelvic side wall in a fold of the broad ligament, traverses the inguinal canal, and ends in the labium majus. **The round ligaments are of little supportive value in preventing uterine prolapse** but help to keep the uterus anteverted. **The uterosacral ligaments** are condensations of the endopelvic fascia that arise from the sacral fascia and insert into the posteroinferior portion of the uterus at about the level of the isthmus. These ligaments contain sympathetic and parasympathetic nerve fibers that supply the uterus. They provide important support for the uterus and are also significant in precluding the development of an enterocele. **The cardinal ligaments (Mackenrodt)** are the other important supporting structures of the uterus that prevent prolapse. They extend from the pelvic fascia on the lateral pelvic walls and insert into the lateral portion of the cervix and vagina, reaching superiorly to the level of the isthmus. **The pubocervical ligaments** pass anteriorly around the bladder to the posterior surface of the pubic symphysis.

In addition, there are four peritoneal folds. Anteriorly, **the vesicouterine fold** is reflected from the level of the uterine isthmus onto the bladder. Posteriorly, **the rectouterine fold** passes from the posterior wall of the uterus, to the upper fourth of the vagina, and thence onto the rectum. The pouch between the cervix and vagina anteriorly and rectum posteriorly forms a cul-de-sac, called the pouch of Douglas. Laterally, the **two broad ligaments** each pass from the side of the uterus to the lateral wall of the pelvis. Between the two leaves of each broad ligament are contained the fallopian

tube, the round ligament, and the ovarian ligament, in addition to nerves, blood vessels, and lymphatics. **The fold of broad ligament containing the fallopian tube is called the mesosalpinx.** Between the end of the tube and ovary and the pelvic side wall, where the ureter passes over the common iliac vessels, is the infundibulopelvic ligament, which contains the vessels and nerves for the ovary. The ureter may be injured when this ligament is ligated during a salpingo-oophorectomy procedure if it is not clearly identified first.

The anatomic position of the uterus may vary within the pelvic cavity as palpated during a pelvic examination. With respect to the horizontal plane on the surface of the examination table, the straight line axis extending from the cervix to the fundal end of the uterine corpus may be in one of three positions. The uterus may tilt in a forward position (anteverted), it may be only slightly forward and in mid-position, or it may tilt in a backward direction (retroverted). Additionally, the fundal portion of the uterus may fold forward (anteflexed) or backward (retroflexed). Most of the time this variation in position is normal and without clinical significance. On occasion the identification of this anatomic variation is important. For example, extreme flexion (ante or retro) may make insertion of an instrument or of an intrauterine device (IUD) higher risk. A retroverted and retroflexed uterus may also be a finding in a woman with pelvic adhesions due to endometriosis or pelvic inflammation due to infection. Figure 3-9 illustrates the potential positions of the uterus within the pelvis.

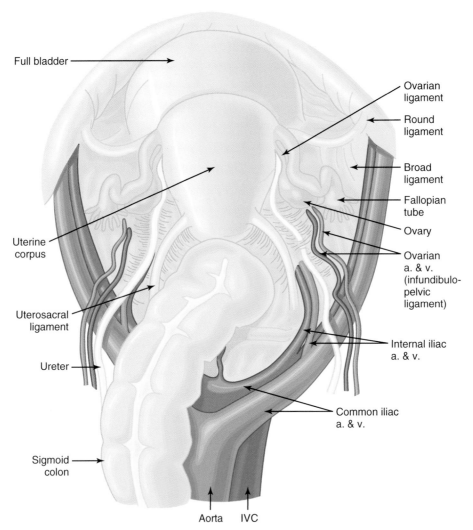

Full bladder

Ovarian ligament

Round ligament

Broad ligament

Fallopian tube

Ovary

Ovarian a. & v. (infundibulo-pelvic ligament)

Uterine corpus

Uterosacral ligament

Ureter

Internal iliac a. & v.

Common iliac a. & v.

Sigmoid colon

Aorta   IVC

FIGURE 3-8 View of the internal genital organs in the female pelvis. *IVC,* Inferior vena cava.

FALLOPIAN TUBES

The oviducts are bilateral muscular tubes (about 10 cm in length) with lumina that connect the uterine cavity with the peritoneal cavity. They are enclosed in the medial four-fifths of the superior aspect of the broad ligament. The tubes are lined by a ciliated, columnar epithelium that is thrown into branching folds. That segment of the tube within the wall of the uterus is referred to as the **interstitial portion.** The medial portion of each tube is superior to the round ligament, anterior to the ovarian ligament, and relatively fixed in position. This nonmobile portion of the tube has a fairly narrow lumen and is referred to as the **isthmus.** As the tube proceeds laterally, it is located anterior to the ovary; it then passes around the lateral portion of the ovary and down toward the cul-de-sac. The **ampullary and fimbriated portions** of the tube are suspended from the broad ligament by the mesosalpinx and are

quite mobile. The mobility of the fimbriated end of the tube plays an important role in fertility. The ampullary portion of the tube is the most common site of ectopic pregnancies.

Normal Embryologic Development of the Ovary

The earliest anatomic event in gonadogenesis is noted at approximately 4 weeks' gestational age (i.e., 4 weeks from conception), when a thickening of the peritoneal, or coelomic, epithelium on the ventromedial surface of the urogenital ridge occurs. A bulging **genital ridge** is subsequently produced by rapid proliferation of the coelomic epithelium in an area that is medial, but parallel, to the mesonephric ridge. Prior to the 5th week, this indifferent gonad consists of germinal epithelium

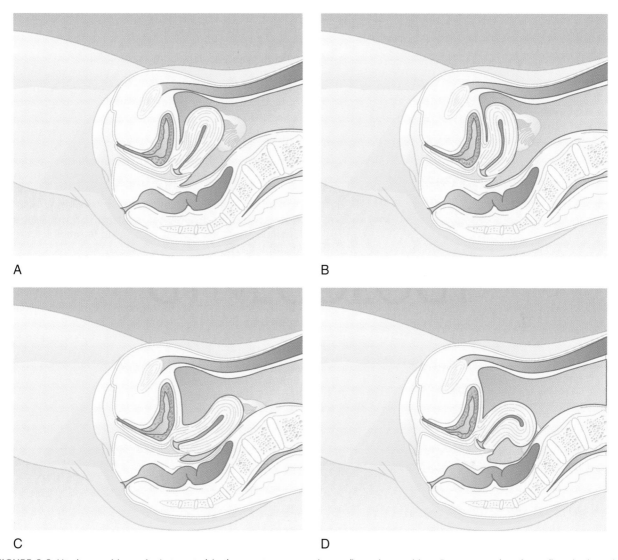

A

B

C

D

FIGURE 3-9 Uterine positions: **A,** Anteverted is the most common (normal) uterine position; **B,** anteverted and anteflexed when the uterine fundus is further forward toward the bladder; **C,** retroverted when the uterus is tilted backward toward the rectum. This position is not always abnormal but could indicate endometriosis affecting the uterosacral ligaments; and **D,** retroverted and retroflexed when there is an additional backward angle of the uterine fundus. A retroverted and retroflexed uterine position is more likely to be associated with endometriosis (see Chapter 25).

surrounding the internal blastema, a primordial mesenchymal cellular mass designated to become the ovarian medulla. After 5 weeks, projections from the germinal epithelium extend like spokes into the mesenchymal blastema to form **primary sex cords.** Soon thereafter in the 7th week, a testis can be identified histologically if the embryo has a Y chromosome. In the absence of a Y chromosome, definitive ovarian characteristics do not appear until somewhere between the 12th and 16th weeks.

As early as 3 weeks' gestation, relatively large primordial germ cells appear intermixed with other cells in the endoderm of the yolk sac wall of the primitive hindgut. These germ cell precursors migrate along the hindgut dorsal mesentery (Figure 3-10) and are all contained in the mesenchyme of the undifferentiated urogenital ridge by 8 weeks' gestation. Subsequent replication of these cells by mitotic division occurs, with maximal mitotic activity noted up to 20 weeks' gestation and cessation noted by term. These oogonia, the end result of this germ cell proliferation, are incorporated into the cortical sex cords of the genital ridge.

Histologically, the first evidence of follicles is seen at about 20 weeks, with germ cells surrounded by flattened cells derived from the cortical sex cords. These flattened cells are recognizable as granulosa

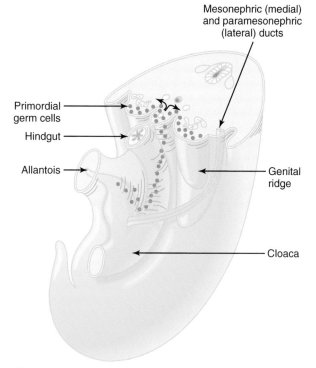

Mesonephric (medial)
and paramesonephric
(lateral) ducts

Primordial
germ cells

Hindgut

Allantois

Genital
ridge

Cloaca

FIGURE 3-10 Migratory path of primordial germ cells from the yolk sac, along the hindgut mesentery, to the urogenital ridge at approximately 5 weeks.

cells of coelomic epithelial origin and theca cells of mesenchymal origin. The oogonia enter the prophase of the first meiotic division and are then called **primary oocytes** (see Chapter 4). It has been estimated that more than 2 million primary oocytes, or their precursors, are present at 20 weeks' gestation, but only about 300,000 primordial follicles are present by 7 years of age.

Regression of the primary sex cords in the medulla produces the **rete ovarii,** which are found histologically in the hilus of the ovary along with another testicular analogue called **Leydig cells,** which are thought to be derived from mesenchyme. Vestiges of the rete ovarii and of the degenerating mesonephros may also be noted at times in the mesovarium or mesosalpinx. Structural homologues in males and females are shown in Table 3-1.

Anatomy of the Ovaries

The ovaries are oval, flattened, compressible organs, approximately $3 \times 2 \times 2$ cm in size. They are situated on the superior surface of the broad ligament and are suspended between the ovarian ligament medially and the suspensory ligament of the ovary or infundibulopelvic ligament laterally and superiorly. Each occupies a position in the ovarian fossa (of Waldeyer), which is a

TABLE 3-1

STRUCTURAL HOMOLOGUES IN MALES AND FEMALES			
Primordia	Female	Male	Major Determining Factors
Gonadal			
Germ cells	Oogonia	Spermatogonia	Sex chromosomes
Coelomic epithelium	Granulosa cells	Sertoli cells	
Mesenchyme	Theca cells	Leydig cells	
Mesonephros	Rete ovarii	Rete testis	
Ductal			
Paramesonephric (müllerian) duct	Fallopian tubes Uterus Superior ⅔ of vagina Gartner duct	Hydatid testis	Absence of Y chromosome
Mesonephric (wolffian) duct Mesonephric tubules	Epoöphoron Paroöphoron	Vas deferens Seminal vesicles Epididymis Efferent ducts	Testosterone Müllerian inhibiting factor
External Genitalia			
Urogenital sinus	Vaginal contribution Skene glands Bartholin glands	Prostate Prostatic utricle Cowper glands Penis Corpora spongiosa Scrotum	Presence or absence of testosterone, dihydrotestosterone, and 5α-reductase enzyme
Genital tubercle Urogenital folds Genital folds	Clitoris Labia minora Labia majora		

shallow depression on the lateral pelvic wall just posterior to the external iliac vessels and anterior to the ureter and hypogastric vessels. In endometriosis and salpingo-oophoritis, the ovaries may be densely adherent to the ureter. Generally, the serosal covering and the tunica albuginea of the ovary are quite thin, and developing follicles and corpora lutea are readily visible.

The blood supply to the ovaries is provided by the long ovarian arteries, which arise from the abdominal aorta immediately below the renal arteries. These vessels course downward and cross laterally over the ureter at the level of the pelvic brim, passing branches to the ureter and the fallopian tube. The ovary also receives substantial blood supply from the uterine artery through the uterine-ovarian arterial anastomosis. **The venous drainage from the right ovary is directly into the inferior vena cava, whereas that from the left ovary is into the left renal vein** (Figure 3-11).

Anatomy of the Ureters

The ureters extend 25 to 30 cm from the renal pelves to their insertion into the bladder at the trigone. Each descends immediately under the peritoneum, crossing the pelvic brim beneath the ovarian vessels just anterior to the bifurcation of the common iliac artery. In the true pelvis, the ureter initially courses inferiorly, just anterior to the hypogastric vessels, and stays closely

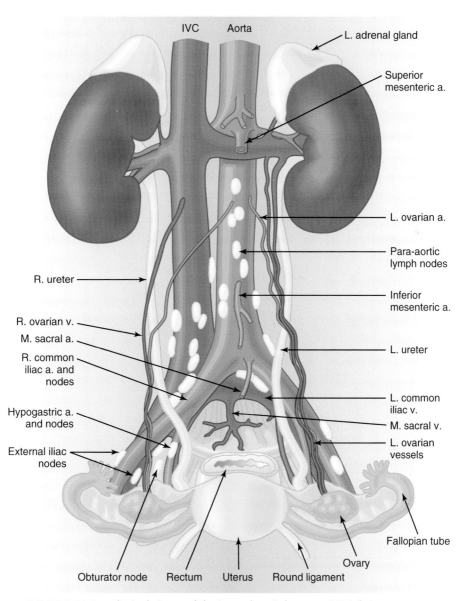

FIGURE 3-11 Lymphatic drainage of the internal genital organs. *IVC,* Inferior vena cava.

attached to the peritoneum. It then passes forward along the side of the cervix and beneath the uterine artery toward the trigone of the bladder.

Lymphatic Drainage

The lymphatic drainage of the vulva and lower vagina is principally to the inguinofemoral lymph nodes and then to the external iliac chains (see Figure 3-11). The lymphatic drainage of the cervix takes place through the parametria (cardinal ligaments) to the pelvic nodes (the hypogastric, obturator, and external iliac groups) and then to the common iliac and para-aortic chains. The lymphatic drainage from the endometrium is through the broad ligament and infundibulopelvic ligament to the pelvic and para-aortic chains. The lymphatics of the ovaries pass via the infundibulopelvic ligaments to the pelvic and para-aortic nodes (see Figure 3-11).

Anatomy of the Bony Pelvis

The bony pelvis (Figure 3-12) is made up of the **two paired innominate bones and the sacrum.** The symphysis pubis is formed anteriorly at the attachment of both innominate bones. The sacrum has five to six vertebrae that are fused in the adult. **The sacrum articulates posteriorly with each innominate bone at the sacroiliac joints. The sacrum also articulates inferiorly with the coccyx and superiorly with the fifth lumbar vertebra.** The true (lesser) pelvis is formed by the sacrum and coccyx posteriorly and by the pubis anteriorly and ischium laterally. The true pelvis contains the pelvic organs; the uterus, vagina, bladder, fal-

lopian tubes, ovaries, and part of the rectum and anus. The false (greater) pelvis is bounded by the lumbar vertebrae posteriorly, iliac fossae bilaterally, and the abdominal wall anteriorly.

The bony pelvis is particularly important during pregnancy and labor. It is clinically important to determine the adequacy of the pelvis for vaginal birth by performing pelvimetry. This may be done during a pelvic examination or using computed tomography, which is more accurate (see Chapter 8).

Anatomy of the Lower Abdominal Wall

Because most intraabdominal gynecologic operations are performed through lower abdominal incisions, it is important to review the anatomy of the lower abdominal wall with special reference to the muscles and fasciae. After transecting the skin, subcutaneous fat, superficial fascia (Camper), and deep fascia (Scarpa) the anterior rectus sheath is encountered (Figure 3-13). **The rectus sheath is a strong fibrous compartment formed by the aponeuroses of the three lateral abdominal wall muscles.** The aponeuroses meet in the midline to form the linea alba and partially encase the two rectus abdominis muscles. The composition of the rectus sheath differs in its upper and lower portions. Above the midpoint between the umbilicus and the symphysis pubis, the rectus muscle is encased anteriorly by the aponeurosis of the external oblique and the anterior lamina of the internal oblique aponeurosis and posteriorly by the aponeurosis of the transversus abdominis and the posterior lamina of

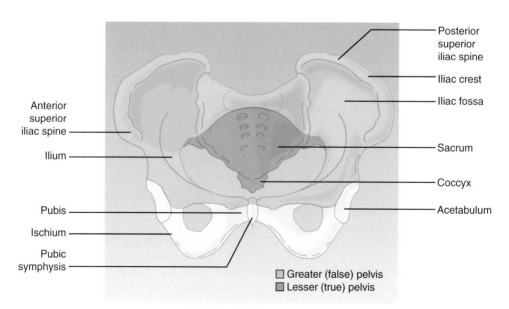

FIGURE 3-12 The bony pelvis.

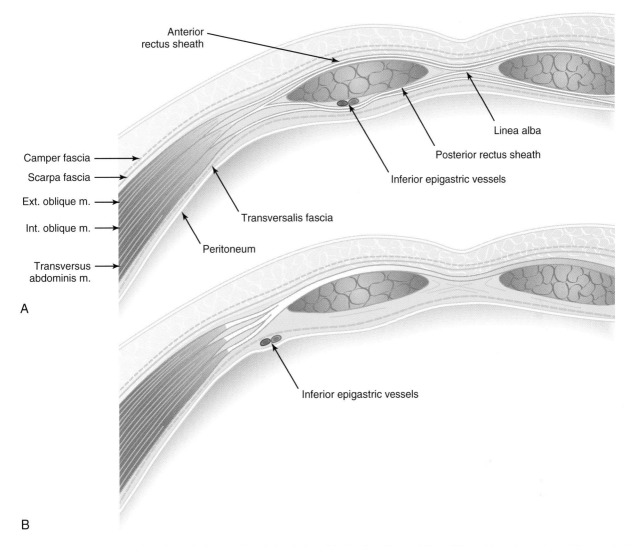

Anterior
rectus sheath

Camper fascia

Scarpa fascia

Ext. oblique m.

Int. oblique m.

Transversus
abdominis m.

Linea alba

Posterior rectus sheath

Inferior epigastric vessels

Transversalis fascia

Peritoneum

A

Inferior epigastric vessels

B

FIGURE 3-13 Transverse section through the anterior abdominal wall just below the umbilicus (A) and just above the pubic symphysis (B). Note the absence of the posterior rectus sheath in B.

the internal oblique aponeurosis. **In the lower fourth of the abdomen, the posterior aponeurotic layer of the sheath terminates in a free crescentic margin, the semilunar fold of Douglas.**

Each rectus abdominis muscle, encased in the rectus sheath on either side of the midline, extends from the superior aspect of the symphysis pubis to the anterior surface of the fifth, sixth, and seventh costal cartilages. A variable number of tendinous intersections (three to five) crosses each muscle at irregular intervals, and any transverse rectus surgical incision forms a new fibrous intersection during healing. The muscle is not attached to the posterior sheath and, following separation from the anterior sheath, can be retracted laterally, as in the Pfannenstiel

incision. **Each rectus muscle has a firm aponeurosis at its attachment to the symphysis pubis, and this tendinous aponeurosis can be transected if necessary to improve exposure, as in the Cherney incision,** and resutured securely during closure of the abdominal wall.

The **inferior epigastric arteries** arise from the external iliac arteries and proceed superiorly just lateral to the rectus muscles between the transversalis fascia and the peritoneum. They enter the rectus sheaths at the level of the semilunar line and continue their course superiorly just posterior to the rectus muscles. In a transverse rectus muscle–cutting (Maylard) incision, the epigastric arteries can be retracted laterally or ligated to allow a wide peritoneal incision.

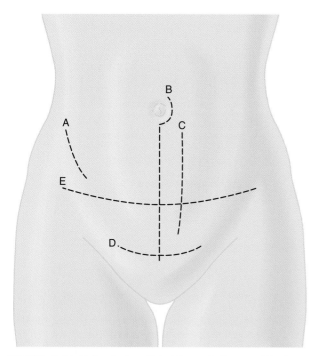

FIGURE 3-14 Abdominal wall incisions: McBurney **(A)**, lower midline **(B)**, left lower paramedian **(C)**, Pfannenstiel or Cherney **(D)**, and transverse, Maylard or Bardenheuer **(E)**.

Abdominal Wall Incisions

The most commonly used lower abdominal incision in gynecologic surgery is the Pfannenstiel incision (Figure 3-14). Although it does not always give sufficient exposure for extensive operations, it has cosmetic advantages in that it is generally only 2 cm above the symphysis pubis, and the scar is later covered by the pubic hair. Because the rectus abdominis muscles are not cut, eviscerations and wound hernias are extremely uncommon. **For extensive pelvic procedures (e.g., radical hysterectomy and pelvic lymphadenectomy), a transverse muscle–cutting incision (Bardenheuer or Maylard) at a slightly higher level in the lower abdomen gives sufficient exposure.** In addition, the skin incision falls within the lines of Langer, so a good cosmetic result can be expected.

When it is anticipated that upper abdominal exploration will be necessary, such as in a patient with suspected ovarian cancer, a midline incision through the linea alba or a paramedian vertical incision is indicated.

Female Reproductive Physiology

JOSEPH C. GAMBONE

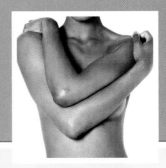

- The female reproductive cycle (menstrual cycle) may be viewed as four separate physiologic cycles (hypothalamic, pituitary, ovarian, and endometrial) but is actually a highly complex and integrated event. This 28 (±7) day cycle allows for the maturation and release of an oocyte (usually only one) that if fertilized may implant in a receptive endometrium. If fertilization and implantation do not occur, the end result is menstruation.
- Communication between the hypothalamus, which releases gonadotropin-releasing hormone (GnRH) in pulses, and the pituitary gland is essential to permit the pituitary to respond to changes in ovarian hormones (estradiol and progesterone) and other factors. This essential communication results in both negative and positive feedback for the release of the pituitary gonadotropins, luteinizing hormone (LH) and follicle-stimulating hormone (FSH). These gonadotropins, also released in pulses, stimulate follicular growth in the ovary (FSH) such that one dominant follicle releases an oocyte in response to a midcycle surge in LH. Other growth factors and peptides such as inhibin-A, inhibin-B, and activin act systemically and locally to control follicular growth.

- After oocyte release, the dominant (graafian) follicle becomes the corpus luteum and secretes both estradiol (E2) and progesterone (P4). The endometrium responds to E2 with growth or proliferation before ovulation and to P4 and E2 after ovulation with maturation that allows for implantation if fertilization occurs. The corpus luteum continues to maintain the uterine lining, stimulated by human chorionic gonadotropin (hCG) from the placental tissue if a pregnancy occurs.
- Fertilization and implantation begin with normal sperm function and penetration of the oocyte in the fallopian tube. Fertilization restores the diploid number of chromosomes and determines the sex of the zygote. The fertilized ovum reaches the endometrium about 3 days after ovulation and after another several days the blastocyst implants.
- As the blastocyst burrows into the endometrium, the trophoblastic strands branch to form the primitive villi. The villi are first distinguished about the 12th day after fertilization and are the essential structures of the placenta. The placenta is the life-support system for the developing fetus for the rest of pregnancy.

Reproductive Cycle

Each female reproductive cycle (menstrual cycle) represents a complex interaction between the hypothalamus, pituitary gland, ovaries, and endometrium. Cyclic changes in the gonadotropins, luteinizing hormone (LH), and follicle-stimulating hormone (FSH) and sex steroid hormones, mainly estradiol (E2) and progesterone (P4), induce functional as well as morphologic changes in the ovary, resulting in follicular maturation, ovulation, and corpus luteum formation. Similar changes at the level of the endometrium allow for successful implantation of the fertilized ovum or a physiologic shedding of the menstrual endometrium when an early pregnancy does not occur. By convention, the normal cycle begins on the first day of menstrual bleeding and ends just before the first day of the next menses. The average length of each cycle is 28 (±7) days.

The reproductive cycle can be viewed from the perspective of each of four physiologic components (Table 4-1). The cyclic changes within the hypothalamic-pituitary axis, ovary, and endometrium are sequentially approached in this chapter, as if they were four separate cycles, but these endocrine events occur in concert in a uniquely integrated fashion. The chapter also includes a discussion of spermatogenesis, fertilization, implantation, and placentation.

TABLE 4-1

ENDOCRINE COMPONENTS OF THE REPRODUCTIVE (MENSTRUAL) CYCLE

Component	Activity	Phases	Comment(s)
Hypothalamic (arcuate nucleus)	Produces pulses of GnRH from the arcuate nucleus. GnRH has a very short half-life of 2-4 min. Action requires frequent pulses. GnRH is sometimes referred to as LH-RH because it generally causes a greater release of LH.	Frequency of pulses is variable among individuals. Pulses are more frequent and lower amplitude in follicular phase and less frequent but higher amplitude in luteal phase (see Figure 4-4). The hypothalamic component changes the least on a daily basis.	Permits the other components of the cycle to act and react. If pathology or medications (e.g., hormonal contraceptives or GnRH analogues) disrupt pulses, the entire cycle stops. When GnRH is given in a continuous infusion (no pulses) downregulation inhibits LH and FSH release.
Pituitary (anterior)	Produces pulses of LH and FSH from the anterior portion of gland. LH half-life is 30 min, FSH half-life is several hours.	Negative feedback initially with strong positive feedback resulting in LH surge and ovulation.	Surge of LH at midcycle triggers ovulation, maturing the oocyte and releasing it from the follicle.
Ovarian	Theca cells produce androgens in response to LH. Granulosa cells aromatize androgens to estrogens in response to FSH (see Figure 4-3). Ovarian inhibins (A and B) inhibit and activin stimulates gonadotropins.	Follicular, ovulatory, and luteal phases. Average overall cycle length is 28 ($\pm$7) days. Luteal phase is generally constant at 12 to 14 days. Follicular phase may vary.	LH triggers ovulation at midcycle. LH then stimulates the corpus luteum to produce P4 and some E2. With pregnancy, placental hCG rescues the corpus luteum by mimicking LH.
Endometrial	Estradiol (E2) from the ovary stimulates growth (proliferation) and progesterone (P4) from the corpus luteum converts endometrium to secretory and withdrawal of E2 and P4 leads to menstruation (see Figures 4-7 and 4-8).	Menstrual, proliferative, and secretory phases. The endometrial component changes the most on a daily basis. Histology may be used to "date" the endometrium and determine day of cycle.	Menstruation is the only visible component. Because it is visible, it is where the cycle is said to start but menstruation actually represents the end of the previous cycle.

FSH, Follicle-stimulating hormone; *GnRH,* gonadotropin-releasing hormone; *hCG,* human chorionic gonadotropin; *LH,* luteinizing hormone; *LH-RH,* luteinizing hormone–releasing hormone.

Hypothalamic-Pituitary Axis

PITUITARY GLAND

The pituitary gland lies below the hypothalamus at the base of the brain within a bony cavity (sella turcica) and is separated from the cranial cavity by a condensation of dura mater overlying the sella turcica (diaphragma sellae). The pituitary gland is divided into two major portions, the neurohypophysis and the adenohypophysis (Figure 4-1). **The neurohypophysis, which consists of the posterior lobe (pars nervosa), the neural stalk (infundibulum), and the median eminence, is derived from neural tissue and is in direct continuity with the hypothalamus and central nervous system. The adenohypophysis, which consists of the pars distalis (anterior lobe), pars intermedia (intermediate lobe), and pars tuberalis, which surrounds the neural stalk, is derived from ectoderm.**

The arterial blood supply to the median eminence and the neural stalk (pituitary portal system) represents a major avenue of transport for hypothalamic secretions to the anterior pituitary.

The neurohypophysis serves primarily to transport oxytocin and vasopressin (antidiuretic hormone) along neuronal projections from the supraoptic and paraventricular nuclei of the hypothalamus to their release into the circulation.

The anterior pituitary contains different cell types that produce six protein hormones: follicle-stimulating hormone (FSH), luteinizing hormone (LH), thyroid-stimulating hormone (TSH), prolactin, growth hormone (GH), and adrenocorticotropic hormone (ACTH).

The gonadotropins, FSH and LH, are synthesized and stored in cells called **gonadotrophs,** whereas TSH is produced by **thyrotrophs.** FSH, LH, and TSH are glycoproteins, consisting of α and β subunits. The α subunits of FSH, LH, and TSH are identical. The same α subunit is also present in human chorionic gonadotropin (hCG). The β subunits are individual for each hormone. The half-life for circulating LH is about 30 minutes, whereas that of FSH is several hours. The difference in half-lives may account, at least in part, for the differential secretion patterns of these two gonadotropins.

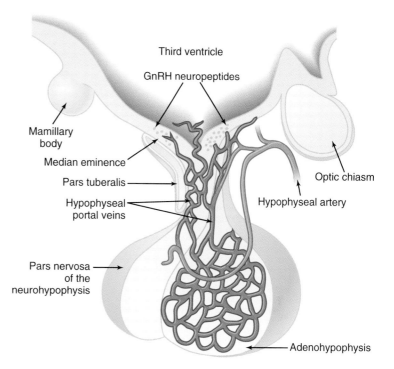

FIGURE 4-1 Hypothalamic-pituitary portal circulatory system. The pulses of gonadotropin-releasing hormone (GnRH) from the arcuate nucleus are transported to the anterior pituitary gland by way of this circulatory system. An interruption or significant alteration of GnRH pulses will cause the reproductive cycle to stop.

Prolactin is secreted by **lactotrophs.** Unlike the case with other peptide hormones produced by the adenohypophysis, **pituitary release of prolactin is under tonic inhibition by the hypothalamus.** The half-life for circulating prolactin is about 20 to 30 minutes. In addition to its lactogenic effect, prolactin may directly or indirectly influence hypothalamic, pituitary, and ovarian functions in relation to the ovulatory cycle, particularly in the pathologic state of chronic hyperprolactinemia (see Chapter 33).

GONADOTROPIN SECRETORY PATTERNS

A normal ovarian cycle can be divided into a follicular and a luteal phase (Figure 4-2). The follicular phase begins with the onset of menses and culminates in the preovulatory surge of LH. The luteal phase begins with the onset of the preovulatory LH surge and ends with the first day of menses.

Decreasing levels of estradiol and progesterone from the regressing corpus luteum of the preceding cycle initiate a rise of FSH by a negative feedback mechanism, which stimulates follicular growth and estradiol secretion. A major characteristic of follicular growth and estradiol secretion is explained by the two-gonadotropin (LH and FSH) two-cell (theca and granulosa cell) theory of ovarian follicular development. According to this theory, there are separate cellular functions in the ovarian follicle wherein LH stimulates theca cells to produce androgens (androstenedione and testosterone) and FSH then stimulates the granu-

losa cells to convert these androgens into estrogens (androstenedione to estrone and testosterone to estradiol) as depicted in Figure 4-3. Initially, at lower levels of estradiol, there is a negative feedback effect on the release of LH from the pool of gonadotropins in the pituitary gonadotrophs. When estradiol levels rise later in the follicular phase (>200 picograms for >50 hours), there is a positive feedback on the release of gonadotropins, resulting in the LH surge and ovulation. The latter occurs 36 to 44 hours after the onset of this midcycle LH surge. With pharmacologic doses of progestins contained in contraceptive pills, there is a profound negative feedback effect on gonadotropin-releasing hormone (GnRH) so that none of the gonadotropin pool is released. Hence, ovulation is blocked (see Chapter 27).

During the luteal phase, both LH and FSH are significantly suppressed through the negative feedback effect of elevated circulating estradiol and progesterone. This inhibition persists until progesterone and estradiol levels decline near the end of the luteal phase as a result of corpus luteal regression, should pregnancy fail to occur. The net effect is a slight rise in serum FSH, which initiates new follicular growth for the next cycle. The duration of the corpus luteum's functional regression is such that menstruation generally occurs 14 days after the LH surge in the absence of pregnancy. When pregnancy occurs, the corpus luteum is "rescued" by hCG which acts like LH and progesterone production continues.

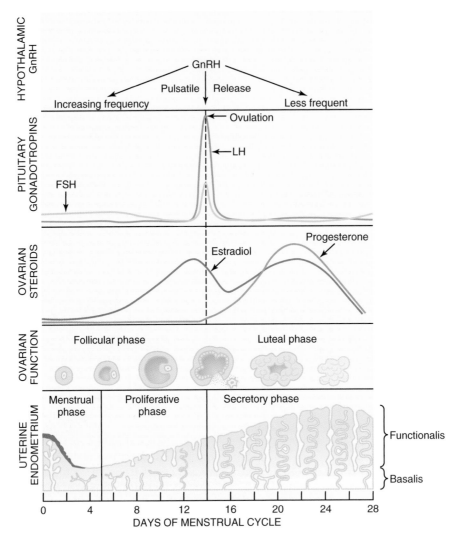

FIGURE 4-2 Hormone activity and levels during a normal menstrual cycle. All four components of the cycle (hypothalamic, pituitary, ovarian, and endometrial) are represented in the figure. These components work in a highly integrated way in a cycle that represents one of the most complex endocrine/end organ systems in physiology. *FSH*, Follicle-stimulating hormone; *GnRH*, gonadotropin-releasing hormone; *LH*, luteinizing hormone.

HYPOTHALAMUS

Five different small peptides or biogenic amines that affect the reproductive cycle have been isolated from the hypothalamus. All exert specific effects on the hormonal secretion of the anterior pituitary gland. They are **GnRH, thyrotropin-releasing hormone (TRH), somatotropin release-inhibiting factor (SRIF) or somatostatin, corticotropin-releasing factor (CRF), and prolactin release-inhibiting factor (PIF).** Only GnRH and PIF are discussed in this chapter.

GnRH is a decapeptide that is synthesized primarily in the arcuate nucleus. It has a very short half-life of 2 to 4 minutes. It is responsible for the synthesis and release of both LH and FSH. Because it usually causes the release of more LH than FSH, it is less commonly called LH-releasing hormone (LH-RH) or LH-releasing

factor (LRF). **Both FSH and LH appear to be present in two different forms within the pituitary gonadotrophs. One is a releasable form and the other a storage form.** GnRH reaches the anterior pituitary via the hypophyseal portal vessels and stimulates the synthesis of both FSH and LH, which are stored within gonadotrophs. Subsequently, GnRH activates and transforms these molecules into releasable forms. GnRH can also induce immediate release of both LH and FSH into the circulation. Receptors for GnRH have been found in other tissues including the ovary, suggesting that GnRH may have a direct effect on ovarian function as well.

GnRH is secreted in a pulsatile fashion throughout the menstrual cycle as depicted in Figure 4-4. The frequency of GnRH release, as assessed indirectly by

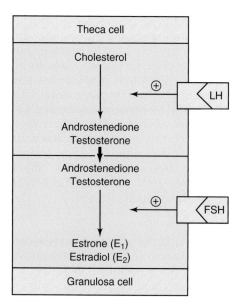

FIGURE 4-3 The two-gonadotropin (LH and FSH), two-cell (theca cell on top and granulosa cell below) theory of follicular development. Each cell is theorized to perform separate functions; LH stimulates the production of androgens (androstenedione and testosterone) in the theca cell and FSH stimulates the aromatization of these androgens to estrogens (estrone and estradiol) in the granulose cell. *FSH*, Follicle-stimulating hormone; *LH*, luteinizing hormone.

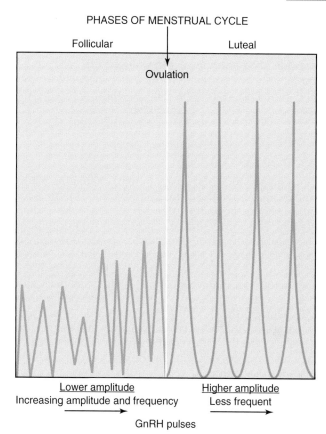

FIGURE 4-4 The pulsatile release of gonadotropin-releasing hormone (GnRH) during the normal menstrual cycle.

measurement of LH pulses, varies considerably among individuals. GnRH pulses in the follicular phase are more frequent and of lower amplitude, whereas in the luteal phase the pulses occur less frequently but are of higher amplitude.

Intravenous and subcutaneous administration of exogenous pulsatile GnRH has been used to induce ovulation in selected women who are not ovulating as a result of hypothalamic dysfunction. **A continuous (nonpulsatile) infusion of GnRH results in a reversible inhibition of gonadotropin secretion through a process of "downregulation" or desensitization of pituitary gonadotrophs.** This represents the basic mechanism of action for the GnRH analogues (nonapeptides, containing only nine amino acids) that have been successfully used in the therapy of such ovarian hormone-dependent disorders as endometriosis, leiomyomas (fibroids), hirsutism, and precocious puberty. There are both agonistic and antagonistic analogues of GnRH.

Several mechanisms control the secretion of GnRH. **Estradiol appears to enhance hypothalamic release of GnRH and may help induce the midcycle LH surge by increasing GnRH release or by enhancing pituitary responsiveness to the decapeptide. Gonadotropins have an inhibitory effect on GnRH release.** Catecholamines may play a major regulatory role as well. Dopamine is synthesized in the arcuate and periventricular nuclei and may have a direct inhibitory effect on GnRH secretion via the tuberoinfundibular tract that projects

onto the median eminence. Serotonin also appears to inhibit GnRH pulsatile release, whereas norepinephrine stimulates it. Endogenous opioids suppress release of GnRH from the hypothalamus in a manner that may be partially regulated by ovarian steroids.

The hypothalamus produces PIF, which exerts chronic inhibition of prolactin release from the lactotrophs. A number of pharmacologic agents (e.g., chlorpromazine) that affect dopaminergic mechanisms also influence prolactin release. Dopamine itself is secreted by hypothalamic neurons into the hypophyseal portal vessels and inhibits prolactin release directly within the adenohypophysis. Based on these observations, it has been proposed that hypothalamic dopamine may be the major PIF. In addition to the regulation of prolactin release by PIF, the hypothalamus may also produce prolactin-releasing factors (PRF) that can elicit large and rapid increases in prolactin release under certain conditions, such as breast stimulation during nursing. Neither PIF nor PRF has been clearly characterized biochemically as of 2014. TRH serves to stimulate prolactin release as well. This phenomenon may explain the association between primary hypothyroidism (with secondary TRH elevation) and hyperprolactinemia. **The precursor protein for GnRH, called GnRH-associated peptide (GAP), has been**

identified to be both a potent inhibitor of prolactin secretion and an enhancer of gonadotropin release. These findings suggest that this GnRH-associated peptide may also be a physiologic PIF and could explain the inverse relationship between gonadotropin and prolactin secretions seen in many reproductive states.

Ovarian Cycle

ESTROGENS

During early follicular development, circulating estradiol levels are relatively low. About 1 week before ovulation, levels begin to increase, at first slowly, then rapidly. The conversion of testosterone to estradiol in the granulosa cell of the follicle occurs through an enzymatic process called aromatization and is depicted in Figure 4-3. The levels generally reach a maximum 1 day before the midcycle LH peak. After this peak and before ovulation, there is a marked and precipitous fall. During the luteal phase, estradiol rises to a maximum 5 to 7 days after ovulation and returns to baseline shortly before menstruation. Estrone (E1, a weaker estrogen) secretion by the ovary is considerably less than secretion of estradiol but follows a similar pattern. Estrone is largely derived from the conversion of androstenedione through the action of the enzyme aromatase (Figure 4-5).

PROGESTINS

During follicular development, the ovary secretes only very small amounts of progesterone and 17α-hydroxyprogesterone. The bulk of the progester- one comes from the peripheral conversion of adrenal pregnenolone and pregnenolone sulfate. Just before ovulation, the unruptured but luteinizing graafian follicle begins to produce increasing amounts of progesterone. At about this time, a marked increase also occurs in serum 17α-hydroxyprogesterone. The elevation of basal body temperature is temporally related to the central effect of progesterone. As with estradiol, secretion of progestins by the corpus luteum reaches a maximum 5 to 7 days after ovulation and returns to baseline shortly before menstruation. Should pregnancy occur, progesterone levels, and therefore basal body temperature, remain elevated.

ANDROGENS

Both the ovary and the adrenal glands secrete small amounts of testosterone, but most of the testosterone is derived from the metabolism of androstenedione, which is also secreted by both the ovary and the adrenal gland. Near midcycle, an increase occurs in plasma androstenedione, which reflects enhanced secretion from the follicle. During the luteal phase, a second rise occurs in androstenedione, which reflects enhanced secretion by the corpus luteum. The adrenal gland also secretes androstenedione in a diurnal pattern similar to that of cortisol. The ovary secretes small amounts of the very potent dihydrotestosterone (DHT), but the bulk of DHT is derived from the conversion of androstenedione and testosterone. The majority of dehydroepiandrosterone (DHEA) and virtually all DHEA sulfate (DHEA-S), which are weak androgens, are secreted by the adrenal glands, although small amounts of DHEA are secreted by the ovary.

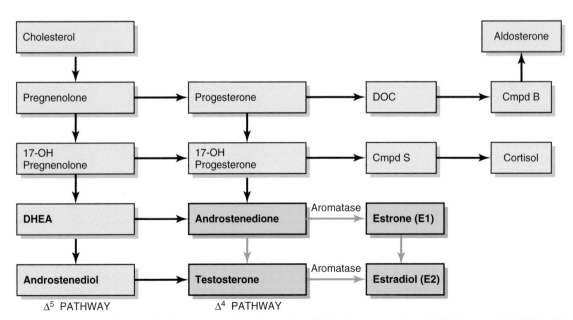

FIGURE 4-5 Steroidogenic pathways showing aromatization in red. *Cmpd B,* Corticosterone; *Cmpd S,* 11-deoxycortisol; *DHEA,* dehydroepiandrosterone; *DOC,* desoxycorticosterone; *OH,* hydroxylase.

SERUM-BINDING PROTEINS

Circulating estrogens and androgens are mostly bound to specific sex hormone–binding globulins (SHBG) or to serum albumin. The remaining fraction of sex hormones is unbound (free), and this is the biologically active fraction. It is unclear whether steroids bound to serum proteins (e.g., albumin) are accessible for tissue uptake and utilization. The synthesis of SHBG in the liver is increased by estrogens and thyroid hormones but decreased by testosterone.

PROLACTIN

Serum prolactin levels do not change strikingly during the normal menstrual cycle. Both the serum level of prolactin and prolactin release in response to TRH are somewhat more elevated during the luteal phase than during the mid-follicular phase of the cycle. This suggests that high amounts of circulating estradiol and progesterone may enhance prolactin release. **Prolactin release varies throughout the day with the highest levels occurring during sleep.**

Prolactin may participate in the control of ovarian steroidogenesis. Prolactin concentrations in follicular fluid change markedly during follicular growth. The highest prolactin concentrations are seen in small follicles during the early follicular phase. Prolactin concentrations in the follicular fluid may be inversely related to the production of progesterone. In addition, hyperprolactinemia may alter gonadotropin secretion. Despite these observations, the physiologic role of prolactin during the normal menstrual cycle has not been clearly established.

FOLLICULAR DEVELOPMENT

The number of oocytes is maximal in the fetus at 6 to 7 million at 20 weeks' gestation. Significant atresia (physiologic loss) of oogonia occurs so that at birth, only 1 to 2 million remain in both ovaries. At puberty (with ongoing atresia) between 300,000 and 400,000 oocytes are available for ovulation with only 400 to 500 actually ovulating. **After puberty, primordial follicles undergo sequential development, differentiation, and maturation until a mature graafian follicle is produced. The follicle then ruptures, releasing the ovum. Subsequent luteinization of the ruptured follicle produces the corpus luteum.**

At approximately 8 to 10 weeks of fetal development, oocytes become progressively surrounded by precursor granulosa cells, which then separate themselves from the underlying stroma by a basal lamina. **This oocyte-granulosa cell complex is called a primordial follicle.** The follicular cells become cuboidal and the stromal cells around the follicle become prominent. This process, which takes place in the fetal ovary at between 20 and 24 weeks' gestation, results in a **primary follicle.** As granulosa cells proliferate, a clear gelatinous material surrounds the ovum, forming the **zona pellucida.** This larger unit is called a **secondary follicle.**

In the adult ovary, **a graafian follicle** forms as the innermost three or four layers of rapidly multiplying granulosa cells become cuboidal and adherent to the ovum **(cumulus oophorus).** In addition, a fluid-filled antrum forms among the granulosa cells. As the liquor continues to accumulate, the antrum enlarges and the centrally located primary oocyte migrates eccentrically to the wall of the follicle. The innermost layer of granulosa cells of the cumulus, which are in close contact with the zona pellucida, become elongated and form the **corona radiata.** The corona radiata is released with the oocyte at ovulation. Covering the granulosa cells is a thin basement membrane, outside of which connective tissue cells organize themselves into two coats: the **theca interna** and **theca externa.**

During each cycle, a cohort of follicles is recruited for development. Among the many developing follicles, only one (the dominant follicle) usually continues differentiation and maturation into a follicle that ovulates. The remaining follicles undergo atresia. On the basis of in vitro measurement of local steroid levels, growing follicles can be classified as either estrogen-predominant or androgen-predominant. **Follicles greater than 10 mm in diameter are usually estrogen-predominant, whereas smaller follicles are usually androgen-predominant.** Mature preovulatory follicles reach mean diameters of approximately 18 to 25 mm. Furthermore, in estrogen-predominant follicles, antral FSH concentrations continue to rise while serum FSH levels decline beginning at the mid-follicular phase. In smaller, androgen-predominant follicles, antral fluid FSH values decrease while serum FSH levels decline; thus, the intrafollicular steroid milieu appears to play an important role in determining whether a follicle undergoes maturation or atresia. Additional follicles may be "rescued" from atresia by administration of exogenous gonadotropins.

Follicular maturation is dependent on the local development of receptors for FSH and LH. FSH receptors are present on granulosa cells. Under FSH stimulation, granulosa cells proliferate and the number of FSH receptors per follicle increases proportionately. Thus, the growing primary follicle is increasingly more sensitive to stimulation by FSH; as a result, estradiol levels increase. Estrogens, particularly estradiol, enhance the induction of FSH receptors and act synergistically with FSH to increase LH receptors.

During early stages of folliculogenesis, LH receptors are present only on the theca interna layer. LH stimulation induces steroidogenesis and increases the synthesis of androgens by thecal cells. In nondominant follicles, high local androgen levels may enhance follicular atresia. However, in the follicle destined to reach ovulation, FSH induces the formation of aromatase enzyme and its receptor within the granulosa cells. As a result, androgens produced in the theca interna of the dominant follicle diffuse into the granulosa cells and are aromatized into estrogens. **FSH also enhances the induction of LH receptors on the granulosa cells of the follicle that is destined to ovulate.** These are essential for the appropriate response to the LH surge, leading to the final stages of maturation, ovulation, and the luteal phase production of progesterone. Thus, **the presence of greater numbers of FSH receptors and granulosa cells and increased induction of aromatase enzyme and its receptors may differentiate between the follicle of the initial cohort that will eventually ovulate and those that will undergo atresia.**

Growth factors such as insulin, insulin-like growth factor (IGF), fibroblast growth factor (FGF), and epidermal growth factor (EGF) may also play significant mitogenic roles in folliculogenesis, including enhanced responsiveness to FSH. Ovarian peptide hormones, inhibin-A, inhibin-B, and activin, have roles in gonadotropin regulation. Both forms of inhibin act to inhibit FSH, whereas activin stimulates FSH release and potentiates its action in the ovary. Ovarian granulosa cells also produce müllerian inhibiting hormone (MIH), levels of which now provide a more accurate assessment of ovarian reserve and potential female fertility (see Chapter 34).

OVULATION

The preovulatory LH surge initiates a sequence of structural and biochemical changes that culminate in ovulation. **Before ovulation, a general dissolution of the entire follicular wall occurs, particularly the portion that is on the surface of the ovary.** Presumably this occurs **as a result of the action of proteolytic enzymes.** With degeneration of the cells on the surface, a stigma forms, and the follicular basement membrane finally bulges through the stigma. When this ruptures, the oocyte, together with the corona radiata and some cells of the cumulus oophorus are expelled into the peritoneal cavity, and ovulation takes place.

Ovulation is now known from ultrasonic studies to be a gradual phenomenon, with the collapse of the follicle taking from several minutes to as long as an hour or more. The oocyte adheres to the surface of the ovary, allowing an extended period during which the muscular contractions of the fallopian tube may bring it in contact with the tubal epithelium. Probably both muscular contractions and tubal ciliary movement contribute to the entry of the oocyte into, and the transportation along, the fallopian tube. Ciliary activity may not be essential, because some women with immotile cilia also become pregnant.

At birth, primary oocytes are in the prophase (diplotene) stage of the first meiotic division. They continue in this phase until the next maturation division occurs (years later) in conjunction with the midcycle LH surge. **A few hours preceding ovulation, the chromatin is resolved into distinct chromosomes, and meiotic division takes place with unequal distribution of the cytoplasm to form a secondary oocyte and the first polar body. Each element contains 23 chromosomes, each in the form of two monads.** The second maturation spindle forms immediately and the oocyte remains at the surface of the ovary. No further development takes place until after ovulation and fertilization have occurred. At that time, and before the union of the male and female pronuclei, another division occurs to reduce the chromosomal component of the egg pronucleus to 23 single chromosomes (22 plus X or Y), each composed of the one monad. The ovum and a second polar body are thus formed. The first polar body may also divide.

LUTEINIZATION AND CORPUS LUTEUM FUNCTION

After ovulation and under the influence of LH, the granulosa cells of the ruptured follicle undergo luteinization. These luteinized granulosa cells, plus the surrounding theca cells, capillaries, and connective tissue, form the corpus luteum, which produces copious amounts of progesterone and some estradiol. **The normal functional life span of the corpus luteum is about 9 to 10 days.** After this time it regresses, and unless pregnancy occurs, menstruation ensues and the corpus luteum is gradually replaced by an avascular scar called a *corpus albicans*. The events occurring in the ovary during a complete cycle are shown in Figure 4-6.

Histophysiology of the Endometrium

The endometrium is uniquely responsive to the circulating progestins, androgens, and estrogens. It is this responsiveness that gives rise to menstruation and makes implantation and pregnancy possible.

Functionally, the endometrium is divided into two zones: (1) the **outer portion,** or **functionalis,** which undergoes cyclic changes in morphology and function during the menstrual cycle and is sloughed off at menstruation; and (2) the **inner portion,** or **basalis,** which remains relatively unchanged during each menstrual cycle and, after menstruation, provides stem cells for the renewal of the functionalis. **Basal arteries** are regular blood vessels found in the basalis, whereas **spiral arteries** are specially coiled blood vessels seen in the functionalis.

The cyclic changes in histophysiology of the endometrium can be divided into three stages: the menstrual phase, the proliferative or estrogenic phase, and the secretory or progestational phase.

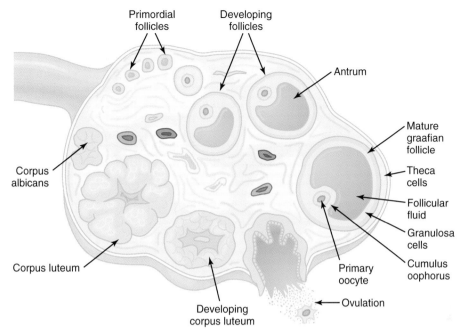

FIGURE 4-6 Schematic representation of the sequence of events occurring in the ovary during a complete follicular cycle. (Adapted from Yen SC, Jaffe R, editors: *Reproductive endocrinology,* Philadelphia, 1978, Saunders.)

MENSTRUAL PHASE

Because it is the only portion of the cycle that is visible externally, the first day of menstruation is taken as day 1 of the menstrual cycle. The first 4 to 5 days of the cycle are defined as the menstrual phase. **During this phase, there is disruption and disintegration of the endometrial glands and stroma, leukocyte infiltration, and red blood cell extravasation.** In addition to this sloughing of the functionalis, there is a compression of the basalis due to the loss of ground substances. Despite these degenerative changes, early evidence of renewed tissue growth is usually present at this time within the basalis of the endometrium.

PROLIFERATIVE PHASE

The proliferative phase is characterized by endometrial proliferation or growth secondary to estrogenic stimulation. Because the bases of the endometrial glands lie deep within the basalis, these epithelial cells are not destroyed during menstruation.

During this phase of the cycle, the large increase in estrogen secretion causes marked cellular proliferation of the epithelial lining, the endometrial glands, and the connective tissue of the stroma (Figure 4-7). Numerous mitoses are present in these tissues and there is an increase in the length of the spiral arteries, which traverse almost the entire thickness of the endometrium. By the end of the proliferative phase, cellular proliferation and endometrial growth have reached a maximum, the spiral arteries are elongated and convo-

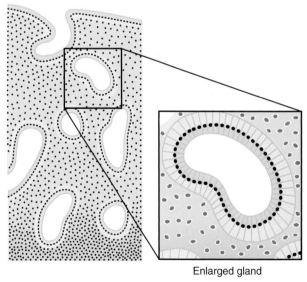

Enlarged gland

FIGURE 4-7 Early proliferative phase endometrium. Note the regular, tubular glands lined by pseudostratified columnar cells.

luted, and the endometrial glands are straight, with narrow lumens containing some glycogen.

SECRETORY PHASE

Following ovulation, progesterone secretion by the corpus luteum stimulates the glandular cells to secrete glycogen, mucus, and other substances. The glands become tortuous and the lumens are dilated

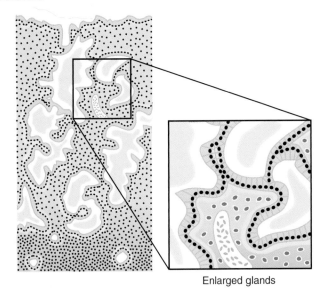

Enlarged glands

FIGURE 4-8 Late secretory phase endometrium. Note the tortuous, saw-toothed appearance of the endometrial glands with secretions in the lumens. The stroma is edematous and necrotic during this stage, leading to sloughing of the endometrium at the time of menstruation.

and filled with these substances. The stroma becomes edematous. Mitoses are rare. The spiral arteries continue to extend into the superficial layer of the endometrium and become convoluted (Figure 4-8).

The marked changes that occur in endometrial histology during the secretory phase permit relatively precise timing (dating) of secretory endometrium.

If pregnancy does not occur by day 23, the corpus luteum begins to regress, secretion of progesterone and estradiol declines, and the endometrium undergoes involution. About 1 day before the onset of menstruation, marked constriction of the spiral arterioles takes place, causing ischemia of the endometrium followed by leukocyte infiltration and red blood cell extravasation. It is thought that these events occur secondary to prostaglandin production by the endometrium. The resulting necrosis causes menstruation or sloughing of the endometrium. Ironically, menstruation, which clinically marks the beginning of the menstrual cycle, is actually the terminal event of a physiologic process that enables the uterus to be prepared to receive another conceptus. The four components of the "integrated" female reproductive cycle are summarized in Table 4-1.

Spermatogenesis, Sperm Capacitation, and Fertilization

Fertilization, or conception, is the union of male and female pronuclear elements. Conception normally takes place in the fallopian tube, after which the fertil-

ized ovum continues to the uterus, where implantation occurs and development of the conceptus continues.

Spermatogenesis requires about 74 days. Together with transportation, a total of about 3 months elapses before sperm are ejaculated. The sperm achieve motility during their passage through the epididymis, but sperm capacitation, which renders them capable of fertilization in vivo, does not occur until they are removed from the seminal plasma after ejaculation. Interestingly, sperm aspirated from the epididymis and testis can be used to achieve fertilization in vitro employing intracytoplasmic injection techniques directly into the ooplasm.

Estrogen levels are high at the time of ovulation, resulting in an increased quantity, decreased viscosity, and favorable electrolyte content of the cervical mucus. These are the ideal characteristics for sperm penetration. **The average ejaculate contains 2 to 5 mL of semen; 40 to 300 million sperm may be deposited in the vagina, 50-90% of which are morphologically normal.** Fewer than 200 sperm achieve proximity to the egg. Only one sperm fertilizes a single egg released at ovulation.

The major loss of sperm occurs in the vagina following coitus, with expulsion of the semen from the introitus playing an important role. In addition, digestion of sperm by vaginal enzymes, destruction by vaginal acidity, phagocytosis of sperm along the reproductive tract, and further loss from passage through the fallopian tube into the peritoneal cavity all diminish the number of sperm capable of achieving fertilization.

Those sperm that do migrate from the alkaline environment of the semen to the alkaline environment of the cervical mucus exuding from the cervical os are directed along channels of lower-viscosity mucus into the cervical crypts where they are stored for later ascent. Two waves of passage to the tubes may occur. **Uterine contractions, probably facilitated by prostaglandin in the seminal plasma, propel sperm to the tubes within 5 minutes.** Some evidence indicates that these sperm may not be as capable of fertilization as those that arrive later largely under their own power. Sperm may be found within the peritoneal cavity for long periods, but it is not known whether they are capable of fertilization. **Ova are usually fertilized within 12 hours of ovulation.**

Capacitation is the physiologic change that sperm must undergo in the female reproductive tract before fertilization. Human sperm can also undergo capacitation after a short incubation in defined culture media without residence in the female reproductive tract, which allows for in vitro fertilization (see Chapter 34).

The acrosome reaction is one of the principal components of capacitation. The acrosome, a modified lysosome, lies over the sperm head as a kind of "chemical drill-bit" designed to enable the sperm to burrow its way into the oocyte (Figure 4-9). The overlying

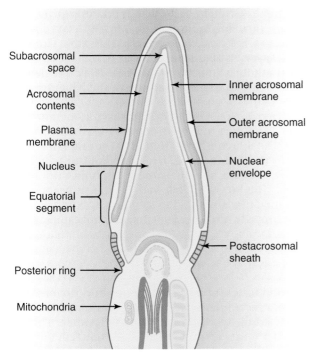

Subacrosomal space

Acrosomal contents

Plasma membrane

Nucleus

Equatorial segment

Posterior ring

Mitochondria

Inner acrosomal membrane

Outer acrosomal membrane

Nuclear envelope

Postacrosomal sheath

FIGURE 4-9 The sperm head.

plasma membrane becomes unstable and eventually breaks down, releasing **hyaluronidase,** a neuraminidase, and **corona-dispersing enzyme. Acrosin,** bound to the remaining inner acrosomal membrane, may play a role in the final penetration of the zona pellucida. The latter contains species-specific receptors for the plasma membrane. After traversing the zona, the postacrosomal region of the sperm head fuses with the oocyte membrane, and the sperm nucleus is incorporated into the ooplasm. This process triggers release of the contents of the cortical granules that lie at the periphery of the oocyte. This cortical reaction results in changes in the oocyte membrane and zona pellucida that prevent the entrance of further sperm into the oocyte.

The process of capacitation may be inhibited by a factor in the semen, thus preserving maximum release of enzyme to allow effective penetration of the corona and zona pellucida surrounding the oocyte. The cellular investments of the oocyte may further activate the sperm, thus facilitating penetration to the oocyte membrane. The corona is not required for normal fertilization to occur, as its removal has no effect on the rate or quality of fertilization in vitro. The major function of these surrounding granulosa cells and their intercellular matrix may be to serve as a sticky mass that causes adherence to the ovarian surface and to the mucosa of the tubal epithelium.

Following penetration of the oocyte, the sperm nucleus decondenses to form the male pronucleus, which approaches and finally fuses with the female pronucleus at syngamy to form the zygote. **Fertiliza-**

tion restores the diploid number of chromosomes and determines the sex of the zygote. In couples with infertility resulting from severe sperm abnormalities, fertilization and subsequent pregnancy can be successfully achieved after the injection of a single sperm, with or without its tail, into the cytoplasm of the oocyte (see Chapter 34).

Cleavage, Morula, Blastocyst

Following fertilization, cleavage occurs. This consists of a rapid succession of mitotic divisions that produce a mulberry-like mass known as a morula. **Fluid is secreted by the outer cells of the morula, and a single fluid-filled cavity develops, known as the blastocyst cavity.** An inner-cell mass can be defined, attached eccentrically to the outer layer of flattened cells; the latter becomes the trophoblast. The embryo at this stage of development is called a **blastocyst,** and the zona pellucida disappears at about this time. A blastocyst cell can be removed and tested for genetic imperfections without harming further development of the conceptus.

Implantation

The fertilized ovum reaches the endometrial cavity about 3 days after ovulation.

Hormones influence egg transportation. Estrogen causes "locking" of the egg in the tube, and progesterone reverses this action. Prostaglandins have diverse effects. Prostaglandin E relaxes the tubal isthmus, whereas prostaglandin F stimulates tubal motility. It is unknown whether abnormalities of egg transportation play a role in infertility, but in animal studies, acceleration of ovum transportation causes a failure of implantation. Additional cytokines may be released by the tubal epithelium and embryo to enhance embryo transportation and development and to signal the impending implantation in the endometrium.

Initial embryonic development primarily occurs in the ampullary portion of the fallopian tube with subsequent rapid transit through the isthmus. This process takes approximately 3 days. **On reaching the uterine cavity, the embryo undergoes further development for 2 to 3 days before implanting.** The zona is shed and the blastocyst adheres to the endometrium, a process that is probably dependent on the changes in the surface characteristics of the embryo, such as electrical charge and glycoprotein content. A variety of proteolytic enzymes may play a role in separating the endometrial cells and digesting the intercellular matrix.

Initially, the wall of the blastocyst facing the uterine lumen consists of a single layer of flattened cells. The thicker opposite wall has two zones: the **trophoblast** and the **inner cell mass (embryonic disk).** The latter differentiates at 7.5 days into a thick plate of **primitive** "dorsal" ectoderm and an underlying layer of "ventral" endoderm. A group of small cells appears between the embryonic disk and trophoblast. A space develops within them, which becomes the amniotic cavity.

Under the influence of progesterone, decidual changes occur in the endometrium of the pregnant uterus. The endometrial stromal cells enlarge and form polygonal or round decidual cells. The nuclei become round and vesicular, and the cytoplasm becomes clear, slightly basophilic, and surrounded by a translucent membrane. During pregnancy, the decidua thickens to a depth of 5 to 10 mm. The **decidua basalis** is the decidual layer directly beneath the site of implantation. **Integrins,** a class of proteins involved in cell-to-cell adherence, peak within the endometrium at the time of implantation and may play a significant role. Additional growth factors act in a synergistic fashion to enhance the implantation process. The **decidua capsularis** is the layer overlying the developing ovum and separating it from the rest of the uterine cavity. The **decidua vera** (parietalis) is the remaining lining of the uterine cavity (Figure 4-10). The space between the decidua capsularis and decidua vera is obliterated by the 4th month with fusion of the capsularis and vera.

The decidua basalis enters into the formation of the basal plate of the placenta. The spongy zone of the decidua basalis consists mainly of arteries and dilated veins. The decidua basalis is invaded extensively by trophoblastic giant cells, which first appear as early as the time of implantation. Minute levels of hCG appear in the maternal serum at this time. The **Nitabuch layer** is a zone of fibrinoid degeneration where the trophoblast meets the decidua. When the decidua is defective, as in placenta accreta, the Nitabuch layer is absent.

When the free blastocyst contacts the endometrium after 4 to 6 days, the syncytiotrophoblast, a syncytium of cells, differentiates from the cytotrophoblast. At about 9 days, lacunae, irregular fluid-filled spaces, appear within the thickened trophoblastic syncytium. This is soon followed by the appearance of maternal blood within the lacunae, as maternal tissue is destroyed and the walls of the mother's capillaries are eroded.

Placenta

As the blastocyst burrows deeper into the endometrium, the trophoblastic strands branch to form the solid, primitive villi traversing the lacunae. The villi, which are first distinguished about the 12th day after fertilization, are the essential structures of the definitive placenta. Located originally over the entire surface of the ovum, the villi later disappear except over the most deeply implanted portion, the future placental site.

Embryonic mesenchyme first appears as isolated cells within the cavity of the blastocyst. When the cavity is completely lined with mesoderm, it is termed the **extraembryonic celom.** Its membrane, the **chorion,** is composed of trophoblast and mesenchyme. When the solid trophoblast is invaded by a mesenchymal core, presumably derived from cytotrophoblast, secondary villi are formed.

Maternal venous sinuses are tapped about 15 days after fertilization. By the 17th day, both fetal and maternal blood vessels are functional, and a placental circulation is established. The fetal circulation is completed when the blood vessels of the embryo are connected with chorionic blood vessels that are formed from cytotrophoblast. Proliferation of cellular trophoblasts at the tips of the villi produces cytotrophoblastic columns that progressively extend through the peripheral syncytium. Cytotrophoblastic extensions from columns of adjacent villi join together to form the cytotrophoblastic shell, which attaches the villi to the decidua. By the 19th day of development, the cytotrophoblastic shell is thick. Villi contain a central core of chorionic mesoderm, where blood vessels are developing, and an external covering of syncytiotrophoblasts or syncytium.

By three weeks, the relationship of the chorion to the decidua is evident. The greater part of the chorion, denuded of villi, is designated the **chorion laeve** (smooth chorion). Until near the end of the third

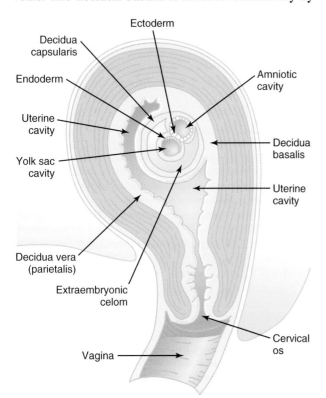

Ectoderm

Decidua capsularis

Endoderm

Uterine cavity

Yolk sac cavity

Amniotic cavity

Decidua basalis

Uterine cavity

Decidua vera (parietalis)

Extraembryonic celom

Cervical os

Vagina

FIGURE 4-10 Early stage of implantation.

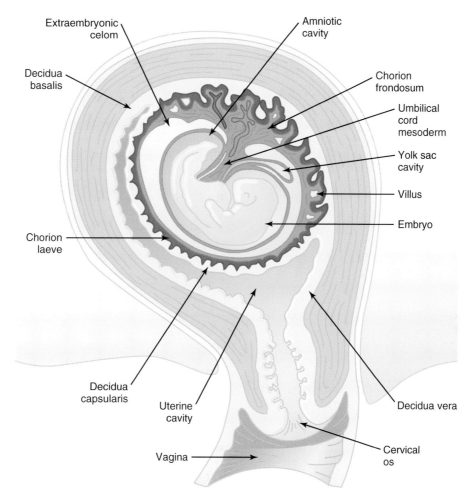

FIGURE 4-11 Relationship of the chorion to the placenta.

month, the chorion laeve remains separated from the amnion by the **extraembryonic celomic cavity.** Thereafter, amnion and chorion are in intimate contact. The villi adjacent to the decidua basalis enlarge and branch **(chorion frondosum)** and progressively assume the form of the fully developed human placenta (Figure 4-11). **By 16 to 20 weeks, the chorion laeve contacts and fuses with the decidua vera, thus obliterating most of the uterine cavity.**

Amniotic Fluid

Throughout normal pregnancy, the amniotic fluid compartment allows the fetus room for growth, movement, and development. Without amniotic fluid, the uterus would contract and compress the fetus. **In cases of leakage of amniotic fluid early in the first trimester, the fetus may develop structural abnormalities including facial distortion, limb reduction, and abdominal wall defects secondary to uterine compression.**

Toward mid-pregnancy (20 weeks), the amniotic fluid becomes increasingly important for fetal pulmonary development. The latter requires a fluid-filled respiratory tract and the ability of the fetus to "breathe" in utero, moving amniotic fluid into and out of the lungs. **The absence of adequate amniotic fluid during mid-pregnancy is associated with pulmonary hypoplasia at birth, which is often incompatible with life.**

The amniotic fluid also has a protective role for the fetus. It contains antibacterial activity and acts to inhibit the growth of potentially pathogenic bacteria. During labor and delivery, the amniotic fluid continues to serve as a protective medium for the fetus, aiding dilation of the cervix. The premature infant, with its fragile head, may benefit most from delivery with the amniotic membranes intact (en caul). In addition, the amniotic fluid may serve as a means of communication for the fetus. Fetal maturity and readiness for delivery may be signaled to the maternal uterus via fetal urinary hormones excreted into the amniotic fluid.

PART 2

Obstetrics

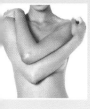
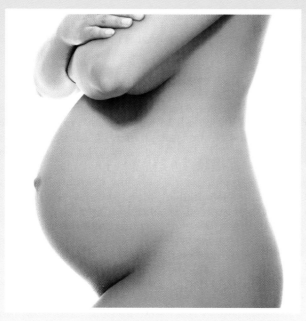

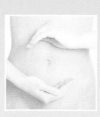
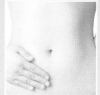

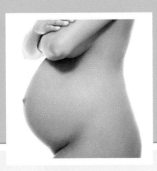

CHAPTER 5

Endocrinology of Pregnancy and Parturition

JOSEPH C. GAMBONE   •   CALVIN J. HOBEL

CLINICAL KEYS FOR THIS CHAPTER

- The hormonal and nonhormonal changes that occur during pregnancy and parturition are regulated through a physiological mechanism referred to as the fetoplacental unit. A series of hormones and transmitters are produced by each of the components of this unit, and they have multiple effects within and between the fetus, the placenta and the mother.
- The fetal component of the fetoplacental unit plays the major role in the regulation of pregnancy and parturition. Most of the activity in the fetal component takes place in the fetal adrenal gland which is larger than the fetal kidney by mid-gestation. The fetal zone of the fetal adrenal gland primarily secretes androgens during fetal life and these androgens act as precursors for estrogen production in the placenta. The overall role of the fetal adrenal is not completely understood.
- The placental trophoblasts are the source of human chorionic gonadotropin (hCG), which "rescues" the corpus luteum very early in pregnancy. The placenta also produces large amounts of steroid and peptide hormones. Because the placenta lacks the enzyme 17α-hydroxylase, it cannot convert progesterone to estrogen. The placenta instead uses androgens from the fetal adrenal as precursors for the production of estrogens that are needed to maintain the pregnancy. In addition to estrogens, progesterone and the corticosteroid, cortisol, are produced in the placenta. Peptide hormones include human placental lactogen (hPL), corticotropin-releasing hormone (CRH), and prolactin. Other important hormones and transmitters include oxytocin, relaxin, prostaglandins, leukotrienes, and parathyroid hormone–related peptide.
- Maternal adaptation and regulation of pregnancy and parturition start with the secretion of 17-hydroxyprogesterone (17-OHP) from the ovarian corpus luteum. If the maternal ovary is deficient in progesterone production, the pregnancy is likely to miscarry. Placental function assures adequate amounts of estrogen (mostly estriol or E3) to increase uterine blood flow for uterine growth, and progesterone to maintain the quiescent state of the uterus throughout most of the gestational period. The absence of myometrial gap junctions facilitates the action of progesterone.
- Labor (which initiates the parturition process) is a release from the state of functional uterine quiescence maintained during pregnancy. This quiescence is due, in large part, to the lack of gap junctions before the onset of labor and the actions of progesterone. Three additional phases of parturition follow the first phase of quiescence, as follows. Phase 1: activation is initiated by uterine stretch and fetal hypothalamic-pituitary-adrenal (HPA) activity. Phase 2: stimulation most likely begins with placental production of CRH. This phase continues with cervical ripening, uterine contractility, and decidual/fetal membrane activation. Phase 3: involution involves expulsion of the fetus with a dramatic increase in oxytocin release and a decrease in parathyroid hormone–related peptide (PTHrP) expression. This phase also involves placental separation and continued uterine contractions.

Women undergo major endocrinologic and metabolic changes that establish, maintain, and end pregnancy. The aim of these changes is the safe delivery of an infant that can survive outside of the uterus. The maturation of the fetus and the adaptation of the mother are regulated by a variety of hormones and transmitters (Table 5-1). This chapter deals with the properties, functions, and interactions of the most important of these hormonal and nonhormonal substances as they relate to pregnancy and parturition.

Fetoplacental Unit

The concept of the fetoplacental unit is based on observations of the interactions between hormones of fetal, placental, and maternal origin. **The fetoplacental**

TABLE 5-1

HORMONES AND TRANSMITTERS OF PREGNANCY AND PARTURITION

Hormone/Transmitter	Source	Function(s)	Clinical Comments
Human chorionic gonadotropin (hCG)	Placental trophoblastic tissue	Prevents regression of (rescues) the corpus luteum of pregnancy; increases T-cells that affect immunity	A likely regulator of a process that provides immune tolerance for the fetus; other trophic activities
Human placental lactogen (hPL)	Placenta	Antagonizes maternal glucose use so more is available for the fetus	Low values found in pregnancy loss; normal levels may increase risk of gestational diabetes
Corticotropin-releasing hormone (CRH)	Placenta	Stimulates fetal adrenocorticotropic hormone (ACTH) secretion, which allows the fetal adrenal to secrete DHEA-S for progesterone production; CRH may facilitate vasodilation	Fetal cortisol stimulates placental CRH release and fetal ACTH secretion; elevated levels may predict an increased risk of preterm birth
Prolactin	Maternal and fetal (late pregnancy) anterior pituitary glands	Stimulation of postpartum milk production	May play a role in fetal adrenal growth, as well as fluid and electrolyte membrane transfer
Progesterone (P4)	Placenta; precursors come from the maternal circulation	Prevents uterine contractions; suppresses gap junction formation	Maintains uterine quiescence
17-Hydroxyprogesterone (17-OHP)	Corpus luteum	Supports early pregnancy until placental production of P4 begins	Corpus luteum function is essential in early pregnancy
Estrogens Estriol (E3), estrone (E1), and estradiol (E2)	Placenta; conversion of androgens (DHEA, DHEA-S) from the fetal adrenal into estrogens	Estriol (E3) is the main estrogen of pregnancy; it increases uterine blood flow and prepares the breast for lactation	Placenta cannot convert progesterone to estrogen; lacks the enzyme 17α-hydroxylase; has role in lung surfactant production
Androgens Dehydroandrosterone (DHEA) and its sulfate (DHEA-S) Dihydrotestosterone (DHT)	During pregnancy, androgens originate mostly in the fetal adrenal cortex	DHEA production is favored, and is a precursor for placental estrogen production	Fetal testis produces testosterone, which is converted to DHT; this is needed for development of male external genitalia; hCG stimulates testosterone production
Cortisol	Derived from circulating cholesterol	Plays a major role in the activation of labor by increasing placental release of CRH and prostaglandins	Late in pregnancy, cortisol promotes the production of lung surfactant
Oxytocin	Maternal hypothalamus and posterior pituitary	Can cause uterine contractions; possible effects on emotion and well-being	Related to uterine contractions, but not the natural initiation of labor; facilitator of childbirth and breastfeeding
Relaxin	Corpus luteum and placenta	Primary function is to promote implantation; also causes uterine relaxation	Too much relaxin can result in a shortened cervix and increased risk of premature labor; too little can interfere with implantation
Prostaglandins PGE$_2$ PGF$_{2\alpha}$	Placental production from arachidonic acid	Thought to play a major role in the initiation of labor	Not true hormones; act at or close to the site of production; prostaglandin synthetase inhibitors can prolong labor
Leukotrienes	Placental production from arachidonic acid	Initiate changes in the endometrium that allow for implantation	Not true hormones; act at or close to the site of production
Parathyroid hormone–related peptide (PTHrP)	Uterus and other organs	Relaxes the uterus and allows for stretch without contractions	Allows for fetal growth during pregnancy; gene that activates PTHrP is off during parturition

unit largely controls the endocrinologic events of the pregnancy. Although the fetus, the placenta, and the mother all provide input, the fetus appears to play the most active and controlling role in its growth and maturation, and probably also in the events that lead to parturition.

FETUS

The adrenal gland is the major endocrine component of the fetus. In mid-pregnancy, it is larger than the fetal kidney. The fetal adrenal cortex consists of an outer definitive, or adult, zone and an inner, fetal, zone. The definitive zone later develops into the three components of the adult adrenal cortex: the zona fasciculata, the zona glomerulosa, and the zona reticularis. During fetal life, the definitive zone secretes primarily glucocorticoids and mineralocorticoids. **The fetal zone, at term, constitutes 80% of the fetal gland and primarily secretes androgens during fetal life.** It involutes following delivery and completely disappears by the end of the first year of life. The fetal adrenal medulla synthesizes and stores catecholamines, which play an important role in maintaining fetal homeostasis. The overall role of the fetal adrenal during fetal growth and maturation is not completely understood.

PLACENTA

The placenta, which functions as an "extra brain" during pregnancy, is unique because it contains genes from both the mother and father. In addition, it is the source of a brain peptide, corticotropin-releasing hormone (CRH), which has a very important regulatory role in pregnancy. Thus, the placenta produces both steroids and peptide hormones in amounts that vary with gestational age. Precursors for progesterone synthesis come from the maternal circulation. **Because of the lack of the enzyme 17α-hydroxylase, the human placenta cannot directly convert progesterone to estrogen** but must use androgens, largely from the fetal adrenal gland, as its source of precursor for estrogen production.

MOTHER

The mother adapts to pregnancy through major endocrinologic and metabolic changes. **The ovarian corpus luteum produces progesterone (mostly 17-hydroxyprogesterone) in early pregnancy** until its production shifts to the placenta. **The maternal hypothalamus and posterior pituitary produce and release oxytocin,** which causes uterine contractions and milk letdown. **The anterior pituitary produces prolactin,** which stimulates milk production. Several important changes in maternal metabolism are described later in the chapter.

Hormones

The fetoplacental unit produces a variety of hormones to support the maturation of the fetus and the adaptation of the mother.

PEPTIDE HORMONES

Human Chorionic Gonadotropin

Human chorionic gonadotropin (hCG) is secreted by trophoblastic cells of the placenta and maintains pregnancy. This hormone is a glycoprotein with a molecular weight of 40,000 to 45,000 and **consists of two subunits: alpha (α) and beta (β).** The α subunit is shared with luteinizing hormone (LH) and thyroid-stimulating hormone (TSH). **The specificity of hCG is related to its β subunit (β-hCG),** and a radioimmunoassay that is specific for the β subunit allows positive identification of hCG. Newer immunoassays for hCG are able to accurately measure low levels of hCG based on the entire molecule and not just the beta subunit. The presence of hCG at times other than pregnancy signals the presence of an hCG-producing tumor, usually a hydatidiform mole, choriocarcinoma, or embryonal carcinoma (a germ cell tumor).

During pregnancy, hCG begins to rise 8 days after ovulation (9 days after the midcycle LH peak). This provides the basis for virtually all immunologic or chemical pregnancy tests. With continuing pregnancy, hCG values peak at 60 to 90 days and then decline to a moderate, more constant level. **For the first 6 to 8 weeks of pregnancy, hCG maintains the corpus luteum and thereby ensures continued progesterone output until progesterone production shifts to the placenta.** Titers of hCG may be abnormally low in patients with an ectopic pregnancy or threatened abortion and abnormally high in those with trophoblastic disease (e.g., moles or choriocarcinoma). This hormone may also regulate steroid biosynthesis in the placenta and the fetal adrenal gland, and stimulate testosterone production in the fetal testicle. Early pregnancy is characterized by an increase in regulatory T cells (Tregs), which are known to facilitate maternal immune tolerance of the fetus. Recent animal research has shown that hCG acts as a central regulator of this immune tolerance during pregnancy.

Human Placental Lactogen

Human placental lactogen (hPL) originates in the placenta. It is a single-chain polypeptide with a molecular weight of 22,300, and it resembles pituitary growth hormone and human prolactin in structure. Maternal serum concentrations parallel placental weight, rising throughout gestation to maximum levels in the last 4 weeks. At term, hPL accounts for 10% of all placental protein production. Low values are found with threatened abortion and intrauterine fetal growth restriction.

Human placental lactogen antagonizes the cellular action of insulin and decreases maternal glucose utilization, which increases glucose availability to the fetus. This may play a role in the pathogenesis of gestational diabetes.

Corticotropin-Releasing Hormone

During pregnancy the major source of CRH is the placenta and it can be measured as early as 12 weeks' gestation, when it passes into the fetal circulation. This 41-amino acid peptide stimulates fetal adrenocorticotropic hormone (ACTH) secretion, which in turn stimulates the fetal adrenal to secrete dehydroepiandrosterone sulfate (DHEA-S), an important precursor of estrogen production by the placenta. The fetal adrenal gland early in pregnancy does not have the enzymes to produce cortisol, but as gestational age increases, it becomes more capable. **Fetal cortisol stimulates placental CRH release, which then stimulates fetal ACTH secretion, completing a positive feedback loop that plays an important role in the activation and amplification of labor, both preterm and term.** Elevated levels of CRH in mid-gestation have been found to be associated with an increased risk of subsequent spontaneous preterm labor.

Prolactin

Prolactin is a peptide from the anterior pituitary with a molecular weight of about 20,000. Normal nonpregnant levels are approximately 10 ng/mL. **During pregnancy, maternal prolactin levels rise in response to increasing maternal estrogen output that stimulates the anterior pituitary lactotrophs. The main effect of prolactin is stimulation of postpartum milk production.** In the second half of pregnancy, prolactin secreted by the fetal pituitary may be an important stimulus of fetal adrenal growth. Prolactin may also play a role in fluid and electrolyte shifts across the fetal membranes.

STEROID HORMONES

Progesterone

Progesterone is the most important human progestogen. **In the luteal phase, it induces secretory changes in the endometrium and in pregnancy, higher levels induce decidual changes. Up to the sixth or seventh week of pregnancy, the major source of progesterone (as 17-hydroxyprogesterone) is the ovarian corpus luteum.** Thereafter, the placenta begins to play the major role. **If the corpus luteum of pregnancy is removed before 7 weeks and continuation of the pregnancy is desired, progesterone should be given to prevent spontaneous abortion.** Circulating progesterone is mostly bound to carrier proteins, and less than 10% is free and physiologically active.

The myometrium receives progesterone directly from the venous blood draining the placenta. **Proges-terone prevents uterine contractions and may also be involved in establishing an immune tolerance for the products of conception.** Progesterone also suppresses gap junction formation, placental CRH expression, and the actions of estrogen, cytokines, and prostaglandin. This steroid hormone therefore plays a central role in maintaining uterine quiescence throughout most of pregnancy.

The fetus inactivates progesterone by transformation to corticosteroids or by hydroxylation or conjugation to inert excretory products. However, the placenta can convert these inert materials back to progesterone. Steroid biochemical pathways are shown in Figure 5-1.

Estrogens

Both fetus and placenta are involved in the biosynthesis of estrone, estradiol, and estriol. **Cholesterol is converted to pregnenolone in the placenta. This precursor is converted into DHEA-S largely in the fetal, and to a lesser extent the maternal, adrenals.** The DHEA-S is further metabolized by the placenta to estrone (E1) and, via testosterone, to estradiol (E2). **Estriol (E3), the most abundant estrogen in human pregnancy, is synthesized in the placenta from 16α-hydroxy-DHEA-S, which is produced in the fetal liver from adrenal DHEA-S.** Placental sulfatase is required to deconjugate 16α-hydroxy-DHEA-S before conversion to E3 (Figure 5-2). Steroid sulfatase activity in the placenta is high, except in rare cases of sulfatase deficiency.

Estrogens have essential roles during pregnancy and parturition. They increase uterine blood flow which allows for necessary uterine growth. They help to prepare the breast tissue for lactation and they stimulate the production of hormone-binding globulins in the liver. They also play a role, along with cortisol, in lung surfactant production.

A sudden decline of estriol in the maternal circulation may indicate fetal compromise in a neurologically intact fetus. Anencephalic fetuses lack a hypothalamus and have hypoplastic anterior pituitary and adrenal glands; thus, estriol production is only about 10% of normal.

Androgens

During pregnancy, androgens originate mainly in the fetal zone of the fetal adrenal cortex. Androgen secretion is stimulated by ACTH and hCG, the latter being effective primarily in the first half of pregnancy, when it is present in high concentration. The fetal adrenal favors production of DHEA over testosterone and androstenedione. **Fetal androgens enter the umbilical and placental circulation and serve as precursors for estrone, estradiol, and estriol** (see Figure 5-1).

The fetal testis also secretes androgens, particularly testosterone, which is converted within target cells to **dihydrotestosterone** (DHT), which is required for the

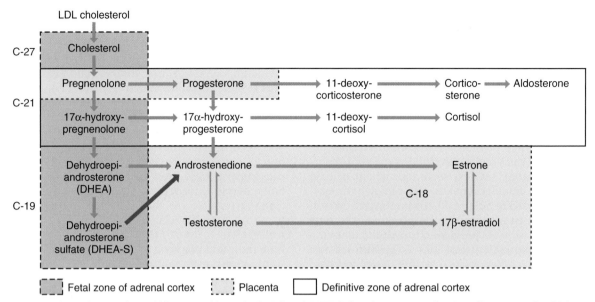

FIGURE 5-1 Main pathways of steroid hormone biosynthesis. Adrenal DHEA is largely transported as its sulfate, DHEA-S, which can also be formed from steroid sulfates starting with cholesterol sulfate. *LDL,* Low-density lipoprotein.

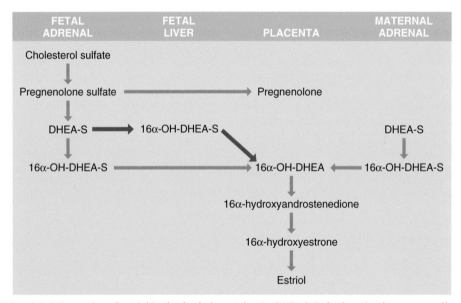

FIGURE 5-2 Formation of estriol in the fetal-placental unit. *DHEA-S,* Dehydroepiandrosterone sulfate.

development of male external genitalia. The main trophic stimulus appears to be hCG.

Glucocorticoids

Cortisol is derived from circulating cholesterol (see Figure 5-1). Maternal plasma cortisol concentrations rise throughout pregnancy and are the primary stimulus for CRH production by the placenta. The diurnal rhythm of cortisol secretion persists during pregnancy unless the patient has significant psychosocial stress, which elevates the morning and late afternoon cortisol level at which time the diurnal rhythm is lost. The plasma level of transcortin rises in pregnancy, probably stimulated by estrogen, and the plasma-free cortisol concentration doubles.

Both the fetal adrenal and the placenta participate in cortisol metabolism. The fetal adrenal is stimulated by ACTH, originating from the fetal pituitary, to produce both cortisol and DHEA-S. In contrast to DHEA-S, which is produced in the fetal zone, cortisol originates in the definitive zone (see Figure 5-1). Toward the end of pregnancy **cortisol promotes differentiation of type II alveolar cells and the biosynthesis and release of surfactant into the alveoli.** Surfactant decreases the force required to inflate the lungs. Insufficiency of surfactant leads to respiratory distress in the premature infant, which can cause death. **Cortisol also plays an important role in the activation of labor,** increasing the release of placental CRH and prostaglandins.

OTHER HORMONES AND TRANSMITTERS

Oxytocin

The oxytocic prohormone, which originates in the supraoptic and paraventricular nuclei of the maternal hypothalamus, migrates down the nerve fibers, and oxytocin accumulates at the nerve endings in the posterior pituitary. Oxytocin is a nonapeptide which is released from the posterior pituitary by various stimuli, such as distention of the birth canal and mammary stimulation. **Oxytocin causes uterine contractions, but impairment of oxytocin production, as in diabetes insipidus, does not interfere with normal labor.** Fluctuations in circulating oxytocin levels before the onset of labor do not correspond to changes in uterine activity. **Maternal serum oxytocin levels rise only during the first stage of labor.** Oxytocin can be administered to induce labor, especially in term pregnancies, or to increase the frequency and strength of contractions during spontaneous labor.

Recently, oxytocin has been shown to affect regions of the brain involved in emotional, cognitive, and social behaviors. The impact on "pro-social" behaviors includes positive effects on relaxation, trust, and psychological stability. If confirmed, these effects could help during labor, childbirth, and aftercare.

Relaxin

Relaxin is a peptide hormone that originates mostly from the ovarian corpus luteum. The placenta also produces relaxin and it reaches its peak concentration in the maternal circulation at the 10th week of pregnancy and then declines. **Relaxin is associated with the softening of the cervix,** which is one of the anatomical signs of pregnancy. **Its primary function appears to be in promoting implantation of the embryo by facilitating angiogenesis.** During hyperstimulation of the ovaries of women undergoing in vitro fertilization (IVF), the ovaries produce excessive levels of relaxin. This excess of relaxin has been shown to be associated with shortening of the cervix and an increased risk of preterm labor.

Prostaglandins and Leukotrienes

Prostaglandins are a family of ubiquitous, biologically active lipids that are involved in a broad range of physiologic and pathophysiologic responses. **They are not true hormones** in that they are not synthesized in one gland and transported via the circulating blood to a target organ. Rather, they are synthesized at or near their site of action. **Prostaglandin E$_2$ (PGE$_2$) and pros-**taglandin F$_{2\alpha}$ (PGF$_{2\alpha}$), prostacyclin, and thromboxane A$_2$ are synthesized in the endometrium, myometrium, the fetal membranes, decidua, and placenta. PGE$_2$ and PGF$_{2\alpha}$ cause contraction of the uterus.** Their receptors in the myometrium are downregulated during pregnancy. Prostaglandins can also cause contraction of other smooth muscles, such as those of the intestinal tract. Hence, when used pharmacologically, prostaglandins may give rise to undesirable side effects such as nausea, vomiting, and diarrhea. The amniotic fluid concentrations of PGE$_2$ and PGF$_{2\alpha}$ rise throughout pregnancy and increase further during spontaneous labor. Levels are lower in women who require oxytocin for induction of labor than in women going into spontaneous labor. Administration of PGE$_2$ or PGF$_{2\alpha}$ by various routes induces labor or abortion at any stage of gestation. **Various synthetic prostaglandin derivatives are currently in use to terminate pregnancy at any stage and to induce labor at term.**

Prostaglandins are thought to play a major role in the initiation and control of labor. Prostaglandin synthesis begins with the formation of arachidonic acid, an obligatory precursor of the prostaglandins of the "2" series (i.e., PGE$_2$, PGF$_{2\alpha}$). Arachidonic acid is stored in esterified form as glycerophospholipid in the trophoblastic membranes. The initial step is the hydrolysis of glycerophospholipids, which is catalyzed by phospholipase A$_2$ or C. **Phospholipase A$_2$ preferentially acts on chorionic phosphatidyl ethanolamine to release arachidonic acid** (Figure 5-3). Free arachidonic acid does not accumulate. Labor appears to be accompanied by a cascade of events in the chorion, amnion, and decidua that release arachidonic acid from its stored form and convert it to active prostaglandins. 17β-Estradiol stimulates several enzymes active in the synthesis of prostaglandins from arachidonic acid.

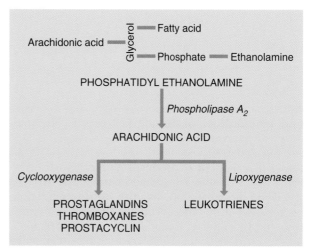

FIGURE 5-3 Diagram of prostaglandin and leukotriene biosynthesis.

There are two cyclooxygenase isoenzymes referred to as COX-1 or PGHS-1, and COX-2 or PGHS-2. These isoenzymes originate from separate genes. COX-1 is expressed in quiescent cells, whereas COX-2 is inducible. It is expressed at sites of inflammation upon cell activation, and potentiates the inflammatory process. COX-1 mRNA expression is low in fetal membranes and does not change with gestational age, whereas COX 2 mRNA expression in the amnion increases with gestational age.

Increased phospholipase A_2 activity may lead to premature labor. Endocervical, intrauterine, or urinary tract infections are often associated with premature labor. Many of the organisms producing these infections have phospholipase A_2 activity, which could produce free arachidonic acid, followed by prostaglandin synthesis, which could trigger labor.

Prostaglandin synthetase inhibitors can prolong gestation. Nonsteroidal antiinflammatory drugs (NSAIDs) inhibit phospholipase A_2, whereas aspirin-like drugs inhibit cyclooxygenase. Because PGE_2 keeps the ductus arteriosus open, premature closure of the ductus may occur after ingestion of NSAIDs or aspirin in large amounts or for a prolonged period of time, resulting in fetal pulmonary hypertension and death.

An additional pathway for arachidonic acid metabolism is the conversion of arachidonic acid to leukotrienes (see Figure 5-3). Both prostaglandins and leukotrienes induce decidualization, which means that they initiate changes in the endometrium during early pregnancy to facilitate implantation of the fertilized ovum.

Although $PGF_{2\alpha}$ is more potent in producing uterine contractile activity, PGE_2 is the most potent prostaglandin for ripening the cervix by inducing changes in the connective tissue. Hence, PGE_2 and its synthetic derivatives are clinically useful for cervical ripening before the induction of labor or abortion.

Changes in Maternal Metabolism

Maternal metabolism adapts to pregnancy through endocrinologic regulation as described below.

ANGIOTENSIN-ALDOSTERONE

Aldosterone is a mineralocorticoid synthesized in the zona glomerulosa of the adrenal cortex. The main source in pregnancy is the maternal adrenal. The fetal adrenal and the placenta do not participate significantly in aldosterone production, although the fetal adrenal is capable of synthesizing it. Aldosterone secretion is regulated by the renin-angiotensin system. Increased renin formed in the kidney converts angiotensinogen (renin-substrate) to angiotensin I, which is further metabolized to angiotensin II, which in turn stimulates aldosterone secretion. Aldosterone stimulates the absorption of sodium and the secretion of potassium in the distal tubule of the kidney, thereby maintaining sodium and potassium balance. The concentration of renin-substrate (a plasma protein), rises in pregnancy. It is thought that the high concentrations of progesterone and estrogen present during pregnancy stimulate renin and renin-substrate formation, thus giving rise to increased levels of angiotensin II and greater aldosterone production. Aldosterone secretion rates decline in pregnancy-induced hypertension and, in some cases, may fall below nonpregnant levels.

CALCIUM METABOLISM

Although calcium absorption is increased in pregnancy, total maternal serum calcium declines. The fall in total calcium parallels that of serum albumin, because approximately half of the total calcium is bound to albumin. Ionic calcium, the physiologically important calcium fraction, remains essentially constant throughout pregnancy because of increased maternal production of parathyroid hormone. The latter facilitates the transfer of calcium across the placenta to the fetus for adequate bone development, and at the same time the mobilization of calcium from the mother's skeleton to maintain adequate calcium homeostasis. In late pregnancy, coinciding with maximal calcification of the fetal skeleton, increased serum parathyroid hormone levels enhance both maternal intestinal absorption of calcium and bone resorption.

Calcium ions are actively transported across the placenta, and fetal serum levels of total as well as ionized calcium are higher than maternal levels in late pregnancy. High fetal ionic calcium suppresses fetal parathyroid hormone production and parathyroid hormone does not cross the placenta. Furthermore, calcitonin production is stimulated, thus providing the fetus with ample calcium for calcification of the skeleton. In the first 24 to 48 hours postpartum, the total serum calcium concentration in the neonate usually falls, while the phosphorus concentration rises. Both adjust to adult levels within 1 week.

Parturition

Parturition means childbirth, and labor is the physiologic process by which a fetus is expelled from the uterus to the outside world.

BIOCHEMICAL BASIS OF CONTRACTION

Muscle contraction is brought about by the sliding of actin and myosin filaments fueled by adenosine triphosphate (ATP) and calcium. While skeletal muscle requires innervation, contraction of smooth muscles such as the myometrium is triggered primarily by hormonal stimuli. Hormonal receptors have been found in the myometrial cell membrane.

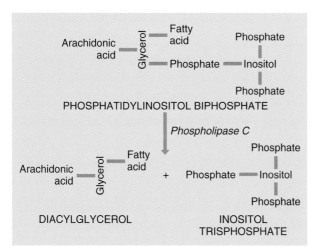

FIGURE 5-4 Diagram of inositol trisphosphate formation.

The binding of oxytocin and prostaglandins to their respective receptors activates phospholipase C, which hydrolyzes phosphatidylinositol bisphosphate, a lipid present in the cell membrane, to inositol trisphosphate and diacylglycerol (Figure 5-4). Inositol trisphosphate induces release of calcium from the sarcoplasmic reticulum, an intracellular calcium storage area. The resulting high intracellular free calcium concentration enables the myofibrils of the myometrium to contract. Subsequently, the calcium is pumped back into the sarcoplasmic reticulum with the help of ATP, and more calcium may enter from the extracellular fluid through both voltage-operated and receptor-operated channels that open briefly. **The maintenance of adequate maternal calcium levels is important because low maternal serum calcium levels have been observed in women at risk for cesarean delivery.**

Unlike the heart, in which the bundle of His is present, no anatomic structures for synchronization of contractions have been found in the uterus; however, recently it has been observed that vitamin D deficiency during pregnancy is associated with myometrial dysfunction and a greater risk of cesarean delivery. Uterine contractions spread as current flows from cell to cell through areas of low resistance. Such areas are associated with gap junctions, which become especially prominent at parturition. **Estradiol and prostaglandins promote the appearance of gap junctions,** whereas progesterone opposes this action of estradiol.

HORMONAL CONTROL OF GESTATIONAL LENGTH AND INITIATION OF LABOR

Gestational length is under the hormonal control of the fetus. Each species has not only a unique gestational length, but also unique mechanisms for controlling that length. Thus, although animal models provide important insights, they do not provide specific infor-mation concerning the control of the human gestational length or the mechanisms that control the initiation of labor.

Animal Models

Most studies have been conducted in sheep, where the fetus appears to control the onset of labor. The fetal hypothalamus stimulates the fetal pituitary to secrete ACTH, which brings about a surge of cortisol from the fetal adrenal. The cortisol surge induces the placental enzyme 17α-hydroxylase and the formation of androgens, which are precursors of estrogen (see Figure 5-1), while simultaneously decreasing progesterone formation. The rise in the estrogen-to-progesterone ratio leads to (1) greater secretion of prostaglandins; (2) formation of myometrial gap junctions, which provide areas of low resistance to current flow and increase coordinated uterine contractions; (3) cervical ripening; and (4) the onset of labor. Administered ACTH, glucocorticoids, or dexamethasone can also initiate parturition. Removal of the fetal pituitary or adrenal, both of which are required for the cortisol surge, will result in prolonged pregnancy.

In a breed of Guernsey cows with a genetic defect resulting in fetal pituitary and adrenal dysfunction, pregnancy is prolonged, and normal vaginal delivery does not occur. **In the rabbit, parturition directly follows a decline in progesterone production secondary to a decline in corpus luteum function.** Abortion can be prevented by administration of progesterone.

The Human

Based upon animal and human research, the process of normal spontaneous human parturition can be divided into four stages.

PHASE 0: QUIESCENCE. Throughout the majority of pregnancy, the uterus remains relatively quiescent. Myometrial activity is inhibited during pregnancy by various substances, but **progesterone appears to play a central role in maintaining uterine quiescence.** Recently, it has been shown that various organs such as the lung, heart, bladder, and uterus are modulated by parathyroid hormone–related peptide (PTHrP), which is produced in each of these organs. This peptide hormone is stimulated by stretch, and during pregnancy PTHrP relaxes the uterus to facilitate fetal growth. At delivery, the gene that regulates PTHrP is turned off, allowing the uterus to contract and to begin the involution process. This reduces the risk of postpartum hemorrhage. Rare uterine contractions that occur during the quiescent phase are of low frequency and amplitude and are poorly coordinated; these are commonly referred to as **Braxton-Hicks contractions** in women. The poor coordination of these contractions is primarily due to an absence of gap junctions in the pregnant myometrium.

PHASE 1: ACTIVATION. Normally, the signals for myometrial activation can come from uterine stretch as a result of fetal growth, or from activation of the fetal hypothalamic-pituitary-adrenal (HPA) axis as a result of fetal maturation. Uterine stretch has been shown in animal models to increase gap junctions and contraction-associated proteins in the myometrium. It is currently thought that once fetal maturity has been reached (as determined by as yet unknown mechanisms), the fetal hypothalamus increases CRH secretion, which in turn stimulates ACTH expression by the fetal pituitary and cortisol and androgen production by the fetal adrenals. Recent data from pregnant mice suggest that the fetus signals the initiation of labor by secreting a major lung surfactant protein, SP-A, into the amniotic fluid.

These data support a critical role for the fetal HPA axis in the initiation of parturition, because surfactant protein synthesis is stimulated by glucocorticoids. The role of PTHrP may also be important in lung development and the onset of parturition. **The concept of a role for the fetal lung in the initiation of parturition is particularly attractive because the fetal lung is the last major organ to mature.**

PHASE 2: STIMULATION. Phase 2 involves a progressive cascade of events leading to a common pathway of parturition, and involving uterine contractility, cervical ripening, and decidual/fetal membrane activation. **This cascade probably begins with placental production of CRH.** Placental CRH synthesis is stimulated by glucocorticoids, in contrast to the inhibitory effect of glucocorticoids on maternal hypothalamic CRH synthesis. Placental CRH enters into the fetal circulation and, in turn, promotes fetal cortisol and DHEA-S production. This positive feedback loop is progressively amplified, thereby driving the process forward from fetal HPA activation to parturition and the placental production of estrogens.

For most of pregnancy, uterine quiescence is maintained by the action of progesterone. At the end of pregnancy in most mammals, maternal progesterone levels fall and estrogen levels rise. In human and nonhuman primate pregnancies, the concentrations of progesterone and estrogens continue to rise throughout pregnancy until delivery of the placenta. A functional progesterone withdrawal may occur in women and nonhuman primates by alterations in progesterone receptor (PR) expression. **There are two progesterone receptors (PRA and PRB) in the human myometrium.** In contrast to PRB, which increases progesterone action, **PRA inhibits progesterone action. The ratio of PRA to PRB in the myometrium in labor is increased, which in effect results in a progesterone withdrawal.**

Functional progesterone withdrawal results in functional estrogen predominance, in part as a result of the increase in placental production of estrogen. The expression of estrogen receptor (ER) isoform, ERα, is normally suppressed by progesterone but as the expression of PR-A increases relative to that of PR-B, so does the expression of ERα in the laboring myometrium. The rising expression of ERα facilitates increased estrogen action. Increasing levels of estrogen also enhance expression of many estrogen-dependent contraction associated proteins (CAPs), including connexin 43 (gap junctions), oxytocin receptor, prostaglandin receptors, cyclooxygenase-2 (COX-2, which results in prostaglandin production), and myosin light-chain kinase (MLCK, which stimulates myometrial contractility and labor).

The progressive cascade of biological processes leads to a common pathway of parturition, involving cervical ripening, uterine contractility, and decidual/fetal membrane activation. **Cervical ripening is largely mediated by the actions of prostaglandins, uterine contractility by the actions of gap junctions and myosin light-chain kinase,** and **decidual/fetal membrane activation by the actions of enzymes such as metalloproteinases,** which ultimately lead to rupture of the membranes.

PHASE 3: INVOLUTION. During expulsion of the fetus, there is a dramatic increase in the release of maternal oxytocin which facilitates the initiation of the final phase of labor. It is thought that some of the increase in oxytocin comes from the fetal pituitary as a result of compression of the fetal head as it passes through the pelvis. Within a short time after the expulsion of the fetus from the uterus the effect of PTHrP decreases which facilitates the return of normal nonpregnant uterine contractility. This decrease accounts for the increased sensitivity of the uterus to oxytocin. **Phase 3 involves placental separation and continued uterine contractions.** Placental separation occurs by cleavage along the plane of the decidua basalis. Uterine contraction is essential to prevent bleeding from large venous sinuses that are exposed after delivery of the placenta, and is primarily effected by oxytocin. This is further supported by oxytocin let down during early breast feeding.

Maternal Physiologic and Immunologic Adaptation to Pregnancy

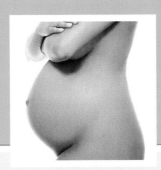

BRIAN J. KOOS • CALVIN J. HOBEL

CLINICAL KEYS FOR THIS CHAPTER

- The hemodynamic changes associated with pregnancy begin at 6 weeks' gestation and are associated with sodium and water retention. The mechanisms for these changes are secondary to elevations in the production of aldosterone, prostaglandins, atrial natriuretic peptide, and nitric oxide that reduce arterial vascular tone. This is followed by formation of arterial-venous shunts, due to invasion of the trophoblasts into the maternal spiral arteries. This invasion, completed at 22 weeks' gestation, allows maternal blood to flow easily into the intervillous placental space and to supply the fetus with adequate nutrition and with exchanges of oxygen and carbon dioxide.

- After complete invasion of the placenta into the spiral arteries, both the systolic and diastolic blood pressure fall (diastolic more than systolic). Toward the end of pregnancy, both diastolic and systolic pressures begin to increase. The gradual increase in the size of the fetus results in mechanical changes in the maternal circulatory and respiratory systems. For the respiratory system, the enlarging fetus and uterus increase the maternal minute ventilation needed to support the increase in oxygen consumption of the fetus and placenta. Maternal renal metabolic requirements are also increased.

- Renal changes during pregnancy play an important role in maintaining maternal-fetal homeostasis. The glomerular filtration rate (GFR) increases early in pregnancy and is maintained for the duration of the pregnancy. Renal function is important for the maintenance of intra vascular volume, and the kidneys are able to decrease or increase sodium tubular reabsorption to maintain sodium balance.

- The placenta receives a significant amount of the cardiac output from the mother and the fetus returns at least 60% of its cardiac output to the placenta, suggesting that the placenta plays a vital role in the metabolic regulation of fetal homeostasis. The fetus has the advantage of having fetal hemoglobin that is capable of transferring greater amounts of oxygen than adult hemoglobin. The fetus, with a higher temperature and lower pH, can shift the oxygen-dissociation curve to the right, while the lower maternal temperature and higher maternal pH shifts the maternal curve to the left. This allows adequate oxygen transfer from the mother to the fetus and is referred to as the double Bohr effect.

- At no other time in the reproductive life of a woman is there an immune challenge as robust as the innate immune system in pregnancy. This system is an inflammatory response during early pregnancy followed by an adaptive immune response, T-lymphocyte helper cell-2 (Th-2), in mid-pregnancy that is designed to prevent rejection of the fetus. The mechanism by which tolerance occurs is complex, and depends upon an organized regulation between Th-1 and Th-2 immunity.

Maternal physiologic adjustments to pregnancy are designed to support the requirements of fetal homeostasis and growth, without unduly jeopardizing maternal well-being. This is accomplished by remodeling maternal cardiovascular, respiratory, renal, and endocrinologic systems to deliver energy and growth substrates to the fetus, while removing inappropriate heat and waste products.

The uterus appears to be a privileged immunologic sanctuary for the fetus and placenta during pregnancy. The pregnant mother's own immunologic defense system remains intact, while allowing an antigenically dissimilar fetus to grow and thrive. At the present time, it is not completely understood how this maternal-fetal immunologic compatibility is regulated.

Normal Values in Pregnancy

The normal values for several hematologic, biochemical, and physiologic indices during pregnancy differ markedly from those in the nonpregnant range and may also vary according to the duration of pregnancy. These alterations are shown in Table 6-1.

Cardiovascular System

CARDIAC OUTPUT

The hemodynamic changes associated with pregnancy are summarized in Table 6-2. **Retention of sodium and water during pregnancy accounts for a total body water increase of 6 to 8 L,** two-thirds of which is located in the extravascular space. **The total sodium accumulation averages 500 to 900 mEq** by the time of delivery. **The total blood volume increases by about 40% above nonpregnant levels, with wide individual variations.** The plasma volume rises as early as the sixth week of pregnancy, and reaches a plateau by about 32 to 34 weeks' gestation, after which little further change occurs. The increase averages 50% in singleton pregnancies, and approaches 70% with a twin gestation. The red blood cell mass begins to increase at the start of the second trimester, and continues to rise

TABLE 6-1

COMMON LABORATORY VALUES IN PREGNANCY			
Test	Normal Range (Nonpregnant)	Change in Pregnancy	Timing
Serum Chemistries			
Albumin	3.5-4.8 g/dL	↓ 1 g/dL	Most by 20 wk, then gradual
Calcium (total)	9-10.3 mg/dL	↓ 10%	Gradual fall
Chloride	95-105 mEq/L	No significant change	Gradual rise
Creatinine (female)	0.6-1.1 mg/dL	↓ 0.3 mg/dL	Most by 20 wk
Fibrinogen	1.5-3.6 g/L	↑ 1-2 g/L	Progressive
Glucose, fasting (plasma)	65-105 mg/dL	↓ 10%	Gradual fall
Potassium (plasma)	3.5-4.5 mEq/L	↓ 0.2-0.3 mEq/L	By 20 wk
Protein (total)	6.5-8.5 g/dL	↓ 1 g/dL	By 20 wk, then stable
Sodium	135-145 mEq/L	↓ 2-4 mEq/L	By 20 wk, then stable
Urea nitrogen	12-30 mg/dL	↓ 50%	1st trimester
Uric acid	3.5-8 mg/dL	↓ 33%	1st trimester, rise at term
Urine Chemistries			
Creatinine	15-25 mg/kg/day (1-1.4 g/day)	No significant change	
Protein	Up to 150 mg/day	Up to 250-300 mg/day	By 20 wk
Creatinine clearance	90-130 mL/min/1.73 m^2	↓ 40-50%	By 16 wk
Serum Enzymatic Activities			
Amylase	23-84 IU/L	↑ 50-100%	
Transaminase			
Glutamic pyruvic (SGPT)	5-35 mU/mL	No significant change	
Glutamic oxaloacetic (SGOT)	5-40 mU/mL	No significant change	
Hematocrit (female)	36-46%	↓ 4-7%	Bottoms at 30-34 wk
Hemoglobin (female)	12-16 g/dL	↓ 1.5-2 g/dL	Bottoms at 30-34 wk
Leukocyte count	4.8-10.8 × 10^3/mm^3	↑ 3.5 × 10^3/mm^3	Gradual
Platelet count	150-400 × 10^3/mm^3	Slight decrease	
Serum Hormone Values			
Cortisol (plasma)	8-21 g/dL	↑ 20 g/dL	
Prolactin (female)	25 ng/mL	↑ 50-400 ng/mL	Gradual, peaks at term
Thyroxine (T$_4$), total	5-11 g/dL	↑ 5 g/dL	Early sustained
Triiodothyronine (T$_3$), total	125-245 ng/dL	↑ 50%	Early sustained

Data from Main DM, Main EK: *Obstetrics and gynecology: a pocket reference,* Chicago, 1984, Year Book, p 7.

TABLE 6-2

CARDIOVASCULAR CHANGES IN PREGNANCY

Parameter	Amount of Change	Timing
Arterial blood pressures		
Systolic	↓ 4-6 mm Hg	All bottom at 20-24 wk, then rise gradually to prepregnancy values at term
Diastolic	↓ 8-15 mm Hg	
Mean	↓ 6-10 mm Hg	
Heart rate	↑ 12-18 beats/min	1st, 2nd, 3rd trimesters
Stroke volume	↑ 10-30%	1st and 2nd trimesters, then stable until term
Cardiac output	↑ 33-45%	Peaks in early 2nd trimester, then stable until term

Data from Main DM, Main EK: *Obstetrics and gynecology: a pocket reference*, Chicago, 1984, Year Book, p 18.

throughout pregnancy. By the time of delivery, it is 20-35% above nonpregnant levels. **The disproportionate increase in plasma volume compared with the red cell volume results in hemodilution with a decreased hematocrit reading, sometimes referred to as physiologic anemia of pregnancy.** If iron stores are adequate, the hematocrit tends to rise from the second to the third trimester.

Cardiac output rises by the tenth week of gestation, reaching about 40% above nonpregnant levels by 20 to 24 weeks, after which there is little change. The rise in cardiac output, which peaks while blood volume is still rising, reflects increases mainly in stroke volume and, to a lesser extent, in heart rate. With twin and triplet pregnancies, the changes in cardiac output are greater than those seen with singleton pregnancies.

The cardiovascular responses to exercise are altered during pregnancy. **For any given level of exercise, oxygen consumption is higher in pregnant than in nonpregnant women.** Similarly, the cardiac output for any level of exercise is increased during pregnancy, and the maximum cardiac output is reached at lower levels of exercise. It is not clear that any of the changes in hemodynamic responses to exercise are detrimental to mother or fetus, but it suggests that maternal cardiac reserves may be lower during pregnancy, and shunting of blood away from the uterus may occur during or after exercise.

INTRAVASCULAR PRESSURES

Systolic pressure falls only slightly during pregnancy, whereas diastolic pressure decreases more markedly; this reduction begins in the first trimester, reaches its nadir in mid-pregnancy, and returns toward nonpregnant levels by term. These changes reflect the elevated cardiac output and reduced peripheral resistance that characterize pregnancy. Toward the end of pregnancy,

vasoconstrictor tone, and with it blood pressure, normally increase. The normal, modest rise of arterial pressure as term approaches should be distinguished from the development of pregnancy-induced hypertension or preeclampsia. **Pregnancy does not alter central venous pressures.**

Blood pressure, as measured with a sphygmomanometer cuff around the brachial artery, varies with posture. In late pregnancy, arterial pressure is higher when the gravid woman is sitting compared with lying supine. When elevations in blood pressure are clinically detected during pregnancy, it is customary to repeat the measurement with the patient lying on her left side. This practice usually introduces a systematic error. In the lateral position, the blood pressure cuff around the brachial artery is raised about 10 cm above the heart. This leads to a hydrostatic fall in measured pressure, yielding a reading about 7 mm Hg lower than if the cuff were at heart level, as occurs during sitting or supine measurements.

MECHANICAL CIRCULATORY EFFECTS OF THE GRAVID UTERUS

As pregnancy progresses, the enlarging uterus displaces and compresses various abdominal structures, including the iliac veins and inferior vena cava (and probably also the aorta), with marked effects. **The supine position accentuates venous compression,** producing a fall in venous return and hence cardiac output. In most gravid women, a compensatory rise in peripheral resistance minimizes the fall in blood pressure. In up to 10% of gravid women, a significant fall occurs in blood pressure accompanied by symptoms of nausea, dizziness, and even syncope. This **supine hypotensive syndrome** is relieved by changing position to the left side (the venous return is greater when the patient turns to the left side as compared with the right side). The expected baroreflexive tachycardia, which normally occurs in response to other maneuvers that reduce cardiac output and blood pressure, does not accompany caval compression. In fact, **bradycardia is often associated with the syndrome.**

The venous compression by the gravid uterus in the supine position elevates pressure in veins that drain the legs and pelvic organs, thereby exacerbating varicose veins in the legs and vulva and causing hemorrhoids. The rise in venous pressure is the major cause of the lower extremity edema that characterizes pregnancy. The hypoalbuminemia associated with pregnancy also shifts the balance of the other major factor in the Starling equation (colloid osmotic pressure) in favor of fluid transfer from the intravascular to the extracellular space. **Because of venous compression, the rate of blood flow in the lower veins is also markedly reduced, causing a predisposition to thrombosis.** The various effects of caval compression are somewhat mitigated by the development of a paravertebral collateral circulation that permits blood from the lower body to bypass the occluded inferior vena cava.

During late pregnancy, the uterus can also partially compress the aorta and its branches. This is thought to account for the observation in some patients of lower pressure in the femoral artery compared with that in the brachial artery. This aortic compression can be accentuated during a uterine contraction, and may be a cause of fetal distress when a patient is in the supine position. This phenomenon has been referred to as the **Poseiro effect.** Clinically, it can be suspected when the femoral pulse is not palpable.

REGIONAL BLOOD FLOW

Blood flow to most regions of the body increases and reaches a plateau relatively early in pregnancy. Notable exceptions occur in the uterus, kidney, breasts, and skin, in each of which blood flow increases with gestational age. **Two of the major increases (those to the kidney and to the skin) serve purposes of elimination: the kidney of waste material and the skin of heat.** Both processes require plasma rather than whole blood, which points to the importance of the disproportionate increase of plasma over red blood cells in the blood volume expansion during pregnancy.

Early in pregnancy, renal blood flow increases to levels approximately 30% above nonpregnant levels and remains unchanged as pregnancy advances. This change accounts for the increased creatinine clearance and lower serum creatinine level. Engorgement of the breasts begins early in gestation, with mammary blood flow increasing two to three times in later pregnancy. The skin blood flow increases slightly during the third trimester, reaching 12% of cardiac output.

There is little information on the distribution of blood flow to other organ systems during pregnancy. **The uterine blood flow increases from about 100 mL/ min in the nonpregnant state** (2% of cardiac output) **to approximately 1200 mL/min** (17% of cardiac output) **at term.** Uterine blood flow, and thus gas and nutrient transfer, to the fetus is vulnerable. **When maternal cardiac output falls, blood flow to the brain, kidneys, and heart is supported by a redistribution of cardiac output, which shunts blood away from the uteroplacental circulation.** Similarly, changes in perfusion pressure can lead to decreases in uterine blood flow. Because the uterine vessels are maximally dilated during pregnancy, little autoregulation can occur to improve uterine blood flow.

CONTROL OF CARDIOVASCULAR CHANGES

The precise mechanisms accounting for the cardiovascular changes in pregnancy have not been fully elucidated. The rise in cardiac output and fall in peripheral resistance during pregnancy may be explained in terms of the circulatory response to an arteriovenous shunt, represented by the uteroplacental circulation. The elevations in cardiac output and uterine blood flow follow different time courses in pregnancy, however, with the former reaching its maximum in the second trimester and the latter increasing to term.

A unifying hypothesis suggests that the elevations in circulating steroid hormones in combination with increases in production of aldosterone and vasodilators such as prostaglandins, atrial natriuretic peptide, nitric oxide, and probably others, reduce arterial tone and increase venous capacitance. These changes, along with the development of arteriovenous shunts, appear responsible for the increase in blood volume and the hyperdynamic circulation of pregnancy (highflow, low-resistance). The same hormonal changes cause relaxation in the cytoskeleton of the maternal heart, which allows the end-diastolic volume (and stroke volume) to increase.

OXYGEN-CARRYING CAPACITY OF BLOOD

Plasma volume expands proportionately more than red blood cell volume, leading to a fall in hematocrit. Optimal pregnancy outcomes are generally achieved with a maternal hematocrit of 33-35%. Hematocrit readings below 27%, or above 39%, are associated with less favorable outcomes. **Despite the relatively low "optimal" hematocrit, the arteriovenous oxygen difference in pregnancy is below nonpregnant levels.** This supports the concept that the hemoglobin concentration in pregnancy is more than sufficient to meet oxygen-carrying requirements.

Pregnancy requires about 1 g of elemental iron: 0.7 g for mother and 0.3 g for the placenta and fetus. A high proportion of women in the reproductive age group enter pregnancy without sufficient stores of iron to meet the increased needs of pregnancy.

Respiratory System

The major respiratory changes in pregnancy involve three factors: the mechanical effects of the enlarging uterus, the increased total body oxygen consumption, and the respiratory stimulant effects of progesterone.

RESPIRATORY MECHANICS IN PREGNANCY

The changes in lung volume and capacities associated with pregnancy are detailed in Table 6-3. **The diaphragm at rest rises to a level of 4 cm above its usual resting position.** The chest enlarges in transverse diameter by about 2.1 cm. Simultaneously, the subcostal angle increases from an average of 68.5 degrees to 103.5 degrees during the latter part of gestation. The increase in uterine size cannot completely explain the changes in chest configuration, as these mechanical changes occur early in gestation.

As pregnancy progresses, the enlarging uterus elevates the resting position of the diaphragm. This

TABLE 6-3

LUNG VOLUMES AND CAPACITIES IN PREGNANCY

Test	Definition	Change in Pregnancy
Respiratory rate	Breaths/minute	No significant change
Tidal volume	The volume of air inspired and expired at each breath	Progressive rise throughout pregnancy of 0.1-0.2 L
Expiratory reserve volume	The maximum volume of air that can be additionally expired after a normal expiration	Lowered by about 15% (0.55 L in late pregnancy compared with 0.65 L postpartum)
Residual volume	The volume of air remaining in the lungs after a maximum expiration	Falls considerably (0.77 L in late pregnancy compared with 0.96 L postpartum)
Vital capacity	The maximum volume of air that can be forcibly inspired after a maximum expiration	Unchanged, except for possibly a small terminal diminution
Inspiratory capacity	The maximum volume of air that can be inspired from resting expiratory level	Increased by about 5%
Functional residual capacity	The volume of air in lungs at resting expiratory level	Lowered by about 18%
Minute ventilation	The volume of air inspired or expired in 1 min	Increased by about 40% as a result of the increased tidal volume and unchanged respiratory rate

Data from Main DM, Main EK: *Obstetrics and gynecology: a pocket reference,* Chicago, 1984, Year Book, p 14.

results in less negative intrathoracic pressure and a decreased resting lung volume, that is, a decrease in functional residual capacity (FRC). The enlarging uterus produces no impairment in diaphragmatic or thoracic muscle motion. Hence, **the vital capacity (VC) remains unchanged. These characteristics—reduced FRC with unimpaired VC—are analogous to those seen in a pneumoperitoneum** and contrast with those seen in severe obesity or abdominal binding, where the elevation of the diaphragm is accompanied by decreased excursion of the respiratory muscles. Reductions in both the expiratory reserve volume and the residual volume contribute to the reduced FRC.

OXYGEN CONSUMPTION AND VENTILATION

Total body oxygen consumption increases by about 15-20% in pregnancy. Approximately half of this increase is accounted for by the uterus and its contents, and the remainder is mainly related to increased maternal renal and cardiac work. Smaller increments are a result of greater breast tissue mass and increased work of the respiratory muscles.

In general, a rise in oxygen consumption is accompanied by cardiorespiratory responses that facilitate oxygen delivery (i.e., by increases in cardiac output and alveolar ventilation). To the extent that elevations in cardiac output and alveolar ventilation keep pace with the rise in oxygen consumption, the arteriovenous oxygen difference and the arterial partial pressure of carbon dioxide (Pco_2), respectively, remain unchanged. **In pregnancy, the elevations in both cardiac output and alveolar ventilation are greater than those required to meet the increased oxygen consumption.** Hence, despite the rise in total body oxygen consump-

tion, the arteriovenous oxygen difference and arterial Pco_2 both fall. The fall in Pco_2 (to 27-32 mm Hg), by definition, indicates hyperventilation.

The rise in minute ventilation reflects an approximately 40% increase in tidal volume at term; the respiratory rate does not change during pregnancy. During exercise, pregnant subjects show a 38% increase in minute ventilation and a 15% increase in oxygen consumption above comparable levels for postpartum subjects. The mechanism is thought to be secondary to the increase in minute ventilation secondary to increasing levels of progesterone and the increased metabolic rate of both the mother and her fetus(es).

When injected into normal nonpregnant subjects, **progesterone increases ventilation.** The central chemoreceptors become more sensitive to CO_2 (i.e., the curve describing the ventilatory response to increasing CO_2 levels has a steeper slope). **Such increased respiratory sensitivity to CO_2 is characteristic of pregnancy and probably accounts for the hyperventilation of pregnancy.**

In summary, both at rest and with exercise, minute ventilation and, to a lesser extent, oxygen consumption are increased during pregnancy. The respiratory stimulating effect of progesterone is probably responsible for the disproportionate increase in minute ventilation over oxygen consumption.

ALVEOLAR-ARTERIAL GRADIENT AND ARTERIAL BLOOD GAS MEASUREMENTS

The hyperventilation of pregnancy results in a respiratory alkalosis. Renal compensatory bicarbonate excretion leads to a final maternal blood pH of between 7.40 and 7.45. During labor (without conduction anesthesia), the hyperventilation associated with each contraction produces a further transient fall in Pco_2. By the end of the first stage of labor, when cervical dilation is complete, a decrease in arterial Pco_2 persists, even between contractions.

In general, when alveolar Pco_2 falls during hyperventilation, alveolar partial pressure of oxygen (Po_2) shows a corresponding rise, leading to a rise in arterial Po_2. In the first trimester, the mean arterial Po_2 may be 106 to 108 mm Hg. **There is a slight downward trend in arterial Po_2 as pregnancy progresses.** This reflects, at least in part, an increased alveolar-arterial gradient, possibly resulting from the decrease in functional residual capacity or FRC discussed previously, which leads to a ventilation-perfusion mismatch.

DYSPNEA OF PREGNANCY

In general, airway resistance is unchanged or even decreased in pregnancy. **Despite the absence of obstructive or restrictive effects, dyspnea is a common symptom in pregnancy. Some studies have suggested that dyspnea may be experienced by as many as 60-70% of women at some time during pregnancy.** Although the mechanism has not been established, the dyspnea of pregnancy may involve the increased sensitivity to the lower levels of Pco_2.

Renal Physiology

ANATOMIC CHANGES IN THE URINARY TRACT

The urinary collecting system, including the calyces, renal pelves, and ureters, undergoes marked dilation in pregnancy, as is readily seen on intravenous urograms. It begins in the first trimester, is present in 90% of women at term, and may persist until the 12th to 16th postpartum week. Progesterone appears to produce smooth muscle relaxation in various organs, including the ureter. **As the uterus enlarges, partial obstruction of the ureter occurs at the pelvic brim in both the supine and the upright positions.** Because of the relatively greater effect on the right side, some have ascribed a role to the dilated ovarian venous plexus. Ovarian venous drainage is asymmetric, with the right vein emptying into the inferior vena cava and the left into the left renal vein.

RENAL BLOOD FLOW AND GLOMERULAR FILTRATION RATE

Renal plasma flow and the glomerular filtration rate (GFR) increase early in pregnancy. Maximum plateau elevations of at least 40-50% above nonpregnant levels are reached by mid-gestation, and they remain unchanged to term. As with cardiac output, renal blood flow and GFR (clinically measured as the creatinine clearance) reach their peak relatively early in pregnancy, before the greatest expansion in intravascular and extracellular volume occurs. **The elevated GFR is reflected in lower serum levels of creatinine and urea nitrogen,** as noted in Table 6-1.

Pregnancy is associated with large reductions in resistance in the afferent and efferent arterioles of the renal arteries, which appears to involve **vasorelaxation induced by relaxin, endothelin, and nitric oxide.** The resulting rise in renal plasma flow accounts for the hyperfiltration.

RENAL TUBULAR FUNCTION

Although 500 to 900 mEq of sodium is retained during pregnancy, **sodium balance is maintained with exquisite precision.** Despite the large amounts of sodium consumed daily (100 to 300 mEq), only 20 to 30 mEq of sodium is retained every week. Pregnant women, given high or low sodium diets, are able to decrease or increase their sodium tubular reabsorption, respectively, to maintain their sodium and fluid balance.

Pregnant women are also able to maintain their fluid balance with no change in the concentrating or diluting ability of the kidney. Plasma osmolarity is reduced by approximately 10 mOsm/kg of water. **Potassium metabolism during pregnancy remains unchanged,** although about 350 mEq of potassium is retained during pregnancy for fetoplacental development and expansion of maternal red cell mass.

The hyperventilation (low partial pressure of CO_2 in arterial blood [$PaCO_2$]) of pregnancy results in respiratory alkalosis, which is compensated by renal excretion of bicarbonate. As a result, maternal renal buffering capacity is reduced.

FLUID VOLUMES

The maternal extracellular volume, which consists of intravascular and interstitial components, increases throughout pregnancy, leading to a state of physiologic extracellular hypervolemia. The intravascular volume, which consists of plasma and red cell components, increases approximately 50% during pregnancy. Maternal interstitial volume shows its greatest increase in the last trimester.

The magnitude of the rise in maternal plasma volume correlates with the size of the fetus; it is particularly marked in cases of multiple gestation. Multiparous women with poor reproductive histories show smaller increments in plasma volume and GFR when compared with those with a history of normal pregnancies and normal-sized babies.

RENIN-ANGIOTENSIN SYSTEM IN PREGNANCY

Plasma concentrations of renin, renin substrate, and angiotensin I and II are increased during pregnancy. **Renin levels remain elevated throughout pregnancy,** with at least a portion of the renin circulating in a high-molecular-weight form.

The uterus and placenta, like the kidney, **can produce renin,** and extremely high concentrations of renin occur in the amniotic fluid. The physiologic role of uterine renin has not been established. Recently, the renin-angiotensin system has been shown to participate in the regulation of maternal-placental-fetal blood flow that is altered by various disease states such as preeclampsia, obesity, and diabetes.

Homeostasis of Maternal Energy Substrates

The metabolic regulation of energy substrates, including glucose, amino acids, fatty acids, and ketone bodies, is complex and interrelated.

INSULIN EFFECTS AND GLUCOSE METABOLISM

In pregnancy, the insulin response to glucose stimulation is augmented. By the 10th week of normal pregnancy and continuing to term, fasting concentrations of insulin are elevated and those of glucose reduced. Until mid-gestation, these changes are accompanied by enhanced intravenous glucose tolerance (although oral glucose tolerance remains unchanged). **Glycogen synthesis and storage by the liver increases, and gluconeogenesis is inhibited.** Thus, during the first half of pregnancy, the anabolic actions of insulin are potentiated.

After early pregnancy, insulin resistance emerges, so glucose tolerance is impaired. The fall in serum glucose for a given dose of insulin is reduced compared with the response in earlier pregnancy. Elevation of circulating glucose is prolonged after meals, although fasting glucose remains reduced, as in early pregnancy.

A variety of humoral factors derived from the placenta have been suggested to account for the antiinsulin environment of the latter part of pregnancy. Perhaps the most important are cytokines and human placental lactogen (hPL), which antagonizes the peripheral effects of insulin. An increase in levels of free cortisol and other hormones may also be involved in the insulin resistance of pregnancy.

LIPID METABOLISM

The potentiated anabolic effects of insulin that characterize early pregnancy lead to the inhibition of lipolysis. **During the second half of pregnancy, probably as a result of rising hPL levels, lipolysis is augmented, and fasting plasma concentrations of free fatty acids are elevated.** Teleologically, the free fatty acids act as substrates for maternal energy metabolism, whereas glucose and amino acids cross the placenta to the fetus. In the humoral milieu of the second half of the pregnancy, the increased free fatty acids lead to ketone body formation (β-hydroxybutyrate and acetoacetate). **Pregnancy is thus associated with an increased risk of ketoacidosis, especially after prolonged fasting.**

In the context of maternal lipid metabolism, the most dramatic lipid change in pregnancy is the rise in fasting triglyceride concentration.

Placental Transfer of Nutrients

The transfer of substances across the placenta occurs by several mechanisms, including simple diffusion, facilitated diffusion, and active transport. **Low molecular size and lipid solubility promote simple diffusion.** Substances with molecular weights greater than 1000 Daltons, such as polypeptides and proteins, cross the placenta slowly, if at all.

Amino acids are actively transported across the placenta, making fetal levels higher than maternal levels. Glucose is transported by facilitated diffusion, leading to rapid equilibrium with only a small maternal-fetal gradient. **Glucose is the main energy substrate of the fetus,** although amino acids and lactate may contribute up to 25% of fetal oxygen consumption. The degree and mechanism of placental transfer of these and other substances are summarized in Table 6-4.

Other Endocrine Changes

THYROID

The thyroid gland undergoes moderate enlargement during pregnancy. This is not because of elevation of thyroid-stimulating hormone (TSH), which remains unchanged. Placenta-derived human chorionic gonadotropin (hCG) has a TSH-effect on the thyroid gland, which can result in abnormally low levels of TSH in the first trimester, when hCG concentrations are highest.

Circulating thyroid hormone exists in two primary active forms: thyroxine (T_4) and triiodothyronine (T_3). The former circulates in higher concentrations, is more highly protein-bound, and is less metabolically potent than T_3, for which it may serve as a prohormone. Circulating T_4 is bound to carrier proteins, approximately 85% to thyroxine-binding globulin (TBG) and most of the remainder to another protein, thyroxine-binding prealbumin. It is believed that only the unbound fraction of the circulating hormone is biologically active. **TBG is increased during pregnancy because the high estrogen levels induce increased hepatic synthesis.** The body responds by raising total circulating levels of T_4 and T_3 and the net effect is that **the free, biologically active concentration of each hormone is unchanged.** Therefore, clinically, the free T_4 index, which corrects the total circulating T_4 for the amount of binding protein, is an appropriate measure of thyroid function, with the same normal range as in the nonpregnant state.

Only minimal amounts of thyroid hormone cross the placenta. The small amount of thyroid hormone

TABLE 6-4

MATERNAL-FETAL TRANSFER DURING PREGNANCY

Function	Substance	Placental Transfer
Glucose homeostasis	Glucose	Excellent—"facilitated diffusion"
	Amino acids	Excellent—active transport
	Free fatty acids	Very limited—essential free fatty acids only
	Ketones	Excellent—diffusion
	Insulin	No transfer
	Glucagon	No transfer
Thyroid function	Thyroxine	Very poor—diffusion
	Triiodothyronine	Poor—diffusion
	Thyrotropin-releasing hormone	Good
	Thyroid-stimulating immunoglobulin	Good
	Thyroid-stimulating hormone	Negligible transfer
	Propylthiouracil	Excellent
Adrenal hormones	Cortisol	Excellent transfer and active placental conversion of cortisol to cortisone beginning at mid-pregnancy*
	Adrenocorticotropic hormone	No transfer
Parathyroid function	Calcium	Active transfer against gradient
	Magnesium	Active transfer against gradient
	Phosphorus	Active transfer against gradient
	Parathyroid hormone	Not transferred
Immunoglobulins	IgA	Minimal passive transfer
	IgG	Good—both passive and active transport from 7 wk gestation
	IgM	No transfer

Data from Main DM, Main EK: *Obstetrics and gynecology: a pocket reference,* Chicago, 1984, Year Book, p 37.
*At mid-gestation, placental 11β-hydroxysteroid dehydrogenase converts cortisol to cortisone.

that crosses the placenta is converted to reverse T_3 (rT_3) which is metabolically inactive. The fetus does not require thyroid hormone from the mother; it synthesizes thyroid hormone from its own thyroid gland to meet its requirements. The fetus does not require thyroid hormone for thermogenesis in utero and at birth it releases TSH in large amounts to begin the release of thyroid hormones for the purpose of thermogenesis.

ADRENAL

Adrenocorticotropic hormone (ACTH) and plasma cortisol levels are both elevated from 3 months' gestation to delivery. Circulating cortisol is also primarily bound to a specific plasma protein, corticosteroid-binding globulin (CBG) or transcortin. **Unlike the level of thyroid hormones, the mean unbound level of cortisol is elevated in pregnancy;** there is also some loss of the diurnal variation that characterizes its concentration in nonpregnant women.

Weight Gain in Pregnancy

The average weight gain in pregnancy uncomplicated by generalized edema is 12.5 kg (28 lb). The components of this weight gain are indicated in Table 6-5. The products of conception constitute only about 40% of the total maternal weight gain.

TABLE 6-5

ANALYSIS OF WEIGHT GAIN IN PREGNANCY

	Increase in Weight (Grams) Up To:			
Tissues and Fluids	10 wk	20 wk	30 wk	40 wk
Fetus	5	300	1500	3400
Placenta	20	170	430	650
Amniotic fluid	30	350	750	800
Uterus	140	320	600	970
Mammary gland	45	180	360	405
Blood	100	600	1300	1250
Interstitial fluid (no edema or leg edema)	0	30	80	1680
Maternal stores	310	2050	3480	3345
Total weight gained	650	4000	8500	12,500

Data from Hytten F, Chamberlain G, editors: *Clinical physiology in obstetrics,* Oxford, 1980, Blackwell Scientific, p 221.

Placental Transfer of Oxygen and Carbon Dioxide

FETAL OXYGENATION

The placenta receives 60% of the combined ventricular output, whereas the postnatal lung receives 100% of

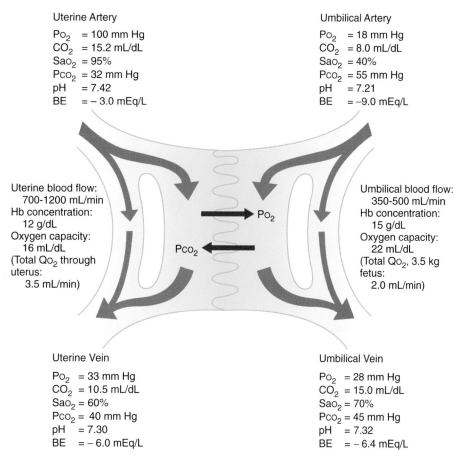

Uterine Artery

P_{O_2} = 100 mm Hg
CO_2 = 15.2 mL/dL
Sa_{O_2} = 95%
P_{CO_2} = 32 mm Hg
pH = 7.42
BE = −3.0 mEq/L

Umbilical Artery

P_{O_2} = 18 mm Hg
CO_2 = 8.0 mL/dL
Sa_{O_2} = 40%
P_{CO_2} = 55 mm Hg
pH = 7.21
BE = −9.0 mEq/L

Uterine blood flow:
  700-1200 mL/min
Hb concentration:
  12 g/dL
Oxygen capacity:
  16 mL/dL
(Total Q_{O_2} through
uterus:
  3.5 mL/min)

P_{O_2}

P_{CO_2}

Umbilical blood flow:
  350-500 mL/min
Hb concentration:
  15 g/dL
Oxygen capacity:
  22 mL/dL
(Total Q_{O_2}, 3.5 kg
fetus:
  2.0 mL/min)

Uterine Vein

P_{O_2} = 33 mm Hg
CO_2 = 10.5 mL/dL
Sa_{O_2} = 60%
P_{CO_2} = 40 mm Hg
pH = 7.30
BE = −6.0 mEq/L

Umbilical Vein

P_{O_2} = 28 mm Hg
CO_2 = 15.0 mL/dL
Sa_{O_2} = 70%
P_{CO_2} = 45 mm Hg
pH = 7.32
BE = −6.4 mEq/L

FIGURE 6-1 Placental transfer of oxygen and carbon dioxide. *BE,* Base excess; *Hb,* hemoglobin. (Adapted from Bonica JJ: *Obstetric analgesia and anesthesia,* ed 2, Amsterdam, 1980, World Federation of Societies of Anesthesiologists, p 29.)

the cardiac output. Unlike the lung, which consumes little of the oxygen it transfers, **a significant percentage of the oxygen derived from maternal blood at term is consumed by placental tissue.** The degree of functional shunting of placental blood past exchange sites is approximately tenfold greater than in the lung. A major cause of this functional shunting is probably a mismatch between maternal and fetal blood flow at the exchange sites, analogous to the ventilation-perfusion inequalities that occur in the lung.

The uteroplacental circulation subserves fetal gas exchange. Oxygen, carbon dioxide, and inert gases cross the placenta by simple diffusion. The rate of transfer is proportional to the difference in gas tension across the placenta and the surface area of the placenta, and the transfer rate is inversely proportional to diffusion distance between maternal and fetal blood. **The placenta normally does not pose a significant barrier to respiratory gas exchange, unless it becomes separated (abruption placenta) or edematous (severe hydrops fetalis).**

The anatomical distribution of uterine and umbilical blood flow and O_2 transfer across the placenta is depicted in Figure 6-1. A **maternal shunt,** which describes the fraction of blood shunted to the myoendometrium and is estimated to constitute 20% of uterine blood flow, is depicted. Similarly, a **fetal shunt,** which supplies blood to the placenta and fetal membranes and accounts for 19% of umbilical blood flow, is shown. The **maternal-to-fetal** P_{O_2} and P_{CO_2} gradients are calculated from measurements of gas tensions in the uterine and umbilical arteries and veins. **The umbilical vein of the fetus, like the pulmonary vein of the adult, carries the circulation's most highly oxygenated blood.** The umbilical venous P_{O_2} of about 28 mm Hg is relatively low by adult standards. This relatively low fetal tension is essential for survival in utero, because a high P_{O_2} initiates physiologic adjustments (e.g., closure of the ductus arteriosus and vasodilation of the pulmonary vessels) that normally occur in the neonate but would be harmful in utero.

Although not involved in respiratory gas exchange, fetal breathing movements are critically involved in lung development and in the development of respiratory regulation. Fetal breathing differs from that in the adult in that it is episodic, sensitive to fetal glucose concentrations, and inhibited by hypoxia. Because of its sensitivity to acute O_2 deprivation, fetal breathing is used clinically as an indicator of the adequacy of fetal oxygenation.

FETAL AND MATERNAL HEMOGLOBIN DISSOCIATION CURVES

Most of the oxygen in blood is carried by hemoglobin in red blood cells. The maximum amount of oxygen carried per gram of hemoglobin, that is, the amount carried at 100% saturation, is fixed at 1.37 mL. The hemoglobin flow rates depend on blood flow rates and hemoglobin concentration. The uterine blood flow at term has been estimated at 700 to 1200 mL/min, with about 75-88% of this entering the intervillous space. The umbilical blood flow has been estimated at 350 to 500 mL/min, with more than 50% going to the placenta (see Figure 6-1).

The hemoglobin concentration of the blood determines its oxygen-carrying capacity, which is expressed in milliliters of oxygen per 100 mL of blood. In the fetus at or near term, the hemoglobin concentration is about 18 g/dL and oxygen-carrying capacity is 20 to 22 mL/dL. The **maternal oxygen-carrying capacity of blood, which is generally proportional to the hemoglobin concentration, is lower than that of the fetus.**

The affinity of hemoglobin for oxygen, which is reflected as the percentage saturation at a given oxygen tension, depends on chemical conditions. As is illustrated in Figure 6-2, **when compared with that in nonpregnant adults, the binding of oxygen by hemoglobin is much greater in the fetus under standard conditions of P_{CO_2}, pH, and temperature.** In contrast, maternal affinity is lower under these conditions, with 50% of hemoglobin saturated with O_2 at a P_{O_2} of 26.5 mm Hg (P_{50}) for mother compared with 20 mm Hg for the fetus.

In vivo, the greater fetal temperature and lower pH shift the O_2-dissociation curve to the right, while the lower maternal temperature and higher pH shift the maternal curve to the left. As a result, the O_2-dissociation curves for the fetal and maternal blood are not too dissimilar at the site of placental transfer. Maternal venous blood probably has an O_2-saturation of about 73% and a P_{O_2} of about 36 mm Hg, and the corresponding values for blood in the umbilical vein are about 63% and 28 mm Hg, respectively. **As the only source of O_2 for the fetus, blood in the umbilical vein has a higher O_2 saturation and P_{O_2} than blood in the fetal circulation** (Figure 6-3). In the presence of a low fetal arterial P_{O_2}, fetal oxygenation is maintained by a high rate of blood flow to fetal tissues, which is supported by a very high cardiac output. This feature, along with the lower P_{50} of fetal blood, results in normal O_2 delivery to fetal organs.

The decrease in the affinity of hemoglobin for oxygen produced by a fall in pH is referred to as the Bohr effect. Because of the unique situation in the

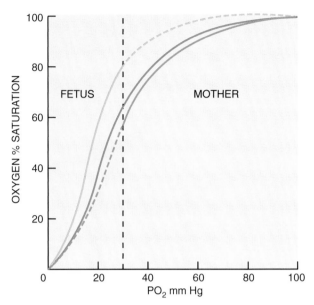

FIGURE 6-2 The oxygen dissociation curve for fetal blood compared with maternal blood. The central continuous curve is for normal adult blood under standard conditions. A vertical line at an oxygen partial pressure of 30 mm Hg divides the curves. The fetal curve normally operates below that level and the maternal curve above it. (Adapted from Hytten F, Chamberlain G, editors: *Clinical physiology in obstetrics*, ed 2, Oxford, 1991, Blackwell, p 418.)

placenta, a double Bohr effect facilitates oxygen transfer from mother to fetus. When CO_2 and fixed acids are transferred from fetus to mother, the associated rise in fetal pH increases the fetal red blood cells' affinity for oxygen uptake. The concomitant reduction in maternal blood pH decreases oxygen affinity and promotes its unloading of oxygen from maternal red cells.

Fetal Circulation

Several anatomic and physiologic factors must be noted in considering the fetal circulation (Table 6-6 and Figure 6-3).

The normal adult circulation is a series circuit with blood flowing through the right heart, the lungs, the left heart, the systemic circulation, and finally the right heart. In the fetus, the circulation is a parallel system with the cardiac outputs from the right and left ventricles directed primarily to different vascular beds. For example, the right ventricle, which contributes about 65% of the combined output, pumps blood primarily through the pulmonary artery, ductus arteriosus, and descending aorta. Only a small fraction of right ventricular output flows through the pulmonary circulation. The left ventricle supplies blood mainly to the tissues supplied by the aortic arch, such as the brain. **The fetal circulation is a parallel circuit characterized by channels (ductus venosus, foramen ovale, and**

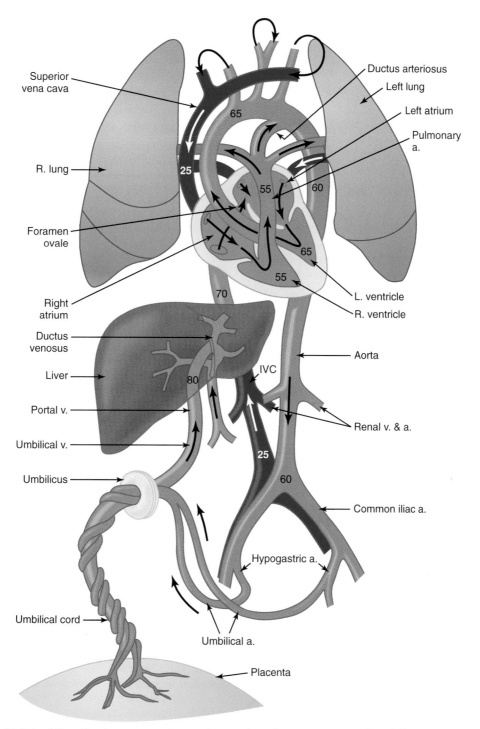

FIGURE 6-3 The fetal circulation. Numbers represent approximate values of percentage saturation of blood with oxygen in utero. *IVC,* Inferior vena cava. (Adapted from Parer JJ: Fetal circulation. In Sciarra JJ, editor: *Obstetrics and gynecology, vol 3: maternal and fetal medicine,* Hagerstown, Md, 1984, Harper & Row, p 2.)

TABLE 6-6

COMPONENTS OF THE FETAL CIRCULATION

Fetal Structure	From/To	Adult Remnant
Umbilical vein	Umbilicus/ductus venosus	Ligamentum teres hepatis
Ductus venosus	Umbilical vein/inferior vena cava (bypasses liver)	Ligamentum venosum
Foramen ovale	Right atrium/left atrium	Closed atrial wall
Ductus arteriosus	Pulmonary artery/descending aorta	Ligamentum arteriosum
Umbilical artery	Common iliac artery/umbilicus	Superior vesical arteries; lateral vesicoumbilical ligaments

Data from Main DM, Main EK: *Obstetrics and gynecology: a pocket reference,* Chicago, 1984, Year Book, p 34.

ductus arteriosus) and preferential streaming, which function to maximize the delivery of more highly oxygenated blood to the upper body and brain, less highly oxygenated blood to the lower body, and very low blood flow to the nonfunctional lungs.

The umbilical vein, carrying oxygenated (80% saturated) blood from the placenta to the fetal body, enters the portal system. A portion of this umbilical-portal blood passes through the hepatic microcirculation, where oxygen is extracted, and thence through the hepatic veins into the inferior vena cava. The majority of the blood bypasses the liver through the ductus venosus, which directly enters the inferior vena cava, which also receives the unsaturated (25% saturated) venous return from the lower body. Blood reaching the heart via the inferior vena cava has an oxygen saturation of about 70%, which represents the most highly oxygenated blood in the heart. Approximately one-third of blood returning to the heart from the inferior vena cava preferentially streams across the foramen ovale into the left atrium, where it mixes with the relatively meager pulmonary venous return. Blood flows from the left atrium into the left ventricle, and then to the ascending aorta.

The proximal aorta, carrying the most highly saturated blood leaving the heart (65%) gives off branches to supply the brain and upper body. Most of the blood returning via the inferior vena cava enters the right atrium, where it mixes with the unsaturated blood returning via the superior vena cava (25% saturated). Right ventricular outflow (O_2 saturation of 55%) enters the aorta via the ductus arteriosus, and the descending aorta supplies the lower body with blood having less O_2 saturation (about 60%) than that flowing to the brain and the upper body.

The role of the ductus arteriosus must be emphasized. Right ventricular output enters the pulmonary trunk, from which its major portion, because of the high vascular resistance of the pulmonary circulation, bypasses the lungs by flowing through the ductus arteriosus to the descending aorta. Although the descending aorta supplies branches to the lower fetal body, the major portion of descending aortic flow goes to the umbilical arteries, which carry deoxygenated blood to the placenta.

CHANGES IN THE ANATOMY OF THE CARDIOVASCULAR SYSTEM AFTER BIRTH

The following changes occur after birth (see Table 6-6):
1. **Elimination of the placental circulation, with interruption and eventual obliteration of the umbilical vessels**
2. **Closure of the ductus venosus**
3. **Closure of the foramen ovale**
4. **Gradual constriction and eventual obliteration of the ductus arteriosus**
5. **Dilation of the pulmonary vessels and establishment of the pulmonary circulation**

The elimination of the umbilical circulation, closure of the vascular shunts, and establishment of the pulmonary circulation will change the vascular circuitry of the neonate from an "in parallel" system to an "in series" system.

Immunology of Pregnancy

Nearly 60 years ago, Peter Medawar recognized the apparent paradox of the immunologic evasion of the semiallogeneic fetus by the mother. He proposed three hypotheses to explain this paradox: (1) anatomic separation of mother and fetus; (2) antigenic immaturity of the fetus; or (3) immunologic "inertness" (tolerance) of the mother. In the intervening years, **it has become apparent that both the mother and her fetus are immunologically aware of each other, and yet tolerance exists for the most part.** Furthermore, while the maternal immune response during pregnancy is qualitatively different, **pregnancy does *not* result in an overall maternal immunosuppression.**

The growth and development of a semiallogeneic conceptus within an immunologically competent mother depends on the manner in which pregnancy alters the immune regulatory mechanisms. Historically, attention in addressing the "Medawar Paradox" has focused exclusively on the mother, but it is now known that **mammalian fetuses are capable of**

mounting immune responses in utero. The interplay between the fetal and maternal immune systems is complex and is an active area of ongoing investigation.

INNATE AND ADAPTIVE IMMUNITY

Mammalian (including human) immune systems have **two fundamental responses: an early "innate" and a later more specific/robust adaptive response.**

The innate immune response is the first line of defense, and includes surface barriers (mucosal immunity), saliva, tears, nasal secretions, perspiration, blood and tissue monocytes/macrophages, natural killer (NK) cells, endothelial cells, polymorphonuclear neutrophils, the complement system, dendritic cells, and the normal microbial flora. **The adaptive immune system is composed of cell mediated (T lymphocytes) and humoral responses (B lymphocytes-antibodies).** Activation of T and consequently B lymphocytes is critical for the development of lifelong immune responses.

Through evolution, innate immune cells have acquired mechanisms that recognize the foreign nature of the inciting antigen and mount a transient protection within hours. There is no need for major histocompatibility complex (MHC) molecules. **The epithelial cell interaction with the antigens induces the release of cytokines and chemokines; which attract the macrophages, dendritic cells, and NK cells.** Macrophages and neutrophils then engulf and lyse the pathogens, and produce cytokines. NK cells play the key role in destroying the virally infected cells. Damaged epithelial cells lead to the activation of complements. Complements can directly kill the microbes by punching holes in their membrane and indirectly by opsonizing them to facilitate their phagocytosis. Complements also promote the inflammatory cell recruitment. **The cytokines released from the immune cells activate the vascular endothelial cells, thereby increasing permeability, and allowing immune effector cells to penetrate into the tissues.**

The critical link between the innate immune response and the adaptive immune response is antigen presentation. Foreign proteins that are phagocytosed are processed intracellularly and then expressed on the cell surface complexed with MHC II. Additionally, the presenting cells provide critical secondary signals (via cell surface molecules) that are permissive for appropriate T cell activation. **Among the most efficient antigen presenting cells are dendritic cells.**

Dendritic cells play a key role in alerting the adaptive immune responses. Immature dendritic cells engulf the pathogens, carry them to the lymph nodes and present them to CD4$^+$ T-lymphocytes. These now activated T cells develop surface receptors for specific foreign antigens and undergo clonal proliferation. **Cytotoxic (activated) T cells can directly kill target**

cells expressing viral antigens together with MHC I. In contrast to antigens presented in the context of MHC II, **a portion of all cellular proteins are expressed on the cell surface of all normal cells in the context of MHC I.** By this mechanism, the immune system can determine if a cell is producing "self" proteins or if the cell has been altered (e.g., by virus) to produce foreign proteins.

Once CD4$^+$ T cells are activated, they can direct an immune response by secreting proteins (cytokines) that activate surrounding cells. By secreting interferon-γ and interleukin-2 (IL-2), a CD4$^+$ T cell induces a cellular immune response via CD8$^+$ "killer" T cells. By secreting IL-4 and IL-5, CD4$^+$ T cells promote B cells to proliferate and differentiate for immunoglobulin (antibody) production. **B cells exposed to antigen for the first time produce IgM.** As the affinity of the immunoglobulin (antibody) increases, the B cell undergoes a genetic rearrangement and may produce a variety of different antibodies. The most specific are usually of the IgG subtype. IgG crosses the placenta and will accumulate in the fetus.

DEVELOPMENT OF FETAL IMMUNITY

The innate immune effector cells first arise from hematopoietic progenitors noted in the blood islands of the yolk sac. By 8 embryonic weeks, the fetal liver becomes the source of these cells, and by 20 weeks, the fetal bone marrow takes over.

Macrophage like cells arise from the yolk sac around 4 weeks, and by 16 weeks, a fetus has the same number of circulating macrophages as adults but they are less functional. The fetus has fewer tissue macrophages. **Immature granulocytes can be found in the fetal spleen and liver by 8 weeks. NK cells are detected in the liver by 8 to 13 weeks and complements 2 and 4 by 8 weeks.** C1, 3, 5, 7, and 9 are found in the serum by 18 weeks. Maternal complements do not cross the placenta into the fetus. The complement system continues to mature after parturition and adult levels are reached by 1 year of age. Skin, one of the main innate barriers, completes its development 2 to 3 weeks after birth.

The cellular component of the adaptive immunity, T cells, are also derived from hematopoietic progenitors that are first seen in the blood islands of the yolk sac by 8 weeks. To differentiate into activated T cells, they must first migrate to the thymus gland. The thymus is a relatively large organ in the fetus, and its sole function appears to be to nurture and develop T cells. After maturation, T cells develop into either CD4 or CD8 types according to the surface receptor expressed. By 16 weeks, the thymus contains T cells in proportion to those found in the adult. **In the newborn, the proportion of CD4 helper T cells and CD8 T cells is similar to that in the adult. However, interferon-γ production is less efficient in fetal CD4 helper T cells.**

Fetal B cells are first detected in the liver by 8 weeks and around the second trimester, B cell production is mostly from the bone marrow. **Fetal B cells secrete IgG or IgA during the second trimester,** but IgM antibodies are not secreted until the third trimester. Cord IgM levels greater than 20 mg/dL suggest an intrauterine infection. **Maternal IgG crosses the placenta as early as the late first trimester, but the efficiency of the transport is poor until 30 weeks.** Significant passive immunity can be transferred to the fetus in this manner and **for this reason premature infants are not as well protected by maternal antibodies. IgM, because of its larger molecular size, is unable to cross the placenta.** The other immunoglobulins (IgA, IgD, and IgE) are also confined to the maternal compartment, but the fetus can make its own IgA and IgM.

Physiologically, newborns have higher neutrophil and lymphocyte counts, and the proportion of lymphocytes and the absolute lymphocyte count are higher in neonates than in adults.

IMMUNOBIOLOGY OF THE MATERNAL-FETAL INTERACTION

Pregnancy poses a special immunologic problem. The embryo must implant and cause a portion (placenta) to invade the uterine lining in order to gain access to the maternal circulation for nutrition and gas exchange. The maintenance of the antigenically dissimilar fetus in the uterus of the mother is of primary importance in obstetrics. The total picture of immune regulation at the maternal-fetal interface is yet to be elucidated, but the following is a synopsis of the current level of understanding.

The primary sites of modulation of the maternal response are the decidua of the uterus, the regional lymphatics, and the placenta. **In the uterus, NK cell–mediated inflammation is necessary for the appropriate attachment and penetration of the fertilized egg into the uterine wall and for early placental development,** whereas increased suppressor T cells, the presence of molecules that inactivate the previously activated maternal lymphocytes (CTLA4), and the absence of B cells provide the needed immune quiescence to allow for successful pregnancy. The placenta, decidua, and the membranes provide the key barrier in protecting the growing fetus from microbial pathogens and toxins circulating in the mother's blood. **The syncytiotrophoblast, that makes up the cell barrier between the fetal and maternal blood in the placenta, does not express classic self/nonself MHC I and II molecules.** Deeper trophoblastic cells do not express MHC II, but some express MHC I, which are not stimulatory. This allows protection from invading microbes but at the same time prevents the destruction of the fetus.

Human leukocyte antigen G (HLA-G) suppresses the adaptive and innate immune responses in the placenta and promotes the release of antiinflammatory cytokines such as IL-10. The soluble forms of HLA-G are found in the blood of pregnant women. HLA-G is thought to act by suppressing the activity of uterine NK cells, which normally destroy cells that *lack* the expression of MHC I.

Understanding the mechanisms of immune regulation is largely derived from the study of autoimmune diseases. Many disease-free individuals possess potentially autoreactive T cells. A variety of mechanisms regulate the response of CD4$^+$ T cells so that they do not react against self-antigens. Naive T helper cells have the potential to become a variety of specialized T cells. There are now four well-recognized possibilities, each with a unique role and ability to cross regulate. T_H1 cells drive cell-mediated immunity by secreting IL-2 and interferon-γ. T_H2 cells drive humoral reactions (antibody/B cell) by secreting IL-4. Regulatory T cells are regulatory subtypes that suppress ongoing cellular immune reactions via cell contact. Lastly, there is a newly described proinflammatory population of T cells (T_H17) that secrete IL-17. **These T_H17 cells, under normal circumstances, are important for the clearance of parasites, bacteria, and fungi, but under pathologic conditions seem to play a crucial role in the development of autoimmune disease.** One of the hallmarks of T cell regulation is the ability of these specialized T cell populations to cross-regulate each other.

IMMUNOLOGIC RESPONSE DURING NORMAL PREGNANCY

The mother's immunologic defense system remains intact during pregnancy. While allowing the fetus to grow, the mother must still be able to protect herself and her fetus from infection and antigenically foreign substances. **The nonspecific (innate) mechanisms of the immunologic system (including phagocytosis and the inflammatory response) are not affected by pregnancy. The specific (adaptive) mechanisms of the immune response (humoral and cellular) are also not significantly affected.** In fact, women with renal transplants do not experience any reduction in serious episodes of acute rejection during pregnancy. No significant change occurs in the leukocyte count. The percentage of B or T lymphocytes is not appreciably altered, nor is there any consistent alteration in their performance during pregnancy. Immunoglobulin levels do not change in pregnancy and vaccine responses are preserved. The main question today, is what are the mechanisms which provide this protection?

There are three reasons to suggest that vitamin D may be an important regulator of the immune system during pregnancy. First, it has been shown that vitamin D deficiency in women who have renal transplants is associated with an increased incidence of infections and an increased risk of kidney rejection. Vitamin D supplementation decreases this risk. It is likely that this applies to pregnant women too. **Second,** both the decidua surrounding the chorion and the placenta have been shown to produce the active form of vitamin D, provided that the mother is not vitamin D deficient of the circulating form of vitamin D (25[OH]D). Thus, the decidua and placenta provide the fetus with a natural mechanism of immune surveillance controlled by the availability of circulating vitamin from the mother. **Third,** recently it has also been shown that the active form of vitamin D stimulates the production of regulatory T cells that suppress the innate inflamma-tory profile that could interfere with the pregnancy, shifting it to the adaptive profile that supports fetal growth and normal pregnancy development.

Pregnant women are at higher risk of severe infection and death from certain pathogens such as viruses (hepatitis, influenza, varicella, cytomegalovirus, polio), bacteria (listeria, streptococcus, gonorrhea, salmonella, leprosy), and parasites (malaria, coccidioidomy-cosis) compared with nonpregnant women. Vitamin D supplementation during pregnancy, therefore, may be important not only to reduce the risk of immunologic fetal rejection, but also to help prevent infection.

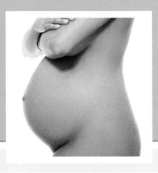

Antepartum Care

Preconception and Prenatal Care,
Genetic Evaluation and Teratology,
and Antenatal Fetal Assessment

CALVIN J. HOBEL • JOHN WILLIAMS III

CLINICAL KEYS FOR THIS CHAPTER

- Preconception counseling is an important component of preventive care for couples that are considering pregnancy. It can identify risks related to family history, maternal medical conditions, and fetal and maternal chromosomal/genetic disorders that may result in congenital abnormalities. A simple screening tool called *Before Pregnancy* is available electronically at StudentConsult.com to facilitate the process of preconception assessment and counseling.

- Adequate prenatal care, including nutritional counseling, is essential for obtaining the best pregnancy outcomes. Early pregnancy complications, secondary to factors related to the mother, her fetus, or the placenta, occur in some pregnancies. Early recognition and management of these problems is vital for the success of the pregnancy. During follow-up visits, it is important to reassure women that their pregnancy is progressing normally or initiate appropriate testing when necessary.

- Traditionally, women older than 34 years of age have been advised to have prenatal testing because they are at increased age-related risk for having offspring with chromosomal and genetic abnormalities and the risk of the more invasive techniques is less than the risk of finding abnormalities. Recently, microarray comparative genomic hybridization (microarray-CGH) has been introduced into clinical practice. There are many submicroscopic chromosomal abnormalities that can now be detected with microarray-CGH that are not maternal age-related. Current guidelines therefore recommend that prenatal diagnostic testing with amniocentesis or

- chorionic villus sampling (CVS) be offered to all pregnant women regardless of their age.

- A number of noninvasive tests are available for screening for fetal chromosomal abnormalities. These include second-trimester maternal serum screening (Quad-Screen), which offers a trisomy 21 detection rate of 81%; first-trimester serum screening combined with ultrasonic measurement of nuchal translucency and visualization of nasal bone, which has a Down syndrome detection rate of 93%, and integrated first- and second-trimester screening, which increases the detection rate to 95%. Recently, noninvasive prenatal testing (NIPT) using cell-free fetal DNA from maternal plasma has been introduced. This less invasive type of prenatal testing has been reported to have a detection rate of >99% for trisomy 21 and trisomy 18. False positive rates for these screening tests have been reported and they should not be considered diagnostic. CVS or amniocentesis is required for confirmation (see Chapter 17).

- Evaluation of fetal well-being during pregnancy starts with the mother's "kick count." When <10 fetal movements are detected in 1 hour on two separate occasions, nonstress testing (NST) and ultrasonic assessment should be performed. When the amniotic fluid index (AFI), determined by ultrasonic measurement, is combined with fetal movements, an NST, and evaluation of fetal tone, the assessment is referred to as a biophysical profile. These techniques have largely replaced the contraction stress test for antenatal fetal assessment.

Pregnancy, to many women, is one of the greatest experiences of their lives. Even before conceiving, a woman may contemplate or ask whether her child will be normal at birth and whether pregnancy will be safe for her. Preconception and prenatal counseling by the well-informed health care professional can offer a sense of security to these women and deliver some of the most cost-effective preventive measures in all of health care. The purpose of this chapter is to provide the reader with a basic understanding of the appropriate evaluation and the optimal care that should be provided when a woman is thinking of trying to conceive, or has become pregnant.

Preconception Care

Ideally, "prenatal care" should begin before pregnancy. Organogenesis begins early in pregnancy and placental development starts with implantation, about 7 days after conception. **Poor placental development has been linked to preeclampsia, preterm birth, and intrauterine growth restriction (IUGR), all of which are associated with low birth weight (<2500 grams), and may play a role in fetal programming of chronic diseases later in life.** This is known as the **Barker hypothesis** (see Chapter 1). In addition, **obesity has become a world-wide problem** associated with metabolic dysregulation, and must be addressed before pregnancy if outcomes are to be improved.

By the time most pregnant women have their first prenatal visit, it is too late to address the risk of low birth weight and obesity, and to reduce the risk of some birth defects. The growing recognition of the importance of women's health before pregnancy has drawn increasing attention to the need for more effective and timely preconception care. **Several models of preconception care have been developed.** According to one model, the major components of preconception care include 12 risk assessments and 6 health promotions and these are summarized in Table 7-1. To cover each of the 18 components would require multiple visits to a health care provider, and this is often not acceptable to young women.

The major problem associated with the implementation of preconception care is a lack of consensus on the necessary components of the care. **For some, preconception care means a single prepregnancy check-up a few months before couples attempt to conceive.** A single visit, however, may be inadequate to address some problems such as smoking cessation or attaining and maintaining a healthy weight.

For others, preconception care should become an important part of comprehensive well-woman care, universally implemented from prepubescence to menopause. In practice, however, asking providers to squeeze more into their already hurried visits may not be practical, and some components (e.g., genetic screening or laboratory testing) may not be indicated for every woman. Absence of any preconception care will miss all of those pregnancies that are unintended at the time of conception (50% in the United States) but are continued despite a lack of planning.

In order to address these issues, *Before Pregnancy* is available electronically at StudentConsult.com and may be used to evaluate women who are planning a pregnancy. **This type of preconception care should be started, especially in high-risk women (e.g., women with obesity, diabetes, or hypertension), 6 months to 1 year before conception is attempted.** A more ambitious goal is for all women to participate, because not all "at risk" women will be identified by obvious existing comorbidities.

Prenatal Care

The three basic components of prenatal care are (1) early and continuing risk assessment, (2) health promotion, and (3) medical and psychosocial interventions and follow-up. Risk assessment includes a complete history, a physical examination, laboratory tests, and assessment of gestational age and well-being of the mother and her fetus(es). Health promotion consists of providing information on proposed care, enhancing general knowledge of pregnancy and parenting, and promoting and supporting healthful behaviors. Interventions include the management and treatment of any existing illness, provision of social and financial resources if required, and referral to and consultation with other specialized providers.

THE FIRST PRENATAL VISIT

The first prenatal visit provides an opportunity to review medical, reproductive, family, genetic, nutritional, and psychosocial histories. Women whose health may be seriously jeopardized by the pregnancy, such as those with Eisenmenger syndrome or a history of peripartum cardiomyopathy, should be counseled about the option of terminating the pregnancy. Reproductive histories that include preterm birth, low birth weight, preeclampsia, stillbirth, congenital anomalies, and gestational diabetes are important to record because of the substantial risk of recurrence. Women with prior cesarean delivery should be asked about the circumstances of the delivery, and discussion about options for the mode of delivery for the current pregnancy should be initiated. Additionally, **the importance of screening women for domestic violence cannot be overemphasized.** As many as 8-10% of pregnant women are physically abused during pregnancy, making domestic violence more common than preeclampsia, diabetes, IUGR, and preterm birth.

Standardized forms have been developed to facilitate overall prenatal risk assessment, and this technology has been incorporated into electronic health records at some institutions. **A complete physical examination should be performed including assessment of the patient's body mass index (BMI).** A woman's BMI can increase between pregnancies by 20-30% because of excessive weight gain in the first pregnancy. Clinicians should be familiar with physical findings associated with normal pregnancy, such as systolic murmurs, exaggerated splitting and S_3 during cardiac auscultation, or spider angiomata, palmar erythema, linea nigra, and striae gravidarum on

TABLE 7-1

ELEMENTS OF PRECONCEPTION COUNSELING AND CARE

Major Components of Preconception Care	Risk Assessment
Reproductive life plan	Ask your patient if she plans to have any (more) children, and how long she plans to wait until she (next) becomes pregnant. Help her develop a plan to achieve those goals.
Past reproductive history	Review prior adverse pregnancy outcomes, such as fetal loss, birth defects, low birthweight, and preterm birth, and assess ongoing biobehavioral risks that could lead to recurrence in a subsequent pregnancy.
Past medical history	Ask about past medical history, such as rheumatic heart disease, thromboembolism, or autoimmune diseases that could affect future pregnancy. Screen for ongoing chronic conditions such as hypertension and diabetes.
Medications	Review current medication use. Avoid category X drugs and most category D drugs unless potential maternal benefits outweigh fetal risks (see Box 7-3). Review use of over-the-counter medications, herbs and supplements.
Infections and immunizations	Screen for periodontal, urogenital, and sexually transmitted infections as indicated. Discuss TORCH (toxoplasmosis, other, rubella, cytomegalovirus, and herpes) infections and update immunization for hepatitis B, rubella, varicella, Tdap (combined tetanus, diphtheria and pertussis), human papillomavirus, and influenza vaccines as needed.
Genetic screening and family history	Assess risk of chromosomal or genetic disorders based on family history, ethnic background, and age. Offer cystic fibrosis screening. Discuss management of known genetic disorders (e.g., phenylketonuria, thrombophilia) before and during pregnancy.
Nutritional assessment	Assess anthropometric (body mass index), biochemical (e.g., anemia), clinical, and dietary risks.
Substance abuse	Ask about smoking, alcohol, drug use. Use T-ACE (tolerance, annoyed, cut down, eye opener) or CAGE (cut-down, annoyed, guilty, eye-opener) questions to screen for alcohol and substance abuse.
Toxins and teratogens	Review exposures at home, neighborhood, and work. Review Material Safety Data Sheet and consult local Teratogen Information Service as needed.
Psychosocial concerns	Screen for depression, anxiety, intimate-partner violence, and major psychosocial stressors.
Physical examination	Focus on periodontal, thyroid, heart, breasts, and pelvic examination.
Laboratory tests	Check complete blood count, urinalysis, blood type and antibody screen, rubella, syphilis, hepatitis B, HIV, cervical cytology; screen for gonorrhea, chlamydia, and diabetes in selected populations. Consider thyroid-stimulating hormone.

Major Components of Preconception Care	Health Promotion
Family planning	Promote family planning based on a woman's reproductive life plan. For women who are not planning on getting pregnant, promote effective contraceptive use and discuss emergency contraception.
Healthy weight and nutrition	Promote healthy prepregnancy weight through exercise and nutrition. Discuss macro- and micronutrients including 5-a-day and daily intake of multivitamin containing folic acid (see www.fns.usda.gov/5day).
Health behaviors	Promote such health behaviors as nutrition, exercise, safe sex, effective use of contraception, dental flossing, and use of preventive health services. Discourage risk behaviors such as douching, nonseatbelt use, smoking, alcohol and substance abuse.
Stress resilience	Promote healthy nutrition, exercise, sleep, and relaxation techniques; address ongoing stressors such as intimate partner violence; identify resources to help your patient develop problem-solving and conflict resolution skills, positive mental health, and relational resilience.
Healthy environments	Discuss household, neighborhood, and occupational exposures to metals, organic solvents, pesticides, endocrine disruptors, and allergens. Give practical tips such as how to reduce exposures during commuting or picking up dry cleaning.
Interconception care	Promote breastfeeding, back-to-sleep, positive parenting behaviors, and reduce ongoing biobehavioral risks.

inspection of the skin. During the breast examination, clinicians **should initiate discussion about breast-feeding.** A pelvic examination should be performed, and the appearance and length of the cervix and the status of the last **Papanicolaou (Pap) smear should be documented, or a new Pap smear obtained.**

Prenatal laboratory testing should be undertaken as outlined in Table 7-1 if not done during preconception care. Screening for, and treatment of asymptomatic bacteriuria significantly reduces the risk of pyelonephritis and preterm delivery.

Women who are Rh negative should receive Rh$_0$(D) immune globulin (Rh$_0$-GAM) at 28 weeks' gestation and postpartum, and at any point of care when sensitization may occur (e.g., threatened abortion or invasive procedures such as amniocentesis and chorionic villus sampling [CVS]). **Rubella vaccination is contraindicated during pregnancy,** and pregnant women who are found to be seronegative should be vaccinated immediately postpartum. **Testing for syphilis is mandated by law in virtually all states.** Early diagnosis and treatment of syphilis can reduce perinatal morbidity. Women who test negative for **hepatitis B surface antigen** and are at high risk for hepatitis B infection (e.g., health care workers) are candidates for vaccination before and during pregnancy. Infants born to women who test positive for hepatitis B surface antigen should receive both hepatitis B immune globulins (HBIG) and hepatitis B vaccine within 12 hours of birth, followed by two more injections of hepatitis B vaccine in the first 6 months of life. With the increasing incidence of whooping cough (pertussis) and serious complications in young children, secondary vaccination with Tdap (tetanus, diphtheria and acellular pertussis) vaccine should be given, ideally between 27 and 36 weeks of pregnancy.

Voluntary and confidential **human immunodeficiency virus (HIV) counseling and testing** should be offered and documented in the medical record. Diagnosis and treatment significantly reduce the risk of vertical transmission. Other tests such as screening for sexually transmitted infections (STIs) like **gonorrhea and chlamydia are generally considered routine.** All pregnant women at high risk for **tuberculosis** (TB) should be screened with a purified protein derivative (PPD) skin test when they begin prenatal care. For women who have received BCG (bacillus Calmette-Guérin) immunization (which can cause a positive test in the absence of TB), a blood test is available called the Interferon Gamma Release Assay (IGRA). A positive test implies that the person has been infected with TB bacteria. HIV and other perinatal (TORCH) infections are also discussed in Chapter 22.

Additionally, the clinician should use the first prenatal visit to confirm pregnancy and determine viability, estimate gestational age and due date, diagnose and deal with early pregnancy loss, provide genetic counseling and information about teratology, and provide advice on alleviating unpleasant symptoms during pregnancy. Information about nutrition, behavioral changes to expect, and the benefits of breastfeeding should be provided as prenatal care progresses. **Clinical pelvimetry should be performed sometime before labor begins** (see Chapter 8).

Confirming Pregnancy and Determining Viability

About 30-40% of all pregnant women will have some bleeding during early pregnancy (e.g., **implantation bleeding**), which may be mistaken for a period. Therefore, a pregnancy test should be performed in all women of reproductive age who present with abnormal vaginal bleeding.

The pregnancy test detects human chorionic gonadotropin (hCG) in the serum or the urine. The most widely used standard is the First International Reference Preparation (1st IRP). The hCG molecule is first detectable in serum 6 to 8 days after ovulation. A titer of less than 5 IU/L is considered negative, and a level above 25 IU/L is a positive result. Values between 6 and 24 IU/L are considered equivocal, and the test should be repeated in 2 days. A concentration of about 100 IU/L is reached about the date of expected menses. Most qualitative urine pregnancy tests can detect hCG above 25 IU/L.

It is important to differentiate a normal pregnancy from a nonviable or ectopic gestation. In the first 30 days of a normal gestation, the level of hCG doubles every 2.2 days. In patients whose pregnancies are destined to abort, the level of hCG rises more slowly, plateaus, or declines.

The use of transvaginal ultrasonography has improved the accuracy of predicting viability in early pregnancies. Using transvaginal ultrasonography, the gestational sac should be seen at 5 weeks' gestation or a mean hCG level of about 1500 IU/L (1st IRP). The fetal pole should be seen at 6 weeks or a mean hCG level of about 5200 IU/L. Fetal cardiac motion should be seen between 6 and 7 weeks or a mean hCG level of about 17,500 IU/L. **The presence of a gestational sac of 8 mm (mean sac diameter) without a demonstrable yolk sac, 16 mm without a demonstrable embryo, or the absence of fetal cardiac motion in an embryo with a crown-rump length of greater than 5 mm indicates probable embryonic demise.** When there is any doubt about these measurements, it is best to repeat the evaluation in 1 week before terminating the pregnancy. Using pulse wave Doppler of the heart to determine heart rate is not recommended.

INCIDENCE OF EARLY PREGNANCY LOSS

Because the incidence of conception is unknown, the incidence of spontaneous abortion (miscarriage) cannot be determined with certainty. **Spontaneous abortion occurs in 10-15% of clinically recognizable pregnancies.** The term *biochemical pregnancy* refers to the presence of hCG in the blood of a woman 7 to 10 days after ovulation but in whom menstruation occurs when expected. In other words, conception has occurred, but spontaneous loss of the gestation takes place without prolongation of the menstrual cycle. When both clinical and biochemical pregnancies are considered, evidence would suggest that **more than 50% of all conceptions are lost, the majority in the 14 days following conception.**

Real-time ultrasonography has been used extensively to monitor the intrauterine events of the first trimester of pregnancy. **If a live, appropriately growing fetus is present at 8 weeks' gestation, the fetal loss rate over the next 20 weeks (up to 28 weeks) is in the order of 3%.**

TYPES OF SPONTANEOUS ABORTION

The terms and definitions in the remainder of this chapter refer only to clinically recognizable pregnancies.

Threatened Abortion

The term *threatened abortion* **is used when a pregnancy is complicated by vaginal bleeding before the 20th week.** Pain may not be a prominent feature of threatened abortion, although a lower abdominal dull ache sometimes accompanies the bleeding. Vaginal examination at this stage usually reveals a closed cervix. Approximately one-third of pregnant women have some degree of vaginal bleeding during the first trimester, and **25-50% of threatened abortions eventually result in loss of the pregnancy.** Current research suggests that there is a continuum of risk between threatened abortion and preterm birth. Thus, the use of ultrasound to assess the location of the placenta and the length of the cervix may provide a baseline to help assess changes after 20 weeks, and may help formulate a plan of management to prevent early preterm birth (see Chapter 12).

Inevitable Abortion

In the case of inevitable abortion, **a clinical pregnancy is complicated by both vaginal bleeding and cramp-like lower abdominal pain.** The cervix is frequently partially dilated, contributing to the inevitability of the process.

Incomplete Abortion

In addition to vaginal bleeding, cramp-like pain, and cervical dilation, an incomplete abortion involves **the passage of some of the products of conception,** often described by the woman as looking like pieces of skin or liver.

Complete Abortion

In complete abortion, after **passage of all the products of conception,** the uterine contractions and bleeding abate, the cervix closes, and the uterus is smaller than the period of amenorrhea would suggest. Ultrasound can be used to assess the presence of retained placental tissue if excessive bleeding continues. In addition, the symptoms of pregnancy are no longer present, and the pregnancy test becomes negative.

Missed Abortion

The term *missed abortion* is used when **the fetus has died but is retained in the uterus,** usually for more than 6 weeks. Because **coagulation problems may develop,** fibrinogen levels should be checked weekly until the fetus and placenta are expelled (spontaneously) or removed surgically.

Recurrent Abortion

Three successive spontaneous abortions usually occur before a patient is considered to be a recurrent aborter. Many clinicians feel that two successive first-trimester losses or a single second-trimester spontaneous abortion is justification for an evaluation of a couple for the cause(s) of the pregnancy losses (see genetic evaluation section that follows).

ETIOLOGY OF RECURRENT ABORTION

Although many factors may result in the loss of a single pregnancy, relatively few factors are present consistently in couples who abort recurrently. Cause and effect relationships in individual patients are frequently difficult to determine.

General Maternal Factors

INFECTION. *Mycoplasma, Listeria,* or *Toxoplasma* **should be specifically sought** in women with recurrent abortions because despite being found infrequently, they are all treatable with antibiotics (see Chapter 22).

SMOKING AND ALCOHOL. Maternal smoking and alcohol consumption are associated with an increased incidence of chromosomally abnormal abortions. Women who smoke 20 or more cigarettes daily and consume more than seven standard alcoholic drinks per week have a fourfold increase in their risk of spontaneous abortion. There is a doubling of the risk of spontaneous abortion with as little as two drinks a week.

PSYCHOSOCIAL STRESS. Domestic violence and other forms of stress are associated with a greater risk of pregnancy complications such as spontaneous abortion, preterm birth, and low birth weight.

MEDICAL DISORDERS. Diabetes mellitus, hypothyroidism, and systemic lupus erythematosus (SLE) are associated with recurrent pregnancy loss. The evidence linking diabetes mellitus with spontaneous abortion is not conclusive, and severe hypothyroidism is more often associated with disordered ovulation than spontaneous abortion. **Up to 40% of clinical pregnancies are lost in women with SLE,** and such patients have an increased risk of pregnancy loss before developing the clinical stigmata of the disease (see Chapter 16).

MATERNAL AGE. If a live fetus is demonstrated by ultrasonography at 8 weeks' gestational age, fewer than 2% of these pregnancies will abort spontaneously when the mother is younger than 30 years of age. If, however, she is older than 40 years, the risk exceeds 10%, and it may be as high as 50% at age 45 years. The probable explanation is the increased incidence of chromosomally abnormal fetuses in older women.

Local Maternal Factors

Uterine abnormalities, including cervical incompetence, congenital abnormalities of the uterine fundus (as may result from gestational exposure to diethylstilbestrol) and acquired abnormalities of the uterine fundus, are known to be associated with pregnancy loss.

Cervical incompetence occurs under a number of circumstances but is usually the result of trauma. This occurs most frequently from mechanical dilation of the cervix at the time of termination of pregnancy, but it may also occur at the time of diagnostic curettage. **The diagnosis of cervical incompetence is usually made when a mid-trimester pregnancy is lost with a clinical picture of sudden unexpected rupture of the membranes, followed by painless expulsion of the products of conception.**

There continues to be controversy surrounding cervical incompetence, with some experts suggesting that cervical incompetence is, in most instances, a variant of preterm delivery, occurring at a time when there is an *associated finding* of asymptomatic ascending infection. The question today in terms of the etiology is what comes first. Is it infection that causes the problem or is it some form of metabolic dysregulation that can be identified early and treated to prevent these changes? Chapter 12 covers newer concepts of the cause(s) of early pregnancy loss and preterm birth.

When cervical incompetence is suspected during pregnancy (e.g., history of cervical incompetence in a previous pregnancy or of cone biopsy of the cervix), sequential ultrasonography of the cervix indicating funneling or shortness of the cervix or widening of the lower uterine segment may identify the problem before a pregnancy loss occurs.

A **congenitally abnormal uterus** may be associated with pregnancy loss in both the first and the second trimesters. Surgical correction of the abnormality, particularly with a history of second trimester loss, is frequently successful. Complete evaluation of the congenitally abnormal uterus usually requires laparoscopic, hysteroscopic, and hysterographic examination before any management plan can be made.

The most commonly acquired abnormalities of the uterus with the potential to affect fecundity are **submucous fibroids.** Although these tend to occur more frequently in women in their late 30s, they should be considered when investigating pregnancy loss in all women. Removal of submucous fibroids and intramural fibroids larger than 6 cm are associated with improved fecundity, especially when there is distortion of the endometrial cavity. Subserous fibroids do not appear to affect fecundity.

Intrauterine adhesions result from trauma to the basal layer of the endometrium from previous surgery or infection. When most of the uterine cavity has been obliterated (Asherman syndrome), amenorrhea results. More frequently, fewer intrauterine adhesions (synechiae) are present, menses are reasonably normal, and the lesions are not even suspected until a pregnancy is attempted and lost. Surgical correction of these intrauterine adhesions is recommended to improve fecundity.

Fetal Factors

The most common cause of spontaneous abortion is a significant genetic abnormality of the conceptus. In spontaneous first-trimester abortions, approximately two-thirds of fetuses have significant chromosomal anomalies, with approximately half of these being autosomal trisomies and the majority of the remainder being triploid, tetraploid, or 45,X monosomies. Fortunately, the majority of these are not inherited from either mother or father and are single nonrecurring events. **When seen on ultrasonography before spontaneous abortion, many such pregnancies appear to consist of an empty gestational sac.** When a fetus is present in many late first-trimester and early second-trimester abortions, it is often significantly abnormal, either genetically or morphologically. It seems that nature has a way of identifying some of its major mistakes and causing them to abort.

Placental Factors

The fetus and placenta interact in terms of genetic and neuroendocrine differences. For example, the placental genetic structure is composed of genes from the mother, the father, and even imprinted genes from the parents of both the mother and father. How these interact and support normal development and specific diseases is the subject of intense investigation. For example **the placenta expresses an enzyme 11β-hydroxylase that converts cortisol to inactive corticosterone, which protects the fetus from excessive cortisol when** the mother is stressed. This enzyme is not turned on until 22 to 24 weeks, thus leaving the fetus at risk from maternal stress before this gestational age. In addition, genetic polymorphisms have been identified that limit the amount of this enzyme produced, thus rendering the fetus at risk after 22 to 24 weeks.

Women with obesity during pregnancy have a greater risk of developing leptin (a placental peptide) resistance that leads to a greater risk of fetal IUGR, which in turn programs the fetus for obesity during childhood. Thus, it is important for the student to develop a sound understanding of the role of the placenta in fetal and maternal health.

Chromosomal Factors

Occasionally, fetal chromosomal abnormalities occur as a result of a chromosomal rearrangement (balanced translocation or inversion) in either or both parents. Therefore, karyotyping is important for evaluation of couples suffering from recurrent abortion.

Immunologic Factors

A successful pregnancy depends on a number of immunologic factors that allow the host (mother) to retain a genetically foreign product (fetus) without rejection taking place (see Chapter 6). The precise mechanism of this immunologic anomaly is not fully understood, but the immunologic functioning of some women as explained in more detail in Chapter 6, particularly those who abort recurrently or those who deliver prematurely, is different from that of women who carry pregnancies to term. Briefly the innate immune system is activated in early pregnancy with the production of specific cytokines that prevent early rejection of the fetus. Subsequently during the second half of pregnancy the adaptive portion of the immune system is activated to downregulate the innate immune system to support the developing fetus.

MANAGEMENT

Threatened Abortion

A threatened abortion is best managed by an ultrasonic examination to determine the viability of the fetus. Of those in whom a live fetus is present, 94% will produce a live baby, although the incidence of preterm delivery in these cases may be somewhat higher than in those who do not bleed in the first trimester. Once a live fetus has been demonstrated to the couple on ultrasonography, management consists essentially of reassurance; however they should be encouraged to undergo first-trimester screening for chromosomal abnormalities such as trisomy 13, 18, or 21. There is no need for admission to hospital, nor is there any evidence that bed rest improves the prognosis; however, psychosocial support is important. Recently, there has been evidence that women with vitamin D deficiency are at increased risk of spontaneous abortion, preterm birth

and stillbirth. The mechanism is thought to be related to abnormal uterine muscle function (see Chapter 11).

Incomplete Abortion

Until bleeding has stopped or is minimal, it is best to insert an intravenous line and take blood for grouping and cross-matching, as shock may occur from hemorrhage or sepsis. Once the patient's condition is stable, the remaining products of conception should be evacuated from the uterus using appropriate pain control. These tissues should be sent for pathologic evaluation. An incomplete abortion that is infected must be managed vigorously. Delay in treatment may result in overwhelming sepsis that may lead to excessive hemorrhage, renal and hepatic failure, disseminated intravascular coagulation (DIC), and rarely, death.

Missed Abortion

Suspected missed abortion should be confirmed by ultrasound to minimize the risk of sepsis and DIC, and to reduce the extent of hemorrhage and the degree of pain that accompanies the spontaneous expulsive process. In some studies vitamin D deficiency has been associated with early pregnancy loss. A proposed mechanism is that women with vitamin D deficiency have an altered immune system. Macrophages do not make the antibacterial peptide cathelicidin, which is important in reducing the risk of infection, as well as contributing to abnormal muscular function.

General Management Considerations

When the patient is Rh negative and does not have Rh (anti-D) antibodies, prophylactic Rh_o-GAM should be administered (see Chapter 15). All couples that have had a pregnancy loss should be seen and counseled some weeks after the event. At that time, questions that the couple may have can be answered, the findings of any pathologic studies discussed, and reassurance given about their chances of reproductive success in the future.

Recurrent Abortion

As far as the mother is concerned, it is appropriate to rule out the presence of systemic disorders such as diabetes mellitus, SLE, and thyroid disease, and it is also necessary to test for the presence of a lupus anticoagulant. Paternal and maternal chromosomes should be evaluated, and hysteroscopy or hysterography should be performed to evaluate the uterine cavity.

Over half of couples with recurrent losses will have normal findings during the standard evaluation. With the information now available on the role of vitamin D in the health of women, it is recommended that women also be assessed for vitamin D deficiency.

When a specific etiologic factor is found, appropriate management often leads to reproductive success.

Many of the **congenital abnormalities of the uterus** can now be diagnosed using pelvic ultrasonography and may no longer require laparotomy for repair. **Cervical incompetence** is managed by the placement of a cervical suture (cerclage) at the level of the internal os; this suture is best placed in the first trimester, once a live fetus has been demonstrated on ultrasonography. **The effectiveness of prophylactic cervical cerclage in preventing recurrent loss from cervical incompetence has not been conclusively established** (see Chapter 17).

Estimating Gestational Age and Date of Confinement

Gestational age should be determined during the first prenatal visit. Accurate determination of gestational age may become important later in pregnancy for the management of obstetric conditions such as preterm labor, IUGR, and postdate pregnancy. Clinical assessment to determine gestational age is usually appropriate for the woman with regular menstrual cycles and a known last menstrual period that was confirmed by an early examination. Estimated date of confinement (EDC) or "due date" may be determined by adding 9 months and 7 days to the first day of the last menstrual period.

Ultrasonography may also be used to estimate gestational age. Measurement of **fetal crown-rump length between 6 and 11 weeks' gestation** can define gestational age to within 7 days. At 12 to 20 weeks, gestational age can be determined within 10 days by the average of multiple measurements (e.g., biparietal diameter, femur length, abdominal and head circumferences). Thereafter, measurements become less reliable with advancing gestation (±3 weeks in the third trimester).

Patients Who Require Genetic Counseling

Ideally, couples should receive preconception counseling before they decide to have children, so that genetic disease in the couple or their families may be identified. Traditionally, the major reason couples have been referred for prenatal diagnosis is advanced maternal age. However, **current clinical guidelines recommend that genetic counseling and invasive prenatal diagnostic testing for chromosomal abnormalities be offered to all couples regardless of maternal age.** A woman's choice of whether to have a diagnostic test or a screening test is based on many factors, including the risk that the fetus will be affected with a chromosomal abnormality, the risk of miscarriage from an invasive procedure, and the perceived burden of having

BOX 7-1

INDICATIONS FOR GENETIC COUNSELING AND PRENATAL DIAGNOSIS OTHER THAN AGE

1. A previous child with or a family history of birth defects, chromosomal abnormality, or known genetic disorder
2. A previous child with undiagnosed mental retardation
3. A previous baby who died in the neonatal period
4. Multiple fetal losses
5. Abnormal serum marker screening results
6. Consanguinity
7. Maternal conditions predisposing the fetus to congenital abnormalities
8. A current pregnancy history of teratogenic exposure
9. A fetus with suspected abnormal ultrasonic findings
10. A parent who is a known carrier of a genetic disorder

an affected child. Women's concerns and preferences vary based on their personal beliefs. Therefore, the decision to offer prenatal screening and diagnosis should no longer be based on maternal age alone.

Additional indications for genetic counseling and prenatal diagnosis are listed in Box 7-1.

CONGENITAL AND HEREDITARY DISORDERS

Chromosomal Disorders

Chromosomal abnormalities occur in 0.5% of live births, but the incidence associated with spontaneous abortions is much higher and is estimated to be approximately 50%. The most common chromosomal abnormalities among live born infants are sex chromosomal aneuploidies (e.g., Turner syndrome [45,X], Klinefelter syndrome [47,XXY]), balanced Robertsonian translocations (translocations within group D or between groups D and G), and autosomal trisomies (e.g., Down syndrome; Figure 7-1).

Women older than 34 years are at increased risk of giving birth to children with autosomal trisomies (e.g., trisomy 21, 13, or 18) or sex chromosomal abnormalities (e.g., triple X syndrome, Klinefelter syndrome). The overall risk of Down syndrome (trisomy 21) is 1 per 800 live births. It increases to about 1 per 300 live births for women who are 35 to 39 years of age and to about 1 in 80 for those 40 to 45 years of age. The incidence of Down syndrome diagnosed at the time of CVS or amniocentesis is considerably higher. In women 35 to 39 years of age, the rate is about 1 in 125; in those 40 to 45, it is about 1 in 20. The discrepancy between the rate of occurrence at delivery and that at prenatal diagnosis is believed to be due in part to fetal loss in the second and third trimester.

Ninety-five percent of cases of Down syndrome are due to meiotic nondisjunctional events leading to 47 chromosomes with an extra copy of chromosome number 21, whereas 4% are due to an unbalanced translocation. Parents of a child with translocation

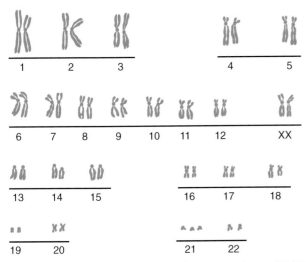

FIGURE 7-1 Karyotype of a patient with Down syndrome (47,XX + 21).

Down syndrome have rearrangements between chromosome 21 and chromosomes 14, 15, 21, or 22. The remaining 1% of individuals with Down syndrome have the mosaic type, which consists of two populations of cells, one with 46 and one with 47 chromosomes.

A couple who has previously had a child with trisomy 21 (Down syndrome) or with a meiotic nondisjunctional type of chromosomal abnormality is believed to be at a small but definite increased risk (about 1%) of giving birth to another child with a chromosomal abnormality and should be referred for prenatal diagnosis.

Approximately 1 in 500 individuals carries a balanced structural chromosomal rearrangement such as a translocation or inversion. Blood chromosomal studies should be performed on a couple after three or more spontaneous abortions because in approximately 3-5% of such couples, one member is a carrier of a balanced rearrangement. The recurrence risk for spontaneous abortions, abnormal offspring, or both is greatly increased among translocation carriers, and it can be estimated according to the type of translocation and which parent carries the translocation. For example, if the mother carries a balanced 14; 21 Robertsonian translocation, the risk for a child with an unbalanced translocation resulting in Down syndrome is 10-15%. However, if the father carries the translocation, the risk for an affected child is 2-3%. These couples should be alerted to the advisability of prenatal diagnosis because of their increased risk for having live born children with unbalanced translocations.

Using fluorescence in situ hybridization (FISH), a labeled chromosome-specific DNA segment or probe is hybridized to metaphase, prophase, or interphase chromosomes and visualized with fluorescent microscopy. FISH analysis has led to the identification of a number of genetic syndromes that could not previously be detected because the chromosomal deletion in these syndromes is beyond the resolution of banded chromosomal analysis. Syndromes that can be identified by FISH analysis include Prader-Willi, Angelman, DiGeorge, and Williams syndromes. Trisomies can also be identified in interphase cells with FISH probes.

Recently, microarray comparative genomic hybridization (microarray-CGH) has been introduced into clinical use. Microarray-CGH is a laboratory technique that quickly scans through the entire genome. With this technique, the patient's DNA and DNA from a normal control are labeled with fluorescent dyes and applied to a microarray chip with oligonucleotide probes. A microarray scanner then measures the fluorescent signals to detect a gain or loss of patient DNA. Microarray-CGH can detect all unbalanced chromosomal abnormalities, including trisomies that are visible with light microscopy, as well as minute chromosomal alterations (micro deletions and micro duplications), also known as copy number variants (CNV) as small as 200 kb. In comparison, deletions and duplications smaller than 5 mb are not visible under standard light microscopy used in karyotyping. It has been shown that 10-15% of children with normal karyotypes who have intellectual disability, autism spectrum disorder, behavioral disorders, or congenital anomalies also have a significant CNV. **In a recent blinded comparison between standard karyotyping and microarray-CGH in women undergoing prenatal diagnosis with CVS or amniocentesis, 1.7% of pregnancies with a normal karyotype and normal ultrasonic findings had a significant CNV.** In the future, microarray-CGH may replace standard karyotype in prenatal diagnostic testing.

Single Gene Disorders

Single gene disorders are relatively uncommon. They follow the laws of mendelian inheritance, and may be passed from generation to generation, as with autosomal dominant disorders, or affect siblings without any family history, as in autosomal recessive disorders. Males may be affected as a result of healthy females transmitting the abnormal gene, as in X-linked recessive disorders.

Autosomal Dominant Disorders

In autosomal dominant disorders, only one abnormal gene is necessary for disease manifestation. The affected individual has a 50% chance of passing the gene and the disorder on to offspring. The unaffected offspring cannot pass on the gene or the disorder. The occurrence and transmission of the genes are not influenced by gender. A spontaneous mutation of genetic material in the germ cells of clinically normal parents can also result in an affected offspring.

The hallmark of autosomal dominant disease is the variable expressivity. It is important to determine whether a child is affected by a spontaneous mutation or is the product of a parent with minimal expression of the same gene. A careful history and physical examination of family members, in addition to biochemical, radiologic, or histologic testing, may be necessary to determine the parents' genetic status.

Some of the common autosomal dominant disorders include tuberous sclerosis, neurofibromatosis, achondroplasia, craniofacial synostosis, adult-onset polycystic kidney disease, and several types of muscular dystrophy.

Autosomal Recessive Disorders

With autosomal recessive disorders, two affected genes must be present for manifestation of the disease. Usually there is no family history, but if a family history exists, siblings of either sex are equally likely to be affected. Consanguineous couples are at an increased risk for having a child who is homozygous for a deleterious recessive gene, with subsequent pregnancies being at 25% risk for producing a similarly affected child.

The majority of autosomal recessive disorders (e.g., Tay-Sachs disease, sickle cell disorders, alpha- and beta-thalassemia, cystic fibrosis, and spinomuscular atrophy, etc.) can be diagnosed prenatally by DNA analysis from amniocytes or chorionic villus cells.

GENETIC SCREENING FOR AUTOSOMAL RECESSIVE DISORDERS

Carrier screening programs for autosomal recessive disorders have traditionally focused on high-risk populations, in which the frequency of heterozygotes is greater than in the general population. Screening for Tay-Sachs disease among Eastern European Jewish and French Canadian populations has proved to be particularly successful in the recognition of couples at 25% risk for having offspring affected with this fatal disease. Table 7-2 lists selected autosomal recessive disorders for which genetic screening has been initiated.

The most common gene carried by North American whites is the cystic fibrosis (CF) gene (carrier frequency, 1/25). With the use of recombinant DNA

technology, the CF gene has been mapped to chromosome 7, and a gene deletion (AF508) has been found in approximately 70% of carriers. More than 1500 mutations have been identified in the CF gene. Genetic counseling is essential in offering CF carrier detection because 15% of carriers (and maybe more depending on ethnic group) remain undetected, and the limitations of the testing must be explained. At present, it is recommended that carrier detection for CF be offered to all pregnant women. Individuals with a family history of CF, partners of identified CF carriers, parents of a fetus with ultrasonic findings of an echogenic bowel, and those who donate sperm should be encouraged to undergo carrier testing.

Sex-Linked Disorders

Sex-linked disorders, caused by recessive genes located on the X chromosome, primarily affect males, whereas unaffected (or mildly affected) females carry the deleterious gene. There is no male-to-male transmission of X-linked disorders. Using gene mapping technology, many sex-linked disorders such as Duchenne muscular dystrophy (DMD) or fragile X syndrome can now be diagnosed by CVS or amniocentesis. X-linked disorders can occur because of new mutations of genetic material as a sporadic event, or from the inheritance of the X-linked recessive gene from the carrier mother.

Fragile X syndrome is an X-linked disorder that is the second most common cause of developmental delay after Down syndrome, and the most common form of inherited cognitive delay. It has an incidence of 1 per 1500 males and 1 per 2500 females. Mental impairment is variable in heterozygous females. The fragile X syndrome is caused by triplet repeat expansion in the long arm of the X chromosome. Using molecular genetic techniques, the number of triplet repeats can be measured in affected individuals to confirm a suspected diagnosis of fragile X or fragile X carrier status. In women who have a family history of developmental delay, genetic counseling is recommended for consideration of fragile X testing in the patient or family member.

Multifactorial Disorders

Many birth defects are inherited in a multifactorial fashion, which means that both genes and the environment play a role. Common multifactorial disorders include cleft lip or palate, neural tube defects (spina bifida or anencephaly), congenital heart defects, and pyloric stenosis.

Neural tube defects occur in about 1 per 1000 births in the United States. In Northern Ireland, Wales, and Scotland, the incidence of neural tube defects is 6 to 8 per 1000 births. Both anencephaly (congenital absence of the forebrain) and spina bifida (open spine)

TABLE 7-2

SELECTED AUTOSOMAL RECESSIVE DISEASES IN DEFINED ETHNIC GROUPS

Disease	Ethnic Group	Carrier Frequency
Sickle cell disease	Blacks	1/10
Cystic fibrosis	Whites	1/25
Tay-Sachs disease	Jews, French Canadians	1/30
Thalassemia	Mediterraneans, Southeast Asians	1/25

are believed to occur before 30 days' gestation because of failure of the neural tube to close. Newborns with anencephaly are stillborn or die within the first few days of life. Newborns with spina bifida have a variable course, depending on the site of the lesion and whether it is a meningocele (herniation of the meninges through an open spinal defect with cord remaining in its usual position) or a myelocele (herniation of the spinal cord). Folic acid has been shown to lower the risk of neural tube defects, and women who have had an infant with a neural tube defect should take vitamins plus **4 mg of folic acid daily before conception. Because neural tube closure is complete by 28 days post-conception, initiating folic acid after the first 28 days has no prophylactic value.**

With **multifactorial disorders in general and with neural tube defects in particular, a couple who has had one affected child has an increased risk of approximately 3% of having another similarly affected child.**

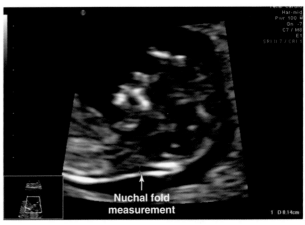

FIGURE 7-2 Ultrasonic image of fetal head at 12 weeks and 0 days showing a lucent area at the posterior aspect of the fetal neck that can be measured. Normal values for this measurement and the risk associated with abnormal measurements are based on gestational age as determined by crown-rump length.

Maternal Ultrasonic and Serum Marker Screening

There are multiple approaches available for maternal screening for fetal aneuploidy. Traditionally, second-trimester screening has been the standard approach. First-trimester aneuploidy screening was introduced in the late 1990s. **First- and second-trimester screening for aneuploidy using cell-free fetal DNA obtained from maternal plasma was introduced in 2012.**

FIRST-TRIMESTER SCREENING

A combination of maternal age, fetal nuchal translucency (NT) thickness and maternal serum-free β-human chorionic gonadotropin (β-hCG) and pregnancy-associated plasma protein-A (PAPP-A) are included in the first-trimester screen. Maternal age alone has only a 30% detection rate. In the early 1990s an association was reported between fetal chromosomal abnormalities and the finding of an abnormally increased nuchal translucency (an echo-free area at the back of the fetal neck) between 10 and 14 weeks' gestational age (Figure 7-2). Increased nuchal translucency has been associated with both chromosomal abnormalities and other congenital anomalies. **Elevated levels of free β-hCG and low levels of plasma protein-A are associated with an increased risk for Down syndrome.** A multicenter study in the United States reported that combining first-trimester maternal serum screening markers with nuchal translucency and maternal age showed a detection rate for Down syndrome of 79%, with a positive screening rate of 5%. Anatomic and radiographic studies have shown absence or hypoplasia of the nasal bones in fetuses with Down syndrome. **Visualization of the nasal bone on first-trimester ultrasound has been shown to**

reduce the risk for Down syndrome, whereas nonvisualization (absence) has been associated with an increased risk.** The addition of nasal bone assessment to nuchal lucency measurement and serum biochemistry can increase the Down syndrome detection rate to 93% with a screen positive rate of 5%.

SECOND-TRIMESTER SCREENING

Traditionally, a woman was offered the serum triple screening test that measures α-fetoprotein (AFP), hCG, and unconjugated estriol (UE3) at 16 to 20 weeks' gestation. Amniotic fluid AFP levels are frequently elevated in blood samples of women carrying fetuses affected with neural tube defects. Approximately 80-85% of all open neural tube defects can be detected by maternal serum AFP (MSAFP). In addition to open neural tube defects, ventral wall defects (gastroschisis or omphalocele) can cause elevations of MSAFP.

If the MSAFP level is elevated, an ultrasound should be done to rule out multiple gestation, fetal demise, or inaccurate gestational age (all of which can give false-positive results). **If none of these factors are present, amniocentesis is recommended to determine the amniotic fluid AFP level and to measure acetylcholinesterase** (AChE). Acetylcholinesterase is a protein that is present only if there is an open neural tube defect.

An association between low maternal serum AFP and Down syndrome has been noted. The combination of low MSAFP, elevated hCG, and low UE3 levels (triple screen) has a detection rate for Down syndrome of approximately 70%, with a positive screen result in approximately 5% of all pregnancies. Low MSAFP, low hCG, and low UE3 levels can also be used to screen for trisomy 18. With the addition of inhibin-A (increased with Down syndrome), the quadruple screen increases the Down syndrome detection rate to 81% with a positive screen result in 5% of pregnancies.

COMBINED FIRST- AND SECOND-TRIMESTER SCREENING

In an attempt to improve the detection rate and minimize the screen positive rate and the number of invasive procedures, a few studies have been conducted to evaluate the concept of combining first- and second-trimester screening. **The approaches that have been proposed include integrated screening and sequential screening.**

INTEGRATED SCREENING. With integrated screening, the first- and second-trimester results are combined into a single risk calculation, and are not reported until after the second-trimester results are available. This approach has been found to have the highest sensitivity and to be the most cost effective.

SEQUENTIAL SCREENING. This involves performance of both first- and second-trimester screening, with disclosure of the first-trimester results for clinical management.

It is not uncommon for one or more of the biomarkers to be abnormal in the presence of a chromosomally normal fetus. An elevated level of β-hCG or AFP and low levels of PAPP-A or estriol (UE3) are associated with complications of pregnancy such as preterm birth, IUGR, and preeclampsia. Thus, these pregnancies require close follow up.

Noninvasive prenatal testing (NIPT) using cell-free fetal DNA from maternal plasma: The quest to develop an early definitive prenatal diagnostic test that is noninvasive has been ongoing for more than 40 years. Initial efforts for noninvasive prenatal diagnosis were directed at isolation of intact fetal cells from maternal blood, which can be achieved as early as 10 weeks' gestational age. However, very few fetal cells are present (1 fetal cell per 10^5 to 10^7 maternal cells), and in most studies, the fetal cell yield has been inconsistent. Although basic work has demonstrated the biologic availability of fetal cells for prenatal diagnosis, a practical technology for consistent recovery and assay has not yet been developed.

The presence of cell-free fetal DNA (ffDNA) in maternal plasma was first reported in 1997. The source of ffDNA is from apoptosis of trophoblast cells that have entered the maternal circulation. **Detection of ffDNA in maternal plasma can be done as early as 9 to 10 weeks.** It comprises 3-10% of total maternal plasma DNA at the end of the first trimester. A variety of methods are available for detection of fetal trisomy with ffDNA. **Detection rates of 99.4%, 99.1%, and 91.7% have been reported for trisomy 21, trisomy 18, and trisomy 13, respectively. Detection rates of 96.2% have been reported for sex chromosome abnormali-** ties (45,X; 47,XXX; 47,XXY; 47,XYY). There are many other cytogenetic abnormalities that may be present in addition to those abnormalities that can be detected with NIPT. **False positive rates for NIPT have been reported** to be as high as 7% for trisomy 21, 36% for trisomy 18, 56% for trisomy 13, and 60% for the sex chromosomal abnormalities. **Thus, a positive NIPT result must be confirmed by a diagnostic test (amniocentesis or CVS).** Diagnostic tests provide a full karyotype analysis. A karyotype is a genome-wide test that evaluates all 23 pairs of chromosomes for size, shape, and banding patterns, to detect numerical and structural chromosomal abnormalities. The karyotype detects a much broader spectrum of chromosomal abnormalities than a specific test for trisomy 21, 18, or 13. Although diagnostic tests are associated with a risk for pregnancy loss, this risk is quite low in the hands of experienced operators.

In summary, NIPT screening can be offered to women who are at risk for fetal aneuploidy. However, it should only be offered to the patient after pretest counseling that includes a discussion of the advantages and disadvantages of screening and diagnostic tests. In addition, a family history should be obtained to determine if the patient needs a prenatal diagnostic test for an inherited genetic disorder.

Genetic counseling is an essential component of screening programs. It provides education and alleviates anxiety in patients with abnormal test results. Patients must be informed of the differences between screening results and diagnostic testing.

Diagnostic Procedures

Recombinant DNA technology coupled with first-trimester fetal tissue sampling has enhanced the growth and development of prenatal diagnosis. Obstetric procedures, such as ultrasonography, amniocentesis, CVS, and cordocentesis (percutaneous umbilical blood sampling [PUBS]) are currently used during prenatal diagnosis. These procedures are described and discussed in Chapter 17.

Teratology

A teratogen is any agent or factor that can cause abnormalities of form or function (birth defects) in an exposed fetus. Such abnormalities include fetal wastage and IUGR, malformations due to abnormal growth and morphogenesis, fetal and placental endocrine disruption, and abnormal central nervous system performance.

It was not until the teratogenic effects of rubella infection were demonstrated in 1941 that any notable consideration was given to environmental factors and their potentially deleterious effects on human pregnancy. In the succeeding decades, the susceptibility of the fetus to many environmental factors has been appreciated.

Probably the best known teratogen is thalidomide, which has been shown to cause phocomelia and other malformations in the offspring of mothers who had been given the drug during pregnancy. It is the only example of a teratogen that, when introduced to the pregnant population, led to a dramatic epidemic of a specific malformation; withdrawal of the drug led to a virtual disappearance of the malformation.

Although drugs are the most obvious source for teratogenic exposure, chemical waste disposal, alcohol, tobacco, cosmetics, and occupational agents contain substances that individuals are exposed to, such as fertilizers and insecticides. Some of these agents are known teratogens, whereas the fetal effects of others are not known.

EXPOSURE

Results of the Collaborative Perinatal Project indicate that more than 900 different drugs are taken by pregnant women in the United States and that 40% of women take medication during the first trimester, when organogenesis is occurring. During the first trimester alone, as many as 32% of pregnant women are exposed to analgesics (mostly aspirin), 18% to immunizing agents, 16% to antimicrobial and antiparasitic agents, and 6% to sedatives, tranquilizers, and antidepressants.

PRINCIPLES OF TERATOLOGY
Fetal Susceptibility

The efficacy of a particular teratogen is, in part, dependent on the genetic makeup of both mother and fetus, as well as on a number of factors related to the maternal-fetal environment. For instance, many congenital abnormalities, such as oral clefts, congenital heart disease, and neural tube defects, are inherited through multifactorial inheritance.

Dose

Depending on the particular teratogen, there may be (1) no apparent effect at a low dose, (2) an organ-specific malformation at an intermediate dose, or (3) a spontaneous abortion at a high dose. Additionally, smaller doses administered over several days may produce a different effect from a single large dose.

Timing

Three stages of teratogenic susceptibility may be identified on the basis of gestational age. Before implantation (1 week postovulation in humans), there is no demonstrable teratogenic insult. The most vulnerable stage is between day 17 to day 56 postconception or from approximately 4 weeks to 10 weeks by gestational age, during the period of organogenesis. **The timing determines which organ system or**

systems are affected. Unfortunately, most women do not realize they are pregnant until this critical period of development is well under way. From about the fourth month of pregnancy to the end of gestation, embryonic development consists primarily of increasing organ size. With the exception of a limited number of tissues (brain and gonads), teratogenic exposure after the fourth month usually causes decreased growth without malformation. Very little attention has been directed toward the role of a combination of factors such as a deficiency in folic acid along with the presence of a drug or chemical substance.

Nature of Teratogenic Agents

Although few agents are known to cause serious malformations in a large proportion of exposed individuals, **there are probably hundreds of potentially teratogenic agents, given the right set of circumstances** (susceptible fetus, embryologically vulnerable period, large teratogenic dose). Furthermore, certain drugs combined with other drugs may be capable of producing malformations, although neither agent would be teratogenic when taken alone.

TERATOGENIC AGENTS

Teratogens may be assigned to three broad categories: (1) drugs and chemical agents, (2) infectious agents, and (3) radiation. The list that follows is far from exhaustive.

Alcohol

The adverse effects of ethyl alcohol on fetal development were not fully realized until the 1970s. The frequency of the fetal alcohol syndrome runs as high as 0.2%, whereas an additional 0.4% of newborns show less severe features of the disorder (Box 7-2).

Antianxiety Agents

Antianxiety agents are currently used by a significant number of pregnant women. Data regarding their teratogenicity are conflicting, although **exposure to meprobamate or chlordiazepoxide has been associated with a greater than fourfold increase in severe congenital anomalies.** Fluoxetine is now the drug of choice for anxiety and depression during pregnancy and is considered safe to continue even in women who breastfeed. The risk of recurrence of significant depression during pregnancy is too great to routinely discontinue treatment during pregnancy. The recent data suggesting that there is an association between vitamin D deficiency and the risk of postpartum depression suggests that supplementation with vitamin D3 during pregnancy may reduce the use of antianxiety agents.

Antineoplastic Agents

Aminopterin and methotrexate, both of which are folic acid antagonists, have been clearly established

BOX 7-2

CLINICAL FEATURES OF FETAL ALCOHOL SYNDROME

Craniofacial

Eyes: Short palpebral fissures, ptosis, strabismus, epicanthic folds, myopia, microphthalmia
Ears: Poorly formed concha, posterior rotation
Nose: Short, hypoplastic philtrum
Mouth: Prominent lateral palatine ridges, micrognathia, cleft lip or palate, faulty enamel
Maxilla: Hypoplastic

Cardiac

Murmurs, atrial septal defect, ventricular septal defect, tetralogy of Fallot

Central Nervous System

Mild-to-moderate mental retardation, microcephaly, poor coordination, hypotonia

Growth

Prenatal-onset growth deficiency

Muscular

Hernias of diaphragm, umbilicus, or groin

Skeletal

Pectus excavatum, abnormal palmar creases, nail hypoplasia, scoliosis

BOX 7-3

ETIOLOGIC FACTORS THAT MAY PLAY A ROLE IN ANTICONVULSANT TERATOGENICITY

Antiepileptic Drugs

Dose, serum levels, metabolism, teratogenicity, metabolic interactions

Genetic Predisposition

Maternal, paternal, and fetal metabolism

Maternal Disease

Teratogenicity, underlying disease, seizures

---

as teratogens. Exposure before 40 days' gestation is lethal to the embryo; later exposure during the first trimester produces fetal effects, including IUGR, craniofacial anomalies, abnormal positioning of extremities, mental retardation, early miscarriage, stillbirth, and neonatal death.

Alkylating agents, including busulfan, chlorambucil, cyclophosphamide, and nitrogen mustard, **have been associated with fetal anomalies** such as severe IUGR, fetal death, cleft palate, microphthalmia, limb reduction anomalies, and poorly developed external genitalia. **During the first trimester, the teratogenic risks may be as high as 30%.**

Anticoagulants

COUMARIN DERIVATIVES. Use of warfarin (Coumadin) during the first trimester is associated with an increased risk of spontaneous abortion, IUGR, central nervous system defects (including mental retardation), stillbirth, and a characteristic syndrome of craniofacial features known as the fetal warfarin syndrome. Embryologically, the most vulnerable time appears to be between 6 and 9 weeks after conception. Warfarin easily crosses the placenta, causing bleeding problems in the fetus, and is excreted in breast milk.

HEPARIN. Heparin has major advantages over Coumadin anticoagulants during pregnancy because it does not cross the placenta. Reported risks include prematurity and fetal demise. Because no specific malforma-

tion syndrome has been described, these abnormalities may be more closely related to the maternal disease necessitating the heparin use.

Anticonvulsants

Approximately 1 in 200 pregnant women is epileptic. Box 7-3 lists the etiologic factors that may play a role in the congenital abnormalities associated with in utero exposure to anticonvulsants. The complexity in providing genetic counseling for pregnant epileptic women is underscored when considering the interactive effects of combined anticonvulsant treatment, the genetic aspects of the disease itself, and the mother's epilepsy. The goals of counseling include providing the patient with the teratogenic risks of her medication, the risk of seizures during pregnancy, and the effect of pregnancy on seizures. From a medication standpoint, the benefits of seizure prevention need to be weighed against the teratogenicity of the drug.

DIPHENYLHYDANTOIN (DILANTIN). A specific syndrome, known as the fetal hydantoin syndrome, has been described, the clinical features of which include craniofacial abnormalities, limb reduction defects, prenatal-onset growth restriction, mental deficiency, and cardiovascular anomalies. Approximately 10% of exposed fetuses demonstrate fetal hydantoin syndrome, whereas an additional 30% may have isolated features of the syndrome.

OXAZOLIDINEDIONE ANTICONVULSANTS. Trimethadione (Tridione) and paramethadione (Paradione), used to treat petit mal epilepsy, have been associated with a characteristic malformation syndrome in exposed fetuses. The clinical features include craniofacial abnormalities, prenatal-onset growth restriction, an increased frequency of mental retardation, and cardiovascular abnormalities. Because of this serious teratogenic potential and because petit mal epilepsy is rare during reproductive years, **oxazolidinedione anticonvulsants are contraindicated during pregnancy.**

VALPROIC ACID. Valproic acid use during pregnancy is associated with a 1-2% risk of open spina bifida.

Other findings reported to be associated with valproic acid exposure include cardiac defects, skeletal defects, and craniofacial malformations.

CARBAMAZEPINE. As with valproic acid, carbamazepine (Tegretol) exposure during pregnancy is associated with an increased risk for fetal spina bifida and is an indication for amniotic fluid AFP analysis. Some studies have reported a specific malformation pattern that includes minor **craniofacial** defects, fingernail hypoplasia, and developmental delay, which are features that would be unlikely to be detected prenatally.

PHENOBARBITAL. The true teratogenicity of phenobarbital is difficult to assess because other drugs are usually taken in combination with this agent, but the risk appears to be very low. **Potential complications of phenobarbital include neonatal withdrawal symptoms and neonatal hemorrhage.**

Hormones

ESTROGEN/PROGESTIN COMBINATIONS. A large number of pregnant women are exposed to progestins or progestin/estrogen combinations because they continue taking birth control pills, unaware that they are pregnant. Recent analyses have failed to confirm any teratogenicity, and the United States Federal Drug Administration (FDA) has removed the product insert warnings. **The main abnormality associated with the use of strongly androgenic progestins during pregnancy is masculinization of the external genitalia in female fetuses, with a risk of up to 2%.**

Miscellaneous Agents

RETINOIDS. Isotretinoin (Accutane) is prescribed for cystic acne or for acne that has not responded to other forms of treatment. **Exposure during pregnancy is clearly associated with a specific malformation pattern that includes central nervous system, cardiovascular, and craniofacial defects (especially ear abnormalities).** The central nervous system findings include hydrocephaly, facial nerve palsies, and cortical blindness. Microcephaly, with severe ear anomalies, microtia, and cleft palate are common findings. **The risk of spontaneous abortion or congenital malformations is greater than 50% in patients who take isotretinoin throughout the first trimester.**

Etretinate, used for severe psoriasis, has been similarly associated with a characteristic malformation pattern. However, unlike isotretinoin, which has a half-life of less than 1 day, etretinate has a half-life of months, leading to a longer risk period even after the agent has been discontinued.

TOBACCO SMOKING. Maternal tobacco smoking interferes with prenatal growth, including birth weight, birth length, and head circumference. The teratogenic effects are related to the extent of maternal exposure to tobacco and include an increased risk for spontaneous abortion, fetal death, neonatal death, and prematurity. Pregnant women should be strongly encouraged to avoid smoking (or second-hand smoke). They should continue to abstain after delivery because second-hand smoke exposure is associated with an increased risk of respiratory diseases in infants and children.

ILLICIT DRUGS. Prenatal cocaine exposure, particularly among chronic abusers, has been associated with fetal malformations, particularly genitourinary tract anomalies, and behavioral abnormalities have also been documented in such fetuses.

INFECTIOUS AGENTS. The exact frequency of significant infection during pregnancy is not known, but it is probably between 15% and 25%. **Viruses, bacteria, and parasites may have serious effects on the fetus, including fetal death, growth delay, congenital malformations, and mental deficiency.** In more recent years, the AIDS epidemic has had a significant impact on pregnancy management. With the now known association between vitamin D deficiency and risk of infections, vitamin D deficiency should be considered as an associated factor in the risk of malformations.

RADIATION. Prenatal ionizing radiation exposure occurs frequently as a result of therapeutic or diagnostic medical and dental procedures. **The medical effects of ionizing radiation are dose-dependent and include teratogenesis, mutagenesis, and carcinogenesis.** The most critical period appears to be from about 2 to 6 weeks after conception. Exposures before 2 weeks will either produce a lethal effect or produce no effect at all. Teratogenicity is still a possibility after 5 weeks, but the risk for deleterious consequences is relatively small. **Diagnostic levels of radiation do not produce a teratogenic risk in the developing fetus.**

Advice during Pregnancy

One of the most important functions of prenatal care is to provide information and support to the woman for self-care. The Cochrane pregnancy and childbirth database (www.cochrane.org) has compiled systematic reviews on the effectiveness of advice and interventions during pregnancy and can be a useful source of information for prenatal care providers. The following sections will examine advice given on alleviating unpleasant symptoms, nutrition, lifestyle, and breastfeeding.

ALLEVIATING UNPLEASANT SYMPTOMS

Nausea and vomiting complicate up to 70% of pregnancies. Eating small, frequent meals, and avoiding greasy or spicy foods may help. Also, having protein snacks at night, saltine crackers at the bedside, and room-temperature sodas are nonpharmacologic approaches that may provide some relief. **Where medication is deemed necessary, antihistamines appear to be the drug of choice,** though no single product has been satisfactorily tested for efficacy and safety. **Vitamin B6 (pyridoxine) and accupressure ("sea sickness arm bands") may be effective.** Patients with dehydration and electrolyte abnormalities from vomiting (hyperemesis gravidarum) should be evaluated for possible secondary causes, and they may need hospitalization for rehydration and antiemetic therapy.

Heartburn affects about two-thirds of women at some stage of pregnancy, resulting from progesterone-induced relaxation of the esophageal sphincter. Avoiding lying down immediately after meals and elevating the head of the bed may help reduce heartburn. When these simple measures fail, antacids, such as calcium carbonate, should be used.

Constipation is a troublesome problem for many women in pregnancy, secondary to decreased colonic motility. Dietary modification, including increased fiber and water intake, can help lessen this problem. Stool softeners may be used in combination with bulking agents. Irritant laxatives should be reserved for short-term use in refractory cases.

Hemorrhoids are caused by increased venous pressure in the rectum. Increased rest, with elevation of the legs, and avoidance of constipation are recommended.

Leg cramps are experienced by almost half of all pregnant women, particularly at night and in the later months of pregnancy. Massage and stretching may afford some relief during an attack. Both calcium and sodium chloride supplementation appear to help reduce leg cramps in pregnancy. Recently, vitamin D deficiency in both men and women has been associated with leg cramps and muscle pain. Because recent evidence suggests at least 40% of women during pregnancy are vitamin D deficient, vitamin D supplementation at 1000 to 2000 IU/day is recommended. Daily requirements are 400 to 600 IU/day, which is the amount of vitamin D in prenatal vitamins, so prenatal vitamins will not correct the deficiency.

Backaches are common during pregnancy and are lessened by avoiding excessive weight gain. Additionally, exercise, sensible shoes, and specially shaped pillows can offer relief. In cases of muscle spasm or strain, analgesics (such as acetaminophen), rest, and heat may lessen the symptoms.

NUTRITIONAL COUNSELING

While the nutritional care plan should be individualized, every woman can benefit from nutritional education that includes counseling on weight gain, dietary guidelines, physical activity, avoidance of harmful substances and unsafe foods, and the importance of breastfeeding.

TABLE 7-3

APPROPRIATE WEIGHT GAIN IN PREGNANCY		
	BMI	Recommended Weight Gain (lb)
Underweight	<19	28-40
Normal	19-25	25-35
Overweight	25-29.5	15-25
Obese	≥30.0	11-20

Institute of Medicine of the National Academies of Science: Weight gain during pregnancy: reexamining the guidelines, May 28, 2009. Available at www.iom.nationalacademies.com/weightgainduringpregnancy.
BMI, Body mass index.

The appropriate weight gain range (based on prepregnancy BMI) during the second and third trimesters of pregnancy is listed in Table 7-3.

Inadequate weight gain has been associated with low birth weight. Women should avoid fasting (>13 hours without food) or skipping meals. This behavior is associated with accelerated ketosis and a greater risk of preterm delivery. They should eat five times per day (breakfast, lunch, afternoon snack, dinner, and bedtime snack). Pregnant women should never skip breakfast. **Excessive weight gain has been associated with fetal macrosomia.** Maternal obesity may occur over time between pregnancies because of the difficulty that some women have returning to prepregnancy body weight. This is especially true when a woman chooses not to breastfeed her infant.

Although weight gain is an important consideration during pregnancy, **the clinician should emphasize the "right amount of nutrition" over the "right amount of weight gain."** Normal pregnancy requires an increase in daily caloric intake of 300 kcal.

LIFESTYLE ADVICE

Women should be advised to rest when tired and reassured that the fatigue usually abates by the fourth month of pregnancy. Normal prepregnancy activity levels are usually acceptable. Advice regarding work should be individualized to the nature of the work, the health status of the woman, and the condition of the pregnancy. Work that requires prolonged standing, shift or night work, and high cumulative occupational fatigue has been associated with an increased risk for low birth weight and prematurity. **Where working conditions involve occupational fatigue or stress, a change in work conditions during pregnancy should be recommended.**

The increase in the use of mobile devices has allowed women to network and access mobile applications **(APPs)** which can provide information about pregnancy. In addition, **establishing a network of friends** before pregnancy allows women to share information about pregnancy, and provide psychosocial support to reduce pregnancy-specific stress.

Women should be advised to continue to exercise during pregnancy, unless there is hypertension, preterm labor, rupture of the membranes, IUGR, an incompetent cervix, persistent second- or third-trimester bleeding, or medical conditions that severely restrict physiologic adaptations to exercise during pregnancy. They should avoid exercising in the supine position after the first trimester, and should modify the intensity of their exercise according to maternal symptoms. **Any type of exercise involving the potential for loss of balance or even mild abdominal trauma should be avoided.**

Travel is acceptable under most circumstances. Prolonged sitting increases the risk of thrombus formation and thromboembolism. Pregnant women should be encouraged to ambulate periodically when taking a long flight or car ride. Support stockings may help reduce lower limb edema and varicose veins. International travel that places the patient at a high risk of exposure to infectious disease should be avoided, whenever possible. When such travel cannot be avoided, appropriate vaccinations should be administered. Specific recommendations are available at www.cdc.gov; select "Traveler's Health." Live attenuated virus vaccinations are generally contraindicated in pregnancy, but inactivated virus vaccines may be acceptable.

Increased, unchanged, and decreased levels of sexual activity can all be normal during pregnancy. Abstinence or condom use may be advisable if there is an increased risk of preterm labor or repeated pregnancy loss, or in women with a history of persistent second- or third-trimester bleeding.

BREASTFEEDING

Breastfeeding has been shown to significantly reduce morbidity and improve cognitive development during infancy and childhood. Providers should initiate discussion with the pregnant woman and her family regarding breastfeeding during the first visit, including possible barriers to breastfeeding, such as previous poor experiences, misinformation, or nonsupportive work environment. Clinicians should emphasize that weight gain during pregnancy is to support fetal growth and for development of a nutritional reserve to support effective breastfeeding. **Breastfeeding for at least 6 months will facilitate complete loss of the required weight gain during pregnancy.** This behavior reduces the risk of postpartum weight retention and the risk of developing obesity. Partners, peers, family members and friends/support groups may also exert an important influence on a woman's decision to breastfeed. Referral to a childbirth preparation class or a lactation consultant may provide additional encouragement to initiate and support breastfeeding.

FOLLOW-UP VISITS

Prenatal visits should be scheduled every 4 weeks until 28 weeks' gestation, every 2 to 3 weeks until 36 weeks, and then weekly until delivery. The schedule of these follow-up visits, however, should be tailored to the needs of individual patients. Women should be screened for depression early in pregnancy, during the third trimester and again postpartum. A simple self-administered 10 question screening tool, the **"Edinburgh Postnatal Depression Scale"** (EPDS), is available at www.fresno.ucsf.edu/pediatrics/downloads/edinburghscale.pdf. **The incidence of depression during pregnancy and the postpartum period is as high as 20%. Multiple studies have shown a significant relationship between vitamin D deficiency and depression.**

During each regularly scheduled visit, the clinician should evaluate blood pressure, weight, urine protein and glucose, uterine size for progressive growth, and fetal heart rate. After the woman reports quickening (first sensation of fetal movement, on average at 20 weeks' gestation) and at each subsequent visit, she should be asked about fetal movement. Between 24 and 34 weeks, women should be taught the warning symptoms of preterm labor (uterine contractions, leakage of fluid, vaginal bleeding, low pelvic pressure, or low back pain). Patients at risk may require additional visits to assess signs and symptoms of preterm labor. Beginning in the late second trimester, they should also be taught to recognize the warning symptoms of preeclampsia (frontal headache, visual changes, hand or facial swelling, epigastric or right upper quadrant pain). Near term, they should be instructed on the symptoms of labor.

Beginning at 28 weeks, systematic examination of the abdomen should be carried out at each prenatal visit to identify the lie (e.g., longitudinal, transverse, oblique), presentation (e.g., vertex, breech, shoulder), and position (e.g., flexion, extension, or rotation of the occiput) of the fetus. This can be accomplished by the maneuvers of Leopold. The **first maneuver** involves palpating the fundus to determine which part of the fetus occupies the fundus. The head is round and hard, whereas the breech is irregular and soft. The **second maneuver** involves palpating either side of the abdomen to determine on which side the fetal back lies. The fetal back is linear and firm, whereas the extremities have multiple parts. The **third maneuver** involves grasping the presenting part between the thumb and third finger just above the pubic symphysis to determine the presenting part. The **fourth maneuver** involves palpating for the brow and the occiput of the fetus to determine fetal head position when the fetus is in a vertex presentation. This is best accomplished with the examiner facing the patient's feet and placing both hands on either side of the lower abdomen just above the inlet. By exerting pressure in the direction of the pelvic inlet, the hand running along the back will bump into the occiput if the head is extended, whereas the hand on the same side of the small parts will bump into the brow if the head is flexed. **If there is a question about the presentation of the fetus a real time ultrasound may be performed.**

Depending on the practice setting and population, either universal or selective **screening for gestational diabetes should be performed between 24 and 28 weeks' gestation. Risk factors for selective screening include family history of diabetes; previous birth of a macrosomic, malformed, or stillborn baby; hypertension; glycosuria; maternal age of 30 years or older; or previous gestational diabetes.** Repeat measurements of hemoglobin or hematocrit levels early in the third trimester have been recommended. Tests for sexually transmitted infections (e.g., syphilis) may also be repeated at 32 to 36 weeks if the woman has specific risk factors for these diseases. The Centers for Disease Control and Prevention recommend **universal screening for maternal colonization of group B streptococcus at 35 to 37 weeks' gestation.** The value of selective ultrasound for specific indications has been clearly established; the value of routine ultrasound in low-risk pregnancies remains undetermined. Ultrasonic examination during pregnancy is not harmful, but **controlled trials have failed to demonstrate that routine ultrasonic examinations for dating in early pregnancy, anatomic survey in mid-pregnancy, or assessment of fetal growth in late pregnancy improve perinatal outcome.**

Assessment of Fetal Well-Being

During the past 20 years, electronic monitoring advances have made the fetus more accessible. They have allowed visualization of the fetus and recording of intrauterine fetal activity. **A combination of maternal self-assessment, nonstress testing (NST), and real-time ultrasonic assessment is used to evaluate fetal well-being.**

MATERNAL SELF-ASSESSMENT OF FETAL WELL-BEING

A simple technique (kick counting) may be used to assess fetal well-being. The mother assesses fetal movement (kick counts) each evening while lying on her left side. She should recognize 10 movements in 1 hour and if she does not, she should retest in 1 hour. If she still does not have 10 fetal movements in 1 hour, she should contact her doctor or present herself (usually to the hospital) for an NST and an ultrasonic assessment.

NONSTRESS TEST ASSESSMENT

The first step in the assessment of fetal well-being is the NST. With the mother resting in the left lateral supine position, a continuous fetal heart rate tracing is obtained using external Doppler equipment. The mother reports each fetal movement, and the effects of the fetal movements on heart rate are determined. **A normal fetus responds to fetal movement with acceleration in fetal heart rate of 15 beats or more per minute above the baseline for at least 15 seconds** (Figure 7-3). If at least two such accelerations occur in a 20-minute interval, the fetus is regarded as being healthy, and the test is said to be reactive. A nonreactive NST is shown in Figure 7-4.

ULTRASONIC ASSESSMENT

The next step in prenatal assessment is to determine the adequacy of amniotic fluid volume by real-time ultrasonography. Reduced fluid (oligohydramnios) suggests fetal compromise. Oligohydramnios can be defined as an amniotic fluid index (AFI) of less than 5 cm. The AFI represents the sum of the linear measurements (in centimeters) of the largest amniotic fluid pockets noted on ultrasonic inspection of each of the four quadrants of the gestational sac. **When amniotic fluid is reduced, the fetus is more likely to become compromised as a result of umbilical cord compression.** Excessive amniotic fluid (polyhydramnios; AFI > 23 cm) can be a sign of poor control in a diabetic pregnancy or an indication that the fetus may have an anomaly.

Fetal breathing (chest wall movements) and fetal movements (stretching and rotational movements) are also used to assess the fetus. A fetus that has at least 30 breathing movements in 10 minutes or 3 body movements in 10 minutes is considered healthy. A combination of a reactive NST, adequate amniotic fluid, adequate fetal breathing, adequate fetal movements, and adequate tone is frequently referred to as a **normal biophysical profile.** Each parameter is given a **score** of 2. A normal profile equals 10. Table 7-4 lists the recommended frequency for biophysical profile testing based on high-risk conditions.

UMBILICAL ARTERY DOPPLER ASSESSMENT

During the ultrasonic assessment, it is relatively easy to assess the fetal umbilical artery vascular resistance. A high systolic/diastolic ratio (S/D) (Figure 7-5) suggests abnormal flow because of increased vascular resistance within the fetal/placental circulation. When the flow becomes very abnormal, diastolic flow ceases and there can be a reversal of flow (Figure 7-6) from the placenta to the fetus. When this occurs the fetus is at high risk and delivery is usually indicated.

PREVENTIVE HEALTH CARE

Management before and during pregnancy presents an opportunity for patient education and the practice of preventive medicine. Childbirth preparation classes for both the patient and her partner are very

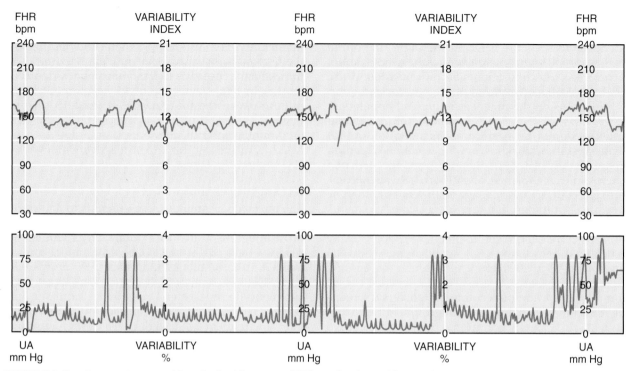

FIGURE 7-3 Reactive nonstress test. Note the fetal heart rate (FHR) accelerations with most fetal movements, denoted by spikes above 75 mm Hg in lower panel. *bpm,* Beats per minute.

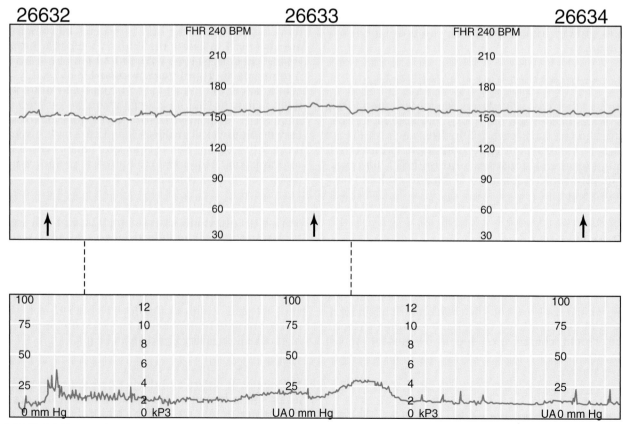

FIGURE 7-4 Nonreactive nonstress test. Note the lack of beat-to-beat variability and the lack of acceleration of the fetal heart rate (FHR) with fetal movements *(arrows). bpm,* Beats per minute.

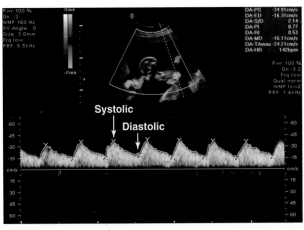

FIGURE 7-5 Fetal umbilical artery Doppler assessment at 31 weeks and 3 days showing a series of Doppler waveforms with systolic (upper) peaks marked with X (+37 cm/sec) and lower X marking diastole (at +21 cm/sec). The systolic-to-diastolic ratio is calculated as 2.14 *(upper right corner),* and normal for this gestational age is <3.2.

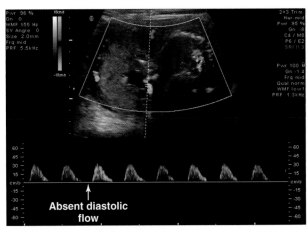

FIGURE 7-6 Fetal umbilical artery Doppler assessment at 26 weeks and 5 days in a case with reduced amniotic fluid (small lucent pocket left of midline with Doppler assessment of cord artery). The systolic-to-diastolic ratio cannot be calculated as in Figure 7-5 because of absent diastolic flow. Only systolic flow can be measured (+30 cm/sec).

TABLE 7-4

RECOMMENDED FREQUENCY FOR BIOPHYSICAL PROFILE TESTING

High-Risk Condition	Frequency
Intrauterine Growth Restriction	
Mild	Weekly
Moderate*	Twice weekly
Diabetes Mellitus	
Class A	Weekly, 37 to 40 wk
	Twice weekly, beyond 40 wk
Class B and worse	Twice weekly, beginning at 34 wk
Post-term pregnancy	Twice weekly, beginning at 42 wk
Decreased fetal movements	Weekly
Other high-risk conditions	Weekly
Maternal or physician concern	Weekly

*For severe intrauterine growth restriction, delivery is usually indicated.

educational, particularly during the first pregnancy. These classes provide an important opportunity for both parents to enhance bonding to the infant before birth. **The presence and encouragement of the baby's father at these classes and during labor and delivery can be most helpful.**

Although preconception, prenatal, and obstetric information is of primary importance, **other topics that may have lifelong relevance can be introduced and emphasized during antepartum care. The pregnancy itself is frequently a strong motivator for women to eliminate potentially harmful habits, such as smoking, or to change dietary patterns** that are associated with an increased incidence of obesity. Therefore, a systematic approach to the dissemination of preventive health care information is generally well received by the pregnant woman.

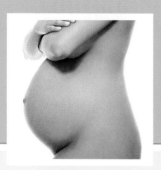

Normal Labor, Delivery, and Postpartum Care

Anatomic Considerations, Obstetric Analgesia and Anesthesia, and Resuscitation of the Newborn

CALVIN J. HOBEL • MARK ZAKOWSKI

CLINICAL KEYS FOR THIS CHAPTER

- Knowledge of the characteristics of the fetal head and maternal pelvis is necessary to understand the dynamic relationship between these two anatomic structures during labor. The fetal head, through a process of molding and flexion followed by internal rotation, passes through the maternal pelvis during the first and second stages of labor. At delivery (expulsion), there is external rotation of the fetal head.

- After the delivery of the fetal head at the end of the second stage of labor, attention must be directed to the management of the third and fourth stages of labor. The third stage of labor is a period when women are at risk for postpartum hemorrhage. Hemorrhage is the leading cause of maternal death worldwide and is among the top three causes of maternal death in the United States. Uterine atony is the leading cause of postpartum hemorrhage, and its prevention and/or early management are essential.

- Women rate pain during labor as one of the most uncomfortable experiences in life. Oxytocin is commonly used to increase the frequency and strength of uterine contractions, which also increases labor pain. Catecholamine release and maternal hyperventilation occur during labor. The resulting vasoconstriction of the uterine arteries decreases uterine blood flow and oxygen dissociation from hemoglobin, causing respiratory alkalosis. Whereas alternative methods offer some degree of pain relief, the gold standard during labor and childbirth is epidural (or combined spinal-epidural) analgesia, which not only provides near-complete relief but also improves uterine blood flow, fetal oxygenation, and the release of stress hormones. Fluid administration before neuraxial analgesia helps prevent hypotension, which, if it does occur, may be treated with small doses of vasopressors.

- Approximately one in three women have a cesarean delivery in the United States. Although the use of general anesthesia for cesarean delivery is very safe, it has increased maternal and neonatal side effects as well as maternal mortality. Most intravenous and inhaled anesthetics cross the placenta. Regional anesthesia (spinal or epidural) is preferable. Some neonatal assistance is required in 10% of births, and vigorous resuscitation is required in 1%. Newborns are ventilated with lower concentrations of oxygen and titrated up as needed to achieve their normal physiologic oxygen saturation of 85-95% in the first minutes of life.

Normal labor is a process that permits a series of extensive physiologic changes in the mother to allow for the delivery of her fetus through the birth canal. **Labor is defined as progressive cervical effacement and dilation resulting from regular uterine contractions that occur at least every 3 minutes and last 30 to 60 seconds each.**

The role of the obstetrician and health care team is to anticipate and manage abnormalities that may occur during either the maternal or fetal birth process. When a decision is made to intervene, it must be considered carefully because each intervention carries not only potential benefits but also potential risks. In the vast majority of cases, the best management may be close observation and, when necessary, cautious intervention.

Anatomic Characteristics of the Fetal Head and Maternal Pelvis

Successful vaginal delivery requires the accommodation, by molding and rotation, of the descending fetal head to the maternal pelvis.

FETAL HEAD

The head is the largest and least compressible part of the fetus. Thus, from an obstetric viewpoint, it is the most important part, whether the presentation is cephalic or breech.

The fetal skull consists of a base and a vault (the cranium). The base of the skull has large, ossified, firmly united, and noncompressible bones. This serves to protect the vital structures contained within the brain stem and its spinal connections.

The cranium consists of the occipital bone posteriorly, two parietal bones bilaterally, and two frontal and temporal bones anteriorly. The cranial bones at birth are thin, weakly ossified, easily compressible, and interconnected only by membranes. These features allow them to overlap under pressure and to change shape to conform to the maternal pelvis, a process known as *molding.*

Sutures

The membrane-occupied spaces between the cranial bones are known as *sutures*. The **sagittal suture** lies between the parietal bones and extends in an anteroposterior direction between the fontanelles, dividing the head into right and left sides (Figure 8-1). The **lambdoidal suture** extends from the posterior fontanelle laterally and serves to separate the occipital from the parietal bones. The **coronal suture** extends from the anterior fontanelle laterally and serves to separate the parietal and frontal bones. The **frontal suture** lies between the frontal bones and extends from the anterior fontanelle to the glabella (the prominence between the eyebrows).

Fontanelles

The membrane-filled spaces located at the point where the sutures intersect are known as *fontanelles*, the most important of which are the **anterior and posterior fontanelles.** Clinically, they are even more useful than the sutures for determining the fetal head position.

The **posterior fontanelle** closes at 6 to 8 weeks of life, whereas the **anterior fontanelle** does not become ossified until approximately 18 months. This allows the skull to accommodate the tremendous growth of the infant's brain after birth.

The anterior fontanelle **(bregma)** is found at the intersection of the sagittal, frontal, and coronal sutures. It is diamond-shaped, measures approximately 2 × 3 cm, and is much larger than the posterior fontanelle. The posterior fontanelle is Y- or T-shaped and is found at the junction of the sagittal and lambdoid sutures.

Landmarks

The fetal skull is characterized by a number of landmarks. From front to back, they include the following (Figure 8-2):
1. **Nasion:** the root of the nose
2. **Glabella:** the elevated area between the orbital ridges
3. **Sinciput (brow):** the area between the anterior fontanelle and the glabella
4. **Anterior fontanelle (bregma):** diamond-shaped
5. **Vertex:** the area between the fontanelles and bounded laterally by the parietal eminences
6. **Posterior fontanelle (lambda):** Y- or T-shaped
7. **Occiput:** the area behind and inferior to the posterior fontanelle and lambdoid sutures

Diameters

Several diameters of the fetal skull are important (see Figures 8-1 and 8-2). The **anteroposterior diameter** presenting to the maternal pelvis depends on the degree of flexion or extension of the head. It is important because the various diameters differ in length. The following measurements are considered average for a term fetus:
1. **Suboccipitobregmatic (9.5 cm):** the presenting anteroposterior diameter when the **head is well flexed,** as in an occipitotransverse or occipitoanterior position; it extends from the undersurface of the occipital bone at the junction with the neck to the center of the anterior fontanelle.

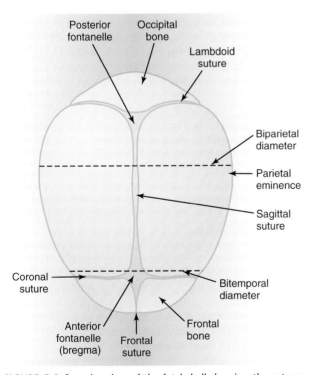

FIGURE 8-1 Superior view of the fetal skull showing the sutures, fontanelles, and transverse diameters.

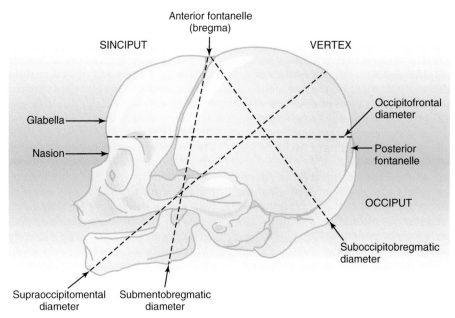

FIGURE 8-2 Lateral view of the fetal skull showing the prominent landmarks and the anteroposterior diameters.

2. **Occipitofrontal (11 cm):** the presenting anteroposterior diameter when the head is deflexed, as in an occipitoposterior presentation; it extends from the external occipital protuberance to the glabella.
3. **Supraoccipitomental (13.5 cm):** the presenting anteroposterior diameter in a brow presentation and the longest anteroposterior diameter of the head; it extends from the vertex to the chin.
4. **Submentobregmatic (9.5 cm):** the presenting anteroposterior diameter in face presentations; it extends from the junction of the neck and lower jaw to the center of the anterior fontanelle.

The transverse diameters of the fetal skull are as follows:
1. **Biparietal (9.5 cm):** the largest transverse diameter; it extends between the parietal bones.
2. **Bitemporal (8 cm):** the shortest transverse diameter; it extends between the temporal bones.

The average circumference of the term fetal head, measured in the occipitofrontal plane, is 34.5 cm.

PELVIC ANATOMY

Bony Pelvis

The bony pelvis is made up of four bones: the sacrum, coccyx, and two innominates (composed of the ilium, ischium, and pubis). These are held together by the sacroiliac joints, the symphysis pubis, and the sacrococcygeal joint. The union of the pelvis and the vertebral column stabilizes the pelvis and allows weight to be transmitted to the lower extremities.

The **sacrum** consists of five fused vertebrae. The anterior superior edge of the first sacral vertebra is called the **promontory,** which protrudes slightly into the cavity of the pelvis. The anterior surface of the sacrum is usually concave. It articulates with the ilium at its upper segment, with the coccyx at its lower segment, and with the sacrospinous and sacrotuberous ligaments laterally.

The **coccyx** is composed of three to five rudimentary vertebrae. It articulates with the sacrum, forming a joint, and occasionally the bones are fused.

The pelvis is divided into the false pelvis above and the true pelvis below the linea terminalis (the edge of the pelvic inlet). The false pelvis is bordered by the lumbar vertebrae posteriorly, an iliac fossa bilaterally, and the abdominal wall anteriorly. Its only obstetric function is to support the pregnant uterus.

The true pelvis is a bony canal and is formed by the sacrum and coccyx posteriorly and by the ischium and pubis laterally and anteriorly. Its internal borders are solid and relatively immobile. The posterior wall is twice the length of the anterior wall. The true pelvis is the area of concern to the obstetrician because its dimensions are sometimes not adequate to permit passage of the fetus.

Pelvic Planes

The pelvis is divided into the following four planes for descriptive purposes (Table 8-1 and Figures 8-3 and 8-4):
1. **The pelvic inlet**
2. **The plane of greatest diameter**
3. **The plane of least diameter**
4. **The pelvic outlet**

These planes are imaginary, flat surfaces that extend across the pelvis at different levels. Except for

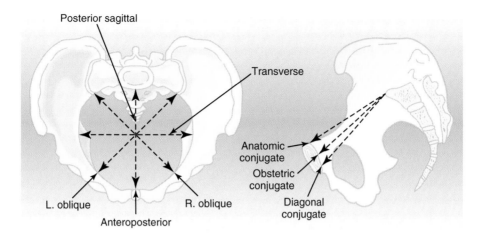

FIGURE 8-3 Pelvic inlet and its diameters.

TABLE 8-1

AVERAGE LENGTH OF PELVIC PLANE DIAMETERS

Pelvic Plane	Diameter	Average Length (cm)
Inlet	True conjugate	11.5
	Obstetric conjugate	11
	Transverse	13.5
	Oblique	12.5
	Posterior sagittal	4.5
Greatest diameter	Anteroposterior	12.75
	Transverse	12.5
Midplane	Anteroposterior	12
	Bispinous	10.5
	Posterior sagittal	4.5-5
Outlet	Anatomic anteroposterior	9.5
	Obstetric anteroposterior	11.5
	Bituberous	11
	Posterior sagittal	7.5

the plane of greatest diameter, each plane is clinically significant.

The **plane of the inlet** is bordered by the pubic crest anteriorly, the iliopectineal line of the innominate bones laterally, and the promontory of the sacrum posteriorly. The fetal head enters the pelvis through this plane in the transverse position.

The **plane of greatest diameter** is the largest part of the pelvic cavity. It is bordered by the posterior midpoint of the pubis anteriorly, the upper part of the obturator foramina laterally, and the junction of the second and third sacral vertebrae posteriorly. The fetal head rotates to the anterior position in this plane.

The **plane of least diameter** is the most important from a clinical standpoint because most instances of arrest of descent occur at this level. It is bordered by the

lower edge of the pubis anteriorly, the ischial spines and sacrospinous ligaments laterally, and the lower sacrum posteriorly. Low transverse arrests generally occur in this plane.

The **plane of the pelvic outlet** is formed by two triangular planes with a common base at the level of the ischial tuberosities. The anterior triangle is bordered by the subpubic angle at the apex, the pubic rami on the sides, and the bituberous diameter at the base. The posterior triangle is bordered by the sacrococcygeal joint at its apex, the sacrotuberous ligaments on the sides, and the bituberous diameter at the base. This plane is the site of a low pelvic arrest.

Pelvic Diameters

The diameters of the pelvic planes represent the amount of space available at each level. The key measurements for assessing the capacity of the maternal pelvis include the following:
1. **The obstetric conjugate of the inlet**
2. **The bispinous diameter of the midplane**
3. **The bituberous diameter of the outlet**
4. **The anteroposterior sagittal diameter of the outlet**

The average lengths of the diameters of each pelvic plane are listed in Table 8-1.

Pelvic Inlet

The pelvic inlet has five important diameters (see Figure 8-3). The anteroposterior diameter is described by one of two measurements. The **true conjugate (anatomic conjugate)** is the anatomic diameter and extends from the middle of the sacral promontory to the superior surface of the pubic symphysis. The **obstetric conjugate** represents the actual space available to the fetus and extends from the middle of the sacral promontory to the closest point on the convex posterior surface of the symphysis pubis.

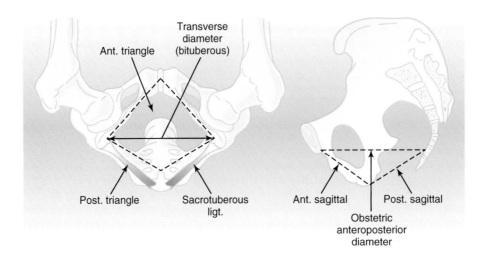

FIGURE 8-4 Pelvic outlet and its diameters.

The **transverse diameter** is the widest distance between the iliopectineal lines. Each **oblique diameter** extends from the sacroiliac joint to the opposite iliopectineal eminence.

The **posterior sagittal diameter** extends from the anteroposterior and transverse intersection to the middle of the sacral promontory.

Plane of Greatest Diameter

The plane of greatest diameter has two noteworthy diameters. The **anteroposterior diameter** (see Figure 8-4) extends from the midpoint of the posterior surface of the pubis to the junction of the second and third sacral vertebrae. The **transverse diameter** is the widest distance between the lateral borders of the plane.

Plane of Least Diameter (Midplane)

The plane of least diameter has three important diameters. The **anteroposterior diameter** extends from the lower border of the pubis to the junction of the fourth and fifth sacral vertebrae. The **transverse (bispinous) diameter** extends between the ischial spines. The **posterior sagittal diameter** extends from the midpoint of the bispinous diameter to the junction of the fourth and fifth sacral vertebrae.

Pelvic Outlet

The pelvic outlet has four important diameters (see Figure 8-4). The **anatomic anteroposterior diameter** extends from the inferior margin of the pubis to the tip of the coccyx, whereas the **obstetric anteroposterior diameter** extends from the inferior margin of the pubis to the sacrococcygeal joint. The **transverse (bituberous) diameter** extends between the inner surfaces of the ischial tuberosities, and the **posterior sagittal diameter** (not listed) extends from the middle of the transverse diameter to the sacrococcygeal joint.

PELVIC SHAPES

Based on the general bony architecture, the pelvis may be classified into four basic types (Figure 8-5): gynecoid, android, anthropoid, and platypelloid.

Gynecoid

The gynecoid pelvis is the classic female type of pelvis and is found in approximately **50% of women.** It has the following characteristics:

1. Round at the inlet, with the widest transverse diameter only slightly greater than the anteroposterior diameter
2. Sidewalls straight
3. Ischial spines of average prominence
4. Large **sacrospinous notch** (depicted in Figure 8-5)
5. Well-curved sacrum
6. Spacious subpubic arch with an angle of approximately 90 degrees

These features create a cylindrical shape that is spacious throughout. The fetal head generally rotates into the occipitoanterior position in this type of pelvis.

Android

The android pelvis is the typical male type of pelvis. It is found in **less than 30% of women** and has the following characteristics:

1. Triangular inlet with a flat posterior segment and the widest transverse diameter closer to the sacrum than in the gynecoid type
2. Convergent sidewalls with prominent spines
3. Shallow sacral curve
4. Long and narrow (small) sacrospinous notch (noted in Figure 8-5 in a gynecoid pelvis)
5. Narrow subpubic arch

This type of pelvis has limited space at the inlet and progressively less space as the fetus moves down the

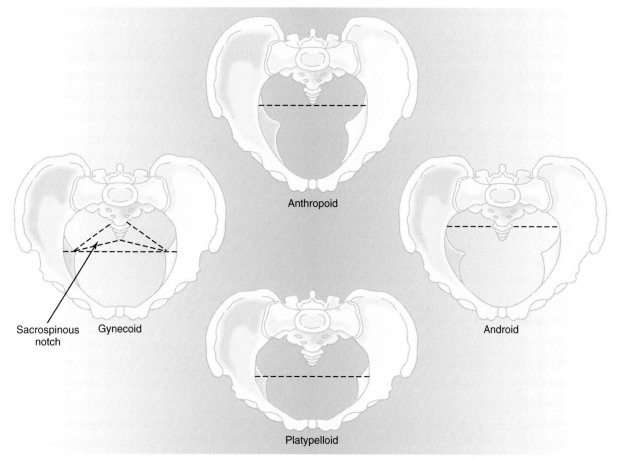

FIGURE 8-5 The four basic pelvic types. The *dashed lines* indicate the transverse diameter of the **inlet**. Note that the widest diameter of the inlet is posteriorly situated in an android or anthropoid pelvis. The gynecoid pelvis illustrates the location of the sacrospinous notch, present in all pelvic types.

pelvis, because of the funneling effect of the sidewalls, sacrum, and pubic rami. Thus, the amount of space is restricted at all levels. The fetal head is forced to be in the occipitoposterior position to conform to the narrow anterior pelvis. Arrest of descent is common at the midpelvis.

Anthropoid

The anthropoid pelvis resembles that of the anthropoid ape. It is found in **approximately 20% of women** and has the following characteristics:
1. A much larger anteroposterior than transverse diameter, creating a long, narrow oval at the inlet
2. Sidewalls that do not converge
3. Ischial spines that are not prominent but are close, because of the overall shape
4. Variable, but usually posterior, inclination of the sacrum
5. Small sacrospinous notch
6. Narrow, outwardly shaped subpubic arch

The fetal head can engage only in the anteroposterior diameter and usually does so in the occipitoposte-

rior position because there is more space in the posterior pelvis.

Platypelloid

The platypelloid pelvis is best described as being a flattened gynecoid pelvis. It is found in **only 3% of women,** and it has the following characteristics:
1. A short anteroposterior and wide transverse diameter, creating an oval-shaped inlet
2. Straight or divergent sidewalls
3. Posterior inclination of a flat sacrum
4. A wide bispinous diameter
5. Long but small sacrospinous notch
6. A wide subpubic arch

The overall shape is that of a gentle curve throughout. The fetal head has to engage in the transverse diameter.

ENGAGEMENT

Engagement occurs when the widest diameter of the fetal presenting part has passed through the pelvic inlet. In cephalic presentations, the widest diameter is biparietal; in breech presentations, it is intertrochanteric.

The station of the presenting part in the pelvic canal is defined as its level above or below the plane of the ischial spines. The level of the ischial spines is assigned as "zero" station, and each centimeter above or below this level is given a minus or plus designation, respectively.

In the majority of women, the bony presenting part is at the level of the ischial spines when the head has become engaged. The fetal head usually engages with its sagittal suture in the transverse diameter of the pelvis. The head position is considered to be **synclitic** when the biparietal diameter is parallel to the pelvic plane and the sagittal suture is midway between the anterior and posterior planes of the pelvis. When this relationship is not present, the head is considered to be **asynclitic** (Figure 8-6).

There is a distinct advantage to having the head engage in asynclitism in certain situations. In a synclitic presentation, the biparietal diameter entering the pelvis measures 9.5 cm; when the parietal bones enter the pelvis in an asynclitic manner, however, the presenting diameter measures 8.75 cm. Therefore, asynclitism permits a larger head to enter the pelvis than would be possible in a synclitic presentation.

CLINICAL PELVIMETRY

The diameters that can be clinically evaluated can be assessed at the time of the first prenatal visit to screen for obvious pelvic contractions, although some obstetricians believe that it is better to wait until later in pregnancy, when the soft tissues are more distensible and the examination is less uncomfortable and possibly more accurate.

The clinical evaluation is started by assessing the pelvic inlet. The pelvic inlet can be evaluated clinically for its anteroposterior diameter. The obstetric conjugate can be estimated from the diagonal conjugate, which is obtained during clinical examination (see Figure 8-3).

The diagonal conjugate is approximated by measuring from the lower border of the pubis to the sacral promontory, using the tip of the second finger and the point where the base of the index finger meets the pubis (Figure 8-7). The obstetric conjugate is then estimated by subtracting 1.5 to 2 cm, depending on the height and inclination of the pubis. Often the middle finger of the examining hand cannot reach the sacral promontory; thus, the obstetric conjugate is considered adequate. If the diagonal conjugate is greater than or equal to 11.5 cm, the anteroposterior diameter of the inlet is considered to be adequate.

The anterior surface of the sacrum is then palpated to assess its curvature. The usual shape is concave. A flat or convex shape may indicate anteroposterior constriction throughout the pelvis.

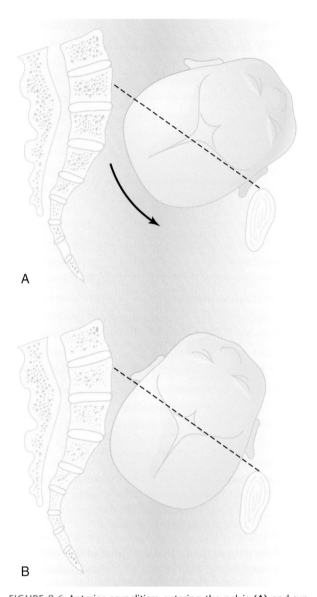

A

B

FIGURE 8-6 Anterior asynclitism entering the pelvis (**A**) and synclitism in the pelvis (**B**). The *curved arrow* shows the direction to correct asynclitism, and the *dashed lines* show the axis that defines synclitism.

The midpelvis cannot be measured accurately clinically in either the anteroposterior or transverse diameter. A reasonable estimate of the size of the midpelvis, however, can be obtained as follows. **The pelvic sidewalls can be assessed to determine if they are convergent rather than having the normal, almost parallel, configuration.** The ischial spines are palpated carefully to assess their prominence, and several passes are made between the spines to approximate the bispinous diameter. The length of the sacrospinous ligament is assessed by placing one finger on the ischial spine and one finger on the sacrum in the midline. The average length is three fingerbreadths. If the sacrospinous

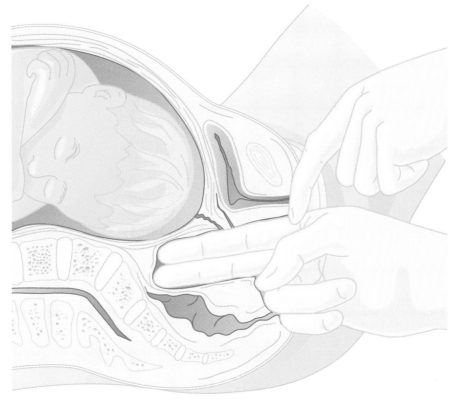

FIGURE 8-7 Clinical estimation of the diagonal conjugate diameter of the pelvis.

notch that is located lateral to the ligament can accommodate two-and-one-half fingers, the posterior midpelvis is most likely of adequate dimensions. A short ligament suggests a forward inclination of the sacrum and a narrowed sacrospinous notch.

Finally, the pelvic outlet is assessed. This is done by first placing a fist between the ischial tuberosities. An 8.5-cm distance is considered to indicate an adequate transverse diameter. The posterior sagittal measurement should also be greater than 8 cm. The infrapubic angle is assessed by placing a thumb next to each inferior pubic ramus and then estimating the angle at which they meet. An angle of less than 90 degrees is associated with a contracted transverse diameter in the midplane and outlet.

Radiologic Assessment of the Pelvis

When an accurate measurement of the pelvis is indicated, nuclear magnetic resonance imaging (MRI) may be used. The advantage of MRI over x-ray or computed tomography for pelvic assessment is the lack of ionizing radiation exposure.

Indications
1. **Clinical evidence or obstetric history suggestive of pelvic abnormalities**
2. **A history of pelvic trauma**

It should always be questioned whether the results obtained by radiologic assessment will have sufficient influence on the patient's management to make the investigation worthwhile.

PREPARATION FOR LABOR

Before actual labor begins, a number of preparatory physiologic events usually occur.

Lightening

Two or more weeks before labor, the fetal head in most primigravid women settles into the brim of the pelvis. In multigravida, this often does not occur until early in labor. **Lightening** may be noted by the mother as a flattening of the upper abdomen and an increased prominence of the lower abdomen.

False Labor

During the last 4 to 8 weeks of pregnancy, the uterus undergoes irregular contractions that normally are painless. Such contractions appear unpredictably and sporadically and can be rhythmic and of mild intensity. In the last month of pregnancy, these contractions may occur more frequently, sometimes every 10 to 20 minutes, and with greater intensity. **These Braxton Hicks contractions are considered false labor in that they are not associated with progressive cervical**

dilation or effacement. They may serve a physiologic role in preparing the uterus and cervix for true labor.

Cervical Effacement

Before the onset of parturition, the cervix is frequently noted to soften as a result of increased water content and collagen lysis. Simultaneous effacement, or thinning of the cervix, occurs as the internal os of the cervix is taken up into the lower uterine segment (Figure 8-8, B). Consequently, patients often present in early labor with a cervix that is already partially effaced. As a result of cervical effacement, the mucous plug within the cervical canal may be released. The onset of labor may thus be heralded by the passage of a small amount of blood-tinged mucus from the vagina (**"bloody show"**).

Induction and Augmentation of Labor

Induction of labor is the process whereby labor is initiated by artificial means after appropriate assessment of the mother and fetus and an explanation to the patient of the indications for induction. In the case of high-risk pregnancies, induction is necessary to reduce the risk of morbidity to the mother and her fetus. In general, induction of labor is not used for the convenience of the mother or her family, and it should not be done before 38 weeks' gestation because of the possibility of neonatal morbidity. **Augmentation** is the artificial stimulation of labor that has begun spontaneously (see Chapter 11).

Cervical effacement and softening (ripening) occur before the onset of spontaneous labor. Cervical ripening frequently has not occurred before a decision to induce labor, yet the success of induction is dependent on these changes in the cervix.

Several mechanical and pharmacologic approaches may be used to promote cervical ripening before the actual induction of uterine contractions. Currently approved pharmacologic treatments include intravaginal application of prostaglandin E_2 using a vaginal insert (on a string) called **Cervidil,** which can be removed quickly if the medication causes hyperstimulation. **Cytotec,** a synthetic prostaglandin E_1 analogue, has also been approved for cervical ripening. One 25-μg tablet placed intravaginally effectively initiates cervical ripening. **Although prostaglandin administration has been demonstrated to shorten the duration of labor induction, the impact on cesarean delivery rates due to failed induction has been minimal.**

Other methods of cervical ripening may include intrauterine placement of a Foley catheter into the cervix and inflation of the balloon with 10 cc of saline.

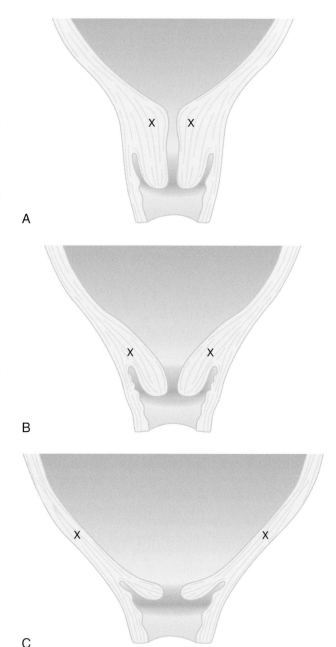

FIGURE 8-8 **A,** The absence of cervical effacement before labor (*X* shows the location of the internal os in a normal cervix). **B,** Cervical os *(X)* being progressively taken up into the lower segment of the uterus (about 50% effaced). **C,** Cervical os *(X)* fully taken up (cervix is completely effaced).

Manual separation of the chorioamnion from the lower uterine segment—referred to as "stripping the membranes"—does not necessarily speed up the onset of labor. **Artificial rupture of the membranes is not recommended** as a method to induce labor.

In addition to cervical ripening, induction of labor requires the initiation of effective uterine contractions. **Oxytocin** is identical to the natural pituitary peptide, and it **is the only drug approved for induction and augmentation of labor.** Pitocin is the synthetic preparation.

The physician must be fully aware of the indications and contraindications for the use of induction and augmentation of labor (Table 8-2). The most common contraindication has been prior uterine surgery in which there has been complete transection of the uterine wall. However, **a previous lower transverse incision is no longer considered a contraindication to a trial of labor.** This is referred to as *vaginal birth after cesarean,* or VBAC.

TECHNIQUE FOR INDUCTION AND AUGMENTATION OF LABOR

A hospital obstetric service must establish guidelines for the proper use of oxytocin for induction and augmentation of labor. In general, an assessment and plan of management should be outlined in the patient's medical record. It is helpful to assess the likelihood of success by a careful pelvic examination to determine the **Bishop score,** which is used to evaluate the status of the cervix and the station of the fetal head (Table 8-3). A high score (9 to 13) is associated with a high likelihood of a vaginal delivery, whereas a low score (<5) is associated with a decreased likelihood of success (65-80%). Before induction is begun, the patient's blood must be typed and screened for antibodies. A blood specimen should be held in the laboratory in case crossmatching becomes necessary. **Continuous electronic monitoring of the fetal heart rate and uterine activity is required during induction.** An internal uterine catheter for monitoring uterine pressure is suggested if intensity cannot be adequately assessed.

Oxytocin Infusion

Several principles should be followed when oxytocin is used to induce or augment labor:

1. **Oxytocin must be given intravenously** to allow it to be discontinued quickly if a complication such as uterine hypertonus or fetal distress develops. Because oxytocin has a half-life of 3 to 5 minutes, its physiologic effect will diminish quickly (within 15 to 30 minutes) after discontinuation.

2. **A dilute infusion must be used and "piggybacked" into the main intravenous (IV) line** so that it can be stopped quickly if necessary, without interrupting the main IV route.

3. **The drug is best infused with a calibrated infusion pump** that can be easily adjusted to deliver the required infusion rate accurately.

TABLE 8-2

INDICATIONS AND CONTRAINDICATIONS FOR INDUCTION AND AUGMENTATION OF LABOR

Induction	Augmentation
Indications	
Maternal	
Preeclampsia	Abnormal labor (in the presence of inadequate uterine activity)
Diabetes mellitus	Prolonged latent phase
Heart disease	Prolonged active phase
Fetoplacental	
Prolonged pregnancy	
Intrauterine growth restriction	
Abnormal fetal testing	
Rhesus type incompatibility	
Fetal abnormality	
Premature rupture of membranes	
Chorioamnionitis	
Contraindications	
Maternal	
Absolute Contracted pelvis	Same contraindications as for maternal and fetoplacental

Relative
  Prior uterine surgery
  Classic cesarean delivery
  Complete transection of uterus
    (myomectomy, reconstruction)
  Overdistended uterus	

Fetoplacental	
Preterm fetus without lung maturity	
Acute fetal distress	
Abnormal presentation	

TABLE 8-3

BISHOP SCORE TO ASSESS LIKELIHOOD OF SUCCESSFUL INDUCTION OF LABOR

Physical Findings	Rating			
	0	1	2	3
Cervix				
Position	Posterior	Mid	Anterior	—
Consistency	Firm	Medium	Soft	—
Effacement (%)	0-30	40-50	60-70	≥80
Dilation (cm)	0	1-2	3-4	≥5
Fetal Head				
Station	−3	−2	−1	+1

4. **The induction of labor for a specific indication generally should not exceed 72 hours.** In patients with a low Bishop score, it is not unusual for an induction to progress slowly. If the cervix effaces and dilates, it is recommended that the membranes be ruptured on the third day. If adequate progress is not made within 12 hours of rupturing the membranes, a cesarean delivery may be performed.

5. **If adequate labor is established, the infusion rate and the concentration may be reduced,** especially during the second stage of labor. Adherence to this principle avoids the risks of hyperstimulation and fetal distress, which frequently occur once labor has been established.

Substantial variation exists regarding the initial dose, incremental dose, and time interval between dose increments when oxytocin is used for labor induction and augmentation. Well-performed clinical studies have supported both low-dose (1 to 30 mU/min) and high-dose (4 to 40 mU/min) protocols, as shown in Table 8-4. It is not surprising that many protocols use moderate doses of oxytocin. Generally, intervals between dose increments should be no less than 20 minutes to permit time for steady-state plasma levels of oxytocin to be achieved and to prevent an increased risk of uterine hyperstimulation.

COMPLICATIONS. The use of oxytocin for the induction and augmentation of labor can cause three major complications. First, an excessive infusion rate can cause **hyperstimulation** and thereby cause fetal distress from ischemia. In rare situations, a tetanic contraction can occur, which can lead to **rupture of the uterus.** Second, because oxytocin has a structure similar to that of antidiuretic hormone, it has an intrinsic **antidiuretic effect** and will increase water reabsorption from the glomerular filtrate. **Severe water intoxication with convulsions and coma can occur** rarely when oxytocin is infused continuously for more than 24 hours. Third,

prolonged infusion of oxytocin can result in **uterine muscle fatigue** (nonresponsiveness) and **postdelivery uterine atony** (hypotonus), **which can increase the risk of postpartum hemorrhage.**

STAGES OF LABOR

There are four stages of labor, each of which is considered separately. These stages in actuality are definitions of progress during labor, delivery, and the puerperium (Table 8-5).

The **first stage** lasts from the onset of true labor to complete dilation of the cervix. The **second stage** spans from complete dilation of the cervix to the birth of the baby. The **third stage** lasts from the birth of the baby to delivery of the placenta. The **fourth stage** spans from delivery of the placenta to stabilization of the patient's condition, usually at about 6 hours postpartum.

First Stage of Labor as Defined by the Friedman Labor Curve

There is currently controversy about how to define the progress of normal labor. Because the purpose of this chapter is to define normal labor, we will use the standard definitions provided by Friedman in 1978 (Figure 8-9). The Friedman labor curve, as well as a recently suggested modification, is covered in Chapter 11.

PHASES. The first stage of labor consists of two phases: a latent phase, during which cervical effacement and early dilation occur, and an active phase, during which more rapid cervical dilation occurs (see Figure 8-9). Although cervical softening and early effacement may occur before labor, during the first stage of labor the entire cervical length (cervical os) is retracted into the lower uterine segment (see Figure 8-8).

LENGTH. The length of the first stage may vary in relation to parity; primiparous patients generally experience a longer first stage than do multiparous patients (see Table 8-5). Because the latent phase may overlap considerably with the preparatory phase of labor, its duration is highly variable. It may also be influenced by other factors, such as sedation and stress. The active phase begins when the cervix is dilated 4 cm in the presence of regularly occurring uterine contractions. The recent guidelines proposed by Zhang and colleagues regarding labor curves (see Chapter 11) suggest that the active phase may not begin until 6-cm dilation. **The minimal dilation during the active phase of the first stage is nearly the same for normal primiparous and multiparous women: 1 and 1.2 cm/hr, respectively.** If progress is slower than this, evaluation for uterine dysfunction, fetal malposition, or cephalopelvic disproportion should be undertaken.

MEASUREMENT OF PROGRESS. During the first stage, the progress of labor may be measured in terms of cervical

TABLE 8-4		
METHOD OF OXYTOCIN INFUSION FOR INDUCTION AND/OR AUGMENTATION OF LABOR		
	Low-Dose Protocol	**High-Dose Protocol**
Starting dose	1 mU/min	4 mU/min
Increment	1 mU/min	4 mU/min
Interval	20 min	20 min
Limited by	5 contractions in 10 min	7 contractions in 15 min
Maximal dose	20-30 mU/min	40 mU/min

Solution: 10 U of oxytocin in 1000 mL of 5% dextrose or balanced salt solution (10 mU/mL).
Administration: Piggyback into main intravenous line; administer solution by infusion pump.

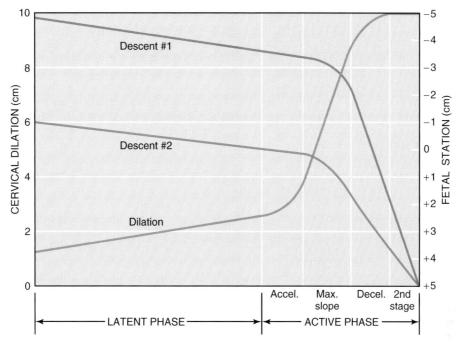

FIGURE 8-9 Cervical dilation and descent of the fetal head during labor. The first descent curve represents a fetus with a floating presenting part at the onset of labor, whereas the second represents a fetus with the presenting part fixed in the pelvis before labor. (Modified from Friedman EA: *Labor: clinical evaluation and management,* ed 2, East Norwalk, CT, 1978, Appleton-Century-Crofts, p 41.)

TABLE 8-5

CHARACTERISTICS OF NORMAL LABOR

Characteristics	Primipara	Multipara
Duration of first stage	6-18 hr	2-10 hr
Rate of cervical dilation during active phase	1 cm/hr	1.2 cm/hr
Duration of second stage	30 min to 3 hr	5-30 min
Duration of third stage	0-30 min	0-30 min

effacement, cervical dilation, and descent of the fetal head. The clinical pattern of the uterine contractions alone is not an adequate indication of progress. After completion of cervical dilation, the second stage commences. Thereafter, only the descent, flexion, and rotation of the presenting part are available to assess the progress of labor.

CLINICAL MANAGEMENT OF THE FIRST STAGE. Certain steps should be taken in the clinical management of the patient during the first stage of labor.

Maternal Position. The mother may ambulate, provided that intermittent monitoring ensures fetal well-being and the presenting part is engaged in patients with ruptured membranes. **If she is lying in bed, the lateral recumbent position should be encouraged** to

ensure adequate perfusion of the uteroplacental unit. When the patient is supine (on her back), the weight of the uterus and fetus can compress the vessels supplying the uterus.

Administration of Fluids. Because of decreased gastric emptying during labor, **oral fluids are best avoided.** However, fasting results in the more rapid development of ketosis in pregnant women. Placement of a 16- to 18-gauge venous catheter is advisable during the active phase of labor. It has been shown that **giving at least 125 mL/hr of 10% dextrose (D) in normal saline (NS),** compared with 5% D/NS or just NS, **results in significantly shorter labor.** Thus, the IV route is used to hydrate the patient with crystalloids and provide calories during labor, to administer oxytocin after the delivery of the placenta, and for the treatment of any unanticipated emergencies.

Investigations. Every woman admitted in labor should have a hematocrit or hemoglobin measurement and a blood clot held in the event that a cross-match is needed. Blood group, rhesus (Rh) type, and an antibody screen should be done if these are not known. It is also important to know the hepatitis B status of the mother so that a pediatrician can be notified if the mother is positive. Additionally, a voided urine specimen should be checked for the presence of protein and glucose.

Maternal Monitoring. Maternal pulse rate, blood pressure, respiratory rate, and temperature should be recorded every 1 to 2 hours during normal labor and more frequently if indicated. Fluid balance, particularly urine output and fluid intake, should be monitored carefully.

Analgesia. Adequate analgesia is important during the first stage of labor (see later in this chapter).

Fetal Monitoring. **The fetal heart rate should be evaluated by auscultation with a DeLee stethoscope, by external monitoring with Doppler equipment, or by internal monitoring with a fetal scalp electrode.** In uncomplicated pregnancies, continuous electronic fetal monitoring is not necessary, as several studies have demonstrated that intermittent auscultation of the fetal heart rate, when performed in conjunction with a 1:1 nurse-to-patient ratio, results in comparable outcomes and may reduce the risk of cesarean delivery. Continuous fetal heart rate monitoring provides a record of the labor and may be preferred for documentation and medicolegal reasons. **In patients with no significant obstetric risk factors, the fetal heart rate should be auscultated or the electronic monitor tracing evaluated at least every 30 minutes in the active phase of the first stage of labor and at least every 15 minutes in the second stage of labor. In patients with obstetric risk factors, the fetal heart rate should be auscultated or the electronic monitoring tracing evaluated at least every 15 minutes during the active phase of the first stage of labor (immediately following a uterine contraction) and at least every 5 minutes during the second stage.**

Uterine Activity. Uterine contractions should be monitored every 30 minutes by palpation for their frequency, duration, and intensity. **For high-risk pregnancies, uterine contractions should be monitored continuously along with the fetal heart rate.** This can be achieved electronically using either an external tocodynamometer or an internal pressure catheter in the amniotic cavity. The latter is particularly of value when a patient's labor is being augmented with oxytocin (Pitocin). When an internal catheter is not used, the strength of uterine contractions should be monitored by palpation every 15 minutes.

Vaginal Examination. During the latent phase, particularly when the membranes are ruptured, vaginal examinations should be done sparingly to decrease the risk of an intrauterine infection. **In the active phase, the cervix should be assessed approximately every 2 hours to determine the progress of labor.** Cervical effacement and dilation, the station and position of the presenting part, and the presence of molding or caput in vertex presentations should be recorded.

Amniotomy. The artificial rupture of fetal membranes may increase uterine activity and may provide information on the volume of amniotic fluid and the presence or absence of meconium; however, current opinion suggests that keeping the membranes intact may be of value in supporting the normal progress of labor and **preventing umbilical cord compression or cord prolapse if the presenting part is not engaged.**

Second Stage of Labor

At the beginning of the second stage, the mother usually has a desire to bear down with each contraction. This abdominal pressure, together with the uterine contractile force, combines to expel the fetus. During the second stage of labor (Figure 8-10, *A*), **fetal descent must be monitored carefully** to evaluate the progress of labor. Descent is measured in terms of progress of the presenting part through the birth canal.

In cephalic presentations, the shape of the fetal head may be altered during labor, making the assessment of descent more difficult. **Molding** is the alteration of the relationship of the fetal cranial bones to each other as a result of the compressive forces exerted by the bony maternal pelvis. Some molding is normal. If cephalopelvic disproportion is present, the amount of molding will be more pronounced. **Caput** is a localized, edematous swelling of the scalp caused by pressure of the cervix on the presenting portion of the fetal head. The development of both molding and caput can create a false impression of fetal descent.

The second stage generally takes from 30 minutes to 3 hours in primigravid women and from 5 to 30 minutes in multigravida.

MECHANISIM OF LABOR. Six movements of the baby enable it to adapt to the maternal pelvis: descent, flexion, internal rotation, extension, external rotation, and expulsion (see Figure 8-10). These movements are discussed here for both an occipitoanterior and occipitoposterior position at engagement. The mechanism of labor for other than vertex presentations is covered in Chapter 13.

Descent. Descent is brought about by the force of the uterine contractions, maternal bearing-down (Valsalva) efforts, and, if the patient is upright, gravity.

Flexion. Partial flexion exists before labor as a result of the natural muscle tone of the fetus. During descent, resistance from the cervix, walls of the pelvis, and pelvic floor causes further flexion of the cervical spine, with the baby's chin approaching its chest. **In the occipitoanterior position, the effect of flexion is to change the presenting diameter from the occipitofrontal to the smaller suboccipitobregmatic** (see Figure 8-2). In the occipitoposterior position, complete flexion may not occur, resulting in a larger presenting diameter, which may contribute to a longer labor.

Internal Rotation. In the occipitoanterior position, the fetal head, which enters the pelvis in a transverse or oblique diameter, rotates so that the occiput turns anteriorly toward the symphysis pubis. Internal rotation probably occurs as the fetal head meets the muscular sling of the pelvic floor. It is often not accomplished until the presenting part has reached the level of the

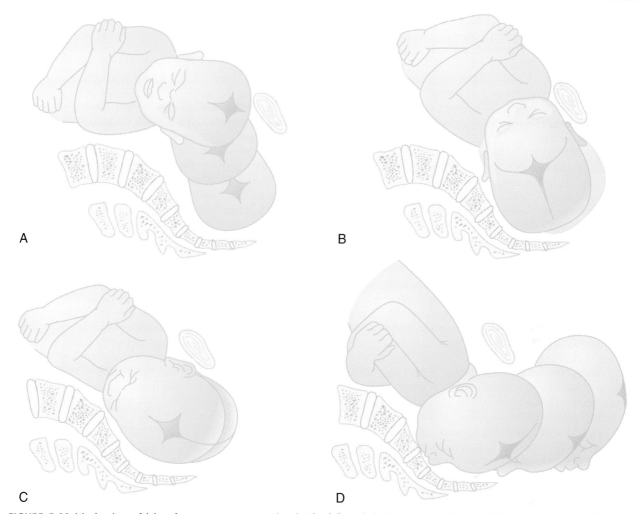

A

B

C

D

FIGURE 8-10 Mechanism of labor for a vertex presentation in the left occipitotransverse position. **A,** Flexion and descent. **B** and **C,** Continued descent and commencement of internal rotation. **D,** Completion of internal rotation to the occipitoanterior position followed by delivery of the head by extension.

ischial spines (zero station) and therefore is engaged. In the occipitoposterior positions, the fetal head may rotate posteriorly so that the occiput turns toward the hollow of the sacrum.

Extension. The flexed head in an occipitoanterior position continues to descend within the pelvis. Because the vaginal outlet is directed upward and forward, extension must occur before the head can pass through it. As the head continues its descent, there is bulging of the perineum followed by crowning (see Figure 8-10, *D*). **Crowning** occurs when the largest diameter of the fetal head is encircled by the vulvar ring. At this time, the vertex has reached station +5. When indicated, an incision in the perineum (**episiotomy**) may aid in reducing perineal resistance. **Current management is to allow the fetus to deliver without an episiotomy when possible.** Good clinical judgment is needed to avoid traumatic tears that may

be more difficult to repair when they occur without an episiotomy. The head is born by rapid extension as the occiput, sinciput, nose, mouth, and chin pass over the perineum.

In the **occipitoposterior position,** the head is born by a combination of flexion and extension. At the time of crowning, the posterior bony pelvis and the muscular sling encourage further flexion. The forehead, sinciput, and occiput are born as the fetal chin approaches the chest. Subsequently, the occiput falls back as the head extends and the nose, mouth, and chin are born.

External Rotation. In both the occipitoanterior and occipitoposterior positions, the delivered head now returns to its original position at the time of engagement to align itself with the fetal back and shoulders. Further head rotation may occur as the shoulders undergo an internal rotation to align themselves anteroposteriorly within the pelvis.

Expulsion. Following external rotation of the head, the anterior shoulder delivers under the symphysis pubis, followed by the posterior shoulder over the perineal body and the body of the child.

CLINICAL MANAGEMENT OF THE SECOND STAGE. As in the first stage, certain steps should be taken in the clinical management of the second stage of labor.

Maternal Position. With the exception of avoiding the supine position, the mother may assume any comfortable position for effective bearing down.

Bearing Down. With each contraction, the mother should be encouraged to hold her breath and bear down with expulsive efforts. This is particularly important for patients with regional anesthesia because their reflex sensations may be impaired.

Fetal Monitoring. During the second stage, the fetal heart rate should be monitored continuously or evaluated every 5 minutes in patients with obstetric risk factors. Fetal heart rate decelerations (head compression or cord compression) with recovery following the uterine contraction may occur normally during this stage (see Chapter 9).

Vaginal Examination. Progress should be recorded approximately every 30 minutes during the second stage. Particular attention should be paid to the descent and flexion of the presenting part, the extent of internal rotation, and the development of molding or caput. During the second stage of labor, the retracted cervix is no longer palpable.

Delivery of the Fetus. When delivery is imminent, the patient is usually placed in the lithotomy position, and the skin over the lower abdomen, vulva, anus, and upper thighs is cleansed with an antiseptic solution. Uncomplicated deliveries, particularly in multiparous women, may be carried out with the patient in the **supine position** with the thighs flexed. The **left lateral position** may be used for delivery in patients who desire to deliver in this position, for those with hip or knee joint deformities that prevent adequate flexion, or for patients with a superficial or deep venous thrombosis in one of the lower extremities.

As the perineum becomes flattened by the crowning head, an episiotomy may be performed to prevent perineal lacerations. Some studies show that the performance of episiotomies may result in a higher proportion of lacerations that involve the anal sphincter (third degree) or anal mucosa (fourth degree).

To facilitate delivery of the fetal head, **a Ritgen maneuver** is performed (Figure 8-11). The right hand, draped with a towel, exerts upward pressure through the distended perineal body, first to the supraorbital ridges and then to the chin. This upward pressure, which increases extension of the head and prevents it from slipping back between contractions, is counteracted by downward pressure on the occiput with the left hand. The downward pressure prevents rapid extension of the head and allows a controlled delivery.

Once the head is delivered, the airway is cleared of blood and amniotic fluid using a bulb suction device. The oral cavity is cleared initially, and then the nares are cleared. Suction of the nares is not performed if fetal distress or meconium-stained liquor is present, because it may result in gasping and aspiration of pharyngeal contents. A second towel is used to wipe secretions from the face and head.

After the airway has been cleared, an index finger is used to check whether the umbilical cord encircles the neck. If so, the cord can usually be slipped over the infant's head. If the cord is too tight, it can be cut between two clamps.

Following delivery of the head, the shoulders descend and rotate into the anteroposterior diameter of the pelvis and are delivered (Figure 8-12). **Delivery of the anterior shoulder is aided by gentle downward traction on the externally rotated head. The brachial plexus may be injured if excessive force is used.** The posterior shoulder is delivered by elevating the head. Finally, the body is slowly extracted by traction on the shoulders.

After delivery, blood will be infused from the placenta into the newborn if the baby is held below the mother's introitus. **Delayed cord clamping is recommended for 1 to 2 minutes.** For the preterm infant, in particular, allowing 1 to 2 minutes provides important benefits, such as improvement in circulatory and respiratory function, a reduction in the need for blood transfusion, and reduced risk of intraventricular hemorrhage. After the cord is clamped, the newborn is given to the mother for skin-to-skin contact. If the newborn is preterm and is stable after a brief period of skin-to-skin contact, it is placed under an infant warmer to prevent hypothermia.

Third Stage of Labor

Immediately after the baby's delivery (the end of the second stage of labor), the cervix and vagina should be thoroughly inspected for lacerations, and surgical repair should be performed when necessary. The cervix, vagina, and perineum may be more readily examined before the separation of the placenta, as no uterine bleeding should be present to obscure visualization. Attention is directed to any:

1. **Perineal lacerations that continue to bleed and need repair.** Lacerations, with or without episiotomy, may be classified as follows:
   a. **First degree:** a laceration involving the vaginal epithelium or perineal skin
   b. **Second degree:** a laceration extending into the subepithelial tissues of the vagina or perineum with or without involvement of the muscles of the perineal body

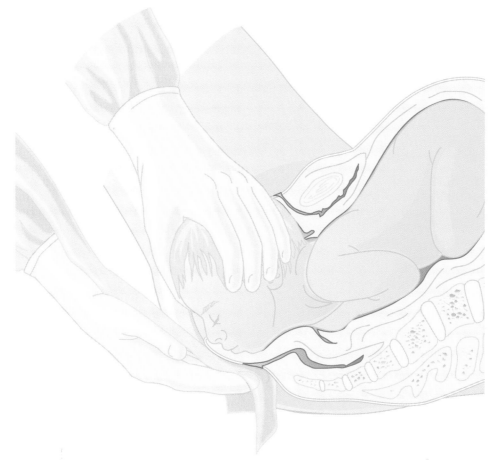

FIGURE 8-11 Ritgen maneuver. The fingers of the right hand, pressing posterior to the rectum, are used to extend the head while counterpressure is applied to the occiput by the left hand to allow a controlled delivery of the fetal head.

   c. **Third degree:** a laceration involving the anal sphincter
   d. **Fourth degree:** a laceration involving the rectal mucosa
2. **Cervical lacerations that are bleeding and need repair.**

DELIVERY OF THE PLACENTA. Separation of the placenta generally occurs within 2 to 10 minutes of the end of the second stage of labor (delivery of the baby). Squeezing the fundus to hasten placental separation is not recommended, because it may increase the likelihood of passage of fetal cells into the maternal circulation. **The initial step in the management of the third stage of labor for prevention of postpartum hemorrhage** is to begin an IV infusion of 40 U of Pitocin in 500 mL of saline at a rate of 10 mL/min for 5 minutes, followed by 1 to 2 mL/min until the patient is transferred to the postpartum unit.

   Signs of placental separation are as follows: (1) **a fresh show of blood** from the vagina, (2) **the umbilical cord lengthens** outside the vagina, (3) **the fundus rises up**, and (4) the **uterus becomes firm and globular.** Only when these signs have appeared should the assistant attempt traction on the cord. With gentle traction and counterpressure between the symphysis and fundus to prevent descent of the uterus into the pelvis, the placenta is delivered.

   The next appropriate step (after Pitocin infusion is started as mentioned above) is the application of uterine massage by either the physician or the nurse in attendance. If the patient is at risk for postpartum hemorrhage (e.g., because of anemia, prolonged oxytocic augmentation of labor, multiple gestation, macrosomia, or polyhydramnios), manual removal of the placenta and manual exploration of the uterus may be necessary.

   Finally, the placenta should be examined to ensure its complete removal (no missing cotyledons) and to detect placental abnormalities. Dilation and curettage may be necessary to evacuate retained placental tissue that is causing hemorrhaging.

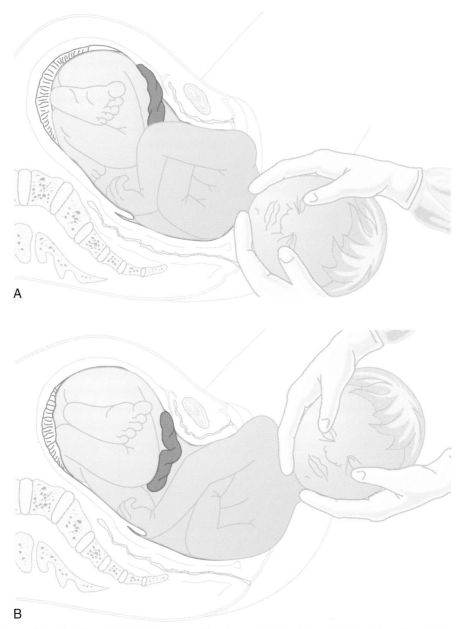

A

B

FIGURE 8-12 Delivery of the shoulders. **A,** Gentle downward traction on the head is applied to deliver the anterior shoulder. **B,** Gentle upward traction is used to deliver the posterior shoulder.

If an episiotomy has been performed (Figure 8-13), it should be repaired as illustrated in Figure 8-14. Absorbable sutures (size 00) should be used, and a rectal examination should be done to ensure that the sutures have not inadvertently transected the rectal mucosa. A third-degree tear (Figure 8-15) should be repaired as shown in Figure 8-16.

Fourth Stage of Labor

The hour immediately following delivery and the first 4 hours postpartum require continued close observa- **tion of the patient** to prevent postpartum hemorrhage. Blood pressure, pulse rate, and uterine blood loss must be monitored closely, and it is important to instruct the patient on massaging the uterus to maintain uterine tone. It is during this time that serious postpartum hemorrhage most commonly occurs, but some women may have frequent bleeding for up to 10 days postpartum, usually because of uterine relaxation, retained placental fragments, **or unrepaired lacerations.** An increase in pulse rate, often out of proportion to any decrease in blood pressure, may indicate hypovolemia.

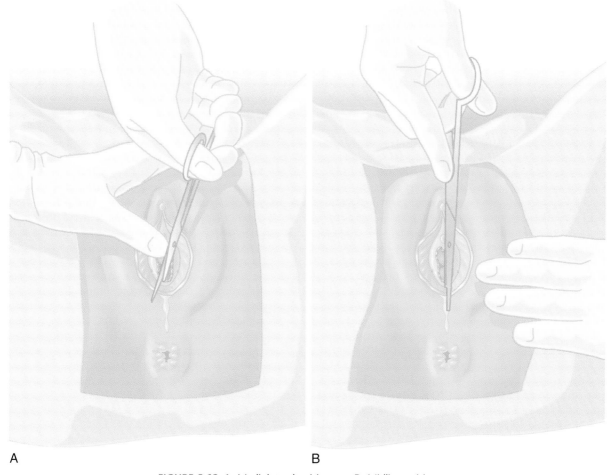

FIGURE 8-13 **A,** Mediolateral episiotomy. **B,** Midline episiotomy.

Puerperium

The puerperium consists of the period following delivery of the baby and placenta to approximately 6 weeks postpartum. During the puerperium, the reproductive organs and maternal physiology return to the prepregnancy state, although menses may not return for much longer.

ANATOMIC AND PHYSIOLOGIC CHANGES

Involution of the Uterus

Through a process of tissue catabolism, the uterus rapidly decreases in weight from about 1000 g at delivery to 100 to 200 g approximately 3 weeks postpartum. The cervix similarly loses its elasticity and regains its prepregnancy firmness. For the first few days after delivery, the uterine discharge (lochia) appears red **(lochia rubra),** because of the presence of erythrocytes. After 3 to 4 days, the lochia becomes paler **(lochia serosa),** and by the tenth day, it assumes a white or yellow-white color **(lochia alba).** Foul-smelling lochia suggests endometritis.

Vagina

Although the vagina may never return to its prepregnancy state, the supportive tissues of the pelvic floor gradually regain their former tone. Women who deliver vaginally should be taught and encouraged to perform Kegel exercises (intermittent tightening of the perineal muscles) to maintain and improve the supportive tissues of the pelvic floor.

Cardiovascular System

Immediately following delivery, there is a marked increase in peripheral vascular resistance because of the removal of the low-pressure uteroplacental circulatory shunt. The cardiac output and plasma volume gradually return to normal during the first 2 weeks of the puerperium. As a result of the loss of plasma volume and the diuresis of extracellular fluid, a marked weight loss occurs in the first week.

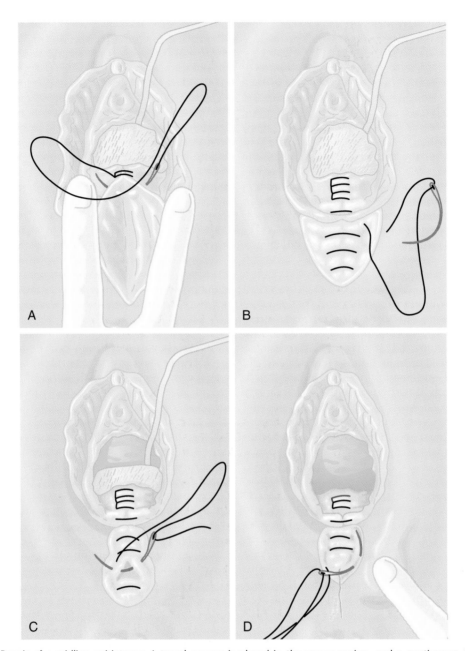

FIGURE 8-14 **A,** Repair of a midline episiotomy. A taped sponge is placed in the upper vagina, and a continuous, locked 00 or 000 absorbable suture is used to close the vaginal epithelium from the apex to the hymeneal ring. **B,** Three interrupted sutures are used to close the deep perineal fascia (of Colles) and underlying levator ani muscles. The vaginal epithelial suture is brought below the skin into the subcutaneous tissue. **C,** The same continuous suture is used to close the superficial fascia down to the anal edge of the episiotomy. **D,** The same suture is used as a subcuticular stitch brought back to the hymeneal ring, where it is doubly tied. The sponge is then removed (which is very important).

Psychosocial Changes

It is fairly common for women to exhibit a mild degree of depression a few days following delivery. The **"postpartum blues"** are probably due to both emotional and hormonal factors. **Recently, a relationship between vitamin D deficiency (<20 ng/mL) or insufficiency (20 to 29 ng/mL) and depression has been reported.** If a patient has symptoms of depression, she should be screened using the Edinburgh Postnatal Depression Scale. Vitamin D supplementation is safe, and at least 2000 to 3000 IU/day can be started following assessment of the level of the vitamin (25[OH]D) in the patient's serum. With understanding and reassurance from both family and physician, the patient's

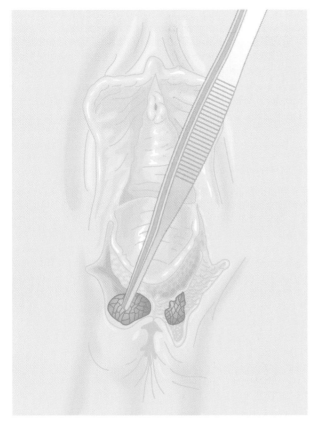

FIGURE 8-15 Third-degree perineal tear extending into the rectum and avulsing the circular rectal sphincter.

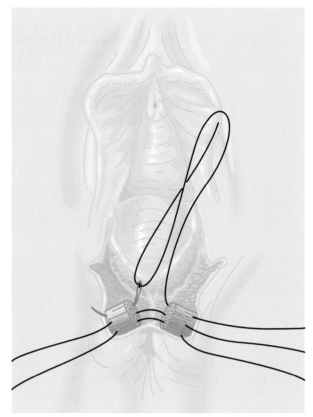

FIGURE 8-16 Repair of a third-degree tear involves approximating the fascia surrounding the rectal sphincter muscle and reapproximating the vaginal tears with locked continuous sutures. The process is then completed in the same way as with a midline episiotomy repair.

postpartum blues usually resolve without consequence. **Any prolonged episodes of depression during or after pregnancy should receive urgent attention.**

Return of Menstruation and Ovulation

In women who do not nurse, menstrual flow usually returns by 6 to 8 weeks, although this is highly variable. Although ovulation may not occur for several months, particularly in nursing mothers, contraceptive use should be emphasized during the puerperium to avoid an undesired pregnancy.

Breastfeeding

There are many advantages to breastfeeding. **First, breast milk is the ideal food for the newborn, is inexpensive, and is usually in good supply. Second, nursing accelerates the involution of the uterus** because suckling stimulates the release of oxytocin, thereby causing increased uterine contractions. **Third,** and probably most important, **there are immunologic advantages for the baby from breastfeeding.** Various types of maternal antibodies are present in breast milk. The predominant immunoglobulin is secretory immunoglobulin A (IgA), which provides protection in the infant's gut by preventing attachment of harmful bacteria (e.g., *Escherichia coli*) to cells on the mucosal surface. This prevents the bacteria from penetrating the bowel wall. It is also thought that maternal lymphocytes pass through the infant's gut wall and initiate immunologic processes that are not yet well understood. **Breastfeeding thereby provides the newborn with passive immunity** against certain infectious diseases until its own immune mechanisms become fully functional by 3 to 4 months. **Fourth, it is a way of transferring appropriate maternal bacteria to the infant's gut.** This also occurs as the infant swallows gut bacteria during its passage through the birth canal, but this does not occur if the baby is delivered by cesarean delivery. For the preterm infant, it is especially desirable to be born vaginally. The normal bacteria obtained assist in the prevention of necrotizing enterocolitis.

LACTATION

Various hormones, such as estrogen, progesterone, human chorionic gonadotropin (hCG), cortisol, insulin, prolactin, and placental lactogen, play an important role in preparing the breasts for lactation. **At delivery, two events are instrumental in initiating lactation. The first is the drop in placental hormones, particularly estrogen.** Before delivery, these hormones interfere with the lactogenic action of prolactin. **Second, suckling stimulates the release of prolactin and oxytocin.** The latter causes contraction of the myoepithelial cells in the alveoli and milk ducts. The suckling stimulus is thought to be important for milk production, as well as for the ejection of colostrum and milk.

On approximately the second day after delivery, **colostrum is secreted.** Its content is composed mostly of protein, fat, and minerals. It is the colostrum that contains secretory IgA. **After about 3 to 6 days, the colostrum is replaced by mature milk.** The content of milk varies considerably, depending on the nutritional status of the mother and the gestational age at the time of delivery. In general, the major components of breast milk are proteins, lactose, water, and fat. The major proteins synthesized in the human breast, which are unique and are not found in cow's milk, are casein, lactalbumin, and β-lactoglobulin. Essential amino acids are delivered via the mother's blood, and some of the nonessential amino acids can be synthesized in the breast. In addition, breast milk is a source of omega-3 fatty acids, which are important for early brain development.

LACTATION SUPPRESSION

When the mother chooses not to breastfeed, lactation suppression is indicated. **The simplest, and probably safest, method to accomplish this is to use a tight-fitting bra.** If breast distention does occur, pumping only makes the situation worse. Ice packs should be applied and the discomfort managed with analgesics.

COMPLICATIONS OF BREASTFEEDING

Cracked Nipples

If the nipples of the breast become fissured, nursing may become difficult. Because fissures are also a portal of entry for bacteria, they should be managed aggressively with a nipple shield and an appropriate cream, such as lanolin or Massé breast cream. Further breastfeeding should be temporarily stopped. Milk can be expressed manually until the nipples heal, at which time breastfeeding can be resumed.

Mastitis

This is an uncommon complication of breastfeeding and usually develops after 2 to 4 weeks. The first symptoms are usually slight fever and chills. These are followed by redness of a segment of the breast, which becomes indurated and painful. **The etiologic agent is usually *Staphylococcus aureus,* which originates from the infant's oral pharynx.** Milk should be obtained from the breast for culture and sensitivity,

and the mother should be started on a regimen of antibiotics immediately. **Because the majority of staphylococcal organisms are penicillinase-producing, a penicillinase-resistant antibiotic, such as dicloxacillin, should be used.** Breastfeeding may be discontinued but is not contraindicated. An appropriate antibiotic should be continued for 7 to 10 days. If a breast abscess ensues, it should be surgically drained. A breast pump can be used to maintain lactation until the infection has cleared if nursing is discontinued.

Drug Passage to the Newborn

Because an infant may ingest up to 500 mL of breast milk per day, maternally administered drugs that pass into breast milk may have a significant effect on the infant. The amount of drug found in breast milk depends on the maternal dose, the rate of maternal clearance, the physicochemical properties of the drug, and the composition of the breast milk with respect to fat and protein. The gestational age of the infant may also be a determinant of the ultimate drug effect. Table 8-6 lists selected drugs with their reported newborn effects.

Interconception Care

Women who have pregnancy complications, such as **preterm birth, preeclampsia, intrauterine growth restriction, gestational diabetes, obesity, and perinatal death,** are at greater risk of having the same problems with subsequent pregnancies. Programs now offer comprehensive **interconception care** to address conditions that have been shown to cause poor outcomes by providing interventions that could mitigate or eliminate any recurrence and/or improve the long-term health of the mother. The rationale for this approach is to provide continuous obstetric care rather than episodic care triggered by another pregnancy. Studies are underway to determine the value of these programs.

Obstetric Analgesia and Anesthesia

The goal of obstetric analgesia and anesthesia is to provide effective pain relief for the mother during the course of labor and delivery that is safe for her and her baby and that has minimal or no adverse effects on the progress and outcome of labor. Anesthetic practices have evolved to include an increased reliance on highly effective and safe regional anesthetic techniques, using low-concentration combinations of narcotics and local anesthetics to minimize the adverse effects of each. Maternal anesthetic risk has also declined because of the increased safety of regional over general anesthesia for cesarean deliveries. **Maternal mortality because of anesthesia has decreased to less than 1 in 500,000 mothers.**

TABLE 8-6

EFFECTS OF MATERNAL DRUG INGESTION ON BREASTFEEDING INFANTS

Drug	Reported Infant Effects
Sedative-Hypnotics	
Diazepam	Sedation
Antipsychotics	
Chlorpromazine	No adverse effects reported
Haloperidol	No adverse effects reported
Nonnarcotic Analgesics	
Acetaminophen	No adverse effects reported
Salicylates	Theoretical risk of platelet dysfunction
Anticonvulsants	
Phenobarbital	Sedation
Phenytoin	Sedation, decreased sucking
Narcotics	
Heroin	May cause addiction
Methadone	Infant death reported
Meperidine	No adverse effects reported
Antibiotics	
Penicillin	May modify bowel flora, cause allergy, or interfere with sepsis workup
Ampicillin	Same as for penicillin
Erythromycin	Same as for penicillin
Nitrofurantoin	Theoretical risk of hemolytic anemia in infants with G6PD deficiency
Tetracycline	Same as for penicillin; theoretical risk of discoloration of teeth and inhibition of bone growth
Digoxin	No adverse effects reported
Thyroid Drugs	
Thyroxine	May interfere with screening for hypothyroidism
Propylthiouracil	Nodular goiter
Antihypertensives	
Methyldopa	No adverse effects reported
Propranolol	No adverse effects reported
Theophylline	One case of infant irritability following maternal administration of a rapidly absorbed oral preparation

G6PD, Glucose-6-phosphate dehydrogenase.

UTERINE BLOOD FLOW

Uterine blood flow at term accounts for 700 to 900 mL/min (about 12% of maternal cardiac output) and is not autoregulated. Regional analgesia or anesthesia may increase uterine blood flow, especially in patients with preeclampsia, by relieving pain and stress and reducing circulating catecholamines. Regional analgesia or anesthesia may also decrease uterine blood flow if

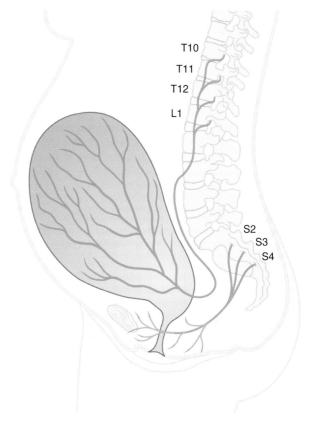

FIGURE 8-17 Pain pathways of parturition: T10 to L1 supply innervation to the uterus, L1 to S4 supply pain pathways to the vagina and deep pelvic structures, and S2 to S4 supply nerve fibers to the pudendal nerve.

hypotension occurs and is not properly and promptly treated. Adequate hydration (e.g., 1000 mL of lactated Ringer solution) 30 to 60 minutes before regional anesthesia helps to improve uterine blood flow and mitigate the risk of hypotension. If hypotension does occur (≥15% below baseline or <100 mm Hg systolic blood pressure), a vasopressor (e.g., 10 mg of IV ephedrine) will typically restore maternal blood pressure and uterine blood flow.

PAIN PATHWAYS

The pain pathways of parturition are shown in Figure 8-17.

ADVERSE EFFECTS OF LABOR PAIN

Maternal hyperventilation during contractions causes respiratory alkalosis that results in (1) a shift of the oxyhemoglobin dissociation curve to the left, (2) increased affinity of maternal hemoglobin for oxygen, and (3) decreased oxygen offloading to the fetus. The cyclic nature of contraction pain may cause a hyperventilation-hypoventilation syndrome whereby the mother blows off so much carbon dioxide during a contraction that she **hypoventilates between contractions** and may even become mildly hypoxemic between contractions. This syndrome is exacerbated by systemic narcotics because they do not adequately relieve the pain of the contraction but do add to the respiratory depression between contractions. **Hypoxemia between contractions** may be attenuated by providing supplemental oxygen. Finally, **labor pain results in increased levels of circulating catecholamines.** The α-adrenergic effects of the catecholamines may reduce uterine blood flow, and the β₂-adrenergic effects may impair uterine contractility.

OPTIONS FOR LABOR PAIN RELIEF

Nonpharmacologic methods include education and psychoprophylaxis (Lamaze method), emotional support, back massage, hydrotherapy, biofeedback, transcutaneous electrical nerve stimulation (TENS), acupuncture, and hypnosis (hypnobirthing). Scientific assessment of these methods has yielded inconsistent results. **In most studies, acupuncture has been found to decrease pain.** These techniques tend to work best early in the first stage of labor, when the pain is least intense, and may decrease pharmacologic usage at that time.

Pharmacologic treatment options include parenteral narcotics, regional analgesia (epidural, spinal, combined spinal-epidural, paracervical, caudal, and pudendal nerve blocks) and inhalational analgesics (nitrous oxide).

Parenteral narcotics have very limited efficacy for the relief of labor pain. They work best in the early first stage, when the pain is primarily visceral and less intense. **All opioids readily cross the placental barrier** and may cause neonatal respiratory depression, depending on the dose and timing relative to delivery. They may also cause decreased fetal heart rate variability (due to narcotic effect) and impaired neonatal breastfeeding. **Fentanyl** and **nalbuphine** are the most commonly used and have short neonatal half-lives. **Remifentanil,** an ultra-short-acting narcotic, may be used for IV patient-controlled analgesia when regional anesthesia is contraindicated. In addition, remifentanil has been used for routine obstetric analgesia in the United Kingdom, with several case reports of associated respiratory arrest.

Neuraxial analgesia (medication injected into the spinal column) is undoubtedly the most effective form of labor pain relief. **Lumbar epidural analgesia is the most common form of neuraxial analgesia,** and its use continues to increase nationally. It may be used to provide pain relief for the first and second stages of labor and, by injecting a higher concentration of local anesthetic, the block may be intensified and extended to provide surgical anesthesia for cesarean delivery or postpartum tubal ligation. There is no fixed cervical dilation at which it is appropriate to provide epidural analgesia, as long as the patient is having regular, painful contractions. Modern epidural management includes an initial bolus of local anesthetic bupivacaine, ropivacaine, or lidocaine, as well as narcotics such as fentanyl or sufentanil to achieve a T10 sensory level, followed by an infusion of a dilute solution of the same agents until delivery. Pain during the first stage of labor is conducted along the sympathetic fibers, entering the spinal cord between T10 and L1. Dilute solutions can be used that permit ambulation, referred to as the "walking epidural." **The goal is to avoid motor block** to minimize any adverse effects on maternal expulsive efforts in the second stage of labor. **Combined spinal-epidural** is a technique that has gained popularity for both labor analgesia and repeat cesarean deliveries. It provides rapid onset of analgesia and/or anesthesia and the prolonged administration capability of an epidural catheter.

A pudendal nerve block anesthetizes somatic afferent nerve fibers entering the spinal cord at sacral segments S2 to S4. It **is usually effective at relieving the perineal pain of the second stage of labor,** as well as the pain of episiotomy and episiotomy repair. It does not affect the ongoing pain of uterine contractions.

ANESTHESIA FOR CESAREAN DELIVERY

The type of anesthesia selected for cesarean delivery is determined by the urgency of the surgery, the presence or absence of a preexisting epidural catheter for labor, the patient's medical condition, pregnancy-related complications, and the presence of any contraindications to regional anesthesia. Absolute and relative contraindications to regional anesthesia are listed in Box 8-1. All patients requiring anesthesia for surgery must have an airway examination, regardless of how urgent the surgery is. A brief history must also be elicited. **If the history or the physical examination suggests that the intubation will be difficult (Box 8-2), then the patient must be given a regional anesthetic or have an awake intubation or the operation must be started with the patient under local anesthesia.**

All patients should be premedicated with a non-particulate antacid. Routine monitors are placed,

---

BOX 8-1

CONTRAINDICATIONS TO REGIONAL ANESTHESIA

Absolute Contraindications

Patient refusal
Coagulopathy
Infection at needle insertion site
Severe hypovolemia with ongoing blood loss

Relative Contraindications (Selected)

Prior back surgery (including Harrington rod placement)
Certain cardiac lesions, especially aortic stenosis
Increased intracranial pressure

BOX 8-2

FACTORS SUGGESTING DIFFICULT INTUBATION

Obesity and/or short neck
Neck flexion and/or extension limitations at atlantooccipital joint
Short chin–hyoid distance (receding chin)
Limited mouth opening
Poor dentition and/or buck teeth
Excess oropharyngeal tissues (see the uvula and tonsillar pillars)
Large tongue

TABLE 8-7

OBSTETRIC ANESTHESIA-RELATED MATERNAL COMPLICATIONS, UNITED STATES, 2004-2009

Complication	Incidence
Arrest	1:128,400
Abscess/meningitis	1:6300
Death	0:257,000
Epidural hematoma	1:251,500
Failed intubation	1:533
High neuraxial block	1:4400
Neurologic Injury	1:36,000
Respiratory arrest	1:10,000

From D'Angelo R, Smiley RM, Riley ET, et al: Serious complications related to obstetric anesthesia. *Anesthesiology* 120:1505–1512, 2014.

TABLE 8-8

COMPARISON OF SPINAL AND EPIDURAL ANESTHESIA

Spinal	Epidural
Advantages	
Faster	Can tailor duration to need
Technically easier	Lower chance of postdural puncture headache
More reliable Defined endpoint	Slower onset Beneficial in patients with cardiac and hypertensive disorders
Minimal chance of patchy block	Faster offset; discharge to room sooner
Denser block	
Lower drug exposure for mother and fetus	
No chance of systemic toxicity	
Disadvantages	
Defined (limited) duration	Slower onset
Higher chance of postdural puncture headache (limited by use of small-bore, pencil-point needles)	Higher risk of systemic toxicity because of accidental intravenous injection
	Risk of high spinal from inadvertent intrathecal or subdural injection
	Risk of "patchy block" from inadequate or asymmetrical dermatomal spread

including a noninvasive blood pressure monitor, electrocardiograph, and pulse oximeter, and adequate left uterine displacement must be instituted. Supplemental oxygen is provided. A crystalloid preload bolus of 10 to 15 mL/kg over 30 to 60 minutes is typically given before regional anesthesia.

For elective or urgent cesarean delivery (nonemergency), regional anesthesia is preferable because the airway is maintained. Complications involving loss of the airway are the leading causes of anesthesia-related maternal mortality and are usually associated with general anesthesia. General anesthesia carries a 1.7-fold higher risk of anesthesia-related maternal mortality than regional anesthesia. Potential complications of obstetric anesthesia are listed in Table 8-7. Women in labor have a higher risk of airway complications than nonpregnant patients because they have (1) a twofold higher chance of failed intubation; (2) a 60% increased oxygen consumption; (3) a decreased functional residual capacity, resulting in a lower oxygen store; and (4) a potentially increased risk of aspiration.

If no epidural is in place, a spinal block is frequently used. A comparison of the characteristics of spinal and epidural anesthesia is shown in Table 8-8.

General anesthesia is employed for cesarean delivery in three situations: (1) there is extreme urgency and no preexisting epidural catheter, (2) there is a contraindication to regional anesthesia, or (3) regional anesthesia has failed (1.7% incidence). When a relative contraindication to regional anesthesia is present, the benefits of regional anesthesia frequently outweigh the risks in the pregnant patient.

The protocol for general anesthesia for cesarean delivery includes **oral administration of nonparticulate antacid** (sodium citrate), routine monitoring and **left uterine displacement, preoxygenation** for at least four vital capacity breaths, and **rapid sequence induction of anesthesia with cricoid pressure** followed by **intubation to prevent passive regurgitation and pulmonary aspiration of gastric contents.** Once the correct position of the endotracheal tube has been confirmed by end-tidal CO_2 and auscultation of the lungs, surgery may begin.

Induction agents used for general anesthesia include **propofol** (most commonly), **thiopental** (not currently available in the United States), **etomidate** (when cardiovascular stability is particularly desirable), and **ketamine** (for patients with hypovolemia or asthma). The muscle relaxant used to facilitate intubation is **succinylcholine** (unless contraindicated), because of its rapid onset and brief duration of action. If contraindicated, vecuronium or rocuronium may be used. **Oxygen delivery is maintained at 50-100% until delivery if the baby is stressed.** Nitrous oxide may be added. After induction, a potent inhalational agent is administered at a modest level (0.5 minimum alveolar concentration) to minimize myometrial relaxation. **Narcotics may be administered after the delivery of the baby** to reduce the need for inhalational anesthesia and provide postoperative pain relief. **The patient must be extubated only when fully awake to minimize the risk of aspiration.**

PATIENTS WHO BENEFIT FROM EARLY ANESTHETIC CONSULTATION

General anesthesia can usually be avoided if an epidural catheter is already in place, so it is helpful to identify those patients who are at increased risk of requiring surgery (e.g., breech presentation, multiple gestation, prematurity, poor fetal heart rate tracing [Categories II and III; see Box 9-1], severe preeclampsia, morbid obesity) and those patients who would pose an especially high anesthetic risk. Such patients should be advised to get an epidural catheter early to avoid the risks of a crash cesarean under general anesthesia. These fetuses may also benefit from the improved uterine blood flow and controlled delivery that epidural analgesia allows.

Mothers who are at particularly high anesthetic risk should receive a prelabor consultation for known significant preexisting medical conditions (e.g., difficult airway [Box 8-2]; significant respiratory, cardiac, hematologic or neurologic disease; spinal surgery; and suspected or known susceptibility to malignant hyperthermia).

UNINTENDED CONSEQUENCES OF REGIONAL ANESTHESIA AND/OR ANALGESIA

Patients who receive epidural analgesia for labor pain have a similar duration of the first stage of labor, but the second stage may be prolonged by 15 minutes on average. Theoretically, a prolongation of the second stage could arise from effects on the release of endogenous oxytocin, prostaglandin $F_{2\alpha}$, and other hormones responsible for the propagation of labor. Prolongation of the second stage could also be due to **impaired ability to push** (unlikely as long as motor block is avoided by appropriate adjustment of the epidural infusion) or to **decreased maternal urge to push** caused by sensory blockade. The latter can usually be overcome by appropriate coaching and decreasing or halting the epidural infusion.

Other side effects and complications of regional anesthesia or analgesia include fever ($0.5°$ C increase), **headache, and backache.** The association with maternal fever may be due to (1) an alteration in the thermoregulatory threshold, (2) interference with peripheral thermoreceptor input to the central nervous system, (3) shifting heat calories from the core to the periphery by vasodilation, (4) an imbalance between maternal heat production and loss (decreased hyperventilation, decreased lower body sweating, and increased shivering), or (5) preexisting increased interleukin-6 and tumor necrosis factor-α levels, which predispose the mother to maternal fever in the presence of regional blocks. The average temperature increase is small, and most women do not develop fever; however, a small subset of women who are predisposed to develop fever do so after epidural administration.

The risk of headache is about 1-2% with spinal anesthesia, and it is less than 1% with an epidural. It occurs when there is an unintended dural puncture ("wet tap"). **Postdural puncture headaches are self-limited, usually resolving within 5 to 7 days.** Cerebrospinal fluid leaks through the hole in the dura, resulting in low intracranial pressure. **The hallmark is a severe _positional_ headache:** little or no headache if supine, but sudden onset of severe headache when sitting upright or standing. The dural hole will heal in about 1 week, or it can be sealed with an epidural blood patch. Symptomatic treatment includes narcotics, nonsteroidal antiinflammatory drugs, caffeine, sumatriptan, and/or an abdominal binder.

There appears to be no association between new-onset, long-term back pain and labor epidural analgesia. The risk of new, chronic back pain in parturients is high (up to 47%), regardless of whether they have had an epidural. Pelvic girdle pain is common during pregnancy and postpartum (>25%), with 26-82% of patients having MRI evidence of levator ani tears or a fracture of the pubic bone.

Resuscitation of the Newborn

Improved surveillance using antenatal and intrapartum fetal heart rate monitoring, real-time ultrasonography, amniocentesis, and umbilical artery Doppler assessments has allowed the clinician to recognize the fetus at risk who may need special care at birth. The goals of an organized approach to neonatal resuscitation are to reverse any intrauterine hypoxia and to prevent postnatal asphyxia, which may result in acute major organ damage and lifelong handicaps.

Preparation for Extrauterine Life

Prematurity is the leading cause of poor neonatal outcome because the fetus has not yet progressed through complete stages of anatomic development and biochemical maturation. Even the fetus delivered at term undergoes changes before and with the onset of labor.

During pregnancy, fetal thyroxine (T_4) is converted to reverse triiodothyronine (T_3), which is metabolically inactive. **Several days before the onset of term labor, cortisol levels increase in the fetus and induce a change in thyroid hormone dynamics. Cortisol induces the enzyme system, allowing the conversion of T_4 to triiodothyronine (T_3), which is metabolically more active and necessary for neonatal thermogenesis.** At birth, there is a surge of thyroid-stimulating hormone, and at no time during life does this hormone reach such high levels as it does 30 minutes after birth. This is followed by a hyperthyroid neonatal state for several days, which is necessary for the newborn to maintain its body temperature.

A second change that occurs with the onset of labor is a change in fetal breathing activity. Fetal breathing, as observed by real-time ultrasonography, is rarely observed once labor is established. This is thought to be associated with a decrease in pulmonary fluid dynamics that may be important for the onset of respiration after delivery, as well as with the retention of surfactant in the lungs.

Finally, labor is a stress to the fetus that stimulates the release of catecholamines. This may be responsible for the mobilization of glucose, lung fluid absorption, alterations in the perfusion of organ systems, and, possibly, the onset of respiration. Only at times of severe stress later in life are catecholamine levels as high as those at birth.

ETIOLOGY OF NEONATAL CARDIORESPIRATORY DEPRESSION

At term, 1% of infants will require vigorous resuscitation (positive pressure ventilation for more than 1 minute), with 10% requiring some assistance. At earlier stages of gestation, almost all infants require some type of supportive care.

FACILITATING NEONATAL ADAPTATION

The American Congress of Obstetricians and Gynecologists and the American Society of Anesthesiologists have made joint statements that **a qualified provider other than the obstetrician or anesthesiologist should be responsible for neonatal resuscitation.** All nurses working in the delivery room should be trained in techniques of neonatal assessment and resuscitation. If risk factors increase the likelihood of delivering an infant with cardiorespiratory depression, a pediatrician trained in neonatal resuscitation should be present.

Following delivery of a normal newborn, the following important steps should occur:

1. Clear the Airway

Descent through the birth canal causes compression of the chest wall, resulting in the discharge of fluid from the mouth and nose. When the head emerges from the vagina, the physician should use a towel or gauze pad to remove secretions from the face. In addition, bulb suction may be used to aspirate secretions from the oropharynx. **Initially, the mouth is suctioned before the nose so that no material is present to aspirate with the first breaths. Deep or vigorous suction should be avoided because posterior pharyngeal stimulation may cause bradycardia from a vagal reflex.** If a moderate amount of meconium is present, placing a nasal tracheal catheter into the oropharynx and applying suction before delivering the body are thought to decrease the risk of meconium aspiration. **If meconium is present and the baby is not vigorous (heart rate >100 beats/min, strong respiratory effort, and good muscular tone), intubation should be performed to suction the trachea after suction of the mouth.**

2. Dry the Newborn

An important part of neonatal adaptation is the initiation of nonshivering thermogenesis. Excessive cooling from exposure of the wet skin is detrimental to all preterm infants and to depressed full-term infants. The newborn should be placed in a preheated environment and dried off with a towel before cutting the cord. This also serves to stimulate the onset of respiration.

3. Clamp the Cord

The umbilical arteries usually close spontaneously within 45 to 60 seconds after birth, whereas the umbilical vein remains patent for 3 to 5 minutes or longer. Delayed cord clamping has been known for decades to confer benefit to the fetus.

4. Ensure Onset of Respiration

The onset of respiration normally occurs within a few seconds after birth. **If respiration has not commenced by 30 seconds, or if the heart rate is less than 100 beats/min, after delayed cord clamping, the infant should be passed off to the resuscitation team to manage the apnea and low heart rate with stimulation, and positive pressure ventilation should be started.** If the baby is delivered at term, 21% oxygen (room air) should be used initially and adjusted upward as measured by pulse oximetry or clinically assessed in terms of nonresponsiveness to resuscitation. **If the infant is preterm, 30-40% oxygen should be used initially** in association with pulse oximetry, and the oxygen concentration should be adjusted to the saturation expected relative to the number of minutes after birth (Figure 8-18). A newborn normally starts with an oxygen saturation of 60-65% at birth (by pulse oximetry), and this increases to 85-95% saturation over the first 10 minutes of life. **Excessive oxygen delivery following hypoxia is associated with retinopathy in about 5-15% of infants, and newborn lung**

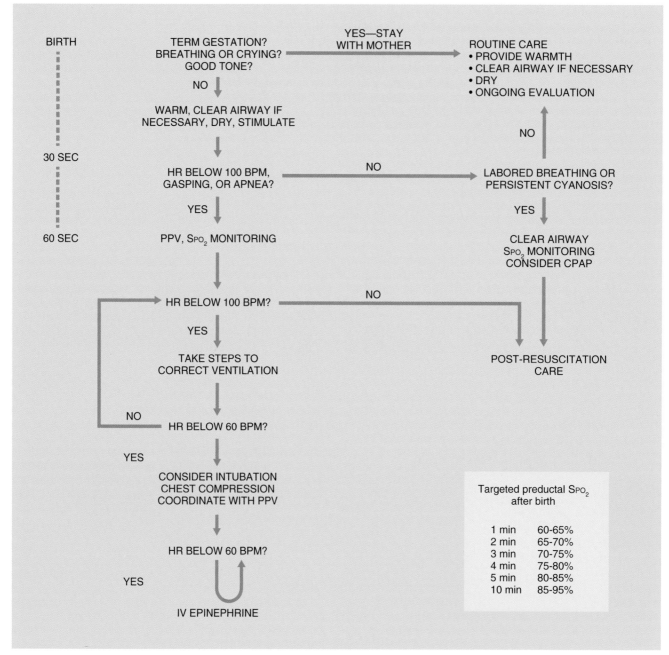

FIGURE 8-18 A time-based approach to the resuscitation of a normal and apneic or cyanotic newborn. *BPM*, Beats per minute; *CPAP*, continuous positive airway pressure; *HR*, heart rate; *IV*, intravenous; *PPV*, positive pressure ventilation; *SPO₂*, peripheral arterial oxygen saturation. (American Academy of Pediatrics, American Heart Association: *Textbook of neonatal resuscitation,* ed 6, Elk Grove Village, IL, and Dallas, TX, 2011, American Academy of Pediatrics and American Heart Association.)

injury (bronchopulmonary dysplasia) may also be a problem. These injuries are especially likely to occur if the infant is preterm.

5. Correct Surfactant Deficiency

For the premature infant, surfactant deficiency is the basic defect responsible for the development of the respiratory distress syndrome. Exogenous surfactant replacement varies from synthetic surfactant to modified or unmodified extracts of natural surfactant. These substances can be given by tracheal injection at birth to prevent the respiratory distress syndrome, or they can be given after the syndrome has developed to reduce its severity and to prevent mortality.

TABLE 8-9

APGAR SCORE FOR DETERMINING THE CONDITION OF A NEWBORN INFANT

Sign	Score		
	0	1	2
1. Heart rate	Absent	<100 beats/min	>100 beats/min
2. Respiratory effort	Absent	Slow, weak cry	Good, strong cry
3. Muscle tone	Limp	Some flexion of extremities	Active motion
4. Reflex irritability (response to stimulation of sole of foot)	None	Grimace	Strong cry
5. Color	Pale, blue	Body, pink; extremities, blue	Completely pink

Apgar Score

The Apgar score is an excellent tool for assessing the overall status of the newborn soon after birth (1 minute) and after a 5-minute period of observation (Table 8-9). A normal Apgar score is 7 or greater at 1 minute and 9 or 10 at 5 minutes.

Resuscitation of the Asphyxiated Infant

During the past 15 years, increasing emphasis has been placed on transferring the mother with a high-risk pregnancy to a tertiary care regional center before labor rather than transferring the sick neonate after delivery.

Ideally, at the time of delivery, **a segment of cord should be doubly clamped to allow blood gas determinations** on cord arterial and venous blood. These measurements serve as a baseline to assess the severity of the neonatal hypoxia and acidosis.

SEQUENCE OF PROCEDURES

A stepwise sequence of procedures is necessary to enable a smooth transition to an adult circulation pattern and a normal metabolic state (see Figure 8-18).

1. Establish an Airway

After placing the newborn in a preheated radiant warmer, the airway should be opened by slightly extending the neck. **In any infant with a high likelihood of asphyxia, suctioning of the airway should be initiated after the delivery of the head.** The asphyxiated neonate usually has meconium present in the upper airway, which may be cleared with an oral suction catheter (DeLee trap) before delivery of the shoulders. **Immediately following the delivery, an endotracheal tube should be inserted** to remove thick mucus or meconium from the trachea and upper airway, unless the infant is vigorous (see above).

2. Initiate Breathing

The indications for positive pressure ventilation include apnea, gasping, and a heart rate less than 100 beats/min. With an established airway, either bag-mask ventilation or ventilation via an endotracheal tube should be initiated at a rate of 40 to 60 breaths/min. Usually, the heart rate increases rapidly after the apnea is corrected, and intermittent bag-mask ventilation with supplemental oxygen can be given until spontaneous respiration commences. In premature infants (<32 weeks), oxygen of 100% or less should be commenced and titrated to an oxygen saturation in the infant of 85-95%.

3. Ensure Cardiac Performance

If cardiac performance is poor (heart rate <60 beats/min after 30 seconds of positive pressure ventilation with oxygen titrated to saturation), external cardiac massage should be initiated. **The best technique for cardiac massage in the newborn is to compress the lower third of the sternum with two thumbs with the hands around the chest.** A compression should occur every half-second, with an interposed ventilation after every third compression (3:1 ratio), resulting in 90 chest compressions and 30 ventilations per minute. The sternum should be depressed to a depth of approximately one-third the anteroposterior diameter of the chest, typically 2 to 2.5 cm in a full-term infant and 1.5 to 2.0 cm in a preterm neonate. Cardiac arrest is rare. **If cardiac massage and artificial ventilation are not successful in reestablishing cardiac function, an endotracheal or IV injection of a dilute solution of epinephrine must be given.** When the heart rate is above 60 beats/min, sternal compression may be discontinued while ventilation is continued.

4. Correct Biochemical Abnormalities

ACIDOSIS. In the case of a very sick newborn, an umbilical arterial catheter should be placed and blood gas analyses performed to monitor the severity of the acidosis and the effectiveness of the resuscitation. Severe

TABLE 8-10

DRUGS USED TO RESUSCITATE THE NEONATE

Medication	Concentration to Administer	Preparation	Dosage and Route	Rate and Precautions
Epinephrine	1:10,000	1 mL	0.01-0.03 mg/kg 0.1-0.3 mL/kg IV or ET	Give rapidly May dilute with normal saline to 1-2 mL if given via ET May give up to 3 times IV dose if given via ET
Volume expanders	PRBC Normal saline Ringer lactate	40 mL	10 mL/kg IV	Give over 5-10 min Give by syringe or IV drip
Sodium bicarbonate	0.5 mEq/mL (4.2% solution)	20 mL or two 10 mL prefilled syringes	2 mEq/kg IV only (4 mL/kg)	Give slowly over at least 2 minutes Give only if infant is being effectively ventilated
Naloxone hydrochloride	0.4 mg/mL	1 mL	0.1 mg/kg (0.25 mL/kg) IV, ET, IM, SC	Giving rapidly is acceptable

ET, Endotracheal tube; *IM,* intramuscular; *IV,* intravenous; *PRBC,* packed red blood cells; *SC,* subcutaneous.

acidosis can be corrected by the infusion of sodium bicarbonate if ventilation is adequate.

ANEMIA. On rare occasions, the newborn may have abnormal perfusion secondary to blood loss (e.g., from vasa previa, abruptio placentae, or a fetomaternal transfusion), which can be corrected only by immediate transfusion with blood (packed red blood cells). A solution of normal saline or lactated Ringer solution can be used to temporarily maintain an adequate vascular volume.

NARCOTIC DEPRESSION. Respiratory depression secondary to medication is unusual with the increased use of conduction anesthesia. If neonatal respiratory depression from excessive use of narcotics is suspected, naloxone (Narcan) is an effective antidote. Intramuscular administration is just as effective as, and easier to administer than, IV dosing. Table 8-10 lists the drugs that are commonly used in resuscitation and their dosages.

HYPOGLYCEMIA. Hypoglycemia can also contribute to unsuccessful resuscitation, especially in infants with intrauterine growth restriction or whose mothers have diabetes. Glucose administration should be considered after the other issues have been addressed. **The use of high concentrations of glucose (e.g., 25-50%) is contraindicated in asphyxiated newborns because the glucose is converted to lactic acid in the absence of oxygen, which may increase the likelihood of brain damage. Concentrated glucose solutions may also cause brain swelling.** If glucose is required, its concentration should not exceed 10%.

OTHER FACTORS. Following a systematic resuscitative effort, other contributing factors must be identified if cardiorespiratory depression persists. **Hypothermia** is one of the most critical aggravating factors, and temperature control must be continuously supported. A **pneumothorax** is not uncommon following a difficult resuscitation. It must be recognized promptly and decompressed with a chest tube. Also, a **diaphragmatic hernia** can result in the displacement of the stomach, bowel, or both into the thoracic cavity. Decreased breath sounds and failure to improve pulmonary function should alert the team to this possibility.

NEONATAL RESPIRATORY FAILURE

Neonates in imminent danger of death from a narrow range of conditions causing hypoxemia and respiratory distress not responsive to conventional forms of therapy are candidates for **extracorporeal membrane oxygenation.** The lives of infants with a congenital diaphragmatic hernia, severe meconium aspiration, or other forms of persistent pulmonary hypertension have been saved using this procedure performed in selected regional centers. Data concerning long-term outcomes of infants treated with extracorporeal membrane oxygenation remain limited. **Carotid artery and/or jugular vein ligation, prolonged anticoagulation, and long-term circulatory bypass are necessary with this procedure, and concerns exist about their long-term consequences.**

LONG-TERM OUTCOME

Low birth weight (<2500 g), whether the result of prematurity or of intrauterine growth restriction, is an independent risk factor for cerebral palsy. By contrast, for infants weighing more than 2500 g, Apgar scores less than or equal to 3 at 5 minutes are generally not associated with an increased risk of cerebral palsy, provided that there is no associated obstetric complication. If both a low Apgar score and an obstetric complication such as severe fetal distress and/or chorioamnionitis are present, there is an increased risk of cerebral palsy.

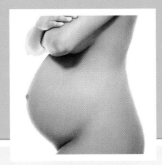

Fetal Surveillance during Labor

CALVIN J. HOBEL • AMY R. LAMB

CLINICAL KEYS FOR THIS CHAPTER

- The most important principle of both fetal and maternal surveillance during labor is that childbirth is a normal process, and the majority of laboring women and their fetuses will have a safe journey. Obstetricians must be aware of each patient's past history and be prepared to monitor the journey based upon maternal and fetal needs during the labor process.
- Simple auscultation of the fetal heart rate in accordance with specific guidelines is acceptable to assess the health of the fetus. Continuous fetal heart rate and uterine activity monitoring have the advantage of providing continuous electronic records throughout the labor process but may not always be necessary.
- The pathophysiology of abnormal fetal heart rate patterns is complex, and both clinical and research findings suggest that hypoxia, acidosis, and inflammation form a

triad of mixed metabolic dysregulation that may increase the risk of early (during delivery) and late (during childhood) physical and mental abnormalities.

- To improve our understanding of the assessment of abnormal and potentially pathologic heart rate patterns, the National Institutes of Health (NIH) has developed a three-tier fetal heart rate interpretation system (normal, intermediate, and abnormal). This is designed to improve the recognition of risk for poor fetal outcomes and to allow implementation of strategies for effective intervention.
- Abnormal fetal heart rate tracings associated with hypoxia, acidosis, and inflammation have five characteristics: (1) absent base line variability, (2) recurrent late decelerations, (3) recurrent variable decelerations, (4) bradycardia, and (5) sinusoidal patterns.

Effective fetal surveillance during labor is an essential element of good obstetric care. On the basis of the antepartum maternal history, physical examination, and laboratory data, 20-30% of pregnancies may be designated high risk, and 50% of perinatal morbidity and mortality occurs in this group. **The remaining 50% of morbidity and mortality occurs in pregnancies that are considered to be normal at the onset of labor.** Although fetal heart rate (FHR) monitoring by auscultation or continuous electronic fetal monitoring (EFM) provides useful information that improves the management of labor and reduces perinatal morbidity and mortality, evidence about its complete adequacy for fetal surveillance is conflicting.

The pathogenesis of abnormal FHR patterns is complex and remains poorly understood. In the past, it was felt that hypoxia was the main cause of abnormal FHR patterns and that continuous EFM and fetal scalp sampling would reliably identify those fetuses at greatest risk. However, a decrease in the incidence of cerebral palsy, one of the most serious complications

associated with pregnancy and childbirth, has not occurred with increased monitoring.

This chapter provides the current concepts and recognized standards for appropriate fetal surveillance during labor.

Methods of Monitoring Fetal Heart Rate

AUSCULTATION OF THE FETAL HEART RATE

The time-honored technique for evaluating the fetus during labor has been auscultation of the FHR. The first step in deciding on the optimal method (auscultation or continuous EFM) is to determine whether a patient has any risk factors. **Auscultation of the fetal heart is performed by listening from the beginning of one contraction to the beginning of the next contraction.** For low-risk patients, a competent nurse should listen every 30 minutes during the first stage of labor and at least every 15 minutes in the second stage of labor. For high-risk patients, the FHR should be assessed every 15 minutes during the first stage of labor and every 5 minutes during the second stage. Some studies have suggested that intermittent auscultation of the fetal heart is comparable to continuous electronic monitoring, in terms of neonatal outcome, if performed at the intervals stated above with a 1 : 1 patient-to-nurse ratio.

CONTINUOUS ELECTRONIC FETAL HEART RATE MONITORING

EFM during labor was developed to detect FHR patterns frequently associated with delivery of infants in a depressed condition. It was reasoned that early recognition of changes in FHR patterns that are associated with hypoxia and umbilical cord compression would serve as a warning that would enable a physician to intervene and prevent fetal death or irreversible brain injury.

Pathophysiology of Abnormal Fetal Heart Rate Patterns

The focus of EFM has been on the recognition that hypoxia leads to a greater risk of acidosis, which can be identified by fetal scalp blood sampling during labor and cord blood gas analysis at delivery. **Today, the cause of abnormal FHR patterns is thought to be more complex and probably related to a combination of hypoxia, acidosis, and inflammation** that subjects all physiologic systems (brain, heart, placenta, blood vessels, and the fetal adrenal gland) to multisystem dysregulation and is associated with a complex array of FHR perturbations. These changes in heart rate are difficult to interpret without better ways to define the most optimal biomarkers that identify the fetus at highest risk. **Important maternal and fetal biomarkers of current research interest are inflammatory markers (such as C-reactive protein) and vitamin D deficiency.**

EFM allows continuous reporting of the FHR, uterine contractions, maternal heart rate, and blood pressure (FHR-UC-MHR-MBP) by means of a monitor that prints results on a two-channel strip chart recorder that can be stored as part of an electronic record. Uterine contractions result in a reduction in blood flow to the placenta, which can cause an interruption in fetal oxygenation and lead to corresponding alterations in the FHR. **The "FHR-UC-MHR-MBP" record can be obtained using external transducers that are placed on the maternal abdomen and arm.** It is important that external palpation of the uterus is carried out to determine the intensity of contractions with this method. **This technique is used in early labor.**

Internal monitoring is carried out by placing a spiral electrode onto the fetal scalp to monitor heart rate and inserting a plastic catheter transcervically into the amniotic cavity to monitor uterine contractions (Figure 9-1). To carry out this technique, the fetal membranes must be ruptured and the cervix must be dilated to at least 2 cm. Caution must be exercised when the decision to rupture the membranes is made,

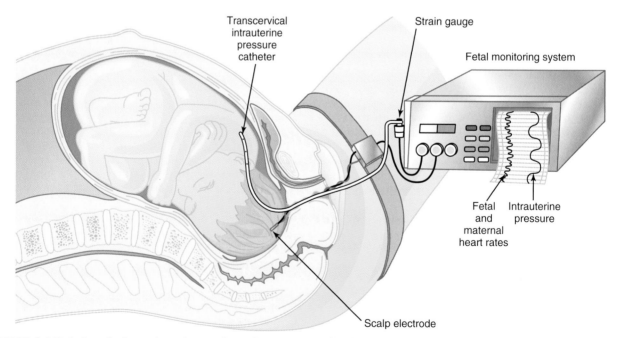

Transcervical intrauterine pressure catheter

Strain gauge

Fetal monitoring system

Fetal and maternal heart rates

Intrauterine pressure

Scalp electrode

FIGURE 9-1 Technique for internal continuous electronic monitoring of both fetal and maternal heart rates, as well as the pressure and frequency of uterine contractions. External monitoring of uterine contractions provides information only about the frequency of contractions.

and it should be performed only when more exact information is needed to monitor a mother or fetus at risk.

Internal monitoring gives better FHR tracings because the rate is computed from the sharply defined R-wave peaks of the fetal electrocardiogram, whereas with the external technique, the rate is computed from the less precisely defined first heart sound obtained with an ultrasonic transducer. However, fetal scalp electrodes should be placed only when the benefit outweighs the risk, and fetal scalp electrodes should always be placed with care. For example, **patients with specific infections (HIV and hepatitis B) should not have a scalp electrode placed.** In addition, when placing a scalp electrode, the presenting part of the fetus must be ascertained to avoid placing the electrode on the face or external genitals if the fetus is presenting as a breech.

The internal uterine catheter allows precise measurement of the intensity of the contractions in millimeters of mercury, whereas the external tocodynamometer measures only frequency and duration, not intensity. The strength of uterine contractions, however, can easily be assessed by abdominal palpation by a trained observer (a nurse or physician).

In the clinical setting, internal and external techniques are often combined by using a scalp electrode for precise heart rate recording and the external tocodynamometer for contractions. This approach minimizes possible side effects from invasive internal monitoring.

Etiology of Hypoxia, Acidosis, and Fetal Heart Rate Changes

The developing fetus presents a paradox. Its arterial blood oxygen tension is only 25 ± 5 mm Hg, as compared with adult values of about 100 mm Hg. The rate of oxygen consumption, however, is twice that of the adult per unit weight, and its oxygen reserve is only enough to meet its metabolic needs for 1 to 2 minutes. Blood flow from the maternal circulation, which supplies the fetus with oxygen through placental exchange of respiratory gases, is momentarily interrupted during a contraction. **A normal fetus can withstand the temporary reduction in blood flow to the placenta without developing hypoxia because sufficient oxygen exchange occurs during the interval between contractions.**

Under normal circumstances, the FHR is determined by the atrial pacemaker. Modulation of the rate occurs physiologically through innervation of the heart by the vagus (decelerator) and sympathetic (accelerator) nerves. A fetus whose oxygen supply is marginal cannot tolerate the stress of contractions and will become hypoxic. **Under hypoxic conditions, chemo-**receptors and baroreceptors in the peripheral arterial circulation of the fetus influence the FHR by giving rise to contraction-related or periodic FHR changes.** Hypoxia, when sufficiently severe, will also result in anaerobic metabolism, resulting in the accumulation of pyruvic and lactic acid and causing fetal acidosis. **The degree of fetal acidosis can be measured by sampling blood from the presenting part. The normal fetal scalp blood pH varies between 7.25 and 7.30. Values below 7.20 are considered to be abnormal (fetal acidosis) but not necessarily indicative of fetal compromise.**

The fetal oxygenation pathway can be interrupted at different locations within the uteroplacental-fetal circulatory loop. For example, impairment of oxygen transportation to the intervillous space may occur as a result of maternal hypertension or anemia; oxygen diffusion may be impaired in the placenta because of infarction or abruption; or the oxygen content in the fetal blood may be impaired because of hemolytic anemia in rhesus (Rh)-isoimmunization. Figure 9-2 summarizes the clinical conditions that may be associated with fetal distress during labor.

It is unrealistic to believe that hypoxia and acidosis are the only markers that determine the ultimate outcome of the fetus and neonate. Other markers of inflammation and the immune system must also play a role. **Current research is focused on vitamin D deficiency and inflammatory markers such as interleukin-6 and C-reactive protein.**

FETAL HEART RATE PATTERNS

The assessment of the FHR depends on an evaluation of the baseline pattern and the periodic changes related to uterine contractions. Table 9-1 gives a comprehensive list of FHR patterns and definitions based upon a workshop sponsored by the National Institute of Child Health and Human Development in 2008.

Baseline Assessment

Baseline assessment of FHR requires the determination of the rate (in beats/min) and the variability. Normal and abnormal rates are listed in Table 9-1. Normal FHR baseline is from 110 to 160 beats/min; tachycardia is a baseline greater than 160 beats/min, and bradycardia is less than 110 beats/min. Baseline variability can be divided into short- and long-term intervals. These are described in the subsections below.

1. **Short-term or beat-to-beat variability.** This reflects the interval between either successive fetal electrocardiographic signals or mechanical events of the cardiac cycle. **Normal short-term variability fluctuates between 6 and 25 beats/min.** Variability below 5 beats/min is considered to be potentially abnormal. When associated with decelerations, a variability of less than 5 beats/min usually indicates severe fetal distress.

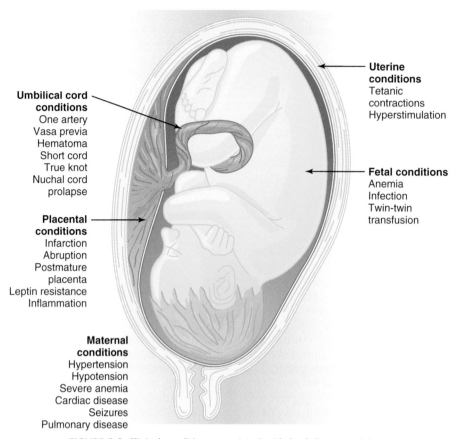

Umbilical cord conditions
One artery
Vasa previa
Hematoma
Short cord
True knot
Nuchal cord
prolapse

Placental conditions
Infarction
Abruption
Postmature
placenta
Leptin resistance
Inflammation

Maternal conditions
Hypertension
Hypotension
Severe anemia
Cardiac disease
Seizures
Pulmonary disease

Uterine conditions
Tetanic
contractions
Hyperstimulation

Fetal conditions
Anemia
Infection
Twin-twin
transfusion

FIGURE 9-2 Clinical conditions associated with fetal distress in labor.

2. **Long-term variability.** These fluctuations may be described in terms of the frequency and amplitude of change in the baseline rate. The normal long-term variability is 3 to 10 cycles per minute. Variability is physiologically decreased during the state of quiet sleep of the fetus, which usually lasts for about 25 minutes until transition occurs to another state. Changes in the long-term variability in prolonged and difficult labors may be a sign of an accumulated risk of metabolic dysregulation.

3. **Decreased beat-to-beat variability.** A prolonged flat baseline is the result of fetal acidosis.

Periodic Fetal Heart Rate Changes

Periodic FHR changes are changes in baseline FHR related to uterine contractions. The responses to uterine contractions may be categorized as follows:

1. **No change.** The FHR maintains the same characteristics it had in the preceding baseline FHR.
2. **Acceleration.** The FHR increases in response to uterine contractions. This is a normal response and is reassuring that the fetal status is normal.
3. **Deceleration.** The FHR decreases in response to uterine contractions. Decelerations may be *early, late, variable,* or *mixed.* All except early decelera-

tions are abnormal and are categorized according to a three-tier FHR interpretation system (Box 9-1).

Types of Patterns

EARLY DECELERATION (HEAD COMPRESSION). This pattern usually has an onset, maximum fall, and recovery that is coincident with the onset, peak, and end of the uterine contraction (Figure 9-3). The nadir of the FHR coincides with the peak of the contraction. This pattern is seen when engagement of the fetal head has occurred. Early decelerations are not thought to be associated with fetal distress. The pressure on the fetal head leads to increased intracranial pressure that elicits a vagal response similar to the Valsalva maneuver in the adult. The vagal reflex can be abolished by the administration of atropine, but this approach is not used clinically.

LATE DECELERATION (UTEROPLACENTAL INSUFFICIENCY). This pattern has an onset, maximal decrease, and recovery that are shifted to the right in relation to the contraction (Figure 9-4). Fetal hypoxia and acidosis are usually more pronounced with severe decelerations. Severe, repetitive late decelerations usually indicate fetal metabolic acidosis, low arterial pH, and increased

TABLE 9-1

ELECTRONIC FETAL MONITORING DEFINITIONS

Pattern	Definition

Baseline	The mean FHR rounded to increments of 5 excluding:
	    Periodic or episodic changes
	    Periods of marked FHR variability
	    Segments of baseline that differ by more than 25 beats/min
	The baseline must be for a minimum of 2 min in any 10-min segment, or the baseline for that time period is indeterminate; in this case, one may refer to the prior 10-min window for determination of baseline
	Normal FHR baseline: 110-160 beats/min
	Tachycardia: FHR baseline is >160 beats/min
	Bradycardia: FHR baseline is <110 beats/min

Baseline variability	Fluctuations in the baseline FHR that are irregular in amplitude and frequency
	Variability is visually quantitated as the amplitude or peak-to-trough in beats per minute
	    Absent: amplitude range undetectable
	    Minimal: amplitude range detectable, but ≤5 beats/min
	    Moderate (normal): amplitude range 6-25 beats/min
	    Marked: amplitude range >25 beats/min

Acceleration	A visually apparent abrupt increase (onset to peak in <30 sec) in the FHR At 32 weeks' gestation and beyond, an acceleration has a peak ≥15 beats/min above baseline, with a duration of 15 sec to 2 min from onset to return Before 32 weeks' gestation, an acceleration has a peak ≥10 beats/min above baseline, with a duration of ≥10 sec but <2 min from onset to return Prolonged acceleration lasts ≥2 min but <10 min in duration If an acceleration lasts ≥10 min, it is a baseline change
Early deceleration	Visually apparent, usually symmetrical, gradual decrease and return of the FHR associated with a uterine contraction A gradual FHR decrease is defined as from the onset to the FHR nadir or ≥30 sec The decrease in FHR is calculated from the onset to the nadir of the deceleration The nadir of the deceleration occurs at the same time as the peak of contraction In most cases, the onset, nadir, and recovery of the deceleration occur after the beginning, peak, and ending of the contraction, respectively
Late deceleration	Visually apparent, usually symmetrical, gradual decrease and return of the FHR associated with uterine contraction A gradual FHR decrease is defined as one of ≥30 sec from the onset to the FHR nadir The decrease in FHR is calculated from the onset to the nadir of the deceleration The decrease is delayed in timing, with the nadir of the deceleration occurring after the peak of the contraction In most cases, the onset, nadir, and recovery of the deceleration occur after the beginning, peak, and ending of contraction, respectively
Variable deceleration	Visually apparent abrupt decrease in FHR An abrupt FHR decrease is defined as one of <30 sec from the onset of the deceleration to the beginning of the FHR nadir The decrease in FHR is calculated from the onset to the nadir of the deceleration The decrease in FHR is ≥15 beats/min, lasting ≥15 sec and <2 min in duration When variable decelerations are associated with uterine contractions, their onset, depth, and duration commonly vary with successive uterine contractions
Prolonged deceleration	Visually apparent decrease in the FHR below the baseline Decrease in the FHR from baseline that is ≥15 beats/min, lasting ≥2 min but <10 min in duration If a deceleration lasts ≥10 min, it is a baseline change
Sinusoidal pattern	Visually apparent, smooth, sine wave–like, undulating pattern in FHR baseline with a cycle frequency of 3-5 per min that persists for ≥20 min

From Macones A, Hankins GDV, Spong CY, et al: The 2008 National Institute of Child Health and Human Development workshop report on electronic fetal monitoring: update on definitions, interpretation, and research guidelines. *Obstet Gynecol* 112:661–666, 2008.
FHR, Fetal heart rate.

BOX 9-1

THREE-TIER FETAL HEART RATE INTERPRETATION SYSTEM

Category I (Normal)

Category I FHR tracings include **all** of the following:
- Baseline rate: 110-160 beats/min
- Baseline FHR variability: moderate
- Late or variable decelerations: absent
- Early decelerations: present or absent
- Accelerations: present or absent

Category II (Intermediate/Possible Early Dysregulation)

Category II FHR tracings include all FHR tracings not categorized as Category I, or Category II tracings may represent an appreciable fraction of those encountered in clinical care. Examples of Category II FHR tracings include any of the following four parameters:
1. Baseline rate
   - Bradycardia not accompanied by absent baseline variability
   - Tachycardia
2. Baseline FHR variability
   - Minimal baseline variability
   - Absent baseline variability not accompanied by recurrent decelerations
   - Marked baseline variability
3. Accelerations
   - Absence of induced accelerations after fetal stimulation
4. Periodic or episodic decelerations
   - Recurrent variable decelerations accompanied by minimal or moderate baseline variability
   - Prolonged deceleration ≥2 min but <10 min
   - Recurrent late decelerations with moderate baseline variability
   - Variable decelerations with other characteristics, such as slow return to baseline, "overshoots," or "shoulders"

Category III (Abnormal)

Category III FHR tracings include either of the following:
- Absent baseline FHR variability and any of the following:
  - Recurrent late decelerations
  - Recurrent variable decelerations
  - Bradycardia
- Sinusoidal pattern

From Macones A, Hankins GDV, Spong CY, et al: The 2008 National Institute of Child Health and Human Development workshop report on electronic fetal monitoring: update on definitions, interpretation, and research guidelines. *Obstet Gynecol* 112:661–666, 2008.
FHR, Fetal heart rate.
Interpretation system: Category I (Normal) = Green, Category II (Intermediate) = Orange, and Category III (Abnormal) = Red.

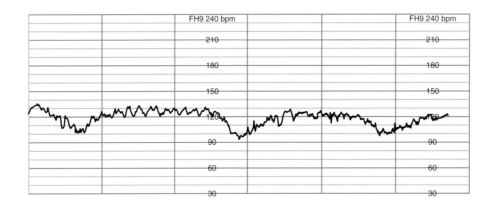
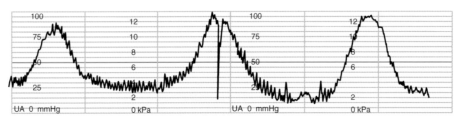

FIGURE 9-3 Early deceleration. Note that the deceleration starts and ends with the uterine contraction. Good beat-to-beat variability is demonstrated.

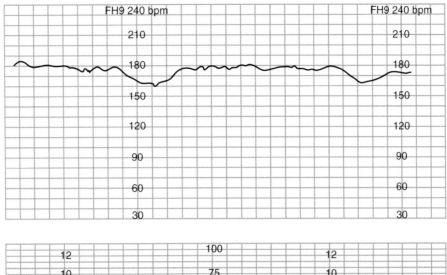

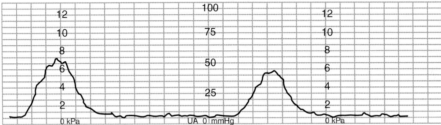

FIGURE 9-4 Late decelerations on electronic fetal monitoring tracing as would be recorded with a severely distressed fetus. Note the fetal tachycardia, lack of beat-to-beat heart rate variability, and the late decelerations *(upper trace)*. Uterine contractions are recorded in the *lower trace.*

base deficit values. The partial pressure of carbon dioxide in the fetal blood is usually in the normal range, and the fetal blood oxygen partial pressure is only slightly below normal because of the Bohr effect—the shift to the left of the oxygen dissociation curve caused by the acidosis.

VARIABLE DECELERATION (CORD COMPRESSION). This pattern has a variable time of onset and a variable form and may be nonrepetitive (Figure 9-5). Variable decelerations are caused by umbilical cord compression. Note that the decelerations have a more rapid drop and more rapid return to normal. This is characteristic of a reflex change, or rapid change, compared with the slower change in both early and late decelerations. Partial or complete compression of the cord causes a sudden increase in blood pressure in the central circulation of the fetus. The bradycardia is mediated via baroreceptors. This reflex can be abolished or ameliorated by atropine (e.g., chemical vagotomy), although this approach is not used clinically. Fetal blood gases indicate respiratory acidosis with a low pH and high carbon dioxide. When cord compression has been prolonged, hypoxia is also present, showing a picture of combined respiratory and metabolic acidosis in fetal blood gases.

The severity of variable decelerations is graded by their duration. When the FHR falls below 80 beats/min

during the nadir of the deceleration, there is usually a loss of the P-wave in the fetal electrocardiogram, indicating a nodal rhythm or a second-degree heart block.

NONPATTERN SIGNS OF FETAL DISTRESS

Fetal Tachycardia

As a baseline change, tachycardia is not a very reliable sign of fetal distress. **In general, fetal tachycardia occurs to improve placental circulation when the fetus is stressed.** Brief periods of tachycardia (15 to 30 minutes) are usually associated with excessive oxytocic augmentation of labor, after which the heart rate returns to baseline when the augmentation is discontinued. **Prolonged periods of tachycardia are usually associated with elevated maternal temperature or an intrauterine infection,** which should be ruled out. The acid-base status is usually normal.

Meconium

Early passage of meconium occurs any time before rupture of the membranes and is classified as trace (+1, +2, +3) and particulate based on its color and viscosity. Trace meconium is lightly stained yellow or greenish amniotic fluid. Meconium of +2 to +3 is dark green or black and is usually thick and tenacious with a pea soup appearance. It is associated with lower 1- and 5-minute Apgar scores and with the risk of meconium aspiration.

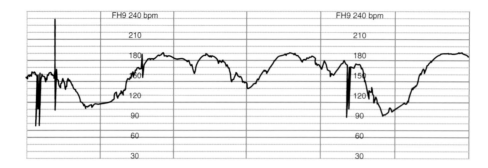

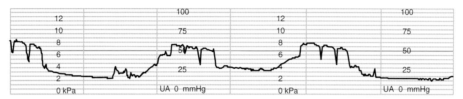

FIGURE 9-5 Umbilical cord compression pattern. Variable decelerations (cord compression) on electronic fetal monitoring traces (six panels [each panel = 60 seconds] beginning on the left side of each tracing) associated with maternal pushing in the second stage of labor. Note in both *upper* and *lower traces* the rapid drop in fetal heart rate with a nadir of 25 seconds, followed by a rapid return toward baseline. In the rightmost panels, the traces also show a decreased beat-to-beat variability with fetal tachycardia, which suggests some fetal distress (Category II-b tracing).

Late passage usually occurs during the second stage of labor, after clear amniotic fluid has been noted earlier. Late passage, which is most often heavy, is usually associated with some event (e.g., umbilical cord compression or uterine hypertonus) late in labor that causes fetal distress.

Strategies for Intervention

In 2008, the National Institute of Child Health and Human Development reported on a series of workshops on EFM with the goal of defining FHR characteristics more clearly to improve the predictive value of monitoring and to allow evidence-based clinical management of intrapartum fetal compromise. Table 9-1 lists the definitions for FHR characteristics, and Box 9-1 displays the three-tier FHR interpretation system.

CATEGORY I FHR (NORMAL)

A normal FHR pattern is strongly predictive of normal fetal acid-base status at the time of observation. The characteristics of Category I tracings are a normal baseline rate, moderate FHR variability, and absence of late or variable decelerations; early decelerations (head compression) may be present or absent. The presence of Category I FHR patterns requires no specific action.

CATEGORY II FHR (INTERMEDIATE/POSSIBLE EARLY DYSREGULATION)

Category II FHR tracings are intermediate and are not predictive of abnormal fetal acid-base status. This cat-

---

BOX 9-2

SUBTYPES OF CATEGORY II FHR TRACINGS

Category II-a: Reduced fetal heart rate variability but without decelerations; risk of fetal acidosis is low
Category II-b: Reduced fetal heart rate variability with mild decelerations; risk of fetal acidosis is moderate
Category II-c: Absence of fetal heart rate variability and deep decelerations; risk of fetal acidosis is high

From Parer JT, Ikeda T: A framework for standardized management of intrapartum fetal heart rate patterns. *Am J Obstet Gynecol* 197:26.e1–e6, 2007.

egory includes changes in (1) baseline rate, (2) baseline FHR variability, (3) accelerations, and (4) periodic or episodic decelerations. There has been an attempt to further subdivide Category II FHR abnormalities to improve the recognition of changes that are most ominous. These subtypes are summarized in Box 9-2.

Strategies for Resuscitation

Because Category II patterns are intermediate, resuscitative measures always depend on the clinical circumstances. **When abnormal patterns are seen, the first step should be a search for the underlying cause.** When the cause is identified, such as maternal hypotension, steps should be taken to correct the problem. In general, a term-sized fetus tolerates Category II FHR patterns better than a preterm fetus. A fetus with additional maternal or fetal risk factors, such as preterm labor, intrauterine growth restriction, preeclampsia, diabetes, or intrauterine infection from chorioamnionitis, may experience metabolic dysregulation sooner than a fetus in a normal parturient with Category I FHR tracings. **The three simple interventions are to (1) change the woman's position to the left lateral recumbent,** or if she is already on her side, switch positions to the other side; **(2) reduce the infusion rate of oxytocin** if this is running; and **(3) increase intravenous fluids** by infusing 1 L of normal saline with either 5% or 10% dextrose to ensure adequate vascular volume and substrate for the fetus and placenta. Studies have shown that this intervention shortens labor in nulliparous women.

Amnioinfusion

A more complex intervention for repetitive variable decelerations (cord pattern) is **amnioinfusion. This is the replacement of amniotic fluid with normal saline infused through a transcervical intrauterine pressure catheter, and it has been reported to decrease both the frequency and severity of variable decelerations.** The use of a double-lumen uterine catheter is recommended because it allows a continuous infusion while measuring uterine tone to guard against overdistention from excessive fluid accumulation. A common technique is to infuse a bolus of up to 800 mL of normal saline at a rate of 10 to 15 mL/min over a period of 50 to 80 minutes. This is followed by a maintenance dose of 3 mL/min until delivery. Overdistention of the uterine cavity can be avoided by maintaining the baseline uterine tone in the normal range and at less than 20 mm Hg. **Amnioinfusion results in reduced cesarean deliveries for fetal distress and fewer low Apgar scores at birth without apparent maternal or fetal distress.**

CATEGORY III FHR (ABNORMAL)

Category III FHR tracings are abnormal and require prompt evaluation because each of the five characteristics (listed in Box 9-1 under Category III FHR patterns) is predictive of abnormal fetal acid-base status. The major issue is to determine the optimal time for intervention, either by vaginal or cesarean delivery, to avoid serious perinatal morbidity and mortality. There are published data to suggest that, in the presence of Category III FHR patterns, the optimal time for delivery is within 30 minutes; thus, the delivery team must act quickly to decide whether there is sufficient time for a vaginal delivery, keeping in mind that it takes at least 30 minutes to prepare for an emergency cesarean delivery. The optimal answer is somewhere between the observations of Category II and the early onset of Category III, so it is sometimes prudent to notify the surgical team that a cesarean delivery may be called when Category II patterns are seen. The degree of fetal acidosis, as determined by fetal scalp blood sampling, to identify the fetus at greatest risk is no longer used by most obstetrical services. Until new biomarkers, such as inflammatory markers, become available, reliance must be placed on FHR categories to determine management.

A review of the five components of the classification of Category III tracings is as follows:
1. **Absent baseline variability** suggests a serious state of metabolic dysregulation.
2. **Recurrent late decelerations** of the FHR have been associated primarily with severely reduced uteroplacental blood flow.
3. **Recurrent variable decelerations** are characteristic of umbilical cord compression and are associated with reduced amniotic fluid volume. They may be related to the loss of the protective effect of intact membranes.
4. **Prolonged bradycardia** is secondary to the failure of the fetus to use its baroreceptive signaling to its cardiovascular centers to control heart rate because of severe metabolic dysregulation.
5. **Sinusoidal patterns** observed on admission suggest the possibility of severe fetal anemia (of unknown cause), and the occurrence of a sinusoidal pattern during labor lasting longer than 20 minutes is suggestive of a severe, acute fetal bleed.

Strategies for Intervention

The simple interventions discussed above for the observations of Category II tracings should have already been implemented, except maybe amnioinfusion. There are four additional procedures that can be used to assess the status of the fetus when Category III FHR patterns are present:
1. **Fetal scalp blood sampling** for pH determination has been used when clinical parameters such as Category III FHR patterns and heavy meconium are present, but it is no longer the standard of practice in many centers. Fetal scalp pH correctly predicts neonatal outcome in 82% of cases as determined by the Apgar score. The false-positive rate is approximately 8%, and the false-negative rate is approximately 10%. Blood is obtained from the fetus by placing an amnioscope transvaginally against the fetal skull (Figure 9-6). Cervical mucus is removed with cotton swabs. Silicone grease is applied to the skull for blood bead formation. A 2 × 2-mm lancet is used for a stab incision, and a drop of blood is aspirated into a long, heparinized capillary tube and sent to the laboratory for pH and base deficit determinations. Table 9-2 lists the normal values for fetal scalp blood samples.
2. **Ultrasonic Doppler velocimetry** for blood flow measurements in umbilical and fetal blood vessels and **percutaneous umbilical blood sampling** have been used antepartum in some centers, but they are generally not feasible methods for labor management.

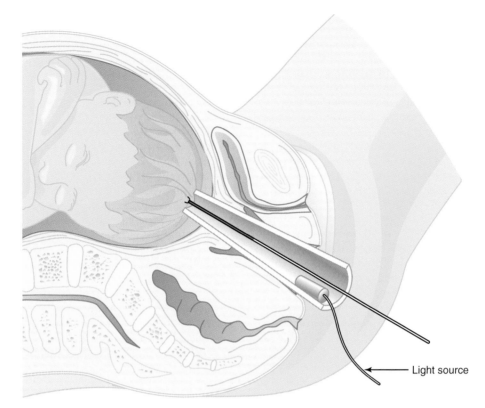

Light source

FIGURE 9-6 This technique of fetal scalp blood sampling via an amnioscope is still used in many centers. After making a small stab incision in the fetal scalp, the blood is drawn off through a long, heparinized capillary tube.

TABLE 9-2

NORMAL RANGES FOR FETAL SCALP AND CORD BLOOD INDICES				
Blood	pH	PCO₂ (mm Hg)	PO₂ (mm Hg)	Base Deficit (mEq/L)
Scalp Blood				
Early labor	7.34-7.38	43-57	20-24	(−0.2)-(0.4)
Active phase	7.34-7.40	36-54	20-24	(−2.0)-(0.0)
Complete cervical dilation	7.26-7.42	36-60	20-24	(−3.3)-(−0.3)
Cord Blood				
Artery	7.22-7.34	32-64	14-22	(−7.8)-(−2.2)
Vein	7.29-7.41	25-53	23-35	(−6.2)-(−1.8)

Data from Hobel CJ: Intrapartum clinical assessment of fetal distress. *Am J Obstet Gynecol* 110:336–342, 1971.
PCO₂, Partial pressure of carbon dioxide in fetal arterial blood; *PO₂*, partial pressure of oxygen in fetal arterial blood.

3. If cervical dilation and station permit, the safest intervention for compression of the umbilical cord is **assisted vaginal delivery.**
4. **Cesarean delivery** is indicated for severe, repetitive decelerations and a FHR tracing indicative of developing acidosis. Another circumstance that may require intervention is a prolonged deceleration. This condition occurs when the FHR falls to 60 to 90 beats/min for more than 2 minutes.

Fetal Assessment at Birth to Document the Status of the Fetus at Risk for Birth Asphyxia

APGAR SCORE

The Apgar scoring system has classically been used to assess the newborn's condition. Over time, however, the Apgar score has come to be used inappropriately to define asphyxia. This is a misapplication because many other conditions (e.g., prematurity, maternal drug administration) can result in low scores that are not reflective of asphyxia. Asphyxia implies hypoxia of sufficient degree to cause metabolic acidosis. Thus, the Apgar score alone cannot be used to define asphyxia. A low Apgar score of less than 5 helps the obstetric team to focus on both cardiovascular and respiratory adaptation (see Table 8-9).

UMBILICAL CORD BLOOD SAMPLING

A more appropriate tool for defining asphyxia is assessment of the fetal and neonatal acid-base status. Normal ranges for these indices are given in Table 9-2. One reasonable protocol for umbilical cord blood pH and blood gas analysis is as follows:

1. Doubly clamp a segment of umbilical cord immediately after birth in all preterm deliveries and in term deliveries where fetal distress is suspected, as well as in cases where the 1- and/or 5-minute Apgar score is low (<7).
2. If a specimen cannot be obtained from the umbilical artery of the cord, obtain a specimen from an artery on the chorionic surface of the placenta.

Controversies about Fetal Monitoring for the Diagnosis and Treatment of Fetal Distress

After more than 40 years of routine use of electronic monitoring for assessment of the FHR during labor, there is significant but incomplete evidence of its effectiveness for improving long-term fetal outcome, particularly in preterm infants. Over the past 40 years, more careful attention to monitoring of the fetus during labor has led to a reduction in the incidence of post-term fetal complications and to an improvement in perinatal mortality rates. The incidence of hypoxic-ischemic encephalopathy in term infants has also decreased. **Preterm births (spontaneous and induced) continue to add to the pool of infants who develop cerebral palsy.**

The improvements in outcome for term infants have not been mirrored by improved prevention of cerebral palsy in preterm infants. There is a pressing need to inform the public, as well as the medical profession, that **cerebral palsy is probably not caused by events during labor such as asphyxia and acidosis.** These intrapartum events appear to play only a small part in the overall incidence of this disorder. Events earlier in pregnancy probably play the major role. **Newer methods must be used to determine the actual prenatal events or unrecognized intrapartum events that increase the risk of preterm birth.** These events could include the subclinical inflammation associated with obesity.

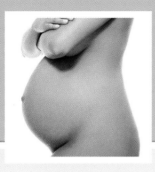

CHAPTER 10

Obstetric Hemorrhage
Antepartum, Intrapartum, and Postpartum

CALVIN J. HOBEL • AMY R. LAMB

CLINICAL KEYS FOR THIS CHAPTER

- Antepartum hemorrhage can be a very serious complication of pregnancy. Hemorrhage may be painless or painful, and the source of the bleeding is usually maternal, but it can rarely be from the fetus. The initial evaluation must be carefully performed to first stabilize the patient, assess the well-being of the fetus, and determine the cause while establishing a plan of management.

- The causes of severe antepartum/intrapartum hemorrhage are usually secondary to abnormal implantation of the placenta. The incidence of placenta previa, the most common type of abnormal placentation, is 0.5%, and bleeding from a **placenta previa** accounts for approximately 20% of all cases of antepartum hemorrhage. The classic presentation of placenta previa is painless vaginal bleeding in a previously normal pregnancy. **Placenta accreta** is a condition that occurs because of excessive invasion of the placental trophoblasts into the myometrium, resulting in failure of placental separation. This usually leads to excessive bleeding when the placenta is manually removed intrapartum. **Abruptio placentae** is due to premature separation of the normally implanted placenta. Placental abruption complicates 0.5-1.5% of all pregnancies (1 in 120 births). Because the bleeding penetrates into the myometrium, it is associated with pain.

- Fetal bleeding may be caused by an abnormal (velamentous) insertion of the umbilical cord between the amnion and chorion and away from the placenta. When the cord insertion and placental edge are close to the cervical opening, changes in the lower uterine segment that occur before labor can cause stretching and bleeding from the cord vessels. With vaginal ultrasound and a simple bedside test to differentiate maternal blood from fetal blood, the source of the bleeding can be diagnosed.

- *Postpartum hemorrhage* is defined as blood loss in excess of 500 mL at the time of vaginal delivery or in excess of 1000 mL for cesarean delivery. Postpartum hemorrhage is a leading cause of maternal mortality worldwide. The prevalence of postpartum hemorrhage is approximately 6% of all deliveries and accounts for 25% of all maternal deaths. Formulating a plan of management based on risk factors for postpartum hemorrhage and using intravenous oxytocin and manual uterine massage after the delivery are key elements of an effective prevention plan for postpartum hemorrhage.

- When postpartum hemorrhage occurs after the patient leaves the labor and delivery area, the obstetric team must reassess the patient to identify the less common causes of delayed postpartum hemorrhage. This requires a careful search for retained products of conception and clotting within the uterus that can keep it from contracting. Other rare causes, such as uterine rupture, must also be considered.

The most common causes of maternal death are hemorrhage, embolism, hypertensive disease, and infection. In this chapter, the causes of obstetric hemorrhage in the late second trimester and the third trimester are discussed. The antepartum causes include placenta previa and accreta, conditions that represent abnormalities of placentation. Placental abruption and fetal causes of bleeding may also present before labor and may result in fetal death.

Postpartum hemorrhage (PPH) is the leading cause of maternal mortality worldwide, and its prevention is an important part of labor management. Uterine atony, genital tract birth trauma, and placental retention are the most common causes of PPH.

Antepartum Hemorrhage

The incidence of bleeding in the late second trimester and the third trimester is between 5% and 8%, because bleeding before 20 weeks (time of potential viability) is usually related to the risk of abortion and the management is less emergent. It is therefore critical for the

CAUSES OF ANTEPARTUM HEMORRHAGE (APH)

Common

Placenta previa
Preterm labor (marginal separation of placenta)

Uncommon

Uterine rupture
Fetal (chorionic) vessel rupture
Cervical or vaginal lacerations
Cervical or vaginal lesions, including cancer
Congenital bleeding disorder
Unknown (by exclusion of the above)

well-being of both the mother and the fetus that the patient who presents with bleeding in the late second trimester and the third trimester be evaluated and managed emergently.

INITIAL EVALUATION

After a complete history has been taken, physical examination is performed, but a pelvic examination is usually postponed until an abdominal ultrasound has been obtained to rule out placenta previa. The differential diagnosis of second- and third-trimester bleeding is listed in Box 10-1.

The vital signs and amount of bleeding should be checked immediately, as should the patient's mental status. The patient's medical history should be checked for known bleeding disorders or liver disease, which predispose the patient to coagulopathy. Once placenta previa has been excluded by abdominal ultrasound, a sterile speculum examination can safely be done to rule out genital tears or lesions (e.g., **cervical cancer**) that may be responsible for the bleeding. If none are identified, a digital examination or pelvic ultrasound may be performed to determine whether cervical dilation is present.

If a patient is bleeding profusely, a team approach to the assessment and management should be instituted to establish hemodynamic stability. This team should include an obstetrician, an anesthesiologist, and nurses who are knowledgeable about the management of a potentially critically ill patient. At least two large-bore peripheral intravenous (IV) lines should be placed, as they allow the most rapid replacement of fluid and blood volume. A central venous pressure line, or preferably a pulmonary artery catheter, is helpful in the management of hypovolemic shock.

A **complete blood count** should be obtained and compared with previous evaluations to help assess the amount of blood loss, although acute blood loss may not be reflected in the hemoglobin level until homeostasis has been reestablished. An assessment of the patient's **coagulation profile** should be done by obtaining a platelet count, serum fibrinogen level, prothrombin time (PT), and partial thromboplastin time. Additionally, the patient should be **typed and cross-hatched for at least 4 units of blood** (packed cells). A rapid but subjective method to test for coagulopathy is to partially fill a "red-top" tube with blood. If a clot does not form, or once formed does not stay clotted, the patient most likely has disseminated intravascular coagulation (DIC).

An important and accurate method of determining the cause of bleeding in the late second trimester and the third trimester is ultrasonography. This evaluation should include not only the location and extent of the placenta (initial ultrasonic assessment to rule out placenta previa) but also an assessment of gestational age, an estimate of fetal weight, determination of the fetal presentation, and screening for fetal anomalies. Uterine activity and the fetal heart rate should be assessed with a monitored strip to rule out labor and to establish fetal well-being (see Chapter 9).

Abnormal Placentation: Placenta Previa and Placenta Accreta

PLACENTA PREVIA

The incidence of placenta previa, the most common type of abnormal placentation, is 0.5%. Approximately 20% of all cases of antepartum hemorrhage are due to placenta previa. Seventy percent of patients with placenta previa present with painless vaginal bleeding in the third trimester, 20% have contractions associated with bleeding, and 10% have the diagnosis made incidentally on the basis of ultrasonography or at term.

Predisposing Factors

Factors that have been associated with a higher incidence of placenta previa include (1) multiparity, which is associated with changes in the size and shape of the uterus, providing more space in the lower uterine segment for implantation; **(2) increased maternal age; (3) prior placenta previa; (4) multiple gestation;** and **(5) cesarean delivery,** which also changes the shape of the lower uterine segment. Patients with a prior placenta previa have a 4-8% risk of having placenta previa in a subsequent pregnancy.

Classification

Placenta previa is classified according to the relationship of the placenta to the internal cervical os (Figure 10-1). **Complete placenta previa** implies that the placenta totally covers the cervical os. A complete placenta previa may be central, anterior, or posterior, depending on where the center of the placenta is located relative to the os. **Partial placenta previa** implies that the placenta partially covers the internal

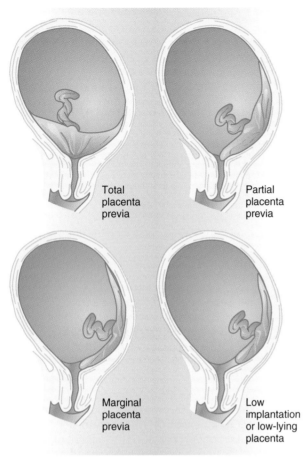

Total placenta previa

Partial placenta previa

Marginal placenta previa

Low implantation or low-lying placenta

FIGURE 10-1 Types of placenta previa.

cervical os. A **marginal placenta previa** is one in which the edge of the placenta extends to the margin of the internal cervical os.

Diagnosis

The classic presentation of placenta previa is painless vaginal bleeding in a previously normal pregnancy. The mean gestational age at onset of bleeding is 30 weeks, with one-third presenting before 30 weeks. Placenta previa is almost exclusively diagnosed on the basis of ultrasonography. Between 4% and 6% of patients have some degree of placenta previa on ultrasonic examination before 20 weeks' gestation. With the development of the lower uterine segment, a relative upward placental migration occurs, with 90% of these resolving by the third trimester. Complete placenta previa is the least likely to resolve, with only 10% of cases resolving by the third trimester. **When placenta previa is diagnosed in the second trimester, a repeat sonogram is indicated at 30 to 32 weeks for follow-up evaluation.**

Transabdominal ultrasonography has an accuracy of 95% for placenta previa detection. If the placenta is implanted posteriorly and the fetal vertex is low, the lower margin of the placenta may be obscured and the diagnosis of placenta previa missed. **Transvaginal ultrasonography can accurately diagnose placenta previa in virtually 100% of cases.**

Management

Once the diagnosis of placenta previa is established, management decisions depend on the gestational age of the fetus and the extent of the vaginal bleeding. **With a preterm pregnancy, the goal is to attempt to obtain fetal maturation without compromising the mother's health.** If bleeding is excessive, delivery must be accomplished by cesarean, regardless of gestational age. When the bleeding episode is not profuse or repetitive, the patient is managed expectantly in the hospital on bed rest. With expectant management, 70% of patients will have recurrent vaginal bleeding before completion of 36 weeks' gestation and will require delivery. **If the patient reaches 36 weeks, fetal lung maturity should be determined by amniocentesis and the patient delivered by cesarean if the fetal lungs are mature.** Elective delivery is preferable, as spontaneous labor places the mother at greater risk for hemorrhage and the fetus at risk for hypovolemia and anemia.

LOW-LYING PLACENTA

A patient with a low-lying placenta (placental margin within 2 cm of the endocervical os) may present in the same way as a patient with placenta previa. It may be difficult to distinguish a low-lying placenta from a marginal placenta previa, but a transvaginal ultrasound is typically diagnostic. **Vaginal delivery is not contraindicated, because during labor the fetal head compresses the edge of the placenta, decreasing the risk of bleeding.** The same level of monitoring should be maintained for maternal hemodynamic stability and fetal well-being.

MATERNAL-FETAL RISKS

Maternal mortality from placenta previa has dropped from 30% to less than 1% over the past 60 years. This has primarily been due to the liberal use of cesarean delivery and careful expectant management. **The rare maternal death is generally associated with complications of cesarean delivery or uncontrolled hemorrhage from the placental site. The lower uterine segment does not contract well, especially after a lower uterine incision.** DIC may also result if a massive hemorrhage or an associated abruption occurs.

The risk of antepartum or intrapartum hemorrhage, or both, is a constant threat to the patient with placenta previa. Bleeding may be exacerbated by an associated placenta accreta or uterine atony. **Placenta previa predisposes the patient to preterm delivery, which poses the greatest risk to the fetus.** As a result of advances in obstetric and neonatal care, the perinatal mortality rate (PMR) for patients with placenta previa has declined over the past decade. **The incidence of malpresentation with placenta previa is 30%, presumably due to the mass effect of the placenta and distortion of the lower uterine segment.**

PLACENTA ACCRETA

Placenta accreta implies an abnormal attachment of the placenta through the uterine myometrium as a result of defective decidual formation (absent Nitabuch layer). This abnormal myometrial attachment of the placental villi is usually superficial (**accreta**), but the villi may invade more deeply into the myometrium (**increta**) or extend through to the uterine serosa (**percreta**). **Two-thirds of patients with this complication require hysterectomy when an attempt to remove the placenta leads to severe hemorrhage intrapartum.** Patients with a history of uterine surgery are at greatest risk of developing an accreta. In fact, **those with prior cesarean delivery have a 10-50% risk of abnormal implantation.** If ultrasonic imaging shows accreta prior to delivery, elective hysterectomy may be performed to prevent hemorrhage. **The etiology of placenta accreta is complex,** but recent evidence suggests the aggressive invasion of the placenta into the spiral arteries is a process unique to primates that has been conserved through evolution. It ensures that invasion of the uterine arteries is complete to maximize fetal access to the maternal circulation for maximal nutrition.

Abruptio Placentae

Abruptio placentae, or premature separation of the normally implanted placenta, complicates 0.5-1.5% of all pregnancies (1 in 120 births). Abruption severe enough to result in fetal death occurs in 1 in 500 deliveries.

PREDISPOSING FACTORS AND PATHOPHYSIOLOGY

Factors associated with an increased incidence of abruption are noted in Box 10-2. The most common of these risk factors is **maternal hypertension,** either chronic or as a result of preeclampsia. **The risk of recurrent abruption is 10% after one abruption and 25% after two.** The etiology may be the opposite of that for placenta accreta. Because abruption is associated with maternal hypertension or preeclampsia, there may be a failure of adequate placental implantation. Its inciting cause is unknown, but placental separation may be due to an inherent weakness or anomaly in the spiral arterioles. **Placental separation is initiated by hemorrhage into the decidua basalis with formation of a decidual hematoma.** The resulting separation of the decidua from the basal plate predisposes to further separation and bleeding, as well as to compression and destruction of placental tissue. Blood may either dissect upward toward the fundus, resulting in a **concealed hemorrhage,** or extend downward toward the cervix, resulting in an external or **revealed hemorrhage.**

DIAGNOSIS AND MANAGEMENT

Clinically, the diagnosis of a placental abruption is entertained if a patient presents with painful vaginal bleeding in association with uterine tenderness, hyperactivity, and increased tone. The signs and symptoms of placental abruption are variable, however. The most common finding is vaginal bleeding, which is seen in 80% of cases. **Abdominal pain and uterine tenderness are present in 66% of cases, fetal distress in 60%, uterine hyperactivity and increased uterine tone in 34%, and fetal death in 15%.**

The diagnosis of placental abruption is made clinically. **Ultrasonography may detect only 2% of abruptions.** Because placental abruption may coexist with a placenta previa, the reason for doing an initial ultrasonic examination is to exclude the previa.

Management of the patient with an abruption includes careful maternal hemodynamic and fetal monitoring, serial evaluation of the hematocrit and coagulation profile, and delivery. **Intensive monitoring of both the mother and the fetus is essential** because rapid deterioration of the condition of either one can occur. Blood products for replacement should always be available, and a large-bore (16- to 18-gauge) IV line must be secured. Red blood cells should be given liberally if indicated. **In the setting of placental abruption, the use of tocolytics or uterine relaxants is not advisable.** Uterine tone must be maintained to control bleeding following delivery, or at least to control the bleeding sufficiently to allow a safe hysterectomy to be performed, if necessary.

MATERNAL-FETAL RISKS

Abruption places the fetus at significant risk of hypoxia and, ultimately, death. **The PMR due to placental abruption is 35%,** and the condition accounts for 15% of third-trimester stillbirths. Fifteen percent of liveborn infants have significant neurologic impairment.

Placental abruption is the most common cause of DIC in pregnancy. This results from release into the maternal circulation of thromboplastin from the disrupted placenta and subplacental decidua, causing a

---

BOX 10-2

RISK FACTORS FOR ABRUPTIO PLACENTAE

Maternal hypertension (chronic or pregnancy-induced)
Placental abruption in a prior pregnancy
Pregnancy after in vitro fertilization (IVF)
Trauma
Polyhydramnios with rapid decompression
Premature rupture of membranes
Short umbilical cord
Folate deficiency
Substance abuse (e.g., cocaine, amphetamines, tobacco)

consumptive coagulopathy. Clinically significant DIC complicates 20% of cases and is most commonly seen when the abruption is massive or fetal death has occurred. **Hypovolemic shock and acute renal failure as a result of massive hemorrhage may be seen with a severe abruption** if hypovolemia is left uncorrected. **Sheehan syndrome** (amenorrhea as a result of maternal postpartum pituitary necrosis) **may be a delayed complication resulting from coagulation within the portal system of the pituitary stalk.** Assessment of pituitary function should be considered in the postpartum follow-up of women after a serious abruption with a coagulation disorder.

Uterine Rupture

Uterine rupture implies complete separation of the uterine musculature through all of its layers, ultimately with all or a part of the fetus being extruded from the uterine cavity. **The overall incidence is 0.5%.**

Uterine rupture may be spontaneous, traumatic, or associated with a prior uterine scar, and it may occur during or before labor or at the time of delivery. **A prior uterine scar is associated with 40% of cases.** With a prior lower-segment transverse incision, the risk for rupture is less than 1%, whereas **the risk with a high vertical (classical) scar is 4-7%.** Sixty percent of uterine ruptures occur in previously unscarred uteri.

DIAGNOSIS AND MANAGEMENT

The signs and symptoms of uterine rupture are highly variable. **Typically, rupture is characterized by the sudden onset of intense abdominal pain.** The patient may or may not have vaginal bleeding, and if it occurs, it can range from spotting to severe hemorrhage. Impending rupture may be heralded by hyperventilation, restlessness, agitation, and tachycardia. After the rupture has occurred, the patient may be free of pain momentarily and then complain of diffuse pain thereafter. The most consistent clinical finding is an abnormal fetal heart rate pattern. **The presenting part may be found to have retracted on pelvic examination, and fetal parts may be more easily palpable abdominally.** Abnormal contouring of the abdomen may be seen. Fetal distress develops commonly, and **fetal death or long-term neurologic sequelae may occur in 10% of cases.**

A high index of suspicion is required, and immediate laparotomy is essential. **In most cases, total abdominal hysterectomy is the treatment of choice,** although debridement of the rupture site and primary closure may be considered in women of low parity who desire more children.

MATERNAL-FETAL RISK

Delay in management of uterine rupture places both mother and child at significant risk. The major risk to the mother is hemorrhage and shock. Although **the associated maternal mortality rate is now less than 1%,** if the mother is left untreated, she will almost certainly die. For the fetus, rapid intervention will minimize morbidity and mortality. **The associated fetal mortality rate is still about 30%.**

Fetal Bleeding

Rupture of a fetal umbilical vessel complicates 0.1-0.8% of pregnancies. **This often results when the cord insertion is velamentous,** implying that the vessels of the cord insert between the amnion and chorion, away from the placenta. The incidence of velamentous cord insertion varies from 1% in singleton pregnancies to 10% in twins and 50% in triplets. **If the unprotected vessels pass over the cervical os, this is termed a *vasa previa*. The incidence of vasa previa is 1 in 5000 pregnancies.** Velamentously inserted vessels need not pass over the os to rupture.

The diagnosis of fetal bleeding is made by performing an Apt test. After obtaining blood from the vagina and putting it into a red-topped test tube, tap water or distilled water is added. The water will lyse blood cells and release hemoglobin into the solution. Adding 1 mL of KOH results in a brown discoloration when the hemoglobin is maternal. If the blood is fetal in origin, the color of the fluid will remain red because the fetal hemoglobin will not be denatured by the KOH. Rupture of a fetal vessel necessitates immediate abdominal delivery. **Vasa previa alone carries a PMR of 50%, which increases to 75% if the membranes rupture.**

Postpartum Hemorrhage

Postpartum hemorrhage (PPH), the leading cause of maternal mortality, is defined as blood loss in excess of 500 mL at the time of vaginal delivery or blood loss in excess of 1000 mL following cesarean delivery. The excessive blood loss usually occurs in the immediate postpartum period, but it can occur slowly over the first 24 hours. **Delayed PPH can occasionally occur, with the excessive bleeding commencing more than 24 hours after delivery.** This is usually due to subinvolution of the uterus and disruption of the placental site "scab" several weeks postpartum or to the retention of placental fragments that separate several days after delivery. The causes of PPH are listed in Box 10-3.

Since 1996, there has been a gradual increase in the incidence of PPH in the United States and other developed countries. This increase has been related to uterine atony. The cause of this increase is not known and is currently under intense investigation.

UTERINE ATONY

The majority of PPH cases (75-80%) are due to uterine atony. The factors predisposing to postpartum uterine

BOX 10-3

CAUSES OF POSTPARTUM HEMORRHAGE

Uterine atony*
Retained placental tissue*
Genital tract trauma
Low placental implantation
Uterine inversion
Coagulation disorders
Amniotic fluid embolism
Retained dead fetus
Inherited coagulopathy
Abruptio placentae (usually ante- or intrapartum)

*Both of these conditions result in retained blood clots and placental fragments, causing uterine stretching and prevention of uterine contractions.

BOX 10-4

FACTORS PREDISPOSING TO POSTPARTUM UTERINE ATONY

History of postpartum hemorrhage*
Prolonged labor*
Grand multiparity (a parity of 5 or more)*
Overdistention of the uterus†
    Multiple gestations
    Polyhydramnios
    Fetal macrosomia
Oxytocic augmentation of labor†
Precipitous labor (one lasting <3 hr)
Magnesium sulfate treatment of preeclampsia†
Chorioamnionitis†
Halogenated anesthetics
Uterine leiomyomata†
Vitamin D deficiency
Genetic and epigenetic factors (maternal, environmental, and fetal)

*High-risk patients (one or more factors).
†Medium-risk patients (one or more factors).

atony are listed in Box 10-4. Recently, several new factors have been identified as potential causes of uterine atony, including **vitamin D deficiency and maternal and fetal genetic factors.** Vitamin D is known to play an important role in muscle function, and muscle is a component of both the uterine and vascular system. Studies have suggested that among patients having a vaginal delivery, 18% of the variation in excessive postpartum bleeding may be attributable to maternal genetic factors, 11% to maternal environmental factors, and 11% to fetal genetic effects.

Most of the blood loss due to uterine atony occurs from the myometrial spiral arterioles and decidual veins that previously supplied and drained the intervillous spaces of the placenta. As the contractions of the partially empty uterus cause placental separation, bleeding occurs and continues until the uterine musculature contracts around the blood vessels and acts as a physiologic-anatomic ligature. **Failure of the uterus** to contract after placental separation (uterine atony) leads to excessive placental site bleeding.

During pregnancy, uterine relaxation is facilitated by progesterone and parathyroid hormone–related peptide (PTHrP). The latter plays an important role in maintaining uterine relaxation during pregnancy (see Chapter 5); however, as soon as the uterus is emptied (delivery of the fetus and placenta), the gene controlling this hormone is turned off and the uterus is allowed to contract more completely. If there is a failure of complete expulsion of the placenta or poor uterine contractility leading to excessive bleeding, the uterus will fill with blood. The distention is thought to reactivate the expression of PTHrP and cause uterine relaxation, thereby leading to excessive hemorrhage.

Management of Patients at Risk for Postpartum Hemorrhage

Because the major cause of PPH is uterine atony, the initial focus should be on prevention of uterine atony by considering the following steps:

1. All women in early labor who have risk factors for PPH should be identified (see Box 10-4) and their hemoglobin checked. For **medium-risk women,** their blood should be typed and screened for irregular antibodies such as Rh and Kell. For **high-risk women,** 2 units of blood should be typed and cross-matched (refer to Stage 0 in Table 10-1).
2. As soon as the fetus has been delivered, an infusion of oxytocin (Pitocin) 10 to 40 U/L IV should be started and maintained during the first 6 hours postpartum.
3. The vagina and perineum should be inspected to rule out any lacerations that could cause excessive bleeding.
4. The placenta should be carefully assessed at delivery to make certain there are no missing cotyledons (lobules of placenta).
5. The uterus should be evaluated by abdominal palpation during the first 1 to 2 hours before transfer to the postpartum unit. The nurses on the postpartum unit should frequently assess the status of uterine contractility, instructing the patient on how to assess uterine firmness and reporting any excessive bleeding. For high-risk patients, continuation of the oxytocin IV infusion during the early postpartum hours should be considered.

DIFFERENTIAL DIAGNOSIS: OTHER LESS COMMON CAUSES OF POSTPARTUM HEMORRHAGE

If the cause of bleeding has not been identified, the management of PPH requires a systematic approach. The fundus of the uterus should be palpated through the abdominal wall to determine the presence or

TABLE 10-1

POSTPARTUM OBSTETRIC HEMORRHAGE CARE SUMMARY

Stage 0 All women in labor or giving birth	Assess for Risk Factors (see Box 10-4) 1. Active management: IV infusion of oxytocin after delivery of the fetus and fundal uterine massage after delivery of the placenta 2. Complete evaluation for missing placental cotyledons and examination of vagina and cervix for lacerations with repair when needed to control bleeding 3. If high risk (history of postpartum hemorrhage plus 1 or more risk factors), consider typing and crossmatching 2 U of PRBCs
Stage 1 Blood loss >500 mL (vaginal delivery) >1000 mL (cesarean delivery)	Begin Hemorrhage Protocol 1. Alert charge nurse and anesthesia staff 2. Type and crossmatch 2 U of PRBCs (if not already done) 3. Increase infusion rate of oxytocin, give methergine and repeat fundal massage 4. Measure blood loss
Stage 2 Total blood loss between 1000 and 1500 mL	Call for Help (Rapid Response Team) 1. Consider complete reexamination of vagina, cervix, and uterine cavity for source of bleeding; if the patient is in the postpartum unit, consider moving her to labor and delivery or the operating room 2. Consider the next level of drugs (carboprost 250 µg IM or misoprostol 800 to 1000 µg per rectum) and request additional laboratory testing (e.g., a coagulation panel) 3. Consider blood transfusion (have 2 U of PRBCs plus 2 U of fresh frozen plasma at the bedside) 4. Consider placement of intrauterine balloon or involve interventional radiology when available for embolization
Stage 3 Total blood loss >1500 mL	Mobilize Surgical Team 1. Consider repeat laboratory tests, including coagulation studies and acid-base gas assessment 2. Transfuse appropriately with PRBCs and platelets 3. Consider B-Lynch suture, uterine artery ligation, or hysterectomy

Modified from the California Maternal Quality Care Collaborative. Available at www.CMQCC.org. Accessed May 10, 2015.
IM, Intramuscular; *IV,* intravenous; *PRBC,* packed red blood cells.

absence of **uterine atony.** Next, a quick but thorough inspection of the vagina and cervix should be performed to ascertain whether any **lacerations** may be compounding the bleeding problem. Any **uterine inversion** or **pelvic hematoma** should be excluded during the pelvic examination. (See Table 10-1, Stages 1 and 2; begin hemorrhage protocol.)

GENITAL TRACT TRAUMA

Trauma during delivery is the second most common cause of PPH. During vaginal delivery, lacerations of the cervix and vagina may occur spontaneously, but they are more common following the use of forceps or a vacuum extractor. The vascular beds in the genital tract are engorged during pregnancy, and bleeding can be profuse. Lacerations are particularly prone to occur over the perineal body, in the periurethral area, and over the ischial spines along the posterolateral aspects of the vagina. The cervix may lacerate at the two lateral angles while rapidly dilating in the first stage of labor. **Uterine rupture may occasionally occur.** At the time of delivery by low transverse cesarean, an inadvertent lateral extension of the incision can damage the ascending branches of the uterine arteries; an extension inferiorly can damage the cervical branches of the uterine artery.

RETAINED PLACENTAL TISSUE

In about one-half of the patients with delayed PPH, placental fragments are present. The uterus is unable to maintain a contraction and involute normally around a retained placental tissue mass. **If retained placental fragments are suspected, ultrasonic assessment of the uterus should be performed. If placental fragments are identified, manual exploration of the uterine cavity** should be performed, with the patient under general anesthesia if necessary. With fingertips together, a gloved hand may be slipped through the open cervix and the hand inserted into the uterus. The endometrial surface should be palpated carefully to identify any retained products of conception, uterine wall lacerations, or partial uterine inversion. If no cause for the bleeding is found, **coagulopathy** must be considered.

LOW PLACENTAL IMPLANTATION

Low implantation of the placenta can predispose the patient to PPH because the relative content of musculature decreases in the lower uterine segment, which may result in insufficient muscular control of placental site bleeding. Verifying a fully drained bladder and the use of uterotonic agents such as oxytocin, methylergonovine, or prostaglandin is usually sufficient. If bleeding continues, surgical management must be considered.

COAGULATION DISORDERS

Peripartum coagulation disorders are high-risk factors for PPH, but fortunately they are quite rare.

Patients with **thrombotic thrombocytopenia** have a rare syndrome of unknown etiology characterized by thrombocytopenic purpura, microangiopathic hemolytic anemia, transient and fluctuating neurologic signs, renal dysfunction, and a febrile course. In pregnancy, the disease is usually fatal.

An **amniotic fluid embolus** is also rare and is associated with an 80% mortality rate. This syndrome is characterized by a fulminating consumption coagulopathy, intense bronchospasm, and vasomotor collapse. It is triggered by an intravascular infusion of a significant quantity of amniotic fluid during a tumultuous or rapid labor in the presence of ruptured membranes. During the process of **placental abruption,** a small amount of amniotic fluid may leak into the vascular system, and the thromboplastin in the amniotic fluid may trigger a consumption coagulopathy.

Patients with **idiopathic thrombocytopenic purpura** have platelets with abnormal function or a shortened lifespan. This causes thrombocytopenia and a tendency to bleed. Circulating antiplatelet antibodies of the immunoglobulin G type may occasionally cross the placenta and result in fetal and neonatal thrombocytopenia as well.

von Willebrand disease is an inherited coagulopathy characterized by a prolonged bleeding time due to factor VIII deficiency. During pregnancy, these patients are likely to have a decreased bleeding diathesis because pregnancy elevates factor VIII levels. In the postpartum period, they are susceptible to delayed bleeding as factor VIII levels fall.

UTERINE INVERSION

Uterine inversion is the "turning inside out" of the uterus in the third stage of labor. It is quite rare, occurring in only about 1 in 20,000 pregnancies. Just after the second stage of labor, the uterus is somewhat atonic, the cervix open, and the placenta attached. **Improper management of the third stage of labor can cause an iatrogenic uterine inversion.** If the inexperienced physician exerts fundal pressure while pulling on the umbilical cord before complete placental separation (particularly with a fundal implantation of the placenta), uterine inversion may occur. As the fundus of the uterus moves through the vagina, the inversion exerts traction on peritoneal structures, which can elicit a profound vasovagal response. The resulting vasodilation increases bleeding and the risk of hypovolemic shock. **If the placenta is completely or partially separated, the uterine atony may cause profuse bleeding, which compounds the vasovagal shock.**

Obstetric Shock and External Bleeding

Hypotension without significant external bleeding may occasionally develop in an obstetric patient. This condition is called obstetric shock. **The causes of obstetric shock include concealed hemorrhage within the uterus, uterine inversion, and amniotic fluid embolism.**

An improperly sutured episiotomy can lead to a concealed PPH. If the first suture at the vaginal apex of the episiotomy incision does not incorporate the cut and retracted arterioles, these can continue to bleed, creating a hematoma that can dissect cephalad into the retroperitoneal space. This may cause shock without external evidence of blood loss. **A soft tissue hematoma, usually of the vulva, may occur following delivery in the absence of any laceration. Uterine rupture** can also occur secondary to blunt abdominal trauma at the time of an automobile accident.

Management of Established Postpartum Hemorrhage and Obstetric Shock

During the diagnostic workup of an established hemorrhage, the patient's vital signs must be monitored closely. However, **young healthy women may tolerate and mask hypovolemia well.** The sensitivity and specificity of the vital signs are not absolute. The estimated blood loss is commonly underestimated, and it should be replaced by quantitated blood loss, where sponges and pads are weighed and measured. Multiple units of packed red blood cells must be typed and cross-matched, and IV crystalloids (such as normal saline or lactated Ringer solution) infused to restore intravascular volume. **Resuscitation with normal saline usually requires a volume of three times the estimated blood loss to replace the intravascular volume. During a massive hemorrhage, morbidity and/or mortality are reduced with an emphasis on early blood product replacement rather than crystalloid-based resuscitation.**

UTERINE ATONY

When uterine atony is determined to be the cause of the PPH, a rapid, continuous IV infusion of dilute oxytocin (40 to 80 U in 1 L of normal saline) **should be given to increase uterine tone.** If the uterus remains atonic and the placental site bleeding continues, 0.2 mg of **ergonovine maleate or methylergonovine** may be given intramuscularly. The ergot drugs are relatively contraindicated in patients with hypertension because the smooth muscle–constricting effects of these drugs may also increase vascular tone and thus increase blood pressure to dangerous levels.

Analogues of prostaglandin $F_{2\alpha}$ given intramuscularly are quite effective in controlling PPH caused by uterine atony. The 15-methyl analogue carboprost (Hemabate) has a more potent uterotonic effect and longer duration of action than the parent compound. The expected time of onset of the uterotonic effect when the 15-methyl analogue is given intramuscularly (0.25 mg) is 5 minutes, with a peak effect around 15 to 20 minutes. When injected into the myometrium, its effect may be more rapid. An alternative next-level drug is misoprostol 800 to 1000 μg per rectum (Table 10-1, Stage 2).

If these pharmacologic treatments fail, **a bimanual compression and massage of the uterine corpus may control the bleeding and cause the uterus to contract.** This was the only method available before the use of uterotonic drugs. Although **packing the uterine cavity is no longer widely practiced,** it may occasionally control PPH and obviate the need for surgical intervention. Alternatively, **a large-volume balloon catheter** has been developed that performs a similar function while maintaining a channel into the uterine cavity, allowing further bleeding to be monitored. If uterine bleeding persists in an otherwise stable patient, an interventional radiologist may be able to **place a percutaneous catheter into the uterine arteries for injection of thrombogenic material to control blood flow and hemorrhaging (see Table 10-1, Stage 2).**

Hysterectomy is a treatment of last resort. If the patient has completed her childbearing, a **supracervical or total abdominal hysterectomy** is the definitive therapy for intractable PPH caused by uterine atony. When reproductive potential is important to the patient, **ligation of the uterine arteries** adjacent to the uterus will lower the pulse pressure. This procedure is more successful in controlling placental site hemorrhage and is easier to perform than bilateral hypogastric artery ligation (see Table 10-1, Stage 3).

GENITAL TRACT TRAUMA

When PPH is related to genital tract trauma, surgical intervention is necessary. When repairing genital tract lacerations, **the first suture must be placed well above the apex of the laceration to incorporate any retracted bleeding arterioles into the ligature.** Repair of vaginal lacerations requires good light and good exposure, and the tissues should be approximated without dead space. A running locked suture technique provides the best hemostasis (Figure 10-2). **Cervical lacerations need not be sutured unless they are actively bleeding.** Large, expanding hematomas of the genital tract require surgical evacuation of clots and a search for bleeding vessels that can be ligated. **Stable hematomas can be observed and treated conservatively.** A retroperitoneal hematoma generally begins in the pelvis. If the bleeding cannot be controlled using a vaginal approach, a laparotomy may be necessary.

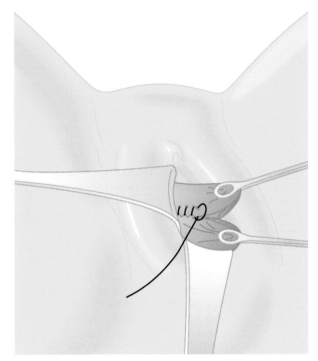

FIGURE 10-2 Suturing a cervical laceration. The first suture must be placed above the apex of the laceration.

An **intraoperative laceration of the ascending branch of the uterine artery** during delivery through a low transverse incision can easily be controlled by the placement of a large suture ligature through the myometrium and broad ligament below the level of the laceration. A **uterine rupture** usually necessitates subtotal or total abdominal hysterectomy, although small defects may be repaired.

RETAINED PRODUCTS OF CONCEPTION

When the placenta cannot be delivered in the usual manner, **manual removal** is necessary (Figure 10-3). This should be performed urgently if bleeding is profuse. Otherwise, it is reasonable to delay for 30 minutes to await spontaneous separation. General anesthesia may be required. Following manual removal of the placenta or placental remnants, the uterus should be scraped with a large curette.

UTERINE INVERSION

The management of a uterine inversion requires quick thinking. The patient rapidly goes into shock, and **immediate intravascular volume expansion with IV crystalloids is required.** An anesthesiologist should be present. When the patient's condition is stable, the partially separated placenta should be completely removed and an attempt made to replace the uterus by placing a cupped hand into the inverted fundus from below

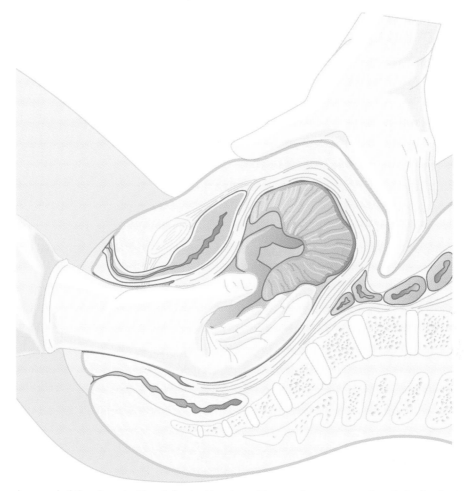

FIGURE 10-3 Manual removal of the placenta. The abdominal hand provides counterpressure on the uterine fundus against the shearing force of the fingers in the uterus.

and elevating it in the long axis of the vagina. If this is unsuccessful, a further attempt should be made using **IV nitroglycerin** (100 μg) **or general anesthesia to relax the uterine muscle.** Once replaced, a dilute infusion of oxytocin should be started to cause the uterus to contract before removing the intrauterine hand. **Rarely, the uterus cannot be replaced from below, and a surgical procedure may be required.** At laparotomy, a vertical incision should be made through the posterior portion of the cervix to incise the constriction ring and allow the fundus to be replaced into the peritoneal cavity. Suturing of the cervical incision completes this procedure.

AMNIOTIC FLUID EMBOLUS

The principal objectives of treatment for amniotic fluid embolism are to support the respiratory system, correct the shock, and replace the coagulation factors. This type of embolism requires immediate cardiopulmonary resuscitation, usually with mechanical venti-lation; rapid volume expansion with an electrolyte solution; positive inotropic cardiac support; placement of a bladder catheter to monitor urine output; correction of the red cell deficit by transfusion with packed red blood cells; and reversal of the coagulopathy with the use of platelets, fibrinogen, and other blood components.

MANAGEMENT OF COAGULOPATHY

When PPH is associated with coagulopathy, the specific defect should be corrected by the infusion of blood products, as outlined in Box 10-5 and Table 10-2. **Patients with thrombocytopenia require platelet concentrate infusions; those with von Willebrand disease require factor VIII concentrate or cryoprecipitate.**

A packed red cell infusion is given to a patient who has bled sufficiently to compromise the delivery of oxygen to the tissues. Therefore, institution of blood transfusion is best judged by symptoms of oxygen deprivation rather than by some empirical hemoglobin

BOX 10-5

LABORATORY EVALUATION OF DISSEMINATED INTRAVASCULAR COAGULATION

Platelet count (normal range 150-450 $\times$ 10^9/L): 1 U of platelets will raise the platelet count by 5-10 $\times$ 10^9/L

Plasma fibrinogen (normal range 175-600 mg/dL): fresh frozen plasma (FFP): 1 U = 1 g of fibrinogen; 4 U of FFP will raise the plasma fibrinogen by 5-10 mg/dL

Cryoprecipitate: 1 bag = 0.25 g of fibrinogen; 16 bags raises the plasma fibrinogen by 5-10 mg/dL

Fibrin split products: Normal range: <0.05 μg/mL (D-dimer method)

TABLE 10-2

BLOOD PRODUCTS USED TO CORRECT COAGULATION DEFECTS

Blood Product	Volume (mL) in 1 U*	Effect of Transfusion
Platelet concentrate	30-40	Increases platelet count by about 5000-10,000
Cryoprecipitate	15-25	Supplies fibrinogen, factor VIII, von Willebrand factor, and fibronectin
Fresh frozen plasma	200	Supplies all factors except platelets (1 g of fibrinogen)
Packed red blood cells	200	Raises hematocrit 3-4%

*Quantity obtained from 1 U (500 mL) of fresh whole blood.

level. No important physiologic impairment has been noted at hemoglobin levels as low as 6 to 8 g/dL (hematocrit of 18-24%). **In general, a 1-U transfusion of packed red blood cells will increase the hemoglobin level by 1 g/dL (and the hematocrit by 3-4%).**

Massive blood replacement (when total blood volume is replaced in a 24-hour period) may be associated with thrombocytopenia, prolonged PT, and hypofibrinogenemia. Thrombocytopenia is the most common abnormality, so platelet transfusion following determination of a low platelet count is not an uncommon scenario. Fresh frozen plasma may be transfused for prolonged PT or hypofibrinogenemia.

In the setting of active bleeding greater than 1000 mL, the hemorrhage care protocol (see Table 10-1) should be activated. Maternal mortality and morbidity have been reduced when a protocol of packed red blood cells, fresh frozen plasma, and platelets, given in a ratio of 6:4:1, is implemented. Treatment should not be delayed while awaiting laboratory results or blood product crossmatching.

Uterine Contractility and Dystocia

CALVIN J. HOBEL • AMY R. LAMB

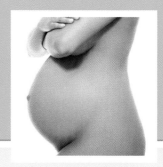

CLINICAL KEYS FOR THIS CHAPTER

- Normal and effective spontaneous labor is dependent upon normal uterine physiology and careful watchful waiting without overly aggressive obstetric management. Dystocia is dysfunctional labor that often has complex origins, and may develop after the normal onset of labor or after the induction of labor for indicated reasons. Metabolic dysregulation before pregnancy or during pregnancy secondary to the mother's health are thought to contribute to the cause(s) of dystocia.
- The uterus is a smooth muscle organ that undergoes dramatic changes to accommodate the developing fetus. Maternal, placental, and fetal hormones play important roles in preparing the uterus to accept a growing and maturing fetus, permitting labor to begin naturally, and allowing the fetus a safe passage and a timely delivery into its new external environment.
- The Friedman labor curve has been the standard used for plotting the progress of labor as defined by cervical dilation over time. More recent studies suggest that the age of women on becoming pregnant has increased and their body mass index (BMI) before pregnancy is significantly higher. These factors, along with excessive weight gain during pregnancy, contribute to abnormalities in the progress of labor during the latent and the active phases. Thus, more attention and time must be spent observing women to avoid the risk of cesarean delivery. Newer parameters for defining dystocia have been proposed as a modification of the Friedman curve.
- Recent studies of the pathogenesis of dystocia have focused on conditions that affect the metabolic dysregulation of normal myometrial function, such as infection and inflammation. These conditions are more common in overweight and obese women. Currently, vitamin D deficiency is related to muscle dysfunction and a greater risk of inflammation, and this deficiency may contribute to the cause(s) of abnormal dystocia.
- Oxytocin for myometrial stimulation in patients with abnormal progress of labor should be used with caution. Other risk factors such as abnormal presentation, excessive size of the fetus (macrosomia), developmental abnormalities of the fetus, and maternal pelvic abnormalities that may increase the risk of dystocia should be recognized and appropriate management initiated. Current evidence indicates that conduction anesthesia does not increase the primary cesarean delivery rate.

Although the definition of **dystocia** is **"difficult childbirth,"** the term is used interchangeably with **dysfunctional labor** and characterizes labor that does not progress normally. Dystocia may be caused by (1) abnormalities of the **"Powers,"** such as ineffective coordinated contractility and uterine expulsive forces; (2) abnormalities of the **"Passenger,"** such as abnormal fetal lie, fetal macrosomia, malpresentation, malposition, or fetal anatomic defects or (3) abnormalities of the **"Passage,"** such as maternal bony pelvic contractures, resulting in mechanical interference with the passage of the fetus through the birth canal.

The cause or causes of abnormal labor should be determined as accurately as possible so that an effective and safe management plan can be developed. The purpose of this chapter is to provide the student with specific metrics that have helped obstetricians understand normal and abnormal labor.

Physiologic Changes of Labor

The pregnant uterus is a large smooth muscle organ consisting of billions of smooth muscle cells. Each smooth muscle cell becomes a contractile element when the intracellular ionic calcium concentration increases to trigger an enzymatic process that results in the formation of the actin-myosin element. Stimulation of oxytocin and/or prostaglandin receptors on the plasma membrane of cells further activates the formation of the actin-myosin element.

Contractions occur in localized areas of the uterus during gestation, but during parturition the entire uterus contracts in an organized way to allow for birth. These coordinated smooth muscle contractions occur as a result of an increase in number and action of special gap junction structures. **Gap junctions are protein channels that form along the interface of two smooth muscle cell membranes and act by promoting the movement of action potentials throughout the myometrium.**

During labor, two distinct segments of the uterus are formed. The **upper segment** actively contracts and retracts to expel the fetus, while the **lower segment,** along with the dilating cervix, becomes thinner and passive and is referred to as the lower uterine segment (LUS).

The pregnant cervix contains collagen, small amounts of smooth muscle, and ground substance and must be structurally altered from a firm, intact sphincter to a soft, pliable, dilated structure through which the fetus can pass at the appropriate time. The collagen fibers are helical strands of amino acids in an intracellular protein matrix of glycosaminoglycan branches (GAGs). The GAGs determine the amount of aggregation of the collagen fibers. Cervical softening involves two changes in the intracellular matrix: a reduction in the number of collagen fibers and an increase in the GAGs, and later decreasing fiber

aggregation. **Several hormones are known to affect cervical softening including prostaglandins (PGs) and relaxin.** Prostaglandin E2 (PGE2) is considered the major hormone causing cervical softening and an increased production of PGE2 coincides with reductions in progesterone levels before parturition. The increase in PGE2 also acts to increase uterine myometrial contractions and uterine pressure and to stimulate the cervix at the onset of labor.

Normal Labor

Labor is diagnosed by regular, painful uterine contractions that increase in frequency and intensity with progressive cervical effacement or dilation.

In early latent phase labor, the cervix softens and effaces with minimal dilation. This is followed by a more rapid active phase of dilation, which is **further subdivided into the acceleration (maximum slope) and deceleration phases.** The descent of the fetal presenting part usually begins during the active phase, accelerating toward the end of the active phase, and climaxing after the cervix is completely dilated. A useful method for assessing the progress of labor and detecting abnormalities in a timely manner is to plot the rate of cervical dilation and descent of the fetal presenting part (Figure 11-1).

Normal cervical dilation and descent of the fetus take place in a progressive manner and occur within

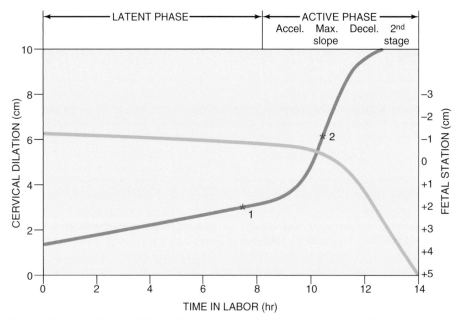

FIGURE 11-1 Graphic plot of cervical dilation *(blue)* and descent of the fetal presenting part *(red)* during labor. *Red star 1* on the *blue line* indicates the beginning of the active phase of labor (as recommended by Cohen and Friedman) and *red star 2* the beginning of the active phase of labor as recommended by Zhang et al. (Revised from Cohen WR, Friedman EA, editors: *Management of labor,* Gaithersburg, Md, 1983, Aspen Publishers, p 13; and Zhang J, Landy HJ, Branch DW, et al: Contemporary patterns of spontaneous labor with normal neonatal outcomes. *Obstet Gynecol* 116:1281–1287, 2010.)

a well-defined time period. **Dysfunctional labor occurs when rates of dilation and descent exceed these time limits.** The phase of labor and the configuration of the abnormal labor curve may indicate the potential causes for the abnormal labor.

Abnormalities of the Latent Phase of Labor

The normal limits of the latent phase of labor extend up to 18 hours for nulliparous patients and up to 10 hours for multiparous patients (see Table 8-5). A latent phase that exceeds these limits is considered prolonged and may be caused by dysfunctional labor, premature or excessive use of sedatives or analgesics, fetal malposition, or abnormal fetal size. A long, closed, firm cervix requires more time to efface and to undergo early dilation than does a soft, partially effaced cervix, but it is doubtful that a cervical factor alone causes a prolongation of the latent phase. **Many patients who appear to be developing a prolonged latent phase are shown eventually to be in false labor or prelabor, with no progressive dilation of the cervix.**

The outcome of a prolonged latent phase is generally favorable for both the mother and the fetus, provided that no other abnormalities of labor subsequently occur.

MANAGEMENT

A prolonged latent phase caused by premature or excessive use of sedation or analgesia usually resolves spontaneously after the effects of the medication have worn off. Therapeutic rest with morphine sulfate or an equivalent drug has been shown to be an effective therapeutic option for women in prolonged latent phase, with about 62% being subsequently admitted in labor, particularly those at term with >50% effacement, about 29% being discharged not in labor, and about 9% being admitted for category II fetal heart rate tracings for continued assessment. Thus, women in true labor wake up in active labor, while those in prelabor stop contracting and can be discharged

If a definitive diagnosis of prolonged latent phase of labor has been made and there are medical reasons to expedite delivery, augmentation of labor by oxytocin may be performed. This is accomplished by the addition of 20 U of oxytocin to 1 L of lactated Ringer solution. A number of protocols have been suggested for the infusion of oxytocin. Oxytocin can be given as "low dose," where the infusion is begun at a rate of 1.0 to 2.0 mU/min and is increased by 1 to 2 mU/min increments every 15 to 40 minutes until the desired frequency and intensity are obtained, or a maximum of 20 to 40 mU/min has been reached. The "high dose" infusion method is begun at a rate of 4 to 6 mU/min with incremental increases of 4 to 6 mU/min every 15

to 40 minutes until uterine contractions of the desired frequency and intensity are obtained or a maximum of 40 mU/min has been reached.

Amniotomy or artificial rupture of the membranes may be considered as part of the management of the latent phase of labor; however, **recent data suggest that amniotomy is associated with an increased risk of cesarean delivery.**

Abnormalities of the Active Phase of Labor

The beginning of the active phase of labor in terms of cervical dilation varies from 3 to 6 cm, depending on either a strict interpretation of the Friedman labor curve (3 cm) or an acceptance of recent evidence that the curve should be modified (up to 6 cm) in certain patients (primarily nulliparous women). There are two clinical reasons for varying the interpretation of the start of the active phase of labor. First, parity plays an important role, and anywhere up to 6 cm is generally considered to be reasonable in a nulliparous woman. Second, recent population studies have demonstrated that **pregnant women are older and heavier now than earlier generations, so the progress of labor is expected to be slower today as a consequence.** The interpretation of the start of the active phase of labor has consequences in terms of defining dystocia, particularly in the nulliparous patient. Thus, because of these factors the onset of the active phase of labor may vary depending on the patient population. Note the differences in the onset of the active phases in Figures 11-1 and 11-2.

After the active phase of labor is deemed to have begun, the rate of dilation progresses more rapidly during normal labor. **Cervical dilation rates of less than 1.2 cm per hour in nulliparous women and 1.5 cm per hour in multiparous women constitute a protraction disorder of the active phase of labor as depicted by the dashed blue line illustrated in Figure 11-2.**

During the latter part of the active phase, the fetal presenting part also descends more rapidly through the pelvis and continues to descend through the second stage of labor as depicted by the red line in Figure 11-1. **A rate of descent of the presenting part of less than 1.0 cm per hour in nulliparous women and 2.0 cm per hour in multiparous women is considered to be a protraction disorder of descent as depicted by the red dashed line in Figure 11-2.**

Figure 11-3 illustrates differences between nulliparous and parous women in terms of the acceptable length of the active phase of labor. Note the marked acceleration in multiparous women, whereas nulliparous women do not accelerate but continue to demonstrate a slower rate of dilation. **A correct interpretation of the beginning of the active phase of labor can have an impact on the frequency of cesarean deliveries for**

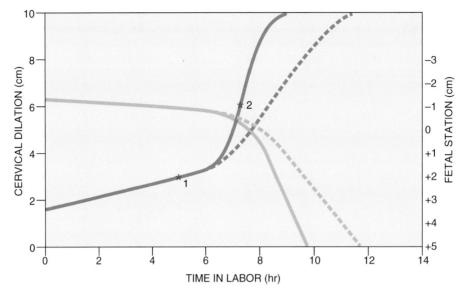

FIGURE 11-2 Normal dilation *(blue)* and descent *(red)* curves of normal labor and curves depicting protracted dilation and descent abnormalities of labor. *Red star 1* on the *blue line* indicates the beginning of the active phase of labor (Friedman) and *red star 2* the beginning of the active phase of labor as recommended by Zhang et al. (Revised from Friedman EA: *Labor: clinical evaluation and management,* ed 2, New York, 1978, Appleton-Century-Crofts, p 65; and Zhang J, Landy HJ, Branch DW, et al: Contemporary patterns of spontaneous labor with normal neonatal outcomes. *Obstet Gynecol* 116:1281–1287, 2010.)

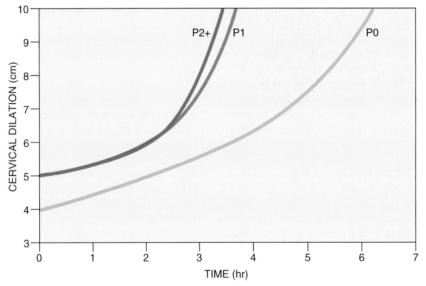

FIGURE 11-3 Average labor curves by parity in singleton, term pregnancies with spontaneous onset of labor, vaginal delivery, and normal neonatal outcomes. *P0,* Nulliparas; *P1,* women of parity 1; *P2+,* women of parity 2 or higher. (Zhang J, Landy HJ, Branch DW, et al: Contemporary patterns of spontaneous labor with normal neonatal outcomes. *Obstet Gynecol* 116:1281–1287, 2010.)

active phase arrest of dilation. By not accounting for a later but normal start of the active phase of labor and not expecting a slower but normal progression of labor in certain patients, more cesarean deliveries may be done unnecessarily.

MANAGEMENT

The American College of Obstetricians and Gynecologists (ACOG) recommends the use of oxytocin for all **protraction and arrest disorders.** Adequate labor is defined as 200 Montevideo units (which is the sum of all the amplitudes of all the contractions in a 10 minute window) as assessed by an intrauterine catheter for at least 2 hours. Arrest of labor should not be diagnosed until the cervix is at least 6 cm dilated. Therefore, a patient having four contractions in 10 minutes, each with an amplitude of 50 mm Hg, should be regarded as having adequate labor. **Amniotomy should**

be considered if rupture of membranes has not occurred spontaneously.

Before deciding to proceed to cesarean delivery in the first stage of labor for abnormal labor progression, it should be ascertained that at least 4 hours of adequate contractions, as defined by 200 Montevideo units per 10 minutes, has occurred. In a nulliparous, singleton term pregnancy, continuing labor for at least 6 hours is still associated with a high likelihood of vaginal delivery, provided that the fetal heart rate is reassuring and there is some progress in labor. **A cesarean delivery is indicated if cephalopelvic disproportion (CPD) is diagnosed.**

ACTIVE MANAGEMENT OF LABOR

Active management of labor has been proposed and utilized in the nulliparous patient as a safe method to lower the incidence of cesarean delivery for dystocia. This strategy of labor management is based on the assessment of the active phase of labor as presented above.

The inclusion criteria and components of the active management of labor are as follows: (1) nulliparous patients should have **spontaneous onset of labor and a singleton fetus in a cephalic presentation;** (2) **prenatal education classes** and intrapartum reassurances to set realistic patient expectations and lower patient anxiety; (3) **constant supervision during labor,** usually by a labor nurse specialist or midwife; (4) **retrospective peer review of all cesarean deliveries;** (5) **no admittance to the labor unit without a clear diagnosis of labor** (this should be based not only on cervical dilation but also on the quality of contractions, which should be regular and painful with at least one of the following: complete cervical effacement, rupture of membranes, or bloody show); (6) **performance of regular examinations for progress of labor based on cervical dilation;** and (7) **the use of medium to high dose oxytocin if the patient fails to demonstrate cervical dilation at a rate of 1 cm/hour or more in the first stage of labor or if there is no descent of the fetal head for 1 hour in the second stage.** Most active management protocols use an initial infusion rate and increments of 4 to 6 mU/min of oxytocin with only 15 minutes between increments to a maximum of 40 mU/min. Performance of an amniotomy on admission is no longer a requirement for the active management of labor.

Many programs using active management of labor have reported a reduction in cesarean delivery rate with no compromise of perinatal outcomes and no cases of uterine rupture.

DYSTOCIA CAUSED BY ABNORMAL PRESENTATION AND POSITION

Presentations other than vertex and positions other than occipitoanterior are considered to be abnormal in the laboring patient. Disorders of the dilation and descent phases of labor occur with increased frequency in cases of abnormal presentation or position because of the altered relationship between the presenting part of the fetus and the maternal pelvis. Fetal malpresentations are discussed further in Chapter 13.

Persistent Occipitotransverse Position

The fetal head normally enters and engages in the maternal pelvis in an occipitotransverse (OT) position and then rotates to an occipitoanterior (OA) position or, in a small percentage of cases, to an occipitoposterior (OP) position. This rotation occurs because the head flexes as the leading part of the vertex encounters the pelvic floor and then rotates to adjust to the shape of the gynecoid pelvis. In a small number of cases, the head fails to flex and rotate and persists in an OT position. This position may be caused by cephalopelvic disproportion; altered pelvic architecture, such as in a patient with a platypelloid or android pelvis; or a relaxed pelvic floor, brought about by epidural anesthesia or multiparity. The diagnosis of a persistent OT position may be difficult at times because of the obscuring of suture lines and fontanelles by the excessive molding and caput formation that often accompany this abnormal position. If the position remains in question, an ultrasonic assessment of the lower abdomen can determine whether or not the face is pointing anterior or posterior, or if the head is flexed or extended.

A persistent OT position with arrest of descent for a period of 1 hour or more is known as transverse arrest. Arrest occurs because of the deflexion that accompanies the persistent OT position, resulting in the larger occipitofrontal diameter (11 cm) becoming the presenting diameter. Until the head undergoes flexion and rotation, further descent cannot take place. Transverse arrest commonly occurs with the vertex at a +2 cm to +3 cm station (which is based on a 5-point scale from zero at the level of the spines to 5 cm when the vertex is beginning to crown before delivery).

The management of transverse arrest at a +2 to +3 station is complex, in part, because at these stations, the widest part of the fetal head is at or above the level of the ischial spines. If the midpelvis is compromised, cesarean delivery is indicated. If the pelvis is judged to be of normal size and the fetus is not macrosomic, oxytocic stimulation of labor may be appropriate if uterine contractions are inadequate.

Manual rotation using the fingers of the examiner's hand or forceps rotation using Kielland forceps may be indicated if the pelvis is of normal size and shape. **Today, forceps rotations are rarely done because of limited training among younger physicians; vacuum extraction, if properly applied, may be attempted.** Forceps rotation and delivery of a persistent OT position at a +2 to +3 station is now referred to as a low forceps procedure. However, because of the marked degree of molding and caput formation that usually occurs in this circumstance, the bony part of the fetal vertex may be at +1 station even though the scalp may be visible at the introitus. Thus what appears to be an uncomplicated low forceps operation may actually be a more difficult midforceps procedure. One method for avoiding this problem is to clinically evaluate the relationship between the fetal head and the sacrum. If the fetal head fills the hollow of the sacrum, the biparietal diameter is usually at or below the spines, and an attempt at forceps delivery can be considered.

Persistent Occipitoposterior Position

The head generally rotates from OT to OA during the descent through the maternal pelvis. Even if the head initially rotates to an OP position, most fetuses will eventually rotate spontaneously during labor to OA, leaving only 5-15% of fetuses with a persistent OP position.

The course of labor in the presence of a persistent OP position is usually normal except for a tendency for the second stage to be prolonged (>2 hours). It is also associated with considerably more discomfort. As with the persistent OT position, the fetal head may become markedly molded with extensive caput formation, which may cause difficulty in diagnosing its correct station and position. **Observation of a prolonged second stage of labor is appropriate, provided that labor continues to be progressive and the fetal heart rate is normal.**

Delivery of the head may occur spontaneously in the OP position, but if the perineum provides undue resistance to delivery, a low forceps-assisted delivery may be required (e.g., using Simpson forceps). In the past, a Kielland forceps rotation was usually performed, but because of a lack of experience and training, **fetuses in the OP position are usually now delivered without rotation. Use of a vacuum extractor with a cup designed for a safe and secure posterior application may be considered.** Sometimes the head will rotate, but it will usually deliver in the OP position. A wide mediolateral episiotomy may be required to lessen the resistance of the outlet. Although routine episiotomies are no longer performed, it is important to perform them when indicated.

DYSTOCIA CAUSED BY ABNORMALITIES OF FETAL STRUCTURE

Macrosomia and Shoulder Dystocia

ACOG defines macrosomia as a fetus weighing 4500 g or more. Large for gestational age is defined as birth weight equal to or above the 90th percentile of fetal weight for a given gestational age. Macrosomia is associated with genetic determinants, maternal diabetes, prepregnancy body mass index (BMI), weight gain during pregnancy, multiparity, male gender, gesta-

tional age greater than 40 weeks, ethnicity, maternal birth weight, maternal height, and maternal age. **Maternal morbidities associated with macrosomia include labor dystocia, shoulder dystocia, and genital trauma,** and there is a corresponding increase in the cesarean delivery rate. **There is also an increased incidence of postpartum hemorrhage and puerperal infection. Both of these conditions have recently been shown to be associated with maternal vitamin D deficiency during pregnancy.** There is increased perinatal morbidity associated with dystocia and birth trauma, especially shoulder dystocia.

An accurate estimate of fetal weight is elusive. **Errors in the estimation of macrosomia by ultrasound may be up to 50%.** Prospective studies have shown that clinical estimates by physicians or patients are as inaccurate as ultrasonic assessments. Suspected macrosomia alone is not an indication for caesarian delivery or induction of labor. Induction of labor has not been shown to improve fetal or maternal outcome. Although the mean duration of labor is prolonged for excessively large fetuses, it is not unusual to encounter unexpected shoulder dystocia after a labor that has been entirely normal up to the moment of delivery.

Shoulder dystocia means difficult delivery of the shoulder. It has been defined as delivery of the shoulder requiring the use of procedures in addition to gentle downward traction on the fetal head or a prolongation of the head-to-body delivery interval to more than 60 seconds.

Shoulder dystocia depends on the size of the maternal pelvis in relation to the size of the fetus and occurs from impaction of the shoulder on the pubic symphysis anteriorly or the sacral promontory posteriorly. The most important risk factors for shoulder dystocia are fetal macrosomia and maternal diabetes. Others include obesity, multiparity, postterm gestation, short stature, previous history of macrosomic birth, and previous history of shoulder dystocia. During labor, risk factors include labor induction, epidural analgesia, prolonged labor, and operative vaginal delivery.

The major neonatal complication of shoulder dystocia is Erb palsy that can be caused by excessive traction on the brachial plexus by the delivery attendant. This is an important malpractice risk in obstetrics. When Erb palsy occurs on the posterior shoulder, the damage could not have been caused by excessive traction, but is most likely due to abnormalities of the sacral promontory applying pressure on the brachial plexus before delivery. Other neonatal complications include **Klumpe palsy,** clavicular fracture, humeral fracture, hypoxia, brain injury, and death. Maternal complications include genital tract lacerations and postpartum hemorrhage.

Shoulder dystocia is recognized at delivery by retraction of the fetal head, which is called the "turtle sign." Shoulder dystocia is not overcome by traction on the fetal head but, instead, by one or more maneuvers designed to displace the anterior shoulder from behind the symphysis pubis. **An initial maneuver that can be attempted is suprapubic pressure,** which involves downward or lateral pressure with the hand over the maternal suprapubic region in an effort to guide the anterior shoulder under or away from the symphysis pubis. The **McRoberts maneuver** may also be employed as an initial or second procedure. In the McRoberts maneuver, the maternal thighs are sharply flexed against the maternal abdomen to reduce the angle between the sacrum and spine, thus freeing the impacted shoulder. Additionally the **"Gaskin" or "all-fours"** maneuver may be attempted. This involves having the mother rotate on to her hands and knees. This position may help to dislodge the shoulder by reducing the angle of the maternal pelvis, and may facilitate easier delivery of the posterior arm. If this is not successful, pressure is applied with the operator's fingers against the scapula of the posterior shoulder in an attempt to rotate (screw) the posterior shoulder upward until it becomes the anterior shoulder. This is known as **"Wood maneuver."** If this maneuver does not correct the problem, a hand is inserted into the vagina and the posterior arm is grasped and pulled across the chest, resulting in delivery of the posterior shoulder and displacement of the anterior shoulder from behind the symphysis pubis. Fracture of the humerus may result from this maneuver, but the bone heals quickly in the neonate. **If none of these maneuvers is successful, one or both clavicles must be fractured,** preferably by pressure on the clavicle directed away from the pleural cavity to prevent traumatic puncture of the lungs.

A maneuver has been described, attributed to **Zavanelli,** to manage shoulder dystocia when previous methods have failed. In this last-resort procedure, the fetal head is manually returned to its prerestitution position, and then slowly replaced into the vagina and then into the uterus by steady upward pressure against the head. Delivery is then accomplished by cesarean delivery. A uterine relaxant may be required to carry out this procedure.

Developmental Abnormalities

Localized abnormalities of fetal anatomy may lead to dystocia. **Internal hydrocephalus** may cause enlargement of the fetal head to the extent that vaginal delivery is not possible. The diagnosis is usually made by ultrasonography performed because of the clinical suspicion. It may be diagnosed as an unexpected finding on ultrasonography performed for another indication.

Several options are available for the delivery of the fetus with hydrocephalus. **Excessive cerebrospinal fluid may be removed** by inserting a needle directly into the ventricular space through the dilated cervix during labor, or transabdominally under ultrasonic guidance before or during labor. **Alternatively, the fetus may be delivered by cesarean** to avoid the risk of infection, which can result from transvaginal or transabdominal drainage. Intrauterine shunting of the fetal ventricular system into the amniotic fluid compartment is still an experimental procedure that has not been shown to have the long-term benefits required to justify its performance.

The accumulation of ascites in the fetal abdomen or enlargement of fetal organs, such as the bladder or liver, may result in unexpected dystocia (because of an enlarged fetal abdomen) after the fetal head has been delivered. Ascites usually occurs as part of hydrops (see Chapter 16), which is defined as fetal fluid retention in two of the following sites: skin, abdomen, pericardial cavity, or pleural cavity. Immune hydrops is usually caused by Rhesus disease, while nonimmune hydrops may be caused by congenital infections, chromosomal abnormalities, or fetal arrhythmias. If any of the above conditions are present, careful ultrasonic evaluation before or during labor should be performed to identify excessive enlargement of the fetal abdomen. Ascitic fluid or urine from a massively enlarged bladder may be removed by transabdominal drainage with a needle before vaginal delivery. Cesarean delivery may be indicated if the fetal abdomen cannot be sufficiently decompressed.

A defect in the fetal lumbosacral vertebrae may result in the protrusion of a meningeal sac (**meningocele**) or a sac containing a portion of the spinal cord (**meningomyelocele**). These defects are usually detected as a result of abnormal serum or amniotic fluid alpha-fetoprotein values or by ultrasonography. If the sac is large, abdominal delivery is advisable to avoid dystocia or rupture of the sac and potential infection. When the sac is small and is covered by fetal skin, as reflected by a normal alpha-fetoprotein value, vaginal delivery is appropriate.

Other potential causes of fetal dystocia include a very large fetal **sacrococcygeal teratoma** and **conjoined twins.**

DYSTOCIA CAUSED BY MATERNAL PELVIC ABNORMALITIES

Cephalopelvic disproportion (CPD) exists if the maternal bony pelvis is not of sufficient size and of appropriate shape to allow the passage of the fetal head (see Chapter 8 on pelvic anatomy and clinical pelvimetry). This problem may occur as a result of contraction of one of the planes of the pelvis. Relative CPD may exist with a normal pelvis, if the fetal head is excessively large or if it is in an abnormal position. Contraction of the maternal pelvis usually occurs at the level of the inlet or midpelvis, but **contraction of the outlet is extremely unusual** unless it is found in association with a midpelvic contraction.

CPD at the level of the pelvic inlet causes a failure of descent and engagement of the head. The finding of an unengaged head in a nulliparous patient at the start of labor indicates an increased likelihood of CPD at the pelvic inlet, but an unengaged fetal head in a multiparous patient in labor is not an unusual occurrence.

The management of a nulliparous patient with an unengaged fetal head in labor should begin with a careful clinical evaluation of the maternal pelvis. If the pelvis is clinically adequate, expectant management with observation of the labor pattern is appropriate. If uterine contractions are ineffective, oxytocic stimulation of labor may be considered.

The occurrence of CPD at the level of the midpelvis occurs more frequently than inlet dystocia because the capacity of the midpelvis is smaller than that of the inlet, and because deflection or positional abnormalities of the fetal head are more likely to occur at that level. The occurrence of bony dystocia at the level of the midpelvis is usually indicated by an arrest of descent of the head at a +1 to +2 station. With CPD and arrest of descent, application of the head to the cervix is poor, resulting in the loss of part of the force needed for cervical dilation. Thus CPD may be associated with a protracted rate of cervical dilation before an arrest of descent is apparent.

DYSTOCIA CAUSED BY CONDUCTION ANESTHESIA

The use of epidural anesthesia for pain control during the first stage of labor has gained wide acceptance. Refinement of the epidural technique has allowed a segmental block and continuous infusion of narcotics and local anesthetics that can be titrated for better pain control, with less interference on the process of labor (see Chapter 8). Epidural anesthesia may reduce pelvic floor muscle tone and increase the incidence of malposition of the fetal head causing persistence of OP position. However, changes in the approach to epidural anesthesia, such as the "walking epidural" may reduce the risk of malpresentation. Current evidence suggests that epidural analgesia does not increase the primary cesarean delivery rate.

Obstetric Complications
Preterm Labor and Delivery, PROM, IUGR, Postterm Pregnancy, and IUFD

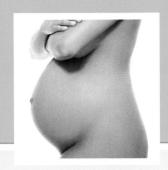

CALVIN J. HOBEL

CLINICAL KEYS FOR THIS CHAPTER

- Prematurity is the leading cause of infant morbidity and mortality. Preterm birth (PTB) is defined as deliveries occurring from 20 weeks up to 37 weeks of gestational age. When preterm birth occurs either spontaneously or in the presence of premature rupture of the membranes (PROM), it must be appropriately managed to prevent early delivery. Premature labor and delivery is best prevented and managed by assessing and treating for infections, assuring fetal lung maturity, and planning a safe delivery as near to term as possible.

- For the past 30 years, infection has been considered the primary cause of premature labor and delivery. Treating infections, however, has not prevented preterm birth, but has decreased the morbidity associated with it. Today, the focus for prevention of preterm labor and delivery is on placental-uterine vascular dysregulation, smoking, and psychosocial and workplace stress. These conditions are associated with the risk of early delivery and poor fetal growth. Assisted reproductive technologies (ARTs) implemented to treat infertility have led to a greater incidence of twinning and higher-order multiples, which has increased the risk of preterm delivery.

- Intrauterine growth restriction (IUGR) is defined as poor fetal growth during pregnancy and reduced size at birth. With IUGR, the infant birth weight is less than the 10th percentile and about 25% of preterm infants are in this category. The causes of IUGR are maternal, placental, and fetal. The main maternal risk factors are poor nutrition, smoking, and metabolic diseases such as hypertension and diabetes. Placental factors are mostly related to failure of proper implantation during early pregnancy. More recently, metabolic dysregulation in women with diabetes has been shown to adversely affect placental function and lead to poor fetal growth. Fetal factors are mostly limited to chronic fetal infections and abnormal development.

- Postterm delivery occurs when there is a failure of the timely onset of labor and the fetus is not delivered at or before 42 weeks' gestation. For the last 30 years, practitioners have recognized that beginning at 41 weeks' gestational age, the risk of fetal distress increases and the fetus fails to continue to grow, increasing the risk of morbidity and mortality. Consequently, fetal assessment techniques have been developed to assess fetal well-being when labor and delivery are delayed. When signs of fetal distress are identified, labor should be induced to rescue the fetus from a potentially hostile environment.

- Intrauterine fetal demise (IUFD) is fetal death between 20 weeks' gestation and the onset of labor. With improved management of IUGR and postterm pregnancies, the incidence of IUFD has decreased dramatically. The remaining causes are often difficult to determine without careful autopsy and genetic studies of the fetus. Management should address the risks to the mother of waiting for spontaneous onset of labor versus the risks of induction of labor. Psychosocial support for the family after delivery is important. It should address concerns about the cause of the fetal death, and how the risk of a similar event can be reduced in the next pregnancy.

About 30% of pregnant women are considered high risk for obstetric complications. A family history of preterm birth, prior obstetric problems such as recurrent early pregnancy loss, preterm birth or fetal demise, and medical problems such as hypertension, diabetes, and obesity are considered to increase the risk for obstetric complications.

This chapter details the causes and treatments for preterm labor and delivery, premature rupture of the membranes (PROM), intrauterine growth restriction (IUGR), postterm pregnancy, and intrauterine fetal demise (IUFD). Despite years of study and research into these problems, their causes are not yet fully understood.

Preterm Labor

Worldwide, preterm labor and delivery are major causes of perinatal morbidity and mortality. **Although fewer than 12% of all infants born in the United States are preterm, their contribution to neonatal morbidity and mortality ranges from 50-70%.** The medical and economic impact of preterm delivery is significant. Major goals of obstetric care should be to reduce the incidence of the condition and to increase the gestational age of infants whose preterm births are unavoidable.

DEFINITION AND INCIDENCE

Preterm birth (PTB) is usually defined as one occurring after 20 weeks and before 37 completed weeks of gestation. Labor that occurs between these gestational ages is defined as preterm labor. Internationally, the lower boundary defining preterm birth varies between 20 and 24 weeks.

Preterm births in the United States increased from 9.8% in 1981 to 12.7% in 2005; however, in the past 6 years, the rate has declined for the seventh straight year to 11.4%. Between 1988 and 2004, the mortality rate for white infants declined by 55% to 5.7 infant deaths per 1000 live births and the mortality rate for black infants declined by 45% to 13.6. In the past 10 years the decline in infant mortality for both races has been less than anticipated. **Because prematurity is the leading cause of infant mortality, the prevention of prematurity has become a high priority.**

ETIOLOGY AND RISK FACTORS

The causes of preterm birth and their estimated frequencies are listed in Table 12-1. **Private patients have a much higher proportion of spontaneous preterm labor, whereas black patients in public institutions have a higher proportion of deliveries due to preterm premature rupture of membranes (PPROM).**

Attempts have been made to define further the spontaneous preterm labor subgroups. Some experts now believe this may be caused by undiagnosed conditions of poor placental implantation, ascending infections via the vagina, or immunologic rejection of uterine and cervical origin. **Recently, genetic thrombophilias have been shown to account for a significant proportion of the uteroplacental problems leading to IUGR and preeclampsia,** the two major reasons for the early induction of labor to avoid fetal death. In the past 10 years, closer surveillance of high risk pregnancies has led to earlier delivery and an increase in the rate of late preterm deliveries (between 34 and 37 weeks), a major contribution to the continued high rate of preterm birth. The decline in preterm birth rate over the past 7 years is thought to be related to the reduced incidence of late preterm birth deliveries.

More women are postponing childbirth as a lifestyle choice, but this is associated with a greater risk of infertility. These women then require assisted reproductive technologies (ARTs) to become pregnant. These technologies are associated with the risk of multiple gestations and the associated increased risks of poor fetal growth and preterm birth. A variety of socioeconomic, psychosocial, and medical conditions have been found to carry an increased risk of preterm delivery in women who postpone childbearing.

Socioeconomic Factors

In the United States, the incidence of preterm deliveries in the black population is twice as high as that in the white population. This factor cannot be viewed as a single entity but probably encompasses other characteristics of the population, such as poor access to, and procurement of, antenatal care, high stress levels, poor nutritional status, and the possibility of genetic differences. In the past 6 years there has been an increase in the incidence of poverty and obesity, which may contribute to the persistence of high levels of preterm birth.

Obstetric, Medical, and Environmental Factors

1. **Recurrent preterm birth:** When one preterm birth has occurred, the relative risk of preterm delivery in the next pregnancy is 3.9, which increases to 6.5 with two previous preterm deliveries.
2. **Second-trimester abortions:** The cause of second-trimester abortions when the fetus is normal is likely to have the same cause as preterm labor (PTL) after 20 weeks. Therefore, these early pregnancy losses are associated with an increased risk for subsequent preterm delivery, especially if a previous preterm birth has also occurred. The risk associated with

TABLE 12-1

PRIMARY CAUSES OF PRETERM BIRTH AND THEIR ESTIMATED FREQUENCY	
Cause	Frequency (%)
Spontaneous preterm labor	35-37
Multiple gestations*	12-15
Preterm premature rupture of membranes (PPROM)	12-15
Late preterm births	50-70
Pregnancy-associated hypertension	12-14
Cervical incompetence/uterine anomalies	12-14
Antepartum hemorrhage	5-6
Intrauterine growth restriction (IUGR)	4-6

*Increased proportion because of advancing maternal age and assisted reproductive technologies (ARTs). ART has increased the incidence of twinning by 50% with a very recent decline due to more elective single embryo transfers.

induced first-trimester abortions is controversial, because they are more likely associated with malformed fetuses that may not have aborted spontaneously. However, if there are repeated first-trimester spontaneous abortions, there is an increased risk of spontaneous loss of a normal fetus because of immunological causes that are poorly understood. Other obstetric factors include multiple gestation and polyhydramnios.

3. **Medical factors:** The major medical factors are hypertension, diabetes, obesity, and genital tract infection. Other factors include bleeding in the first trimester, urinary tract infections, uterine anomalies, and incompetent cervix.

4. **Environmental and behavior factors:** Smoking during pregnancy is associated with an increased risk of preterm birth. Smoking cessation should be considered in any preventative program for preterm birth. Recently, attention has been directed toward maternal employment, physical activity, nutritional status stress, and anxiety as major risk factors for preterm birth. In addition, several papers have associated vitamin D deficiency with a greater risk of preterm birth, preeclampsia, and IUGR.

PATHWAYS THOUGHT TO CAUSE PRETERM BIRTH:

1. Infection (cervical-vaginal-urinary)
2. Placental-vascular
3. Psychosocial stress and work strain (fatigue)
4. Uterine stretch (multiple gestations)

Infection-Cervical Pathway

Bacterial vaginosis has been shown to be associated with preterm delivery, independent of other recognized risk factors. **Treatment of bacterial vaginosis has reduced the incidence of preterm delivery. For many years, it has been known that treatment of asymptomatic and clinical cystitis is associated with a reduced incidence of PTB.** In addition, treating women in preterm labor with antibiotics significantly prolongs the time from the onset of treatment to delivery, compared with that in patients who do not receive antibiotics. Thus, addressing the issue of these relatively asymptomatic infections is an important strategy for preventing preterm birth.

There is a link between vaginal-cervical infections and progressive changes in the cervical length, as measured by vaginal ultrasonography. The relative risk of preterm birth increases significantly from 2.4 for a cervical length of 3.5 cm (50th percentile) to 6.2 for a length of 2.5 cm (10th percentile). **Short cervices appear to be more common in women who have had prior preterm births and pregnancy terminations.**

The most recent test to be developed is cervical and vaginal fetal fibronectin. This substance is a basement membrane protein produced by the fetal membranes. When the fetal membranes are disrupted, as with repetitive uterine activity, and/or in the presence of infection, shortening of the cervix can occur. In the presence of these changes, fibronectin (a protein substance) is secreted into the vagina and can be tested. **A positive fetal fibronectin test at 22 to 24 weeks predicts more than half of the spontaneous preterm births that occur before 28 weeks.** A positive test for fetal fibronectin is significantly associated with a short cervix, vaginal infections, and uterine activity. A negative test is the best predictor of a low risk of preterm delivery.

Placental-Vascular Pathway

The placental-vascular pathway begins early in pregnancy at the time of implantation, when there are important changes taking place at the placental/decidual/myometrial interface. Initially, there are important immunologic changes, with a switch from a Th-1 (helper cell) type of immunity, which may be embryotoxic, to a Th-2 antibody profile, in which blocking antibody production is thought to prevent rejection. At the same time, the trophoblasts are invading the spiral arteries of the decidua and myometrium, assuring that a low resistance vascular connection is established. **All three conditions associated with preterm delivery (spontaneous, PROM, and IUGR) are associated with failure of the trophoblast to properly invade the spinal arteries.** Poor trophoblastic invasion may be caused by placental factors or maternal abnormalities secondary to atherosclerosis. Alterations in both of these early changes are thought to play an important role in the pathophysiology of poor fetal growth, an important component of preterm birth (indicated and spontaneous), fetal growth restriction, and preeclampsia.

The placenta is also an important source of progesterone production that plays an important role in the immune system and in the maintenance of uterine relaxation. The altered placental progesterone production in women at risk of preterm birth is thought to be secondary to placental hormonal dysregulation. Both 17-OH progesterone and vaginal progesterone play an important role in the prevention of preterm birth.

Stress-Strain Pathway

Both mental (cognitive) and work-related stress and strain are postulated to initiate a stress response that increases release of cortisol and catecholamines. The biochemical response to stress is important for the maintenance of metabolic regulation. However, cortisol from the adrenal gland initiates early placental corticotrophin-releasing hormone (CRH) gene expression, and elevated levels of CRH are known to initiate labor at term. Catecholamines released during the stress response not only affect blood flow to the uteroplacental unit, but also cause uterine contractions (norepinephrine). Poor nutrition in the form of reduced calories and/or abnormal patterns of intake (fasting) are known stressors and have been associated with a significantly increased risk of preterm birth. **In support of the stress pathway are the studies that have shown that the rate of change of CRH, a mediator of the stress response, increases significantly in the weeks before the onset of preterm labor. Thus, too much stress (chronic stress) is thought to be toxic and may cause preterm labor.** Stress reduction and psychosocial support are the only current interventions that can be applied to this pathway. Meta-analyses have suggested that psychosocial support via networking between women's social groups can decrease the risk of preterm birth.

Uterine Stretch Pathway

Uterine stretch as a result of increasing volume during normal and abnormal gestations is an important physiological mechanism that facilitates the process of emptying the uterus. In normal pregnancy, the hormone **parathyroid-related protein (PTrP)** plays an important role in relaxing the myometrial tissues, but when stretch exceeds certain limits (e.g., multiple gestations, fetal macrosomia, and polyhydramnios), PTrP fails to keep the uterus relaxed and labor begins. This pathway is common in patients with **polyhydramnios** and those with **multiple gestations,** both of which have an increased risk of preterm birth.

PREVENTION OF PRETERM BIRTH

The ideal time to assess risk factors for premature labor and PTB is before conception. This allows time to identify problems and take measures to mitigate any risk. Unfortunately, very few women are seen before pregnancy for the type of counseling and intervention that would be necessary (see Chapter 7) and it is usually at the first prenatal visit that these measures are initiated. **The important risk factors for PTB are a history of previous PTB, a family history of PTB and child abuse, smoking (including second hand), a history of recurrent early pregnancy losses, previous cervical surgery, obesity, substance abuse, and medical conditions such as hypertension and diabetes.**

For all women, but particularly those who are at high risk for PTB, medical conditions should be managed and appropriate supplementation of folic acid (4 mg/day) and vitamin D (2000 to 3000 IU/day) should be initiated in early pregnancy, in addition to prenatal vitamins. A probiotic supplement should be considered to improve the gut biome. The length of the cervix should be a component of the ultrasonic study at 18 to 20 weeks. **Women with a short cervix (between 10 and 20 mm) should receive vaginal progesterone 200 mg daily from 19 to 20 weeks until 36 weeks.** For women with a history of PTB, 250 mg intramuscular 17OH progesterone caproate weekly, until 36 weeks, or vaginal progesterone, 200 mg daily from 16 to 36 weeks should be initiated.

DIAGNOSIS AND MANAGEMENT OF PRETERM LABOR

The diagnosis of preterm labor between 20 and 37 weeks is based on the following criteria in patients with ruptured or intact membranes: (1) **documented uterine contractions** (4 per 20 minutes or 8 per 60 minutes) and (2) **documented cervical change** (cervical effacement of 80% or cervical dilation of 2 cm or more). Uterine contractions are not a good predictor of preterm labor, but cervical changes are.

Provided that membranes are not ruptured and there is no contraindication to a vaginal examination (e.g., placenta previa), **an initial assessment must be done to ascertain cervical length and dilation and the station and nature of the presenting part.** The patient should also be evaluated for the presence of any underlying correctable problem, such as a urinary tract or vaginal infection. She should be placed in the lateral decubitus position to take the uterine weight off the great vessels, monitored for the presence and frequency of uterine activity, and reexamined for evidence of cervical change after an appropriate interval, unless the preceding criteria for preterm labor have already been met. **During the period of observation, either oral or parenteral hydration (5% dextrose) should be initiated.** Clear liquids of caloric value should be considered. Fasting is not healthy during this phase of management.

With adequate hydration and bed rest, uterine contractions cease in approximately 20% of patients. These patients, however, remain at high risk for recurrent preterm labor.

Because of the role of cervical colonization and vaginal infection in the etiology of preterm labor and PROM, **cultures should be taken for group B *Streptococcus*.** Other organisms that may be important are *Ureaplasma, Mycoplasma,* and *Gardnerella vaginalis.* The latter is associated with bacterial vaginosis, a diagnosis that can be made by the presence of three of four clinical signs (vaginal pH > 4.5, amine odor after addition of a few drops of 10% potassium hydroxide [KOH] on a glass slide, the presence of clue cells, and the presence of a milky discharge).

Antibiotics should be administered to patients who are in preterm labor. For patients who are not allergic to penicillin, a 7-day course of ampicillin and erythromycin may be given. Those allergic to penicillin may be given clindamycin.

Once the diagnosis of preterm labor has been made, the following laboratory tests should be obtained: complete blood cell count, random blood glucose level, serum electrolyte levels, urinalysis, and urine culture and sensitivity. **An ultrasonic examination of the fetus should be performed to assess fetal weight,** document presentation, assess cervical length, and rule out the presence of any accompanying congenital malformation. The test may also detect an underlying etiologic factor, such as twin pregnancy or uterine anomaly.

If the patient does not respond to bed rest and hydration, tocolytic therapy should be instituted, provided that there are no contraindications. Measures implemented at 28 weeks should be more aggressive than those initiated at 35 weeks. Similarly, a patient with advanced cervical dilation on admission requires more aggressive management than one whose cervix is closed and minimally effaced.

UTERINE TOCOLYTIC THERAPY

It is assumed that physiologic events leading to the initiation of labor also occur in preterm labor. The pharmacologic agents presently being used all seem to inhibit the availability of calcium ions, but they may also exert a number of other effects. The agents currently used and their dosages are presented in Box 12-1.

Magnesium Sulfate

In the United States, magnesium sulfate is frequently the drug of choice for initiating tocolytic therapy. Magnesium acts at the cellular level by competing with calcium for entry into the cell at the time of depolarization. Successful competition results in an effective decrease of intracellular calcium ions, resulting in myometrial relaxation.

BOX 12-1

UTERINE TOCOLYTIC AGENTS

Magnesium Sulfate

Solution: Initial solution contains 6 g (12 mL of 50% $MgSO_4$) in 100 mL of 5% dextrose; maintenance solution contains 10 g (20 mL of 50% $MgSO_4$) in 500 mL of 5% dextrose

Initial dose: 6 g over 15 to 20 min, parenterally

Titrating dose: 2 g/hr until contractions cease; follow serum levels (5-7 mg/dL); maximal dose, 4 g/hr

Maintenance dose: Maintain dose for 12 hr, then 1 g/hr for 24 to 48 hr; consider switching to nifedipine (see below)

Nifedipine

Preparation: Oral gelatin capsules of 10 or 20 mg

Loading dose: 30 mg; if contractions persist after 90 min, give an additional 20 mg (second dose); if labor is suppressed, a maintenance dose of 20 mg is given orally every 6 hr for 24 hr and then every 8 hr for another 24 hr

Failure: If contractions persist 60 min after the second dose, treatment should be considered a failure

Prostaglandin Synthetase Inhibitors

Short-term use only

Although magnesium levels required for tocolysis have not been critically evaluated, it appears that the levels needed may be higher than those required for prevention of eclampsia. Levels from 5.5 to 7.0 mg/dL appear to be appropriate. These can be achieved using the dosage regimen outlined in Box 12-1. After the loading dose is given, a continuous infusion is maintained, and plasma levels should be determined until therapeutic levels have been reached. The drug should be continued at therapeutic levels until contractions cease unless the labor progresses. Because magnesium is excreted via the kidneys, adjustments must be made in patients with an abnormal creatinine clearance. Once successful tocolysis has been achieved, the infusion should be continued for at least 12 hours. The infusion rate may then be weaned over 2 to 4 hours and then discontinued. In very high risk patients (advanced cervical dilation or continued labor in very low birth weight cases), the infusion may be continued until the fetus has been exposed to glucocorticoids to enhance lung maturity.

A common minor side effect is a feeling of warmth and flushing on first administration. Respiratory depression is seen at magnesium levels of 12 to 15 mg/dL, and cardiac conduction defects and arrest are seen at higher levels.

In the fetus, plasma magnesium levels approach those of the mother, and a low plasma calcium level may also be demonstrated. The neonate may show some loss of muscle tone and drowsiness, resulting in a lower Apgar score. These effects are prolonged in the preterm neonate because of the decrease in renal clearance.

Long-term parenteral magnesium therapy has been used for control of preterm labor in selected patients. An important side effect seems to be loss of calcium, and it may be important in such patients to institute calcium therapy on a prophylactic basis. Because vitamin D deficiency has been associated with the risk of premature labor, vitamin D supplementation should be considered because vitamin D is required for adequate mobilization of calcium from the skeleton.

Nifedipine

Nifedipine as an oral agent is very effective in suppressing preterm labor with minimal maternal and fetal side effects. It works by inhibiting the slow, inward current of calcium ions during the second phase of the action potential of uterine smooth muscle cells and may gradually replace intravenous magnesium sulfate. The only side effects are headache, cutaneous flushing, hypotension, and tachycardia. The latter two side effects can be partially avoided by making certain the patient is well hydrated and by the use of support stockings, such as thromboembolism-deterrent (TED) hose, to prevent pooling of blood in the lower extremities.

Prostaglandin Synthetase Inhibitors

Prostaglandins induce myometrial contractions at all stages of gestation, both in vivo and in vitro. Because prostaglandins are locally synthesized and possess a relatively short half-life, prevention of their synthesis within the uterus could inhibit labor. **These agents are used on a short-term basis** in circumstances where prostaglandin production may be the inciting factor, as may occur in the presence of uterine fibroids. In the United States **indomethacin is the most commonly used prostaglandin inhibitor; it can be administered both orally and rectally, with some slight delay in absorption from rectal administration as compared with the oral route.** Peak serum levels of indomethacin occur 1.5 to 2 hours after oral administration. Excretion of the intact drug occurs in maternal urine. It can result in oligohydramnios and premature closure of the fetal ductus arteriosus, which in turn may lead to neonatal pulmonary hypertension and cardiac failure. In addition, **indomethacin decreases fetal renal function, and indomethacin-exposed infants have a greater risk of necrotizing enterocolitis, intracranial hemorrhage, and patent ductus arteriosus.** Short-term use may be acceptable, but if patients are given indomethacin, the fetus should be evaluated with ultrasonography for ductus arteriosus flow.

Combined therapy with nifedipine and prostaglandin synthetase inhibitors is currently being used in Australia, Canada, and Europe.

Oxytocin Receptor Antagonists

Atosiban was the first oxytocin receptor antagonist developed. It binds to receptors in the myometrium and other gestational tissues, preventing the oxytocin-induced increase in inositol triphosphate. The latter is the messenger that increases intracellular calcium, and causes myometrial contractions and up-regulation of prostaglandin production. **These agents are not approved for use in the United States.**

Efficacy of Tocolytic Therapy

Although the advent of tocolytic agents has failed to decrease preterm births in large population studies, their use has improved neonatal survival, decreased respiratory distress syndrome (RDS), and increased the birth weight of infants. The benefit of measures to postpone delivery beyond 34 weeks is under investigation, with the thought that the longer the fetus remains in utero the better the outcome.

Antibiotic Therapy

A number of studies have advocated the use of antibiotic prophylaxis in patients with preterm labor. Such patients may have a higher incidence of **subclinical chorioamnionitis** than previously thought.

Diagnostic amniocentesis in patients with idiopathic preterm labor has identified about 15% whose amniotic cavity is colonized with pathogens. It is reasonable to assume that a proportion of the remainder will have occult bacteria in the decidual cell space between the chorion and the myometrium. **The use of prophylactic antibiotics in women with preterm labor may prevent progression from a subclinical infection to clinical amnionitis.**

Contraindications to Tocolytic Therapy

Contraindications include **severe preeclampsia, severe bleeding from placenta previa or abruptio placentae, chorioamnionitis, IUGR, fetal anomalies incompatible with life, and fetal demise.** Because of the low success rate, advanced cervical dilation may also preclude tocolytic therapy, although therapy may delay delivery sufficiently for glucocorticoid administration to accelerate fetal lung maturity. Management of patients should be individualized, and even if the patient's cervix is dilated to 6 cm and infrequent contractions are occurring, it is advisable to employ tocolytics and to administer glucocorticoid therapy.

USE OF GLUCOCORTICOIDS FOR FETAL PULMONARY MATURATION

Antenatal corticosteroid therapy for fetal pulmonary maturation reduces mortality and the incidence of RDS and intraventricular hemorrhage (IVH) in preterm infants. These benefits extend to a broad range of gestational ages (24 to 34 weeks) and are not limited by gender or race. **Treatment consists of 2 doses of 12 mg of betamethasone, given intramuscularly 24 hours apart, or 4 doses of 6 mg of dexamethasone given intramuscularly 12 hours apart.** Optimal benefit begins 24 hours after initiation of therapy and lasts 7 days. Treatment with corticosteroids for less than 24 hours is still associated with significant reductions in neonatal mortality secondary to respiratory distress syndrome and intraventricular hemorrhage, so they should be given unless immediate delivery is anticipated.

LABOR AND DELIVERY OF THE PRETERM INFANT

A certain number of patients will not respond to tocolytic therapy. The goal in these patients should be to conduct both labor and delivery in an optimal manner so as not to contribute to the morbidity or mortality of the preterm infant. All parameters for assessing gestational age and fetal weight must be considered. **With modern neonatal care, the lower limit of potential viability is 24 weeks or 500 g, although these limits vary with the expertise of the neonatal intensive care unit.**

Fetal heart rate patterns characterized as Category II (Intermediate/possibly Early Dysregulation; see Boxes 9-1 and 9-2) that are relatively innocuous in the term fetus may indicate a more ominous outcome for the preterm fetus. The clinician should not wait until

Category III (Abnormal) patterns are observed. In Box 9-2 there are subtype patterns in Category II that may help the clinician to consider immediate delivery to prevent the occurrence of Category III heart rate patterns. **Continuous fetal heart monitoring and prompt attention to abnormal fetal heart rate patterns are extremely important.** Acidosis at birth adversely affects respiratory function by destroying surfactant and delaying its release.

With a vertex presentation, vaginal delivery is preferred, independent of gestational age, provided that fetal acidosis and delivery trauma are avoided. **Use of outlet forceps and an episiotomy to shorten the second stage are advocated.** Some reports recommend cesarean delivery for the very low birth weight baby.

Approximately 23% of infants present as a breech at 28 weeks, compared with about 4% at term. This presentation carries an increased risk of cord prolapse or compression. In addition, cervical entrapment of the after-coming fetal head may occur at delivery because before term the head is proportionally larger than the buttocks. **For the breech fetus estimated at less than 1500 g, neonatal outcome is improved by cesarean delivery.**

Premature Rupture of the Membranes

DEFINITION AND INCIDENCE

Premature rupture of the membranes (PROM) is defined as amniorrhexis (spontaneous rupture of the membranes as opposed to amniotomy) before the onset of labor at any stage of gestation. Preterm PROM (PPROM) should be used to define those patients who are preterm with ruptured membranes, whether or not they have contractions.

ETIOLOGY AND RISK FACTORS

The etiology of PROM remains unclear, but a variety of factors are purported to contribute to its occurrence, including vaginal and cervical infections, abnormal membrane physiology (apoptosis secondary to oxidative stress), incompetent cervix, and nutritional deficiencies.

DIAGNOSIS

Diagnosis of PROM is based on the history of vaginal loss of fluid and confirmation of amniotic fluid in the vagina. Episodic urinary incontinence, leucorrhea, or loss of the mucus plug must be ruled out. **Because of the risk of introducing infection and the usually long latency period from the time of examination until delivery, the examiner's hands should not be inserted into the vagina of a patient who is not in labor, whether preterm or term.** A sterile vaginal speculum examination should be performed to confirm the diagnosis, to assess cervical dilation and length, and if the patient is preterm, to obtain cervical cultures and amniotic fluid samples for pulmonary maturation tests.

On speculum examination, pooling of amniotic fluid in the posterior vaginal fornix can usually be seen. A Valsalva maneuver or slight fundal pressure may expel fluid from the cervical os, which is diagnostic of PROM. **Confirmation of the diagnosis can be made by (1) nitrazine paper test: amniotic fluid will turn blue in the presence of the alkaline amniotic fluid, (2) fern test: placing a sample of amniotic fluid on a microscopic slide left to air dry will show ferning, and (3) AmniSure test: a highly accurate test measuring placental alpha microglobulin-1 (PAMG-1), which is present in high levels in amniotic fluid.** A fluid sample is obtained with a vaginal swab and placed in a test solution and the result read as positive or negative in 5 to 10 minutes. False-positive nitrazine test results occur in the presence of alkaline urine, blood, or cervical mucus. For the fern test, the presence of blood, which is usually seen in patients in early labor, may make the pattern appear to be skeletonized. The AmniSure test is not affected by the presence of blood or infection. As in the case of preterm labor with intact membranes, a complete ultrasonic examination should be carried out to rule out fetal anomalies and to assess gestational age and amniotic fluid volume.

MANAGEMENT

General Considerations

An intact amniotic sac serves as a mechanical barrier to infection, but in addition, amniotic fluid has some bacteriostatic properties that may play a role in preventing chorioamnionitis and fetal infections. **Intact membranes are not an absolute barrier to infection,** because bacterial colonization still occurs in the decidual space/membrane interface in 10% of patients in term labor and in up to 25% of patients in preterm labor.

For preterm fetuses with PPROM, the risks associated with preterm delivery must be balanced against the risks of infection and sepsis. For the mother, the risks include not only the development of chorioamnionitis, but also the possibility of failed induction in the presence of an unfavorable cervix, resulting in subsequent cesarean delivery.

Management is dictated to a large extent by the gestational age at the time of membrane rupture, although **the quantity of amniotic fluid remaining after PPROM may be as important as gestational age in determining pregnancy outcome.**

Ultrasonic definition of oligohydramnios has been standardized. Objective criteria include measurement of the vertical axis of amniotic fluid present in four quadrants, the total being called the **amniotic fluid index (AFI).** A value of less than 5 cm is considered abnormal.

Oligohydramnios associated with PROM in the fetus at less than 24 weeks may lead to the development of pulmonary hypoplasia. Factors that may be responsible include fetal crowding with thoracic compression, restriction of fetal breathing, and disturbances of pulmonary fluid production and flow. The duration of membrane rupture is an important consideration. Constraints placed on fetal movements in utero can also result in a variety of positional skeletal abnormalities, such as talipes equinovarus.

If PROM occurs at 36 weeks or later and the condition of the cervix is favorable, labor should be induced after 6 to 12 hours if no spontaneous contractions occur. In the presence of an unfavorable cervical condition with no evidence of infection, it is reasonable to wait 24 hours before induction of labor to decrease the risk of failed induction and maternal febrile morbidity. The following discussion applies when premature membrane rupture occurs before 36 weeks' gestational age.

Laboratory Tests

In addition to the laboratory tests obtained for the patient in preterm labor, sufficient amniotic fluid can usually be obtained from the vaginal pool for **pulmonary maturation studies.** Because of the higher incidence of chorioamnionitis in association with PROM, amniotic fluid should also be examined with **Gram stain and culture.**

Conservative Expectant Management

Conservative management applies to the care of patients with PPROM who are observed with the expectation of prolonging gestation. **Because the risk of infection appears to increase with the duration of membrane rupture, the goal of expectant management is to continue the pregnancy until the lung profile is mature.** Careful surveillance must be maintained to diagnose chorioamnionitis at an early enough stage to minimize fetal and maternal risks. In its fulminant state, chorioamnionitis is associated with a high maternal temperature and a tender, sometimes irritable, uterus.

In cases of subclinical infection, diagnosis and treatment may be delayed. A combination of factors should alert the clinician to the possibility of chorioamnionitis, including maternal temperature greater than 100.4° F (38° C) in the absence of any other site of infection, fetal tachycardia, a tender uterus, and uterine irritability when noted on nonstress testing while measuring fetal heart rate and uterine activity.

The presence of bacteria by Gram stain or culture of amniotic fluid obtained at amniocentesis correlates with subsequent maternal infection in about 50% of cases and with neonatal sepsis in about 25%. The presence of white blood cells alone in amniotic fluid is less predictive of infection. The decision to perform amniocentesis is based on the gestational age, the presence of early signs of infection, and the AFI as measured by real-time ultrasonography. Recently, investigators have described elevation of inflammatory cytokines in the amniotic fluid and in the fetal circulation in preterm infants who have subsequently developed chronic lung disease during the neonatal period. A similar response may be associated with a greater risk of damage to the preterm baby's brain, thus increasing the risk of cerebral palsy. Therefore, the management of patients with PROM is critical for the prevention of neonatal morbidity. Some centers around the world do not conservatively manage PROM.

Ampicillin or erythromycin significantly prolongs the interval to delivery in patients with PPROM. The neonates delivered from patients receiving prophylaxis also have less morbidity.

Management of Chorioamnionitis

Once chorioamnionitis has been diagnosed, antibiotic therapy should be delayed only until appropriate cultures have been taken. Ampicillin and gentamycin in combination are the drugs of choice. In the penicillin-sensitive patient, cephalosporins may be indicated, noting the 12% incidence of crossover sensitivity. Once antibiotics have been started, labor should be induced. **If the condition of the cervix is unfavorable, and there is evidence of fetal involvement, it may be necessary to perform a cesarean delivery.**

The presence of active genital herpes is an important concern in the presence of ruptured membranes. Herpes infection at a site remote from the cervix and vagina is probably not associated with an increased risk of fetal infection, so the site of infection should be taken into consideration before recommending immediate cesarean delivery.

Tocolytic Therapy

The use of tocolytics to control preterm labor in patients with PROM is controversial. The arguments against their use are that they may mask evidence of maternal infection (e.g., tachycardia) and that contractions associated with the membrane rupture may be indicative of uterine infection. Arguments for their use are that PROM is sometimes initially associated with evidence of uterine contractions, and time is gained for fetal pulmonary maturation. **In the presence of infection, tocolysis is usually unsuccessful.**

Use of Corticosteroids

There is a "natural" decreased incidence of RDS in infants who are born with PPROM 16 to 72 hours after membrane rupture, presumably because of the endogenous release of corticosteroids from the stress of decreased amniotic fluid volume and early infection. Perhaps for this reason, the National Institutes of Health (NIH) guidelines for glucocorticoid therapy recommend they be given to patients with PPROM only up to 32 weeks, rather than up to 34 weeks as recommended when the membranes are intact.

Outpatient Management

Outpatient management is not recommended, unless there is no evidence of infection and a normal AFI after a period of inpatient observation for 2 to 3 days. In this situation, the site of rupture may have closed by overlapping of the amnionic and chorionic membranes. **To be eligible for such management, the patient should be reliable, fully informed regarding the risks involved, and prepared to participate in her own care.** The fetus should be presenting as **a vertex,** and the **cervix should be closed** to minimize the chance of cord prolapse. At home, restricted physical activity should be advised, no coital activity should occur, and the patient should monitor her temperature at least four times per day. Instructions should be given to return immediately if the temperature exceeds 100° F (37.8° C).

The patient should be seen weekly, at which time her temperature should be taken, nonstress testing performed after 28 weeks, and the baseline fetal heart rate and AFI evaluated. Ultrasonic evaluation of fetal growth should also be carried out every 2 weeks. **Any patient with oligohydramnios is not a candidate for outpatient management.**

Labor and Delivery

The same considerations discussed under preterm labor apply to patients with PROM. The decrease in amniotic fluid that is sometimes seen can result in early cord compression and the presence of variable fetal heart decelerations. This is true of both vertex and breech presentations; therefore, there is a necessity for abdominal delivery in a large number of cases.

Tests of Pulmonary Maturity

By far the major determinant of successful extrauterine existence is the ability of the neonate to maintain successful oxygenation. Pulmonary maturation involves changes in pulmonary anatomy in addition to alterations of physiologic and biochemical parameters. **Beginning at about 24 weeks,** the terminal bronchioles divide into three or four respiratory bronchioles. **Type II pneumocytes, which are important in surfactant synthesis, begin to proliferate** during this phase.

Surfactant is required for successful lung function in the fetus and is a complex mixture of phospholipids, neutral lipids, proteins, carbohydrates, and salts. It is important in decreasing alveolar surface tension, maintaining alveoli in an open position at a low internal alveolar diameter, and decreasing intraalveolar lung fluid. **Synthesis takes place in the type II pneumocytes by the incorporation of choline, and signifi-**cant recycling seems to occur by resorption and secretion.

Initially, the important phospholipid was thought to be phosphatidylcholine (lecithin), but it is apparent that other components, such as phosphatidylinositol (PI) and phosphatidylglycerol (PG), are also important. These substances are produced and secreted in increasing amounts as gestation advances, and the continued egress of tracheal fluid into the amniotic fluid results in their increasing presence near term.

Measurement of these substances in the amniotic fluid obtained by amniocentesis allows prediction of the risk of development of RDS in the neonate. **Lecithin (L) levels increase rapidly after 35 weeks, whereas sphingomyelin (S) levels remain relatively constant** after this gestational age. The lecithin and sphingomyelin concentrations are measured by thin-layer chromatography and are expressed as the **L/S ratio.** The presence of blood or meconium in the amniotic fluid will affect the L/S ratio; meconium will decrease it and blood will normalize it to a value of 1.4.

LUNG PROFILE

Using two-dimensional thin-layer chromatography, both PG and PI can be measured. Along with the L/S ratio, these make up the lung profile. RDS is rare when the L/S ratio is greater than 2 and PG is present, whereas when the L/S ratio is less than 2 and no PG is present, more than 90% of infants will develop RDS. **If the L/S ratio indicates pulmonary immaturity (L/S < 2) but PG is present, fewer than 5% of infants develop RDS.** The lung profile offers a more reliable predictor of pulmonary maturity, especially in infants of diabetic mothers. Other advantages of using PG are that contamination with vaginal secretions or blood, as occurs in cases of ruptured membranes and vaginal pool sampling, does not interfere with its detection.

RAPID TESTS FOR FETAL LUNG MATURITY

A rapid test to assess fetal lung maturity, which could then be followed up with the more standard tests, provides a very useful clinical tool. One such test is the **lamellar body number density (LBND) assessment,** which is performed using an electronic cell counter (Coulter). This test can be completed within 2 hours by any hospital clinical laboratory. Normal ranges have been developed and depend on the individual laboratory (maturity ≥ 46,000 µL LBND), and the sensitivity and predictive value are as good if not better than the standard L/S ratio.

Surfactant Therapy

RDS in preterm infants is caused by a lack of surfactant. Surfactant production by type II pneumocytes may be induced by corticosteroids and thyroid-releasing

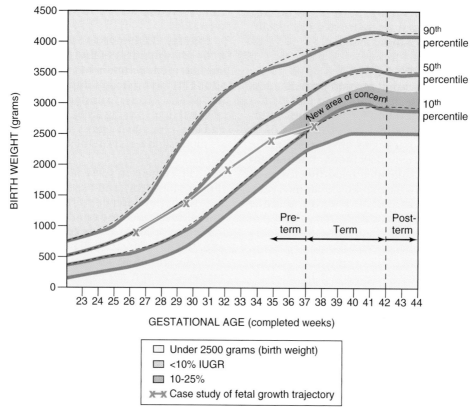

FIGURE 12-1 The birth weight/gestational age growth curve showing three different parameters that describe the characteristics of the fetus at birth. First, the *light pink color* shows that any birth weight below <2500 grams is defined as underweight (low birth weight [LBW]). The *medium pink color* defines those pregnancies <10th percentile and defines fetuses that are classified as intrauterine growth restricted (IUGR). The *dark pink color* defines a new area that defines a fetus that is not LBW but is IUGR based upon the birth weight/ gestational aged growth curve. In addition it defines a group of fetuses who have had normal estimated fetal weight in early pregnancy, but because of complications during pregnancy (see case history in text) have poor fetal growth and become IUGR. This case is classic because it fits the criteria as defined by David Barker when he described the fetal origins for the risk of adult cardiovascular disease secondary to fetal programming in utero. (The birth weight-gestational curve modified using Oken E, Kleinman KP, Rich-Edwards J, et al: A nearly continuous measure of birth weight for gestational age using a United States national reference. *BMC Pediatr* 3:6, 2003.)

hormone, but many premature infants still develop RDS. Several human studies using instillation of surfactant into the pulmonary tree immediately post-delivery have shown dramatic improvements in lung mechanics and infant survival. A wide variety of surfactant preparations are now available, including synthetic surfactants and surfactants derived from animal sources.

Intrauterine Growth Restriction

Intrauterine growth restriction (IUGR) by definition occurs when the birth weight of a newborn infant is below the 10th percentile for a given gestational age. The terms small for gestational age (SGA), low birth weight (<2500 grams), and IUGR should not be used synonymously. The term SGA merely indicates that a fetus or neonate is below a defined reference range of weight for a gestational age, whereas IUGR (<10th percentile) refers to a small group of fetuses or neonates

whose growth potential has been limited by pathologic processes in utero, with resultant increased perinatal morbidity and mortality (Figure 12-1 defines these parameters). **Growth-restricted fetuses are particularly prone to problems such as meconium aspiration, asphyxia, polycythemia, hypoglycemia, and mental retardation. They are at greater risk for developing adult onset conditions such as hypertension, diabetes, and atherosclerosis (see Barker hypothesis in Chapter 1).**

ETIOLOGY

The causes of IUGR can be grouped into three main categories: **maternal, placental, and fetal.** Combinations of these are frequently found in pregnancies with IUGR.

Maternal

Maternal causes include poor nutritional intake, cigarette smoking, drug abuse, early cardiovascular

disease, hypertension, diabetes, obesity (associated with leptin resistance), alcoholism, cyanotic heart disease, and pulmonary insufficiency. In recent years, the **antiphospholipid syndrome** (autoantibody production) has been identified as a cause of IUGR in some women, both with and without hypertension. Antiphospholipid antibodies such as lupus-like anticoagulant and anticardiolipin contribute to the formation of vascular lesions in both the uterine and placental vasculature that may result in impaired fetal growth and demise. Recently, several **hereditary thrombophilias** have been identified, which have been associated with a greater risk for IUGR, abruption, and preeclampsia. These conditions result in vascular lesions within the spinal arteries supplying the placenta. Identification and treatment with low-dose heparin and low-dose aspirin have been shown to reduce the risk of IUGR.

Placental

This category is representative of circumstances in which there is inadequate substrate transfer because of placental insufficiency. **Conditions that lead to this state include essential hypertension, obesity (associated with leptin resistance which leads to placental dysfunction), chronic renal disease, and pregnancy-induced hypertension.** If the latter occurs late in pregnancy and is not accompanied by chronic vascular or renal disease, significant IUGR is unlikely to occur. A small fraction of cases may be attributable to placental or cord abnormalities (e.g., velamentous cord insertion).

Fetal

Examples of fetal causes include **intrauterine infection** (listeriosis and TORCH [toxoplasmosis, other infections, rubella, cytomegalovirus infection, and herpes simplex] agents) and **congenital anomalies. Chapter 22 reviews TORCH infections.**

CLINICAL MANIFESTATIONS

Two types of fetal growth restriction have been described: symmetric and asymmetric. In fetuses with symmetric growth restriction, growth of both the head and the body is inadequate. The head-to-abdominal circumference ratio may be normal, but the absolute growth rate is decreased. Symmetric growth restriction is most commonly seen in association with intrauterine infections or congenital fetal anomalies.

When **asymmetric growth restriction occurs, usually late in pregnancy, the brain is preferentially spared at the expense of abdominal viscera.** As a result, the head size is proportionally larger than the abdominal size. The liver and fetal pancreas undergoes the most dramatic anatomical and biochemical changes. When there is insufficient nutrition to the fetus, caused by either poor maternal nutrition or poor

<table>
<tr><td>BOX 12-2</td></tr>
<tr><td>FACTORS TO BE EVALUATED IN DATING A PREGNANCY</td></tr>
<tr><td>Accuracy of the date of the last normal menstrual period.
Evaluation of uterine size on pelvic examination in the first trimester.
Evaluation of uterine size in relation to gestational age during subsequent antenatal visits (concordance or size-for-dates discrepancy).
Gestational age when fetal heart tones are first heard using a Doppler ultrasonic device (usually at 12-14 weeks).
Date of quickening (usually 18-20 weeks in a primigravida and 16-18 weeks in a multigravida).
Sonographic measurement of fetal length (crown-rump) in the first trimester is most accurate.</td></tr>
</table>

uterine blood flow, the fetal liver fails to store glycogen because of inadequate glucose from the mother. **Changes in the liver are now thought to play an important role in programming the fetus for a greater risk of obesity and diabetes later in life.** The fetal phenotype (small size) is known as the thrifty phenotype, but when born into an environment of plenty, there is increased risk of developing obesity, diabetes, and cardiovascular disease in later life (see Chapter 1).

DIAGNOSIS

Growth restriction may go undiagnosed unless the obstetrician establishes the correct gestational age of the fetus (Box 12-2), identifies high-risk factors from the obstetric data base, and serially assesses fetal growth by fundal height or ultrasonography. **Fetal or neonatal IUGR is usually defined as weight at or below the 10th percentile for gestational age.**

Serial uterine fundal height measurements should serve as the primary screening tool for IUGR. A more thorough sonographic assessment should be undertaken when (1) the fundal height lags more than 3 cm behind expectations or (2) the mother has high-risk conditions such as preexisting hypertension, chronic renal disease, advanced diabetes with vascular involvement, preeclampsia, viral disease, addiction to nicotine, alcohol, or hard drugs, or the presence of serum lupus anticoagulant or antiphospholipid antibodies.

Recently, interest has focused on the prediction of patients at risk for IUGR at mid-pregnancy. Patients with abnormal triple screens (α-fetoprotein [AFP], human chorionic gonadotropin [hCG], and unconjugated estriol [UE3]) who do not have abnormal fetuses by ultrasonography and amniocentesis may be at increased risk for IUGR. In addition, elevations of umbilical artery and uterine artery Doppler assessments (increased resistance) as early as mid-pregnancy have been associated with a greater risk of IUGR as pregnancy progresses.

At present, a number of sonographic parameters are used to diagnose IUGR: (1) biparietal diameter

(BPD), (2) **head circumference**, (3) **abdominal circumference**, (4) **femoral length**, (5) **amniotic fluid volume** (6) **calculated fetal weight**, and (7) **umbilical and uterine artery Doppler.** Of these, **the abdominal circumference is the single most effective parameter for predicting fetal weight because it is reduced in both symmetric and asymmetric IUGR.** Most formulas for estimating fetal weight incorporate two or more parameters to reduce the variance of measurements.

Clinical Example of Fetal Growth Restriction

Using the standard fetal birth weight (vertical axis) and gestational age (horizontal axis) the fetal growth profile in a 34-year-old woman having her second pregnancy is illustrated in Figure 12-1. In this case the patient's first pregnancy was complicated by a fetus with IUGR at term. For the current pregnancy, her weight and blood pressure were normal with a body mass index of 30. At 20 weeks, the estimated fetal weight by ultrasound was at the 50th percentile and genetic markers were normal. Follow-up ultrasound at 26 weeks and 4 days showed a normal fetal weight at the 50th percentile, but by 29 weeks and 5 days, the estimated fetal weight decreased to the 25th percentile, at which time the maternal uterine artery vascular resistance was significantly increased and the fetal umbilical vascular resistance was normal. By 32 weeks, the fetal weight continued to decrease and both maternal uterine artery and the umbilical artery vascular resistance were abnormal, suggesting that this fetus was also going to develop IUGR. Ultrasonic measurements at 34 weeks and 3 days showed continued poor growth and by 37 weeks 3 days, the fetus was at the 10th percentile. Antenatal testing revealed an abnormal heart rate pattern (loss of fetal heart rate variability and a nonreactive fetal heart rate response to stimulation) and a reduced amniotic fluid index. The fetus was delivered by cesarean delivery with a birth weight of 2652 grams. Figure 12-1 illustrates the three different parameters that define how birth weight and gestational age are used to detect abnormalities of fetal growth.

As pregnancy advances, the head circumference remains greater than the abdominal circumference until approximately 34 weeks, at which point the ratio approaches one (see Figure 12-1). **After 34 weeks, the normal pregnancy is associated with an abdominal circumference that is greater than the head circumference.** When asymmetric growth restriction occurs, usually in the third trimester, the BPD is essentially normal, whereas the ratio of head to abdominal circumference is abnormal. **With symmetric growth restriction, the head-to-abdominal circumference ratio may be normal,** but the absolute growth rate is decreased, and estimated fetal weight is reduced (see Figure 12-1).

From 50-90% of infants with manifestations of IUGR at birth can be identified with serial prenatal ultrasonography. The accuracy depends on the quality of the assessments, the criteria used for diagnosis, and the effect of interventions applied when this diagnosis is made. For example, an improvement may be observed in fetal growth after interventions such as work stoppage, bed rest, dietary modification, and curtailment of the use of tobacco, hard drugs, and alcohol.

It is worthwhile to plot out each serial measurement on a standard growth curve. For example, a fetus measuring near the 10th percentile in mid-gestation may continue to grow along that curve (SGA) or, conversely, may fall well below the 10th percentile (IUGR) later in pregnancy (see Figure 12-1).

MANAGEMENT

Prepregnancy

An important part of preventive medicine is to anticipate the risk for women with a prior infant with IUGR, and to consider interventions before a woman plans her next pregnancy. **Improving nutrition and stopping smoking** are two approaches that should improve fetal growth. The patient should be assessed for evidence of early cardiovascular disease as a cause of the IUGR. The assessment should include measurement of biomarkers that define risk for cardiovascular disease such as hemoglobin A1c (HA1c), high-density lipoprotein (HDL), and C-reactive protein (CRP) (risk of diabetes, hypertension, and inflammation). **For women with antiphospholipid antibodies and a past history of giving birth to an infant with IUGR, low-dose aspirin (81 mg/day) in early pregnancy may reduce the likelihood of recurrence.** For patients with one of the hereditary thrombophilias, low-dose heparin (5000 U twice daily), with or without low-dose aspirin (81 mg/day), has also been shown to reduce the risk of recurrent IUGR.

Antepartum

Once a fetus has been identified as having decreased growth, attention should be directed toward modifying any associated factors that can be changed. Because poor nutrition and smoking exert their main effects on birth weight in the latter half of pregnancy, **cessation of smoking and improved nutrition can have a positive impact.** The working woman who becomes fatigued is more likely to have a low-birth-weight infant. **Work leave, or in some cases of maternal disease, hospitalization, will increase uterine blood flow** and may improve the nutrition of the fetus at risk.

The objective of clinical management is to expedite delivery before the occurrence of fetal compromise, but after fetal lung maturation has been achieved. This requires regular fetal monitoring with a twice-weekly nonstress test (NST) and biophysical profile. Most institutions use a modified biophysical profile that includes an NST and AFI. The oxytocin challenge test (OCT) is rarely used because its false-positive rate approaches 50%.

Fetuses clinically suspected of IUGR could be approached as follows:

1. For cases in which results of fetal monitoring are **normal** and ultrasonic findings strongly suggest normal growth, **no clinical intervention** is warranted.

2. **When ultrasonic findings strongly suggest IUGR, delivery is indicated at gestational ages of 34 weeks or later only if abnormal fetal surveillance indicates an increased risk of fetal death. Pulmonary maturity should normally be documented by amniocentesis.** In the presence of severe oligohydramnios, amniocentesis may not be feasible, so delivery should be strongly considered without assessment of lung maturity. These fetuses are at great risk of asphyxia, and the stress associated with IUGR usually accelerates fetal pulmonary maturity.

3. For those cases in which ultrasonic findings are **equivocal** for IUGR, **bed rest, fetal surveillance, and serial ultrasonic measurements at 3-weekly intervals** are indicated to avoid preterm delivery

Assessment of fetal movements (kick counts) each evening while resting comfortably on the left side is a simple technique whereby a pregnant woman can help in the assessment of fetal well-being. If 10 movements are not perceived in 1 hour, a biophysical assessment should be arranged. Some providers instruct their patients, irrespective of their risk, to begin a fetal kick count chart at 28 weeks.

Doppler-derived umbilical artery systolic-to-diastolic ratios are abnormal in IUGR fetuses. Fetuses with growth restriction tend to have increased vascular resistance and to demonstrate low, absent, or reversal of diastolic flow. This noninvasive technique can be used to evaluate high-risk patients, and may help in the timing of delivery when used in conjunction with the modified biophysical profile (see Chapter 7 for more information about Doppler assessment of fetal well-being).

LABOR AND DELIVERY

IUGR per se is not a contraindication to induction of labor, but there should be a low threshold to perform a cesarean delivery because of the poor capacity of the IUGR fetus to tolerate asphyxia. As a result, **during labor, these high-risk patients must be electronically monitored to detect the earliest evidence of fetal distress.**

A combined obstetric-neonatal team approach to delivery is mandatory because of the likelihood of neonatal asphyxia.

After birth, the infant should be carefully examined to rule out the possibility of congenital anomalies and chronic infections. **The monitoring of blood glucose levels is important, because the fetuses do not have adequate hepatic glycogen stores,** and hypoglycemia is a common finding. Furthermore, **hypothermia is not uncommon** in these infants. **Respiratory distress syndrome is more common in the presence of fetal distress,** because fetal acidosis reduces surfactant synthesis and release.

PROGNOSIS

The long-term prognosis for infants with IUGR must be assessed according to the varied etiologies of the growth restriction. If infants with chromosomal abnormalities, autoimmune disease, congenital anomalies, and infection are excluded, **the short-term outlook for these newborns is generally good.** However, poor fetal growth in utero increases the risk for chronic conditions such as hypertension and diabetes later in life (see Chapter 1).

Postterm Pregnancy

The prolonged or postterm pregnancy is one that persists beyond 42 weeks (294 days) from the onset of the last normal menstrual period. **Estimates of the incidence of postterm pregnancy range from 6-12% of all pregnancies.** The incidence of postterm pregnancies has been reduced significantly in the past 10 years because induction before 42 weeks has significantly reduced fetal morbidity secondary to prolonged gestation.

Perinatal mortality is two to three times higher in these prolonged gestations. Much of the increased risk to the fetus and neonate can be attributed to development of the **fetal postmaturity (dysmaturity) syndrome, which occurs when a growth restricted fetus remains in utero beyond term.** Occurring in 20-30% of postterm pregnancies, **this syndrome is related to the aging and infarction of the placenta,** with resulting placental insufficiency. Some of these fetuses meet the criteria for having IUGR and should not have been allowed to advance to term. If there is any evidence of intrauterine hypoxia (such as meconium staining of the umbilical cord, fetal membranes, skin, and nails), perinatal mortality is even further increased.

The fetus with postmaturity syndrome typically has loss of subcutaneous fat, long fingernails, dry, peeling skin, and abundant hair. The 70-80% of postdate fetuses not affected by placental insufficiency continue to grow in utero, many to the point of **macrosomia (birth weight greater than 4000 g). Macrosomia often results in abnormal labor, shoulder dystocia, birth trauma, and an increased incidence of cesarean delivery.**

ETIOLOGY

The cause of postterm pregnancy is unknown in most instances. Prolonged gestation is common in association with an anencephalic fetus. This is probably related to the lack of a fetal labor-initiating factor from the fetal adrenals, which are hypoplastic in anencephalic fetuses. Rarely, prolonged gestation may be associated with **placental sulfatase deficiency** and **extrauterine pregnancy. Paternal genes,** as expressed by the fetus, play a role in the timing of birth.

DIAGNOSIS

The diagnosis of postterm pregnancy is often difficult. The key to appropriate classification and subsequent successful perinatal management is the accurate dating of gestation. It is estimated that **uncertain dates are present in 20-30% of all pregnancies** (see Box 12-2).

MANAGEMENT

Antepartum

The appropriate management revolves around **identifying the low percentage of fetuses with postmaturity syndrome** that are truly at risk of intrauterine hypoxia and fetal demise. When biophysical tests of fetal well-being are available, the timing of delivery for each patient should be individualized. **However, if the gestational age is firmly established at 41 weeks, the fetal head is well fixed in the pelvis, and the condition of the cervix is favorable, labor usually should be induced.**

The two clinical problems that remain are (1) patients with good dates at 42 weeks' gestation with an unripe cervix and (2) patients with uncertain gestational age seen for the first time with a possible or probable diagnosis of prolonged pregnancy.

In the first group of patients, a twice-weekly NST and biophysical profile should be performed. The AFI is an important ultrasonic measurement that should also be used in the management of these patients. The AFI is the sum of the vertical dimensions (in centimeters) of amniotic fluid pockets in each of the four quadrants of the gestational sac. **Delivery is indicated if there is any indication of oligohydramnios (AFI < 5) or if spontaneous fetal heart rate decelerations are found on the NST.** So long as these parameters of fetal well-being are reassuring, labor need not be induced unless the cervical condition becomes favorable, the fetus is judged to be macrosomic, or there are other obstetric indications for delivery.

Some institutions begin weekly testing at 40 weeks to avoid missing the few fetuses that are stressed before 41 weeks. **At 41 weeks' gestation with firm dates, delivery should be initiated by the appropriate route, regardless of other factors,** in view of the increasing potential for perinatal morbidity and mortality.

When the patient presents very late for initial assessment but the gestational age is in question and fetal assessment is normal, an expectant approach is often acceptable. The risk of intervention, with the delivery of a preterm infant, must be considered. The woman herself can participate in the fetal assessment by doing fetal kick counts during the postterm period.

Intrapartum

Continuous electronic fetal monitoring must be employed during the induction of labor. The patient should be encouraged to lie on her left side to assure adequate perfusion of the uterus and **the fetal membranes should be ruptured as early as is feasible so that an internal fetal scalp electrode can be applied and the color of the amniotic fluid assessed.** Cesarean delivery is indicated for fetal distress. It should not be delayed because of the decreased capacity of the postterm fetus to tolerate asphyxia and the increased risk of meconium aspiration. If meconium is present, neonatal asphyxia should be anticipated, and a neonatal resuscitative team should be present at delivery.

Intrauterine Fetal Demise

Intrauterine fetal demise (IUFD) is fetal death after 20 weeks' gestation but before the onset of labor. It complicates about 1% of pregnancies. With the development of newer diagnostic and therapeutic modalities, the management of IUFD has shifted from watchful expectancy to more active intervention.

ETIOLOGY

In more than 50% of cases, the etiology of antepartum fetal death is not known or cannot be determined. Associated causes include IUGR, hypertensive diseases of pregnancy, diabetes mellitus, erythroblastosis fetalis, umbilical cord accidents, fetal congenital anomalies, fetal or maternal infections, fetomaternal hemorrhage, antiphospholipid antibodies, and hereditary thrombophilias.

DIAGNOSIS

Clinically, fetal death should be suspected when the patient reports the absence of fetal movements, particularly if the uterus is small for dates, or if the fetal heart tones are not detected using a Doppler device. Because the placenta may continue to produce hCG, a positive pregnancy test does not exclude an IUFD.

Diagnostic confirmation has been greatly facilitated since the advent of ultrasonography. **Real-time ultrasonography confirms the lack of fetal movement and absence of fetal cardiac activity.**

MANAGEMENT

Fetal demise between 14 and 28 weeks allows for two different approaches: watchful expectancy and induction of labor.

Watchful Expectancy

About 80% of patients experience the spontaneous onset of labor within 2 to 3 weeks of fetal demise. The patient's feeling of personal loss and guilt may create significant anxiety, and this conservative approach may prove unacceptable. Thus, in general, the management of women who fail to go into labor spontaneously is active intervention by induction of labor or dilation and evacuation (D&E).

Induction of Labor

Justifications for such an intervention include the **emotional burden** of carrying a dead fetus on the patient, the slight possibility of **chorioamnionitis,** and the **10% risk of disseminated intravascular coagulation** when a dead fetus is retained for more than 5 weeks in the second or third trimesters.

Vaginal suppositories of prostaglandin E_2 (dinoprostone [Prostin E2]) can be used from the 12th to the 28th week of gestation. Dinoprostone is an effective drug with an overall success rate approaching 97%. Although at least 50% of patients receiving dinoprostone experience nausea and vomiting or diarrhea with temperature elevations, these side effects are transient and can be minimized with premedication (i.e., prochlorperazine [Compazine]). **There have been reported cases of uterine rupture and cervical lacerations,** but with properly selected patients, the drug is safe. The maximum recommended dose is a 20-mg suppository every 3 hours until delivery. **Dinoprostone usage in this range is contraindicated in patients with prior uterine incisions** (e.g., cesarean, myomectomy) because of the unacceptable risk of uterine rupture. Furthermore, prostaglandins are contraindicated in patients with a history of bronchial asthma or active pulmonary disease, although the E series act primarily as bronchodilators. **Misoprostol (Cytotec, a synthetic prostaglandin E_1 analogue)** vaginal tablets have been found to be quite effective with little or no gastrointestinal side effects, and they are less expensive than dinoprostone.

After 28 weeks' gestation, if the condition of the cervix is favorable for induction and there are no contraindications, Cytotec followed by oxytocin are the drugs of choice.

Monitoring of Coagulopathy

Regardless of the mode of therapy chosen, **weekly fibrinogen levels should be monitored during the period of expectant management, along with a hematocrit and platelet count.** If the fibrinogen level is decreasing, even a "normal" fibrinogen level of 300 mg/dL may be an early sign of consumptive coagulopathy in cases of fetal demise. An elevated prothrombin and partial thromboplastin time, the presence of fibrinogen-fibrin degradation products, and a decreased platelet count may clarify the diagnosis.

If laboratory evidence of mild disseminated intravascular coagulation is noted in the absence of bleeding, delivery by the most appropriate means is recommended. If the clotting defect is more severe or if there is evidence of bleeding, blood volume support or use of component therapy (fresh-frozen plasma) should be given before any intervention.

FOLLOW-UP

A search should be undertaken to determine the cause of the intrauterine death. **TORCH and parvovirus studies and cultures for *Listeria* are indicated.** In addition, **all women with a fetal demise should be tested for the presence of anticardiolipin antibodies. Testing for the hereditary thrombophilias should also be considered. If congenital abnormalities are detected, fetal chromosomal studies and total body radiographs should be done, in addition to a complete autopsy.** The autopsy report, when available, must be discussed in detail with both parents. In a stillborn fetus, the best tissue for a chromosomal analysis is the fascia lata, obtained from the lateral aspect of the thigh. The tissue can be stored in saline or Hanks solution. **A significant number of cases of IUFD are the result of fetomaternal hemorrhage,** which can be detected by identifying fetal erythrocytes in maternal blood **(Kleihauer-Betke test).**

The parents may experience feelings of guilt or anger, which may be magnified when there is an abnormal fetus or genetic defect. **Referral to a bereavement support group for counseling** is advisable.

Subsequent pregnancies in a woman with a history of IUFD must be managed as high-risk cases.

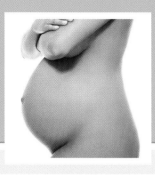

Multifetal Gestation and Malpresentation

CALVIN J. HOBEL

CLINICAL KEYS FOR THIS CHAPTER

- In the United States and other developed countries, multiple gestations have increased, and currently account for at least 3.5% of live births. The two major reasons for this increase have been the use of assisted reproductive technologies (ARTs) to treat infertility, and the increasing maternal age of women having children. Twins are twice as likely in women over the age of 35. Complications of pregnancy such as preeclampsia, preterm birth, poor fetal growth, and monochorionicity significantly increase the risk of perinatal morbidity and mortality in multifetal gestations.

- The prognosis and the risk for morbidity are dependent on zygosity (the genetic makeup of the zygote). Ultrasonographic evaluation of the pregnancy is helpful in determining zygosity. Monozygotic twins (monochorionic) are more likely to involve congenital anomalies, weight discordance, twin-twin transfusion syndrome (TTTS), and other morbidity. Discordant fetal gender confirms dizygotic (two chorions) gestations and visualization of a thick amnio-chorionic septum is suggestive of dizygotic twins. Confirmation of the zygosity may require detailed examination of the placenta at delivery.

- There are significant physiologic adaptations that must occur with multiple gestations. In a normal pregnancy, the maternal blood volume is augmented by 40% (2 L) over the nonpregnant baseline, while in multiple gestations the blood volume increases by 3 L or more. These changes are associated with a significantly increased risk of iron and folate deficiency, and an increase in preeclampsia, hypertension, and maternal respiratory problems such as shortness of breath (dyspnea).

- Management of twin gestations during pregnancy and delivery depends upon the type of problems that develop during pregnancy such as preterm labor, poor fetal growth, hypertensive disorders, and how the fetuses present at the onset of labor. The key is to establish a plan of management that assures a safe delivery at or near term. Generally, if the first twin (twin A) is in a vertex position and the delivery is by the vaginal route, it is appropriate to plan to deliver twin B vaginally. When twin A is breech, the general consensus is that the birth of both twins should be by cesarean delivery.

- Common malpresentations include breech (the most common), face, and brow. Face and brow presentations occur in about 1 in 500 and 1 in 1400 deliveries, respectively. Compound and shoulder presentations are rare, and usually are associated with premature births. Persistent brow presentations almost always require cesarean delivery.

Multiple gestations are defined as any pregnancy in which two or more embryos or fetuses occupy the uterus simultaneously. It is of utmost importance to recognize multiple gestations as a complication of pregnancy. **Because twins deliver at a mean gestational age of about 36 weeks, the perinatal mortality and morbidity for multiple gestations disproportionately exceed that of singleton pregnancies.** Maternal morbidity is also increased, because of the additional physiologic stresses associated with two (or more) fetuses and placentas and a rapidly enlarging uterus.

The term *malpresentation* **encompasses any fetal position other than vertex at delivery, and includes breech, face, brow, compound, and shoulder presentations.** Both fetal and maternal factors contribute to the occurrence of a malpresentation. The most common malpresentation is breech.

Multiple Gestations

Multiple gestations include twins, identical and fraternal, and high-order multiple gestations that consist of three or more fetuses.

TABLE 13-1

THE RELATIONSHIP BETWEEN THE TIMING OF CLEAVAGE AND THE NATURE OF THE MEMBRANES IN TWIN GESTATIONS	
Time of Cleavage*	Nature of Membranes
0-72 hr	Diamniotic, dichorionic
4-8 days	Diamniotic, monochorionic
9-12 days	Monoamniotic, monochorionic

*Time interval between ovulation and cleavage of the egg.

ETIOLOGY AND CLASSIFICATION OF TWINNING

Multiple gestations occur either as the result of the splitting of an embryo (i.e., **identical or monozygotic twinning**) or the fertilization of two or more eggs produced in a single menstrual cycle (i.e., **fraternal or dizygotic twinning**). Because **dizygotic twins** arise from separate eggs, they are structurally distinct pregnancies coexisting in a single uterus, each with its own amnion, chorion, and placenta. **Monozygotic twins** arise from cleavage of a single fertilized egg at various stages during embryogenesis, and thus the arrangement of the fetal membranes and placentas will depend on the time at which the embryo divides (Table 13-1). The earlier the embryo splits, the more separate the membranes and placentas will be. If division occurs within the first 72 hours of fertilization, the membranes will be **diamniotic, dichorionic** with a thick, four-layered intervening membrane. If division occurs after 4 to 8 days of development, when the chorion has already formed, **monochorionic, diamniotic** twins will evolve with a thin, two-layered septum. If splitting occurs after 8 days, when both amnion and chorion have already formed, the result will be **monochorionic, monoamniotic, twins** residing in a single sac with no septum. Of all monozygotic twins, 30% are dichorionic, diamniotic, and 69% are monochorionic, diamniotic. Only 1% of twins are monoamnionic. Because twins share a sac in this type, without an intervening membrane, the risk of umbilical cord entanglement is high, resulting in a net mortality in these twins of almost 50% (Figure 13-1).

INCIDENCE AND EPIDEMIOLOGY

Twins account for approximately 3.5% of all births in the United States. The frequency of **monozygotic** twinning, which depends on a very infrequent biologic event (embryo splitting), is constant in all populations studied at about 1 in 250 births. However, **the frequency of dizygotic twinning, which arises from multiple ovulations in the mother, is strongly influenced by family history, ethnicity, and maternal age.** A family history of dizygotic but not monozygotic twins in the maternal pedigree increases the likelihood of dizygotic twinning in subsequent generations. In western

Nigeria, twinning occurs in 1 of 22 gestations, whereas in the Native American and Inuit populations, twinning is less than one-fifth of that rate. Twins are twice as common in women over 35 as in women at 25 years of age. Given these statistics, approximately **two-thirds of spontaneously conceived twins are fraternal** and one-third are identical (monozygotic). However, in recent years, the incidence of multizygotic multifetal gestation has increased markedly with the more widespread use of ovulation induction agents and the practice of transferring multiple embryos after in vitro fertilization. The incidence of multiple gestations following the use of clomiphene is about 6-8% and about 20-30% following gonadotropin therapy.

DETERMINATION OF ZYGOSITY

The prognosis and expected morbidity of twins is strongly dependent on zygosity: **monozygotic twins are more likely to have congenital anomalies, weight discordance, twin-twin transfusion syndrome, neurologic morbidity, premature delivery, and fetal death.** Thus, **determination of zygosity is the most important next step after multifetal pregnancy has been first diagnosed.**

Ultrasonographic evaluation of the pregnancy is frequently very helpful in determining zygosity. Imaging of discordant fetal gender confirms a dizygotic gestation. Visualization of a thick amnion-chorionic septum is suggestive of dizygotic twins, as is the presence of a "peak" or inverted "V" at the base of the membrane septum (Figure 13-2, *A*). Conversely, in a monochorionic gestation, the dividing membrane is fairly thin (see Figure 13-2, *B*). Because an early embryonic split can infrequently result in dichorionic, diamniotic twins with separate placentas, these findings are not definitive. Similarly, in rare cases of postzygotic genetic events, monochorionic twins may be gender discordant. **Thus, definitive diagnosis of zygosity may require detailed examination of the placenta after delivery.** Thirty percent of twins will be of different sex and are, therefore, dizygotic. Twenty-three percent have monochorionic placentas and are, therefore, monozygotic. Twenty-seven percent will have the same sex, dichorionic placentas, but different blood groupings, and must be, therefore, dizygotic. **Twenty percent will have the same sex, dichorionic placentas, and identical blood groupings. For the latter group, further studies, such as human leukocyte antigen (HLA) typing or DNA analysis,** will be required to **allow determination of zygosity.**

ABNORMALITIES OF THE TWINNING PROCESS

Among monozygotic multiple gestations, abnormalities in the twinning process are relatively common and include conjoined twins, interplacental vascular anastomoses, twin-twin transfusion syndrome (TTTS), fetal malformations, and umbilical cord abnormalities.

MONOCHORIONIC TWIN PLACENTATION   DICHORIONIC TWIN PLACENTATION

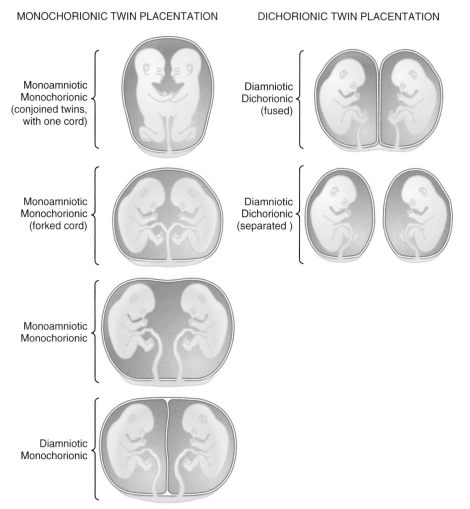

Monoamniotic Monochorionic (conjoined twins, with one cord)

Monoamniotic Monochorionic (forked cord)

Monoamniotic Monochorionic

Diamniotic Monochorionic

Diamniotic Dichorionic (fused)

Diamniotic Dichorionic (separated)

FIGURE 13-1 Diagrammatic representation of the major types of twin placentas found with monozygotic twins. (Redrawn from Benirschke K, Driscoll SG: *Pathology of the human placenta,* New York, 1974, Springer-Verlag, p 263.)

Conjoined Twins

If division of the embryo occurs very late (13 days, after the embryonic disc has completely formed), cleavage of the embryo will be incomplete, resulting in **conjoined twins.** Fortunately, this is a very rare event, occurring **once in 70,000 deliveries.** Conjoined twins are classified according to the anatomic location of the incomplete splitting: **thoracopagus** (anterior), **pygopagus** (posterior), **craniopagus** (cephalic), **or ischiopagus** (caudal). The majority of such twins are thoracopagus. Delivery of conjoined twins frequently requires cesarean delivery, but postnatally, these gestations have a surprisingly optimistic prognosis in many cases. More advanced contemporary imaging has allowed detailed mapping of the shared organs and more successful surgical separations.

Interplacental Vascular Anastomoses

Interplacental vascular anastomoses occur almost exclusively in monochorionic twins at a rate of 90% or more. The most common type is arterial-arterial, followed by arterial-venous and then venous-venous. **Vascular communications between the two fetuses via the placenta may give rise to a number of problems, including abortion, hydramnios, TTTS, and fetal malformations.** Overall, the incidence of both minor and major congenital malformations in twins is twice that of singletons, with the greater incidence of malformations occurring in monochorionic twins.

Twin-Twin Transfusion Syndrome

The presence of unbalanced anastomoses in the placenta (typically arterial-venous connections) leads to a syndrome in which the circulation of one twin perfuses that of the other (i.e., TTTS) in approximately **10% of monozygotic twins.** In this syndrome, arterial blood from the "donor twin" enters the placenta (via the umbilical artery) and is taken up by the umbilical venous system belonging to the "recipient twin," which results in a net transfer of blood from the "donor" to the recipient

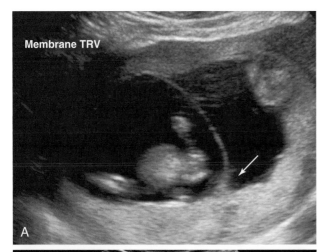

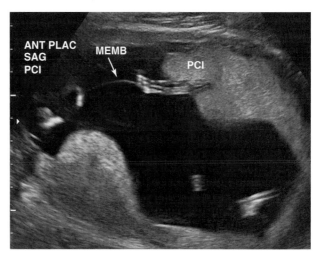

FIGURE 13-3 Ultrasound of a twin-twin transfusion syndrome with one twin *(upper left)* in an amniotic cavity with a reduced fluid volume and a membrane separating this fetus from the second twin in an amniotic cavity with an excessive amount of fluid *(right and lower half of scan image)*. *ANT PLAC*, Anterior placenta; *MEMB*, membrane (amnion); *PCI*, placental cord insertion; *SAG*, sagittal view.

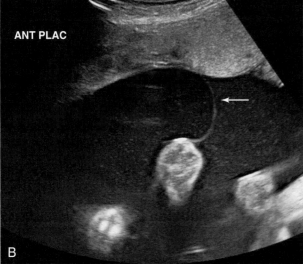

FIGURE 13-2 **A,** Real-time ultrasound with a thick vertical amnion-chorion septum (membrane) separating one twin (left side) from the second twin on the right. The *arrow* (right) points to a "peak" or "inverted V" suggesting dizygotic twins. **B,** Ultrasound of a thin vertical membrane separating one twin on the left side from the second twin on the right suggesting a monochorionic gestational sack. *ANT PLAC,* Anterior placenta; *TRV,* transverse view of membrane.

twin. **Fetal complications include hypovolemia, hypotension, anemia, oligohydramnios, and growth restriction in the donor twin, and hypervolemia, hydramnios, hyperviscosity, thrombosis, hypertension, cardiomegaly, polycythemia, edema, and congestive heart failure in the recipient twin.** Both twins are at risk of demise from the circulatory derangement, and the pregnancy is predisposed to preterm delivery due to overdistention of the uterus with hydramnios.

Twin to twin transfusion is diagnosed using ultrasound. Typically, the donor twin is smaller and may have oligohydramnios, absent bladder, and anemia. The recipient twin, on the other hand, is larger with possible polyhydramnios, cardiomegaly, and ascites or hydrops (Figure 13-3).

Given the poor prognosis of untreated TTTS (approximately 50% survival of any twin), **treatment with either serial amnioncenteses with fluid reduction from the recipient twin's sac, or laser photocoagulation of the anastomotic vessels** on the surface of the placenta, are performed in specialized centers.

Fetal Malformations

Arterial-arterial placental anastomoses can result in fetal structural malformations. In this situation, the arterial blood from the donor twin enters the arterial circulation of the recipient twin, and the reversed blood flow may cause thrombosis within critical organs or atresias due to trophoblastic embolization. The recipient twin, being perfused in a reverse direction with relatively poorly oxygenated blood, fails to develop normally. This so-called **acardiac twin** typically has aplastic and/or dysmorphic anatomical development cephalad of the abdomen, but often has fully formed lower extremities.

Umbilical Cord Abnormalities

Abnormalities of the umbilical cord occur with a higher frequency in twins and are primarily associated with monochorionic twins. Absence of one umbilical artery occurs in about 3-4% of twins, as opposed to 0.5-1% of singletons. **The absence of one umbilical artery is significant because in 30% of such cases, it is associated with other congenital anomalies (e.g., renal agenesis).** Marginal and velamentous umbilical cord insertions also occur more frequently in twins and may cause growth abnormalities, particularly in the third trimester.

Retained Dead Fetus Syndrome

It is not unusual for one twin to die in utero remote from term, whereas the remaining twin and the pregnancy continue to be viable. Over time (after 3 weeks or more in pregnancies that have progressed beyond 20 weeks), the **retained dead fetus syndrome can develop, which involves disseminated intravascular coagulopathy in the mother** as a result of the transfer of nonviable fetal material with thromboplastin-like activity into the maternal circulation. In such cases, the maternal platelet count and fibrinogen levels should be checked once a week to identify possible coagulation abnormalities. The dead fetus will be reabsorbed if the demise occurs before 12 weeks' gestation. Beyond this time, the fetus will shrink and become dehydrated and flattened **(fetus papyraceus).**

ALTERED MATERNAL PHYSIOLOGIC ADAPTATION WITH MULTIPLE FETUSES

A number of normal maternal physiologic responses to pregnancy are exaggerated with multiple gestations. Whereas in normal pregnancy, maternal blood volume is augmented by 40% (2 L over the nonpregnant baseline), in twins this increase may be 3 L or more. **The increased blood volume and demand for iron and folate increase the risk of anemia in the mother** and make the patient less able to tolerate the stresses of infection, labor, and premature labor. **Preeclampsia and gestational hypertension are almost doubled in multifetal gestation.** The increased uterine size associated with multiple fetuses can cause **maternal respiratory embarrassment, orthostatic hypotension due to compression of the vena cava, and compromised renal function due to compression of the ureters.**

DIAGNOSIS

Historical factors such as a maternal family history of dizygotic twinning, the use of fertility drugs, a maternal sensation of feeling larger than with previous pregnancies, or a sensation of excessive fetal movements should raise the suspicion of twins. Physical signs, including excessive weight gain, excessive uterine fundal growth, and auscultation of fetal hearts in separate quadrants of the uterus are suggestive but not diagnostic. An obstetric ultrasound should be performed when a multiple gestation is suspected. **The diagnosis of multiple gestations requires a sonographic examination demonstrating two separate fetuses and heart activities, and can be made as early as 6 weeks' gestation.**

ANTEPARTUM MANAGEMENT

Because of the high risk of preterm birth, intensive antepartum management schemes should be directed at prolonging gestation and increasing birth weight, in order to decrease perinatal morbidity and mortality. The complications of multiple gestations are shown in Box 13-1.

BOX 13-1

COMPLICATIONS OF MULTIPLE GESTATIONS

Maternal

Anemia
Hydramnios
Hypertension
Premature labor
Postpartum uterine atony
Postpartum hemorrhage
Preeclampsia
Cesarean delivery

Fetal

Malpresentation
Placenta previa
Abruptio placentae
Premature rupture of the membranes
Prematurity
Umbilical cord prolapse
Intrauterine growth restriction
Congenital anomalies
Increased perinatal morbidity
Increased perinatal mortality

First and Second Trimesters

Between 16 and 22 weeks, the patient is seen every 2 weeks for ultrasonic cervical length assessment, because **incompetent cervix is more common with multiple gestations.** A suture (cerclage) can be placed in the cervix if marked shortening is noted in the absence of contractions, though the benefit of a cervical cerclage has been under scrutiny recently and is the subject of multiple clinical studies with conflicting findings. **Adequacy of maternal diet is assessed** due to the increased need for overall calories, iron, vitamins, and folate. The Institute of Medicine (IOM) recommends women with twins gain a total of 16.0 to 20.5 kg (35 to 45 lb) during the pregnancy. However, **optimal weight gain is somewhat dependent on prepregnancy maternal body mass index (BMI),** because obese women (BMI > 30) have better outcomes with less weight gain than women who are of normal weight before pregnancy.

Third Trimester

During the third trimester, **prevention of prematurity is of utmost importance.** The cervix is monitored closely with ultrasonic measurements for early effacement and dilation that may precede frank premature labor. A cervical length less than 25 mm at 24 to 28 weeks is associated with a doubling of the risk of premature birth. Interventions to prolong the length of twin pregnancy, such as bed rest, serial uterine activity monitoring, hospitalization, and prophylactic vaginal progesterone, have been carried out but have not been consistently shown to prolong gestation. Nevertheless, most experts utilize a combination of these therapies, individualized for the patient's circumstances.

Discordant fetal growth, which is signified by one fetus flattening its growth rate, is a cause of morbidity and mortality. Fetal growth is monitored by ultrasound every 4 to 6 weeks beginning at 24 weeks, with additional fetal surveillance (e.g., biophysical testing, non-stress fetal heart rate assessment) when fetal growth falls below the normal curve. **The patient should be monitored closely for signs of preeclampsia,** including the development of nondependent edema, urinary protein, and rising arterial blood pressure.

Because twins experience higher rates of stillbirth and growth restriction than singletons, **fetal well-being should be confirmed at least weekly by nonstress testing (NST) or biophysical profile (BPP) assessment from 36 weeks onward,** and earlier in the presence of complications such as intrauterine growth restriction (IUGR), discordant growth, hypertension, or polyhydramnios. Umbilical artery Doppler assessment of fetal well-being is helpful to help determine the timing of delivery to prevent fetal demise if the fetus has IUGR (see Chapter 7). **The contraction stress test (CST) should not be used,** because these pregnancies are already predisposed to preterm labor.

Intrapartum Management

TREATMENT OF PRETERM LABOR

The treatment of preterm labor is discussed elsewhere (see Chapter 12), but multiple gestations present special challenges. **Relative contraindications to tocolysis in these pregnancies include a gestational age of 34 weeks or more, growth failure of one or more fetuses, concerning fetal status on biophysical monitoring, and preeclampsia.** Aggressive tocolysis typically involves use of agents with adverse cardiovascular effects in the mother, such as β-mimetics, magnesium sulfate, and calcium channel blockers. These agents, particularly when combined with antenatal corticosteroid therapy, have been associated with maternal volume overload and congestive heart failure. Box 13-2 provides a list of necessary prerequisites for the management of labor in pregnancies complicated by multiple gestations.

In the special case of monoamniotic twins, birth by cesarean delivery is usually accomplished by 34 to 36 weeks because of the increased risk of lethal cord entanglement. For diamniotic twin pregnancies, delivery management is outlined below.

VERTEX-VERTEX PRESENTATIONS

To choose the safest route of delivery for mother and babies, the presentations of the fetuses must be accurately known. By convention, the presenting twin is designated as twin A and the second twin as twin B.

BOX 13-2

PREREQUISITES FOR THE INTRAPARTUM MANAGEMENT OF MULTIPLE GESTATIONS

A secondary or tertiary care center
A delivery room equipped for immediate cesarean delivery, if necessary
A well-functioning large-bore intravenous line (e.g., 16-gauge) for rapid administration of fluids and blood
Blood available for transfusion
The capability to continuously monitor the fetal heart rates simultaneously
An anesthesiologist who is immediately available to administer general anesthesia should intrauterine manipulation or cesarean delivery be necessary for delivery of the second twin
Two obstetricians scrubbed and gowned for the delivery, one of whom is skilled in intrauterine manipulation and delivery of the second twin
Imaging techniques (i.e., sonography) for determining the precise presentations of the twins
Two pediatricians, one of whom is skilled in the immediate resuscitation of the newborn
An appropriate number of nurses to assist in the delivery and care of the newborn infants

---

Vertex (twin A)-vertex (twin B) occurs 50% of the time, followed by vertex-breech, breech-vertex, and breech-breech.

Vertex-vertex twins are managed similarly to a singleton vertex presentation. Both fetal heart rates should be monitored continuously during labor (Figure 13-4). Oxytocin (Pitocin) can be used to manage hypotonic contractions. After delivery of the first twin, the cord is clamped (identified as twin A) and cut, but cord blood samples are not obtained until the second fetus has been delivered to prevent potential hemorrhage from the undelivered fetus through placental vascular anastomoses. A vaginal examination is then performed to assess the presentation and station of the second twin. If the second twin is still in a vertex presentation, spontaneous delivery is expected. If necessary, forceps or vacuum can be used to assist delivery of a vertex second twin. **Because the second twin is at increased risk of cord prolapse, abruptio placentae, and malpresentation, careful attention to fetal heart monitoring is necessary.**

After delivery of the second fetus, the cord blood samples can be obtained and the placenta delivered. Care should be taken not to disrupt the fetal membranes, as these will often reveal the zygosity of the twins. Following delivery of the placenta, uterine tone should be closely monitored, as the incidence of postpartum atony and hemorrhage is increased in multiple gestations. See Chapter 10 for the prevention of postpartum hemorrhage.

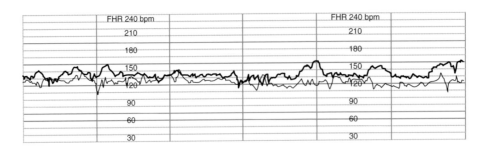

FIGURE 13-4 A fetal heart rate (FHR) tracing of a twin gestation. One twin *(dark tracing)* has accelerations of FHR more marked than those of the second twin *(lighter tracing)*. Both degrees of accelerations indicate a state of "fetal well-being" for both twins.

BOX 13-3

CAUSES OF PERINATAL MORBIDITY AND MORTALITY IN TWINS

Respiratory distress syndrome
Birth trauma
Cerebral hemorrhage
Birth asphyxia
Birth anoxia
Congenital anomalies
Stillbirths
Prematurity

MANAGEMENT OF OTHER PRESENTATIONS

Increased risk of fetal injury exists with delivery of a breech fetus. For this reason, **breech-breech and breech-vertex twins are usually delivered by cesarean delivery.** When delivery of vertex-breech or vertex-transverse twins is contemplated, informed consent by the mother and the skill of the obstetrician are determining factors in choosing between cesarean and vaginal delivery. **Although there is presently no scientific evidence that cesarean delivery is superior for the vertex-breech presentation, difficulty in extracting the breech second twin can result in umbilical cord prolapse, head entrapment, neck injury, and asphyxia.** Unless the obstetrician is comfortable with managing these problems, planned cesarean is the only reasonable choice.

PERINATAL OUTCOME

The high perinatal mortality rate in twin gestations (30 to 50 per 1000 births), approximately five times that in singleton gestations, **is largely attributable to prematurity and congenital anomalies** (Box 13-3). Birth asphyxia is also a significant factor, and thus it is not

surprising that second twins have twice the perinatal mortality of first-born twins. **Compared with singletons, death from complications of birth trauma (with both cesarean and vaginal routes) is four times more frequent with second-born twins and twice as frequent with first-born twins.** Congenital anomalies and stillbirths account for about a third of the perinatal mortality rate. **Stillbirths occur twice as frequently in twins as in singletons.** Cerebral hemorrhage, asphyxia, and anoxia account for one-tenth of the overall perinatal mortality rate.

Twin gestations experience a fourfold increase in cerebral palsy. The increased morbidity in multiple gestations is related to placental and anatomic abnormalities, and trauma associated with the delivery. **Low birth weight** (mean birth weight in twins is 2395 vs. 3377 g for singletons), **prematurity, and IUGR may predispose to permanent brain injury.** Postnatally, twins on average are shorter and lighter than singletons of similar birth weight until 4 years of age.

MULTIPLE GESTATIONS WITH MORE THAN TWO FETUSES

Although higher order multiple gestations (triplets and higher) can result from embryo splitting and polyovulation, **the most frequent cause today is iatrogenic from the use of ovulation induction agents.** The incidence of spontaneous triplets is 1 in 8000 and that of spontaneous quadruplets 1 in 700,000 births. However, because of the widespread use of assisted reproductive technologies, the current estimate of the incidence of triplets is 1 in 3000 births. This rate has tripled in the last two decades. **Recently advanced treatment for infertility, such as in vitro fertilization (IVF) has been focused on a reduction in multiple births.** There has been a significant decrease in twins and higher order multiple births from IVF as a result of embryo freezing at the blastocyst stage (day 5) and elective single embryo transfer.

Prematurity increases as the number of fetuses increases. The average length of gestation is 33 weeks for triplets but only 29 weeks for quadruplets, with mean birth weights 1818 and 1395 g, respectively. Theoretically, delivery of higher order multiples can follow the principles outlined above for twins. However, in contemporary practice, almost all high order multiples are delivered by cesarean delivery to decrease the risk of morbidity in these very premature pregnancies. **The perinatal mortality rate for triplets and quadruplets is 50 to 100 per 1000 births, a rate that is twice that of twins.**

Fetal Malpresentation

Malpresentations of the fetus in utero include breech, face, and brow presentations, with breech the most common and face and brow occurring in about 1 in 500 and 1 in 1400 deliveries, respectively. Compound and shoulder presentations are rare, and usually associated with premature births.

BREECH PRESENTATION

Breech presentation occurs when the fetal buttocks or lower extremities present into the maternal pelvis. **The incidence of breech presentation is 4% of all deliveries.** Before 28 weeks, approximately 25% of fetuses are presenting as a breech. As the fetus grows and occupies more of the uterus, it tends to assume a vertex presentation to accommodate best to the confines and shape of the uterus. By 34 weeks' gestation, most fetuses have assumed the vertex presentation position.

Etiology

The major factor predisposing to breech presentation is prematurity. Approximately 20-30% of all singleton breeches are of low birth weight (<2500 g). However, fetal structural anomalies (e.g., hydrocephalus) may restrict the ability of the fetus to present as a vertex. In breech presentations, the incidence of structural anomalies is greater than 6%, or two to three times that of a vertex. **Other etiologic factors include uterine anomalies** (e.g., bicornuate uterus), **multiple gestation, placenta previa, hydramnios, contracted maternal pelvis, and pelvic tumors** that obstruct the birth canal.

Classification

There are three types of breech presentation: **frank, complete, and incomplete or footling** (Figure 13-5). **Frank breech** occurs when both fetal thighs are flexed and both lower extremities are extended at the knees. **A complete breech** has both thighs flexed and one or both knees flexed (sitting in a "squat" position). **An incomplete (or footling) breech** has one or both thighs extended and one or both knees or feet lying below the buttocks. At term, 65% of breech fetuses are frank, 25% are complete, and 10% are incomplete.

Diagnosis

The diagnosis of breech presentation can often be made by the **Leopold examination** (see Chapter 8), in which the firm fetal head is palpated in the fundal region and the softer, smaller breech occupies the lower uterine segment above the symphysis pubis. In a frank breech in labor, the fetal buttocks, anus, sacrum, and ischial tuberosities can be palpated on vaginal

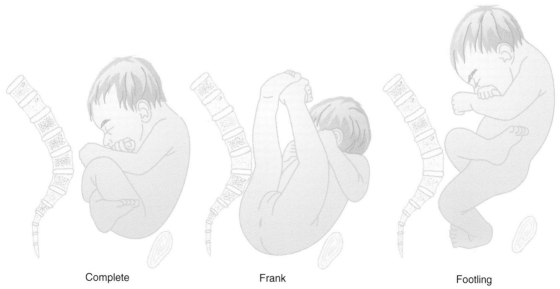

Complete   Frank   Footling

FIGURE 13-5 Types of breech presentation.

examination. With a complete breech, the feet, ankles, and often the buttocks are palpable through the dilated cervix. Vaginal examination of an incomplete breech reveals one or both fetal feet, but ultrasound may be required for definitive diagnosis.

Pregnancy Management

EXCLUDE FETAL AND UTERINE ANOMALIES. If breech presentation is suspected after 34 weeks, the prenatal records and any prior ultrasonic examinations should be reviewed for the presence of uterine myomata, a müllerian anomaly, or fetal structural abnormality. If suspicious, a thorough ultrasonic examination should be performed.

EXTERNAL CEPHALIC VERSION. External cephalic version (ECV) is a procedure in which the obstetrician manually converts the breech fetus to a vertex presentation via external uterine manipulation under ultrasonic guidance. **ECV may be considered in a breech presentation at term before the onset of labor. Version is not carried out before 36 to 37 weeks' gestation** because of the tendency for the premature fetus to revert spontaneously to a breech presentation. The procedure must be carried out in a hospital that is equipped to perform an emergency cesarean delivery because of the small risk of placental abruption or cord compression. The patient should have an intravenous access, and should have nothing by mouth for 8 hours before the version attempt in case emergency delivery is necessary. **Evidence of uteroplacental insufficiency, placenta previa, nonreassuring fetal monitoring, hypertension, intrauterine growth restriction, oligohydramnios, or a history of previous uterine surgery are contraindications to external cephalic version.** The immediate success rate of external version is 35-76%. Though ECV has been shown to decrease the rate of cesarean delivery, perinatal mortality rate has not been affected by this procedure. Only 2% of successful term versions revert to breech.

Labor Management

VAGINAL DELIVERY. Until the publication of randomized trials demonstrating that vaginal breech delivery was associated with increased perinatal mortality compared with planned cesarean, vaginal breech deliveries were performed in selected centers in patients who met strict criteria. These criteria are summarized in Box 13-4. **The standard of care now in most practices is to deliver all breeches by cesarean** to avoid the potential morbidities of umbilical cord prolapse, head entrapment, birth asphyxia, and birth trauma.

ASSISTED BREECH DELIVERY. Because the breech presentation can present in a setting in which cesarean delivery is impossible or unsafe, vaginal delivery of the breech continues to be an important practitioner skill.

BOX 13-4

CRITERIA FOR VAGINAL DELIVERY OF A BREECH PRESENTATION

Fetus must be in a frank or complete breech presentation.
Gestational age should be at least 36 weeks.
Estimated fetal weight should be between 2500 and 3800 g.
Fetal head must be flexed.
Maternal pelvis must be adequately large, as assessed by x-ray pelvimetry* or tested by prior delivery of a reasonably large baby.
There must be no other maternal or fetal indication for cesarean delivery.
Anesthesiologist must be in attendance.
Obstetrician must be experienced.
Assistant must be scrubbed and prepared to guide the fetal head into the pelvis.

*Inlet: anteroposterior (AP) diameter ≥11.0 cm; transverse diameter ≥10.0 cm. Midpelvis: AP ≥11.5 cm, transverse diameter ≥10.0 cm.

Once the fetus has delivered spontaneously to the umbilicus (Figure 13-6, *A*), gentle downward traction is exerted until the scapulae appear at the introitus (see Figure 13-6, *B*). After delivery of the scapulae, the shoulders are delivered by sweeping each arm in turn across the fetal chest until only the fetal head remains undelivered (see Figure 13-6, *C*). Once the shoulders have been delivered, the head is delivered by manual flexion of the fetal head with one hand flexing the head at the base of the skull while the operator's other hand is applied to the fetal maxilla for downward flexion (see Figure 13-6, *D*). Some obstetricians use Piper forceps routinely because this method has been shown to result in delivery of the head with the least amount of trauma to the fetus (see Figure 13-6, *E*).

Cesarean Delivery

During the process of breech vaginal delivery, successively larger parts of the fetus deliver, with the largest part, the fetal head, delivering last. In the very premature infant, the abdomen is much smaller than the head, so the lower extremities, abdomen, and trunk may deliver through an incompletely dilated cervix, leaving the fetal head trapped. This can result in fetal asphyxia and birth trauma. **Premature breech fetuses are thus preferentially delivered by cesarean delivery because of the head-abdominal size disparity.** Cesarean delivery is currently preferred for both preterm and term breech infants, although significant trauma can still occur if care is not taken with delivery of the arms and head.

Complications and Outcome

Even with optimal management, the perinatal mortality of breech fetuses is approximately 25 per 1000 live births versus 12 to 16 per 1000 for nonbreech

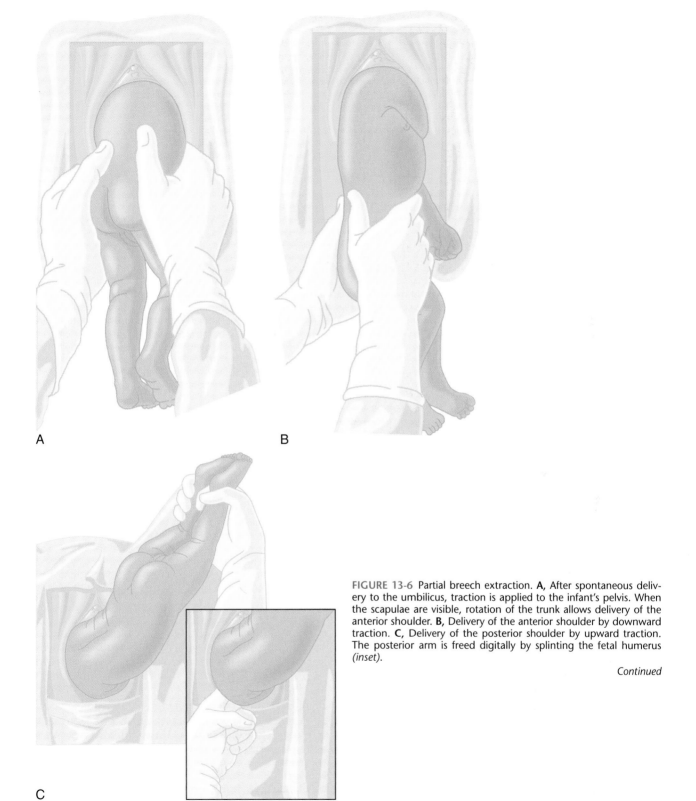

A

B

C

FIGURE 13-6 Partial breech extraction. **A,** After spontaneous delivery to the umbilicus, traction is applied to the infant's pelvis. When the scapulae are visible, rotation of the trunk allows delivery of the anterior shoulder. **B,** Delivery of the anterior shoulder by downward traction. **C,** Delivery of the posterior shoulder by upward traction. The posterior arm is freed digitally by splinting the fetal humerus *(inset).*

Continued

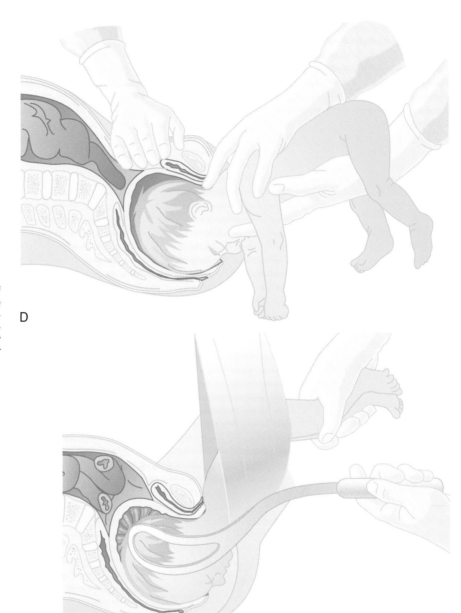

FIGURE 13-6, cont'd **D**, Delivery of the after coming head using the Mauriceau-Smellie-Veit maneuver. Abdominal pressure is applied to maintain flexion of the fetal head. **E**, Delivery of the after coming head using Piper forceps.

fetuses. When prematurity and multiple gestations are excluded, the perinatal mortality for breech fetuses is still significantly higher than for vertex fetuses. **Factors that contribute to increased perinatal morbidity and mortality include lethal congenital anomalies, prematurity, birth trauma, and asphyxia.** Asphyxia typically results from umbilical cord prolapse during labor or entrapment of the aftercoming head. Birth trauma can occur whenever forceful traction is exerted on the fetus and can involve the brachial plexus **(Erb palsy)**, pharynx, and liver.

FACE PRESENTATION

Face presentation occurs when the fetal head is hyperextended such that the fetal face, between the chin and orbits, is the presenting part. **The incidence is about 1 in 500 deliveries.**

Etiology

The etiology of face presentation is somewhat enigmatic. During normal vertex delivery, the fetal head is markedly flexed, with the fetal occiput as the leading part. Factors that permit the fetus to enter the pelvis

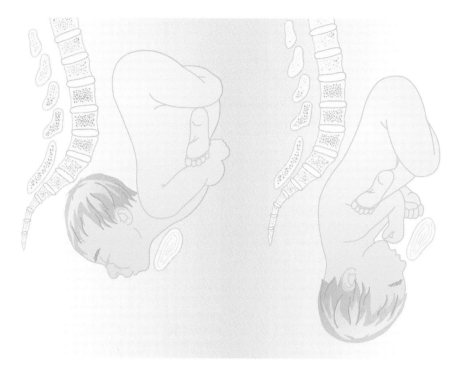

FIGURE 13-7 Spontaneous delivery of a mentum anterior face presentation. Note the flexion of the head under the symphysis pubis. The chin appears first, followed by the nose, brow, vertex, and occiput.

with a markedly extended head include extreme prematurity, high maternal parity, and congenital anomalies such as fetal goiter. In the majority of cases, no etiologic factor is evident.

Diagnosis

The diagnosis of face presentation is usually made at the time of vaginal examination during labor, when the soft tissues of the fetal mouth and nose are noted adjacent to the malar bones and orbital ridges. Face presentation is then confirmed by sonography. Because anencephalic fetuses uniformly present face first, **anencephaly should be ruled out when face presentation is suspected.**

Mechanism of Labor

The position of the presenting face is classified according to the location of the fetal chin (mentum). **Approximately 60% of face presentations are mentum anterior at the time of diagnosis,** whereas 15% are mentum transverse and 25% mentum posterior. The mechanism of labor with a face presentation is similar to the vertex presentation in that the longest diameter (mentum to brow) enters the pelvis transversely. As labor proceeds and the face descends to the midplane, internal rotation occurs into the vertical axis. If the mentum rotates anteriorly under the symphysis pubis, vaginal delivery should be expected. Forceps, but not vacuum, can be applied to assist if prerequisites are met. However, **if the mentum rotates posteriorly, the**

fetal head will be unable to extend farther to complete the expulsive process. Thus, mentum posterior cases and those with persistent mentum transverse must be delivered by cesarean delivery. Because final rotation from mentum transverse may occur only after a significant period of maternal pushing, patience is necessary. Approximately half of the mentoposterior and mentotransverse presentations spontaneously rotate to a mentoanterior position. When spontaneous vaginal delivery (Figure 13-7) or low forceps delivery occurs (Figure 13-8), perinatal morbidity and mortality for face presentations are similar to those for vertex presentations.

Other Presentations

Brow presentation occurs when the presenting part of the fetus is between the facial orbits and anterior fontanelle (Figure 13-9). This type of presentation arises as the result of extension of the fetal head such that it is midway between flexion (vertex presentation) and hyperextension (face presentation). **The incidence is about 1 in 1400 deliveries. With a brow presentation, the presenting diameter is the supraoccipitomental diameter,** which is much longer than the presenting diameter for a face or a vertex presentation.

The intrapartum management is expectant, because the brow presentation is an unstable one. Fifty to 75 percent will convert to either a face presentation, through extension, or a vertex presentation, through

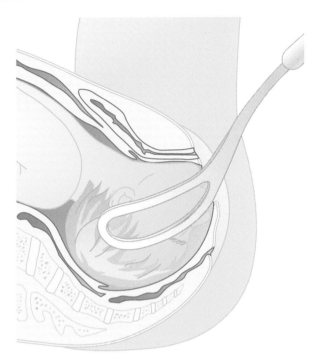

FIGURE 13-8 Simpson forceps applied to a mentum anterior face presentation.

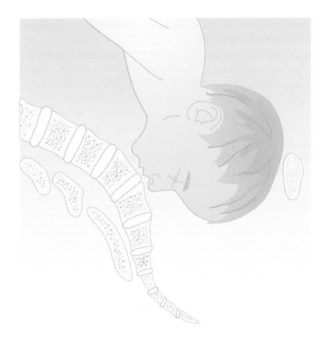

FIGURE 13-9 Brow presentation. Note the large presenting diameter (occipitomental).

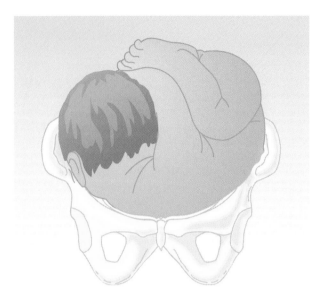

FIGURE 13-10 Shoulder presentation. Note the transverse lie of the fetus with the back down, which cannot be delivered vaginally.

flexion, and will subsequently deliver vaginally. **With a persistent brow presentation, the large presenting diameter makes vaginal delivery impossible, unless the fetus is very small or the maternal pelvis is very large, and delivery must be accomplished by cesarean delivery.** There is an increased incidence of both prolonged labor (30-50%) and dysfunctional labor (30%). As with face presentations, midpelvic delivery and methods to convert the brow presentation to a vertex presentation are contraindicated. **Perinatal morbidity and mortality are similar to those for vertex presentations.**

A **compound presentation** occurs when a fetal extremity (usually the hand) prolapses alongside the presenting part (the head) and both parts enter the maternal pelvis at the same time. This presentation occurs more frequently with premature gestations. The incidence of a hand or arm prolapsing alongside the presenting fetal head is 1 in 700 deliveries and management is expectant. Usually the prolapsed part of the fetus does not interfere with labor. If the arm prolapses, it is best to wait to see if it moves out of the way as the head descends. If it does not, the arm may be gently pushed upward while the head is simultaneously pushed downward by fundal pressure. If the complete extremity prolapses and the fetus then converts to a **shoulder presentation** (Figure 13-10), birth must be accomplished by cesarean delivery.

Hypertensive Disorders of Pregnancy

LONY C. CASTRO • CALVIN J. HOBEL

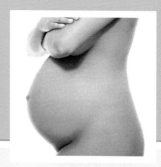

- Preeclampsia (sometimes called *toxemia of pregnancy*) is a multisystem disorder that is thought to arise as a consequence of inadequate cytotrophoblastic invasion of the spiral uterine arteries and failure to establish the normal low resistance uteroplacental circulation. This leads to placental ischemia and the presumptive involvement of secondary mediators responsible for endothelial dysfunction, local and systemic vasospasm, and activation of the coagulation system. Clinical manifestations of preeclampsia reflect this pathophysiology, and the disease begins to resolve with the delivery of the placenta.
- The diagnosis of preeclampsia is based on the presence of new-onset hypertension after 20 weeks' gestation, accompanied by new onset of proteinuria. When evaluating a pregnant woman with new-onset hypertension without proteinuria, preeclampsia can also be diagnosed if there is evidence of one or more of the following abnormalities: thrombocytopenia or disseminated intravascular coagulation (DIC), elevated transaminases or other signs of hepatic injury, central nervous system (CNS) symptoms, an elevated or rising serum creatinine level, or pulmonary edema (Box 14-1).
- Severe hypertension (systolic blood pressure ≥160 mm Hg and/or diastolic blood pressure ≥110 mm Hg) in the setting of preeclampsia requires rapid blood pressure control, usually with parenteral labetalol or hydralazine to prevent CNS hemorrhage or stroke. When preeclampsia is accompanied by new-onset grand mal seizures, it becomes eclampsia. Eclampsia can result in major maternal morbidity, including intracerebral hemorrhage, placental abruption, and preterm birth or fetal death.
- The diagnosis of chronic hypertension requires at least either known hypertension before pregnancy or the development of hypertension before 20 weeks' gestation. Chronic hypertension is generally not treated in pregnancy unless the blood pressure is ≥160/105 mm Hg. Superimposed preeclampsia is diagnosed by the detection of new-onset proteinuria or the development of signs of severe preeclampsia after 20 weeks' gestation in a pregnant woman with chronic hypertension. Management of superimposed preeclampsia is similar to that outlined for preeclampsia.
- *Gestational hypertension* refers to the development of elevated blood pressure without proteinuria or other signs of preeclampsia after 20 weeks' gestation or within 72 hours of delivery that resolves by 12 weeks postpartum. These women must be followed closely, because a significant percentage will go on to develop preeclampsia in the current pregnancy or in a subsequent pregnancy.

The hypertensive disorders of pregnancy (including preeclampsia/eclampsia, chronic hypertension, superimposed preeclampsia, and gestational hypertension) are important contributors to maternal and perinatal morbidity and mortality. The worldwide incidence of these disorders is reported to be about 10%, but regional estimates vary, depending on the population being studied and on the criteria used for diagnosis. Preeclampsia is most easily recognized in pregnant women who present with the "classic triad" of new-onset hypertension, proteinuria, and edema in the latter half of pregnancy. However, this is only one of the ways in which this multisystem disorder can present. Both the mother with preeclampsia and the fetus carried in an affected pregnancy can present with significant multisystem disorders and complications.

The Centers for Disease Control and Prevention states that preeclampsia/eclampsia is one of the leading causes of maternal mortality in the United States. The mortality is primarily due to central

BOX 14-1

CRITERIA FOR SEVERE PREECLAMPSIA

- Severe hypertension (systolic BP ≥160 mm Hg or diastolic BP ≥110 mm Hg) at rest on two occasions at least 4 hr apart*
- Renal insufficiency (serum Cr >1.1 mg/dL or doubling of baseline values)
- Cerebral or visual disturbances
- Pulmonary edema
- Epigastric or right upper quadrant pain
- Elevated liver enzymes (AST or ALT at least two times normal level)
- Thrombocytopenia (platelet count <100,000/μL)

Based on the American College of Obstetricians and Gynecologists Executive Summary: Hypertension in pregnancy, 2013.
ALT, Serum alanine aminotransferase; *AST,* serum aspartate aminotransferase; *BP,* blood pressure; *Cr,* creatinine.
*4-hr delay not required if antihypertensive therapy is initiated.

BOX 14-2

GENERAL CLASSIFICATION OF HYPERTENSIVE DISORDERS OF PREGNANCY

- Preeclampsia/eclampsia
- Chronic hypertension
- Chronic hypertension with superimposed preeclampsia
- Gestational hypertension

Based on the American College of Obstetricians and Gynecologists Executive Summary: Hypertension in pregnancy, 2013.

nervous system (CNS) hemorrhage. Because of this concern, there is an increased emphasis on the use of standardized practice guidelines to manage patients with preeclampsia and other hypertensive disorders, with the aim of decreasing the maternal and perinatal morbidity and mortality that accompany them.

Classification and Definitions

The general classification of hypertensive disorders recommended in 2013 by the American College of Obstetricians and Gynecologists (ACOG) Task Force on Hypertension in Pregnancy reaffirmed the previous classification of hypertensive disorders used in the Working Group Report on High Blood Pressure in Pregnancy issued in 2000 (Box 14-2).

Blood pressure readings vary, depending on maternal position and the gestational age of the pregnancy. Maternal blood pressure tends to be lower in the left lateral decubitus position and higher in the sitting position. In the supine position, some pregnant women will have elevated pressure, whereas others will have supine hypotension due to compression of the vena cava by the uterus. In addition to positional variations, arterial blood pressure normally declines during the

first and second trimesters of pregnancy and rises to prepregnancy levels in the third trimester.

The diagnosis of hypertension should be reserved for pregnant women with a systolic blood pressure ≥140 mm Hg and/or a diastolic blood pressure ≥90 mm Hg. Blood pressure measurements should be taken with the woman in the sitting position after she has rested ≥10 minutes if she is ambulatory. In the hospitalized patient, either sitting or lateral decubitus measurements may be used; however, measurements should be corrected to the level of the right atrium, and consistency of measurement is advised. The length of the blood pressure cuff should be ≥1.5 times the circumference of the upper arm and the fifth Korotkoff sound (disappearance) should be used for the determination of diastolic pressure.

PREECLAMPSIA/ECLAMPSIA

Preeclampsia is a multisystem disorder unique to pregnancy and has varying clinical presentations. The diagnosis is based on the presence of new-onset hypertension in the latter half of gestation, accompanied by new-onset proteinuria and/or other evidence of organ dysfunction. When evaluating a pregnant woman with new-onset hypertension who does not have proteinuria, preeclampsia can be diagnosed if there is evidence of one or more of the following abnormalities: thrombocytopenia or disseminated intravascular coagulation (DIC), elevated transaminases or other signs of hepatic injury, CNS symptoms, an elevated or rising serum creatinine level, or pulmonary edema. Preeclampsia is classically considered to be a disease affecting the first pregnancy, but it also occurs in multiparas, especially if there are predisposing risk factors (see discussion of pathogenesis and risk factors below). Box 14-1 lists the criteria for diagnosing severe preeclampsia.

New-onset hypertension **is defined as the development of hypertension** (systolic blood pressure ≥140 mm Hg or diastolic blood pressure ≥90 mm Hg on two occasions 4 hours apart) **in a woman whose blood pressure readings were previously normal, after the 20th week of pregnancy.** *New-onset proteinuria* **is defined as ≥0.3 g of protein in a timed 24-hour urine collection or a protein/creatinine ratio ≥0.3 after the 20th week of gestation.** This usually correlates with a urinalysis report of ≥30 mg/dL (1+ on dipstick) on a clean-catch urine sample. At each prenatal clinic visit, a pregnant woman's blood pressure, weight, and dipstick urinalysis should be recorded, and she should be assessed for edema. **Rising blood pressures should be of concern,** because they may precede the development of the full preeclamptic syndrome. Similarly, **preeclampsia is often preceded by, or associated with, the development of generalized edema.** Dependent edema (edema of the lower extremities) is very common in normal pregnancies. Hand and facial edema are more likely to be associated with preeclampsia, but they are not diagnostic of the preeclamptic syndrome.

Preeclampsia is often a progressive disease and may have severe features, depending on the severity of the hypertension and the degree to which other organ systems are affected. **Box 14-1 lists specific criteria for the diagnosis of severe preeclampsia.** If any of the symptoms, signs, or laboratory abnormalities listed in Box 14-1 are present in a woman with preeclampsia, it is very likely that she has severe disease, which is associated with much greater maternal and perinatal morbidity.

A variant of severe preeclampsia with particularly high morbidity is the HELLP syndrome. This syndrome occurs in preeclamptic women with evidence of *h*emolysis, *e*levated *l*iver enzymes, and *l*ow *p*latelets (thrombocytopenia). In contrast to more typical presentations of preeclampsia, the patient with HELLP syndrome is more likely to be multiparous, older than 25 years of age, and at less than 36 weeks' gestation. Hypertension may be initially absent in 20% of the patients, whereas 30% will have mild elevations in blood pressure and 50% will have severe elevations.

ECLAMPSIA

Eclampsia is the presence of new-onset grand mal seizures in a woman with preeclampsia that cannot be attributed to other causes. Patients with severe preeclampsia, especially those with CNS symptoms, are at the greatest risk of developing seizures, but the seizures can occur in patients with preeclampsia without other evidence of severe disease. **There is a wide range in the reported frequency and timing of eclamptic seizures. Clinical practices,** including the use of magnesium sulfate intrapartum and postpartum for seizure prophylaxis in women with preeclampsia, as well as the timely recognition and delivery of women with severe preeclampsia, undoubtedly **influence these numbers. In one review of this subject, 38-53% of eclamptic seizures occurred before labor, 18-36% occurred during labor, and 11-44% occurred after delivery** (usually within the first 24 to 48 hours). When evaluating atypical cases of eclampsia (i.e., more than 48 hours postpartum or previous evidence of only mild disease), it is important to consider other causes of seizures, such as underlying seizure disorder; hypertensive encephalopathy; metabolic abnormalities, including hypoglycemia and hyponatremia; and CNS hemorrhage, thrombosis, tumor, or infection.

CHRONIC HYPERTENSION

The diagnosis of chronic hypertension requires at least one of the following: known hypertension before pregnancy or the development of hypertension before 20 weeks' gestation.

Most pregnant women with chronic hypertension will have essential hypertension, but **a small percent-age will have secondary hypertension** that has renal, vascular, endocrinologic, or behavioral causes (e.g., methamphetamine and cocaine use). Most of these conditions can be suspected on the basis of a thorough history and physical examination. Certain endocrinologic disorders, in particular hyperthyroidism, may present for the first time during pregnancy. Depending on the associated symptoms, signs, and response to medication, a workup to determine the etiology of the hypertension may be indicated. **It is not uncommon for the physiologic stress of pregnancy to cause subclinical vascular or renal disease to become manifest.** In these situations, it may be very difficult to differentiate between preeclampsia and an aggravated chronic hypertensive condition. Sometimes only careful postpartum follow-up will indicate the correct diagnosis.

CHRONIC HYPERTENSION WITH SUPERIMPOSED PREECLAMPSIA

Preeclampsia may become superimposed on chronic hypertensive disease. Superimposed preeclampsia can be very difficult to distinguish from poorly controlled chronic hypertension, especially if the woman is not seen until after the 20th week of gestation, but the two conditions are managed differently. In general, superimposed preeclampsia carries a worse prognosis than either condition alone.

The diagnosis of superimposed preeclampsia should be reserved for those women with chronic hypertension who develop new-onset proteinuria ($\geq$0.3 g in a 24-hour collection) after the 20th week of gestation. In pregnant women with preexisting hypertension and proteinuria, the diagnosis of superimposed preeclampsia should be considered if they experience sudden significant increases in blood pressure or proteinuria or the new onset of any of the other signs and symptoms of severe preeclampsia listed in Box 14-1, including thrombocytopenia or abnormally elevated liver enzymes.

GESTATIONAL HYPERTENSION

The diagnosis of gestational hypertension is made if hypertension without proteinuria or other signs of organ dysfunction first appears after 20 weeks' gestation or within 48 to 72 hours of delivery and resolves by 12 weeks postpartum. It is extremely difficult to differentiate this condition from the early stages of preeclampsia. These women must be followed closely because a significant percentage go on to develop proteinuria and the full preeclamptic syndrome at a later stage in pregnancy. Others will have previously unrecognized chronic hypertension. **The diagnosis of gestational hypertension can only be made in retrospect, if the pregnancy has been completed without the development of proteinuria or other evidence of preeclampsia, and if the blood pressure has returned to normal before the 12th week postpartum.**

Preeclampsia/Eclampsia

PATHOGENESIS AND RISK FACTORS

Preeclampsia is called a "disease of theories" because genetic, immunologic, vascular, hormonal, nutritional, and behavioral factors have all been proposed as causes. No single, definitive "cause" has been identified and the origins of the disease are considered to be multifactorial. **Because of the resolution of the preeclampsia after delivery, most attention has been focused on the placenta and the uteroplacental-fetal interface.**

Inadequate uteroplacental perfusion leading to placental ischemia, or hypoxia, appears to be central to the development of the disease. This has been attributed to failure of the cytotrophoblasts to adequately invade the uterine spiral arteries and establish the low-resistance uteroplacental circulation characteristic of normal pregnancy. Placental ischemia could also be due to underlying maternal vascular disease. This could explain the well-documented maternal risk factors for preeclampsia, such as chronic hypertension, advanced maternal age, or methamphetamine use. Immunologically mediated placental vascular damage could explain the higher incidence of preeclampsia in primigravidas and in pregnant women with autoimmune disorders such as the antiphospholipid syndrome. Alternatively, ischemia could be caused by increased metabolic demand in the setting of a multiple gestation, a large singleton fetus, or gestational trophoblastic disease. **When preeclampsia arises in the early second trimester (14 to 20 weeks), a hydatidiform mole or choriocarcinoma should be considered. Other as yet poorly defined genetic and environmental factors will likely be identified that explain the high risk of recurrence of preterm preeclampsia in subsequent pregnancies and the familial association (i.e., increased risk in daughters of women with preeclampsia).**

It is postulated that uteroplacental ischemia results in oxidative and inflammatory stress, with the involvement of secondary mediators leading to endothelial dysfunction, vasospasm, and activation of the coagulation system. The nature of these toxins has not yet been identified, but it may involve production of reactive oxygen and nitrogen species. This is supported by the observation that preeclampsia is increased in pregnant women with underlying conditions, such as obesity and diabetes, that are associated with chronic inflammation and dyslipidemia. A hypoxic placenta may also shed microparticles derived from apoptosis of syncytiotrophoblasts, which can then lead to widespread endothelial injury. Antiangiogenic factors have also been shown to cause systemic hypertension, vascular injury, and activation of the coagulation system. Preeclamptic women have an imbalance in angiogenic and antiangiogenic proteins. Circulating levels of the proangiogenic proteins vascular endothelial growth factor and placental growth factor are decreased, whereas levels of the antiangiogenic proteins soluble fms-like tyrosine kinase 1 (sFlt1) and soluble endoglin are markedly increased. In animal models, overexpression of sFlt1 results in a preeclampsia-like syndrome.

Endothelial dysfunction leads to an imbalance between different classes of locally produced vasoconstrictors and vasodilators. Preeclampsia is associated with a disturbance in prostaglandin production, with a decrease in the ratio of the vasodilators prostaglandin E_2 and prostacyclin to the vasoconstrictor $PGF_{2\alpha}$ and thromboxanes. **Endothelial changes also appear to involve a relative deficiency in the production of nitric oxide, a vasodilator and inhibitor of platelet aggregation, along with increased production of endothelin.** Endothelin is an extremely potent vasoconstrictor and activator of platelets. This shift in the production of locally acting vasoactive substances could enhance vasoconstriction in response to circulating pressor hormones.

The net effect of the above-described processes would be widespread vasoconstriction leading to hypoxic/ischemic damage in different vascular beds, systemic hypertension, activation of the coagulation system, and worsening placental ischemia. The relative severity of the signs and symptoms of preeclampsia in any given individual would vary on the basis of which specific organ system was affected.

PATHOLOGY

Three major pathologic lesions are classically associated with preeclampsia and eclampsia: (1) lack of decidualization of the myometrial segments of the spiral arteries; (2) glomerular capillary endotheliosis; and (3) ischemia, hemorrhage, and necrosis in many organs, presumably secondary to arteriolar constriction.

Under normal circumstances, the invasion of trophoblast results in the replacement of the muscular and elastic layers of the spiral arteries by fibrinoid and fibrous tissue, resulting in large, tortuous, low-resistance channels that extend through the myometrium. In preeclampsia, this change is mostly limited to the decidual segments of the vessels and may result in a 60% reduction in the diameter of the myometrial segment of a spiral artery. **The extent of placental infarction is increased in almost all preeclamptic pregnancies.**

The typical renal lesion of preeclampsia/eclampsia is "glomerular capillary endotheliosis," which is best seen by electron microscopy. This disorder is manifested by marked swelling of the glomerular capillary endothelium and deposits of fibrinoid material in and beneath the endothelial cells. **Arteriolar vasospasm of relatively short duration (1 hour) can cause hypoxia and necrosis of sensitive parenchymal cells.**

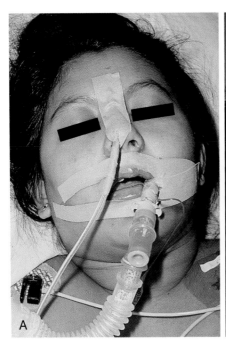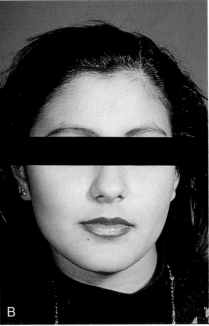

FIGURE 14-1 A postpartum patient after an eclamptic seizure and delivery secondary to severe preeclampsia (A). She experienced confusion, severe headache, and loss of vision before the eclamptic seizure. Note the marked facial edema. Because of the patient's loss of vision, the diagnosis of posterior reversible encephalopathy syndrome was assessed by magnetic resonance imaging, which showed segmental vasoconstriction. The cause is related to loss of autoregulation of the cerebral circulation because of vascular endothelial damage and brain edema. The treatment includes prevention of recurrent seizures with magnesium sulfate, aggressive control of hypertension, and reduction of excessive vascular volume by rapid diuresis with furosemide. Note the patient's status at 6 weeks postpartum (B). (From Sibai BM: Etiology and management of postpartum hypertension-preeclampsia. *Am J Obstet Gynecol* 206:470–475, 2012.)

Vasospasm of longer duration (3 hours) can lead to infarction of vital organs, such as the liver, placenta, and brain. In the liver, periportal necrosis and hemorrhage may occur, with subcapsular hematoma and hepatic rupture being rare complications. In the brain, focal areas of hemorrhage and necrosis may occur. In the retina (the clinical window to the arterial vasculature), vasospasm may be visualized on ophthalmoscopic examination. **Retinal hemorrhage is considered to be an extremely ominous sign** because it may signal similar phenomena in other vital organs.

CLINICAL AND LABORATORY MANIFESTATIONS

Many of the clinical and laboratory manifestations of preeclampsia discussed below can be explained on the basis of endothelial dysfunction, vasospasm, and activation of the coagulation system. This unifying principle may one day lead to the definitive explanation of the causes of preeclampsia.

Weight Gain and Edema

Abnormal weight gain and edema occur early with preeclampsia and reflect an expansion of the extravascular fluid compartment. This expansion is related to the endothelial injury and increased capillary permeability that allow fluid to diffuse from the intravascular to the extravascular space. Thus, many patients with preeclampsia have an increase in total body fluid volume but have intravascular volume depletion. **The hematocrit may also increase, reflecting the relative hypovolemia and hemoconcentration. These "leaky" capillaries predispose women with preeclampsia to pulmonary edema if they are treated with aggressive volume loading. Diuretic therapy is generally not advised unless there is evidence of pulmonary edema.**

Figure 14-1 shows a preeclamptic woman with fluid retention just before delivery (see Figure 14-1, *A*) and at her postpartum visit 6 weeks after delivery (see Figure 14-1, *B*).

Hypertension

The elevation of blood pressure seen in preeclampsia (particularly the increase in diastolic pressure) is a result of generalized vasospasm and an increase in systemic vascular resistance. The blood pressure changes may occur days to weeks after the onset of pathologic fluid retention. Cardiac output in untreated pregnant patients with preeclampsia is not significantly different from that of normal subjects in the last trimester of pregnancy.

Renal Function

Renal blood flow and glomerular filtration rate (GFR) are significantly lower than in patients with a normal pregnancy. The decrease in renal blood flow results from constriction of the afferent arteriolar system. **This afferent vasoconstriction may eventually lead to damage to the glomerular membranes, thereby increasing the permeability of these membranes to proteins and leading to proteinuria.** The renal vasoconstriction and decrease in GFR also account for elevations in serum concentrations of creatinine, blood urea nitrogen, and uric acid.

In the antepartum period, proteinuria may occur days or weeks after the onset of hypertension. If the disease first manifests during labor or in the immediate postpartum period, this progression of events is compressed into hours and sometimes minutes. Renal involvement may progress to significant oliguria and frank renal failure.

Coagulation System

Activation of the coagulation system is often clinically apparent with severe disease. **Thrombocytopenia is the most common abnormality.** Although platelet counts tend to decline even in normal pregnancies, a value <100,000 cells/mm^3 is clearly pathologic and, if accompanied by other signs of preeclampsia, is evidence of severe disease. DIC may occur, especially if there is a placental abruption. **The specific combination of hemolysis, elevated liver function tests, and low platelet levels (the HELLP syndrome)** can occur without clinical manifestations of DIC and **is a sign of severe preeclampsia,** even if blood pressures are normal or only minimally elevated. Women with preexisting thrombophilias, either acquired or inherited, are at increased risk for developing preeclampsia.

Liver Function

In the liver, vasospasm may result in focal hemorrhages and infarctions leading to right upper quadrant or epigastric pain and elevated serum enzyme levels (alanine aminotransferase and aspartate aminotransferase). Hepatic rupture is a rare, ominous complication of preeclampsia that is usually associated with the HELLP syndrome. When significant hemolysis is present, bilirubin levels are often elevated. Elevated alkaline phosphatase levels are frequently seen in pregnancy and are usually not of clinical significance, as they are mostly due to placental production of this enzyme.

Placental Function

Decreased uteroplacental perfusion and ischemia can lead to fetal compromise in the form of intrauterine growth restriction (IUGR), oligohydramnios, or fetal heart rate abnormalities. A commonly accepted clinical sign of inadequate placental perfusion is an umbilical artery Doppler study revealing absent or reversed umbilical artery end diastolic flow. **Extensive placental infarctions can result in retroplacental hemorrhage, or abruption,** which is an important cause of perinatal morbidity and mortality.

Central Nervous System Effects

Cerebral vascular resistance is high in patients with preeclampsia and eclampsia. In patients with hypertension without convulsions, cerebral blood flow may remain within normal limits as a result of autoregulatory phenomena. In patients with convulsions, however, cerebral blood flow and oxygen consumption are significantly lower. **Visual disturbances** such as blurred vision, spots, and scotomata represent degrees of retinal vasospasm. Sudden loss of vision (cortical blindness) is due to occipital lobe ischemia. If the mother is expeditiously stabilized and delivered, full restoration of vision is likely to occur. **A new-onset headache and increased reflex irritability or hyperreflexia are extremely concerning signs of CNS involvement and may predict imminent seizures.**

Evaluation and Management of Preeclampsia

There are three important questions the clinician must ask when managing a woman with preeclampsia. First, does the disease process have severe features? Second, is there evidence of fetal compromise (i.e., IUGR, oligohydramnios, or heart rate abnormalities)? Third, is the fetus mature enough for a reasonably uncomplicated course after delivery?

Delivery is the only definitive cure for preeclampsia, so it is always beneficial for the mother; however, it may result in the delivery of a very preterm neonate. The goal of management is to decrease or prevent the maternal complications of severe preeclampsia while minimizing the neonatal complications arising from prematurity. A woman with preeclampsia, without evidence of fetal compromise, and whose disease does not appear to be severe or progressing will generally not be delivered unless the gestational age is 37 weeks or older, whereas **a woman with severe preeclampsia or eclampsia whose disease presents at or beyond 34 weeks' gestation should usually be delivered after a brief period of stabilization. Severe preeclampsia presenting at less than 34 weeks' gestation may in certain situations be stabilized, and with careful monitoring of the mother and fetus, delivery may be delayed until the pregnancy reaches 34 weeks.**

The initial maternal assessment involves a complete medical history, physical examination, and laboratory evaluation. The evaluation should focus on whether there is any past history of elevated blood pressure or renal disease, either before pregnancy or during previous pregnancies. The patient should be questioned carefully regarding symptoms of severe preeclampsia or its complications, including headache, visual

BOX 14-3

INITIAL LABORATORY EVALUATION FOR A PATIENT WITH PREECLAMPSIA

- CBC, platelet count, LDH: if abnormal, order D-dimers, coagulation panel, and smear
- Renal studies: serum BUN creatinine and uric acid, urinalysis, 24-hr urine for protein and creatinine, or protein/creatinine ratio
- Liver function tests: AST, ALT, and bilirubin

ALT, Serum alanine aminotransferase; *AST,* serum aspartate aminotransferase; *BUN,* blood urea nitrogen; *CBC,* complete blood count; *LDH,* lactate dehydrogenase.

changes, nausea, vomiting, abdominal or epigastric pain, and vaginal bleeding. Her medical record should be reviewed to determine when in the current pregnancy her blood pressure started to rise and when proteinuria developed.

The physical examination should be focused on the assessment of blood pressure, weight gain, edema, fundal height, and reflexes, as well as on a qualitative assessment of urinary protein excretion with a dipstick. In addition, findings consistent with severe preeclampsia, such as epigastric or right upper quadrant tenderness, uterine tenderness, and signs of pulmonary edema, should be sought. If there is severe headache or visual symptoms, an ophthalmic examination may be indicated. The initial laboratory studies recommended are outlined in Box 14-3.

A careful fetal evaluation is also indicated. This should begin with an accurate determination of fetal gestational age based on clinical and sonographic data, if available. Fetal ultrasound should be performed to evaluate fetal growth, amniotic fluid index, and the umbilical artery Doppler resistance index or systolic/diastolic ratio. **A nonstress test (NST) should also be done** to determine if there is evidence of acute fetal compromise.

It is generally advisable to hospitalize patients with a presumed diagnosis of preeclampsia to determine the disease's severity and the maternal and fetal status. After the initial evaluation, if there is no evidence of severe preeclampsia or **fetal compromise, management consists of observation with careful monitoring of both the mother and fetus for progression of the disease. There is no evidence that bed rest is helpful,** although some activity restriction may be indicated. Chronic antihypertensive therapy or diuretic therapy does not prevent the progression to severe disease and is not recommended. Depending on the special circumstances surrounding each case, expectant management can be carried out in the hospital or on an outpatient basis. The mother will require frequent reassessment of symptoms and blood pressure, along with weekly laboratory tests. The fetus needs to be followed with monitoring of fetal activity, heart rate reactivity (NST), and amniotic fluid volume. **The patient**

should be delivered by the time she reaches 37 weeks, or earlier if she develops signs or symptoms of worsening disease or if there is evidence of fetal compromise.

If the initial evaluation is consistent with the diagnosis of severe preeclampsia, the patient should remain hospitalized for the remainder of the pregnancy. After 34 weeks' gestation, stabilization and delivery are appropriate for most patients. For those patients at less than 34 weeks' gestation who have severe preeclampsia, the decision regarding delivery needs to be individualized after carefully considering the risks to the neonate of prematurity versus the potential maternal and fetal risks of continuing the pregnancy. Both the mother and fetus require very close monitoring with maternal laboratory parameters and fetal assessment testing repeated daily or more often if necessary. **In some instances, initial stabilization of the patient with severe preterm preeclampsia with magnesium sulfate for seizure prophylaxis, along with medical control of severe hypertension and corticosteroids for fetal lung maturity, will moderate the disease process and allow delivery to be delayed in the hopes of advancing gestational age.** Either a deterioration in clinical status (e.g., uncontrollable hypertension, deteriorating renal function, pulmonary edema, evidence of HELLP syndrome or coagulopathy, worsening liver function, CNS symptoms, abruption, or abnormal fetal testing) or attainment of a gestational age of 34 weeks is an indication for delivery.

INTRAPARTUM MANAGEMENT OF PREECLAMPSIA

Labor should be induced, and vaginal delivery anticipated, in the absence of any obstetric indications for cesarean delivery, such as failure to progress in labor, nonreassuring fetal status, or nonvertex presentation. The mother and fetus must be carefully monitored during labor and delivery. **Two of the most important maternal issues to be dealt with are seizure prophylaxis and control of hypertension.** Other potential maternal problems that may develop include oliguria, pulmonary edema, and thrombocytopenia or the HELLP syndrome.

If the fetus is growth-restricted or if placental abruption occurs, the fetal heart rate tracing may show evidence of late decelerations, bradycardia, or other signs of fetal compromise necessitating cesarean delivery (see Chapter 9). In most instances, epidural anesthesia is the anesthetic of choice for operative delivery or pain relief during labor, unless there is evidence of coagulopathy.

SEIZURE PROPHYLAXIS

Because of the risk of seizures and their attendant morbidity and even mortality, attention must be given to the level of CNS irritability. Peripheral reflexes, particularly of the patella and ankle, are generally used as determinants of heightened instability. **In patients with preeclampsia, severe headaches, visual changes, sustained clonus, or a positive Chvostek sign can be prodromal symptoms or signs of eclampsia.**

Seizure prophylaxis with magnesium sulfate should be instituted in patients with severe preeclampsia during the initial period of stabilization and again during the intrapartum period, and it should be continued for 24 hours postpartum or until there is evidence of resolution of the disease. **Randomized controlled trials have confirmed that magnesium sulfate is the agent of choice for the prevention and treatment of eclamptic seizures. It is both efficacious for seizure control and associated with low neonatal morbidity.** Both intramuscular (IM) and intravenous (IV) routes are effective for prophylaxis; however, the IM injections can be very painful, and only the IV route is recommended in the United States.

Table 14-1 outlines the protocols for magnesium administration, and Table 14-2 reviews the relationship between serum magnesium concentrations, clinical response, and signs of toxicity, including loss of patellar reflex, warmth and flushing, somnolence and slurred speech, and, most significantly, paralysis and cardiac arrest. Therapeutic levels are generally accepted to be in the range of 4.8 to 9.6 mg/dL, but, to avoid toxicity, levels should not be allowed to rise above 7 to 8 mg/dL. **The magnesium ion is excreted exclusively through the kidneys, so careful monitoring of urine output is essential.** A magnesium overdose can have severe, even fatal, consequences. Magnesium should be given by a controlled infusion pump with a fail-safe mechanism to prevent errors in administration (i.e., inadvertent bolus infusion). **Serial assessments of urine output, deep tendon reflexes, and respirations are important for detecting signs of magnesium toxicity.** These clinical assessments should be supplemented with serial measurements of serum magnesium levels every 6 hours and arterial oxygen saturation via pulse oximetry. In a patient who has oliguria or a serum creatinine ≥1.1, maintenance infusion rates should be halved and serial magnesium levels measured every 2 hours. **Magnesium toxicity can occur even in a patient with apparently normal renal function.** Magnesium toxicity is treated by stopping the infusion and, when severe, administering IV calcium gluconate, 10 mL of a 10% solution, along with resuscitative measures if necessary.

ANTIHYPERTENSIVE THERAPY

Arterial blood pressure ≥160 mm Hg systolic or ≥110 mm Hg diastolic must be treated promptly. In the setting of severe preeclampsia, blood pressures reaching these levels represent a hypertensive emergency. In some women with preeclampsia, even elevations of systolic blood pressure in the 150 to 159 mm Hg range require urgent treatment, especially in those women whose previous systolic blood pressures have been in the 90 to 100 mm Hg range and who now have HELLP syndrome or eclampsia.

The goal of antihypertensive therapy in severe preeclampsia is to stabilize the mother by lowering blood pressure carefully to prevent CNS hemorrhage. In general, the blood pressure should not be lowered to normal levels or to <130/80 mm Hg. **Caution must be exercised not to lower the arterial pressure too much or too rapidly, for either may result in a decreased uteroplacental blood flow and fetal distress, which may necessitate an emergency cesarean delivery in an unstable mother.**

The safest, most efficacious drugs for the acute control of severe hypertension complicating preeclampsia are labetalol and hydralazine. Although hydralazine has theoretical advantages over labetalol in that it is a direct vasodilator and does not induce bronchospasm, rapid bolus infusions are potentially more likely to induce precipitous hypotension. In general, either is acceptable, and use of one or the other will be determined by the individual circumstances. Table 14-3 details the dosages, durations of action, and potential complications of these two drugs.

Oral nifedipine has been used successfully, starting at a dose of 10 mg orally and repeated in 20 to 30 minutes if necessary to a maximum dose of 30 mg. **Nifedipine should be used cautiously to avoid hypotension,** particularly when used in conjunction

TABLE 14-1

ANTICONVULSIVE MAGNESIUM SULFATE THERAPY		
Type of Treatment	**IV***	**IM**
Loading dose in 100 mL of fluid	4-6 g over 15-20 min	5 g in each buttock
Maintenance dose	1-2 g/hr controlled IV	5 g/4 hr infusion

IM, Intramuscular; *IV,* intravenous.
*Only the IV route is recommended in the United States.

TABLE 14-2

CLINICAL CORRELATES OF SERUM MAGNESIUM SULFATE LEVELS	
Clinical Response	**Serum Levels* (mg/dL)**
Loss of patellar reflex	8-12
Warmth and flushing	9-12
Somnolence	10-12
Slurred speech	10-12
Paralysis and respiratory difficulty	15-17
Cardiac arrest	30-35

*Therapeutic range: 4.8-9.6 mg/dL.

TABLE 14-3

EMERGENCY PARENTERAL THERAPY FOR SEVERE HYPERTENSION DURING PREGNANCY

Agent	Action	Dose	Side Effects	Comments
Hydralazine	Direct vasodilator	5 mg IV over 1-2 min, then 5-10 mg IV every 20-40 min until blood pressure is 130-150/80-100 mm Hg. If no response after 20-25 mg, switch to another drug. Alternatively, give continuous IV infusion of 0.5-10 mg/hr.	Headache, tachycardia, flushing, vomiting	Increases cardiac output and probably uterine renal blood flow; has historically been drug of choice for short-term control.
Labetalol hydrochloride	Nonselective α_1-blocker β_1-blocker	Start with 10-20 mg IV bolus. If response is inadequate after 10 min, give 20-80 mg IV every 20-30 min if needed to lower blood pressure to 130-150/80-100 mm Hg. Total dose not to exceed 300 mg. Alternatively, give a continuous IV infusion of 1-2 mg/min.	Nausea, vomiting, heart block, bronchoconstriction, dizziness	Current drug of choice in many centers. Avoid if evidence of asthma or acute heart failure.
Nifedipine	Calcium channel blocker	10-20 mg orally; repeat in 30 min if inadequate response, then 10-20 mg every 2-6 hours if needed to lower blood pressure to 130-150/80-100 mm Hg.	Reflex tachycardia and headaches	

Modification of the Seventh Report of the Joint National Committee on Prevention, Detection, Evaluation, and Treatment of High Blood Pressure (JNC VII), 2004, Tables 21 and 23.
IV, Intravenous.

with magnesium sulfate. Because of the potential for a precipitous drop in blood pressure, short-acting nifedipine is generally not advised in this setting.

MANAGEMENT OF FLUID BALANCE

Accurately recorded intake and output data must be kept to calculate fluid requirements. **Patients with preeclampsia experience vasoconstriction, have interstitial edema, and often demonstrate some degree of reduced intravascular volume, which may reduce urinary output.** In addition, they may be receiving several different therapeutic infusions, such as magnesium sulfate and oxytocin, which have a direct or indirect effect on urinary output.

The most common errors that occur in the management of these patients are fluid volume overload, resulting in pulmonary edema, and excessive volume restriction. Water intoxication is rare with current management. The conservative approach is to replace documented output plus insensible loss with an appropriate electrolyte-containing fluid. Because of the multifaceted pathophysiology of this disease, central hemodynamic monitoring using a pulmonary artery catheter may aid in the management of refractory cases of oliguria or pulmonary edema.

MANAGEMENT OF ECLAMPSIA

Eclampsia is a true obstetric emergency, and all physicians involved in the care of pregnant women should

be prepared to recognize an eclamptic seizure and begin initial resuscitative/stabilization efforts. The management of these patients should be carried out by a team of physicians and well-trained nurses in an isolated labor room, with minimal noise and not too much light. As with any seizure condition, the initial requirement is to protect the patient from injury, clear the airway, and give oxygen by face mask to relieve hypoxia. Blood pressure and pulse oximetry should be recorded every 10 minutes with the patient in the lateral position. A 16- to 18-gauge IV line should be placed for drawing blood and administering drugs and fluids. An indwelling catheter should be placed in the bladder, and laboratory tests should be performed as outlined in Box 14-3.

Pharmacologic stabilization consists of preventing recurrent convulsions and controlling hypertension. Randomized controlled trials have confirmed that magnesium sulfate is the most efficacious drug for preventing recurrent eclamptic seizures and has the best safety profile for the mother and fetus. The administration of IV magnesium sulfate for the treatment of eclamptic seizures is similar to its prophylactic use as outlined in Table 14-1, except that the loading dose is generally increased from 4 to 6 g. The maintenance dose remains 2 g/hr if renal function appears normal. If diazepam (Valium) is used in addition to magnesium sulfate, personnel skilled in intubation should be readily available in case maternal respiratory depression occurs. In general, it is desirable to avoid polypharmacy.

Eclamptic seizures often induce a fetal bradycardia that usually resolves after maternal stabilization and correction of hypoxia, unless there is a placental abruption. It is very important to stabilize the mother before any attempt is made to deliver the infant. Induction of labor or performing a cesarean delivery during the acute phase may aggravate the course of the disease. **Once hypoxia has been corrected, convulsions controlled, and the diastolic blood pressures brought down to the 90 to 100 mm Hg range, delivery should be expedited, preferably by the vaginal route.**

Currently, there is no scientifically proven method for the prevention of preeclampsia that is applicable to the general population of pregnant women. Low-dose aspirin (60 to 80 mg/day beginning at the end of the first trimester) has been studied extensively in over 30,000 women. Its use is currently advised by the ACOG Task Force for women with a history of recurrent preeclampsia or severe preterm preeclampsia, but the risk reduction is likely to be small. Although nutritional interventions have a sound theoretical and experimental basis, it is likely that dietary modifications and weight reduction will have to be implemented before conception in order to be successful. **The current goal is to identify the disease early, monitor its effects on the mother and fetus, stabilize the patient if the disease is severe, and deliver the baby before there is major disease-induced maternal or fetal morbidity.**

MANAGEMENT OF CHRONIC HYPERTENSION

The primary goals of management of chronic hypertension are to control hypertension and detect the development of superimposed preeclampsia in the mother and IUGR in the fetus. In the patient with uncomplicated hypertension whose blood pressures are well controlled and who does not show signs of superimposed preeclampsia or IUGR, the outcome for both the mother and fetus should be good.

When a woman with chronic hypertension is first seen during her pregnancy, it is important to review previous records to determine whether she has essential hypertension or a secondary cause of high blood pressure. If no previous evaluations have been done, it may be appropriate to rule out some of the more common endocrinologic, renal, or cardiovascular causes of hypertension. Baseline laboratory tests similar to those outlined in Box 14-3, with the addition of an electrocardiogram, may be useful. The purpose of these tests is to establish a baseline should the patient later develop superimposed preeclampsia, as well as to look for evidence of end organ dysfunction.

It is important to review the antihypertensive medications being taken and to discontinue any that are potentially teratogenic. **The ACOG Task Force recommends starting antihypertensive therapy if the sys-**tolic blood pressure is ≥160 mm Hg or the diastolic blood pressure is ≥105 mm Hg. There is little evidence that lowering blood pressure below the 140/90 mm Hg range benefits the pregnancy.** In fact, lowering the blood pressure too much may result in decreased uterine perfusion pressure and iatrogenic fetal growth restriction. **In many women, blood pressures will decrease to normal in the second trimester, and no antihypertensive medication will be needed.**

As a general rule, the safest antihypertensive medication should be used at the lowest possible dose needed to keep blood pressure at about 130/80 mm Hg to 140/90 mm Hg. **Methyldopa** is considered to be the safest antihypertensive medication in pregnancy, but **calcium channel blockers** and **labetalol** are also considered to be safe. **Angiotensin-converting enzyme inhibitors, angiotensin II receptor blockers, renin inhibitors, and mineralocorticoid blockers should be avoided at all stages of pregnancy because of potential fetal toxicity.** Beta blockers should be used with caution because they may cause fetal growth restriction and may affect the interpretation of the NST. The risks and benefits of moderate exercise (e.g., walking) or increased periods of rest in the left lateral decubitus position have not been well defined, although they are often recommended.

Because these pregnancies have a high incidence of IUGR, both early and serial ultrasonic examinations are indicated. The early ultrasound (before 12 weeks) is primarily for dating, and the 18- to 22-week ultrasound is for the assessment of fetal anomalies. Serial ultrasonic examinations (every 3 to 4 weeks after 26 to 28 weeks) are of great assistance in detecting IUGR. Depending on the clinical circumstances, periodic fetal monitoring with NSTs and amniotic fluid assessment, supplemented by umbilical artery Doppler studies if there is evidence of IUGR or preeclampsia, may be initiated as early as 26 to 28 weeks and should be commenced by 32 to 34 weeks in all patients with hypertension. **Maternal detection of daily fetal kick counts by the mother in the third trimester** or earlier is an important method of assessing fetal well-being.

A significant increase in hypertension or the development of proteinuria in a previously nonproteinuric patient with chronic hypertension is a likely sign of superimposed preeclampsia. The incidence of superimposed preeclampsia varies from 15-25%. These patients should undergo repeat laboratory evaluation, as outlined in Box 14-3. Management should follow that outlined for severe preeclampsia.

The timing of delivery in the patient with chronic hypertension depends on the clinical circumstances. **For patients without evidence of fetal growth restriction or superimposed preeclampsia, in whom blood pressure is well controlled and who have no other indications for delivery, pregnancy may be allowed to progress until at least 38 weeks' gestation, provided**

that fetal well-being is normal. Any progression beyond the 40th week should be very carefully considered and probably avoided. The presence of IUGR, blood pressure deterioration, or the advent of proteinuria may dictate earlier delivery. **The route of delivery should be vaginal in the absence of other obstetric reasons for cesarean delivery.**

Sequelae and Outcomes

Women with a history of severe preterm preeclampsia are at high risk for recurrent preeclampsia (up to 40%) in a subsequent pregnancy and are the ones most likely to benefit from prepregnancy lifestyle interventions or antepartum use of low-dose aspirin. There is increasing evidence that a history of preeclampsia raises a woman's risk for cardiovascular disease in later life as compared with women who do not experience preeclampsia. Women with gestational hypertension also seem to have a higher incidence of chronic hypertension later in life. **The female offspring of women with preeclampsia experience an increased risk of preeclampsia in their own pregnancies,** providing evidence of a genetic basis for the disease.

Some of the more serious complications of preeclampsia, such as cerebrovascular accidents and renal failure, may have long-term maternal sequelae. Overall, the mortality rate of women with hypertensive disease of pregnancy varies according to the severity of the disease, socioeconomic level, and quality of care received. Although at present there is no proven way of preventing preeclampsia, accessible, high-quality prenatal care should prevent the majority of severe complications associated with the disease.

Fetal and neonatal sequelae are more difficult to determine, because some of the morbidity and mortality associated with these hypertensive syndromes are related to IUGR, prematurity, and acute and chronic fetal distress. All of these may have long-term CNS and cardiovascular effects.

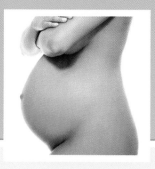

Rhesus Alloimmunization

LONY C. CASTRO • CALVIN J. HOBEL

CLINICAL KEYS FOR THIS CHAPTER

- In this chapter, the term *hydrops fetalis* refers to immune (or rhesus [Rh] antibody-mediated) hydrops fetalis and is synonymous with the older term *erythroblastosis fetalis*. Hydrops fetalis is a form of in utero heart failure. In the setting of Rh alloimmunization, it is characterized by the presence of fetal ascites, pericardial effusion, pleural effusion, subcutaneous edema (best seen as scalp edema), and polyhydramnios. The Rh complex is made up of a number of antigens, including C, D, E, c, d, and e. The vast majority of cases of Rh alloimmunization are due to antibodies to the D antigen.
- Identifying the pregnancy at risk for RhD-mediated hydrops fetalis involves two steps: (1) identifying all RhD-negative pregnant women who have a positive anti-D antibody screen and (2) determining the RhD status of the fetus, either by inference if the father is homozygous for the RhD antigen or by direct assessment of the fetal RhD antigen status through fetal DNA testing. Only pregnancies involving an RhD-negative mother sensitized to the D antigen carrying an RhD-positive fetus are at risk for RhD antibody-mediated hydrops fetalis.
- Once a pregnancy is identified as being at risk for RhD antibody-mediated hydrops fetalis, serial maternal anti-D antibody titers should be obtained. Once titers reach a critical threshold (≥1:16), or if the mother has a history of a previously affected fetus, serial fetal ultrasonography should be performed to detect fetal anemia. These include Doppler studies of the middle cerebral artery (MCA) and fetal imaging for evidence of placentomegaly, hepatomegaly, and hydrops fetalis.
- Treatment and management of an affected fetus involves percutaneous umbilical cord blood sampling (PUBS) for measurement of fetal hemoglobin, intrauterine transfusions, betamethasone to enhance fetal lung maturity, antepartum testing, and assessment of the need for early delivery. These fetuses often require additional treatment for hyperbilirubinemia or anemia in the neonatal period.
- RhD isoimmunization is the only form of isoimmunization that can be prevented with passive immunization. This is done by routinely administering Rh immune globulin to all RhD-negative women who are anti-D–negative at 28 weeks' gestation and within 72 hours of delivery of an RhD-positive fetus. Rh immune globulin should also be given to these women after any episode of antepartum bleeding or trauma.

Rhesus (Rh) alloimmunization is an immunologic disorder that occurs in a pregnant, Rh-negative woman who is carrying an Rh-positive fetus. The immunologic system in the mother is stimulated by fetal cells that cross the placental barrier into the maternal circulation to produce antibodies to the Rh antigen, which then cross the placenta into the fetal circulation and opsonize fetal Rh-positive red cells, resulting in their destruction in the spleen.

One of the earliest signs of fetal anemia caused by Rh alloimmunization is an elevated fetal middle cerebral artery (MCA) Doppler peak systolic velocity. Other early ultrasonic signs are an increase in the size and thickness of the placenta and fetal hepatomegaly. If the hemolysis is allowed to progress untreated, it will result in severe extramedullary hematopoiesis, portal hypertension, hypoalbuminemia, and the progressive development of in utero heart failure or hydrops fetalis. Figure 15-1 shows a fetus severely affected by erythroblastosis fetalis, which should now be completely preventable.

Pathophysiology

The Rh complex is made up of a number of antigens, **including C, D, E, c, d, e, and other variants, such as**

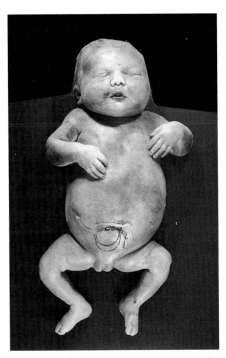

FIGURE 15-1 Fetal hydrops is the most serious condition associated with severe rhesus (Rh) incompatibility (erythroblastosis fetalis) between the mother and fetus. The fetal anemia caused by the blood incompatibility can lead to extramedullary hematopoiesis, portal hypertension, heart failure, and excessive fluid leakage into the extracellular space of the fetus. This can lead to subcutaneous edema, hepatomegaly, ascites, pericardial effusion, and pleural effusion. Note the increased abdominal circumference of the infant in this photograph. The placenta is also enlarged (not pictured) in this condition, and increased fetal renal output (in response to the edema) leads to an increase in amniotic fluid (polyhydramnios). Fetal death is common. This condition should be very rare with preventive measures and modern management of Rh incompatibility.

partial D antigens. More than 90% of cases of Rh alloimmunization are due to antibodies to the D antigen, and this is the only form of alloimmunization that can be prevented with Rh immune globulin prophylaxis. Therefore, this chapter is limited to a discussion of the D antigen, although the same principles apply to other antigen-antibody combinations. A person who lacks the D antigen on the surface of the red blood cells is regarded as being "RhD-negative," and an individual with the D antigen is considered to be "RhD-positive."

About 8% of African Americans are RhD-negative, whereas about 15% of white Americans are RhD-negative. **Only 1-2% of Asian and 1-2% of Native Americans are RhD-negative. When RhD-negative patients are exposed to the RhD antigen, they may become sensitized.** Most cases of sensitization are caused by a placental leak of fetal red blood cells into the maternal circulation (fetomaternal hemorrhage) during pregnancy. The fetal and maternal circulations are normally separated by the placental barrier. Small hemorrhages occur in either direction across the intact placenta throughout pregnancy. With advancing gestational age, the incidence and size of these transplacental (fetomaternal) hemorrhages increase, with the largest hemorrhages usually occurring at delivery. **Most immunizations occur at the time of delivery, and antibodies appear either during the postpartum period or following exposure to the antigen in the next pregnancy.**

Sensitization can also occur if an RhD-negative woman is exposed to RhD-positive blood via mismatched transfusion or hematopoietic stem cell transplantation or by injection with contaminated needles. In rare cases, the "grandmother" theory has been invoked. This theory suggests that an RhD-negative woman may have been sensitized from birth by receiving enough RhD-positive cells from her mother during her own delivery (i.e., a maternal-fetal hemorrhage) to produce an antibody response.

In general, two exposures to the RhD antigen are required to produce any significant sensitization, unless the first exposure is massive. The first exposure leads to primary sensitization, whereas the second causes an anamnestic response leading to the rapid production of immunoglobulins. **The initial response to exposure to the RhD antigen is the production of immunoglobulin M (IgM) antibodies (which cannot cross the placenta) for a short period of time, followed by the production of IgG antibodies that are capable of crossing the placenta. If the fetus has the RhD antigen, these antibodies will coat the fetal red blood cells,** causing them to be destroyed, or hemolyzed, in the spleen. If the hemolysis is mild, the fetus can compensate by increasing the rate of erythropoiesis. If the hemolysis is severe, it can lead to profound fetal anemia, resulting in extramedullary hematopoiesis, portal hypertension, hypoalbuminemia, hyperbilirubinemia, and heart failure (hydrops fetalis), as well as intrauterine fetal death. High bilirubin levels can damage the central nervous system and lead to **neonatal encephalopathy and kernicterus.** Before the widespread use of RhD immune globulin for prevention of RhD isoimmunization, kernicterus was one of the leading causes of cerebral palsy and sensorineural deafness.

If a pattern of mild, moderate, or severe disease has been established with two or more previous pregnancies, the disease tends either to be of the same severity or to become progressively more severe with subsequent pregnancies. **If a woman has a history of fetal hydrops with a previous pregnancy, the risk of hydrops with a subsequent pregnancy is about 90%.** Hydrops usually develops at the same time as or earlier than in the previous pregnancy.

Incidence

Although fetomaternal hemorrhage is very common, the incidence of RhD immunization within 6 months of the delivery of the first RhD-positive, ABO-compatible infant is only about 8%. In addition, the incidence of sensitization with the development of a secondary immune response before the next RhD-positive pregnancy is 8%. Therefore, the overall risk of immunization for the second full-term, RhD-positive, ABO-compatible pregnancy is about one in six pregnancies. The risk of RhD sensitization following an ABO-incompatible, RhD-positive pregnancy is only about 2%. The protection against immunization in ABO-incompatible pregnancies is due to the destruction of the ABO-incompatible cells in the maternal circulation and the removal of the red blood cell debris by the liver.

Fetomaternal hemorrhage may also occur before delivery. Establishment of the fetal circulation occurs at approximately 4 weeks' gestation, and the presence of the RhD antigen has been demonstrated as early as 38 days following conception. Consequently, RhD isoimmunization can occur at any time during pregnancy, from the early first trimester onward. In the first trimester, the most common causes of fetomaternal hemorrhage are spontaneous or induced abortions. **The incidence of immunization following spontaneous abortion is 3.5%, whereas that following induced abortion is 5.5%.** The risk is low in the first 8 weeks, but it rises to significant levels by 12 weeks' gestation. **The risk of immunization following ectopic pregnancy is about 1%. Fetomaternal hemorrhage can also occur in the setting of second- or third-trimester vaginal bleeding, after invasive procedures such as amniocentesis or chorionic villus sampling, after abdominal trauma, or after external cephalic version.** If necessary, the amount of fetal blood entering the maternal circulation after an episode associated with fetomaternal hemorrhage can be estimated using the Kleihauer-Betke test (described in the next section of this chapter). **All pregnant RhD-negative women who are not sensitized to the D antigen should routinely receive prophylactic Rh immune globulin at 28 weeks' gestation, within 72 hours of delivery of an RhD-positive fetus, and at the time of recognition of any of the problems cited above that are associated with fetomaternal hemorrhage.**

Detecting Fetomaternal Hemorrhage

The Kleihauer-Betke test is dependent on the fact that adult hemoglobin is more readily eluted through the cell membrane in the presence of acid than is fetal hemoglobin. The maternal blood is fixed on a slide with ethanol (80%) and treated with a citrate phosphate buffer to remove the adult hemoglobin. After staining with hematoxylin and eosin, the fetal cells can readily be distinguished from the maternal cells. All cells are then counted. The percentage of fetal cells present on the slide is determined and can be used to estimate the extent of the fetomaternal hemorrhage (measured in milliliters of whole blood) on the basis of the following equation:

$$\text{Percentage of fetal cells} \times 5000$$
$$\text{(estimated maternal blood volume in milliliters)}$$

As an example, if the Kleihauer-Betke is reported as 0.2%, then the estimated volume of fetal blood in the maternal circulation would be 0.002×5000, or 10 mL of fetal whole blood. There are a number of different formulas available for estimating the degree of fetomaternal hemorrhage, and all should be viewed as estimates based on their underlying assumptions regarding maternal and fetal blood volume. However, they are of value in determining the amount of Rh immune globulin to administer to prevent sensitization of an RhD-negative woman who is suspected of having a fetomaternal hemorrhage (refer to the "Prevention of RhD Alloimmunization" section later in this chapter).

Recognition of the At-Risk Pregnancy

A blood sample from every pregnant woman should be sent at the first prenatal visit for determination of the blood group and RhD type and for antibody screening. **In RhD-negative patients whose anti-D antibody titers are positive (i.e., those who are RhD-sensitized), the RhD status of the father of the baby should be determined.**

PATERNAL RHD GENOTYPING

If the father is RhD-negative, the fetus will be RhD-negative and hemolytic disease will not occur, so further monitoring is unnecessary. If the father is RhD-positive, his Rh genotype should be determined using quantitative polymerase chain reaction. If he is homozygous for the D antigen, the fetus will be RhD-positive and potentially affected. In this case, the pregnancy must be monitored closely for hemolytic disease. If the father is heterozygous, the fetus has a 50% chance of being RhD-positive, indicating the need for fetal RhD genotyping. Approximately 56% of RhD-positive whites are heterozygous for the RhD antigen. If it is not possible to test the D antigen status and zygosity of the father, it must be assumed that he is D antigen–positive.

TECHNIQUES FOR EVALUATING FETAL RHD STATUS

Fetal RhD status should be determined in RhD-sensitized pregnancies when the father is heterozygous for the RhD antigen or his RhD antigen status is unknown. This can be done noninvasively by testing cell-free fetal DNA in maternal plasma as early as the end of the first trimester. If this testing is inconclusive, amniocentesis can be performed in the second trimester and fetal RhD genotyping can be done using amniocytes. A risk of amniocentesis, as noted earlier, is fetomaternal hemorrhage and worsening of the hemolytic disease. Chorionic villus sampling carries an even greater risk of worsening hemolytic disease if the fetus is RhD-positive, and its use for determining fetal RhD status is discouraged.

MATERNAL RHD ANTIBODY TITER

Maternal anti-D antibody titers are used as a screening tool to estimate the severity of fetal hemolysis in Rh disease. At many centers, anti-D antibody titers are used to help guide decision making regarding the initiation of testing procedures (e.g., MCA Doppler studies and percutaneous umbilical blood sampling). **The American College of Obstetricians and Gynecologists and independent researchers have stated that a fetus in the first immunized pregnancy is not in serious jeopardy when the anti-D antibody titer remains below 1:16.** In patients with a positive titer less than 1:16, repeat titers should be obtained every 2 to 4 weeks. If the titer rises to 1:16 or greater, a detailed ultrasound to detect hydrops and Doppler studies of the MCA are indicated. Titers are not generally useful for following a patient with a history of a previous fetus or neonate with hemolytic disease. In this setting, even if the titers are below the critical threshold, the patient should be followed and evaluated as if her titers were high.

ULTRASONIC DETECTION OF FETAL HEMOLYTIC DISEASE

Ultrasonic examinations of a woman with a fetus at risk for hemolytic disease include MCA Doppler studies and a detailed examination looking for the advent of fetal hydrops. **Serial Doppler assessments of peak systolic velocity in the fetal MCA have proven to be the most valuable tools for detecting fetal anemia.** In at-risk pregnancies, this test should be performed every 1 to 2 weeks from 18 to 35 weeks' gestation. A fetal MCA peak systolic velocity value above 1.5 multiples of the median for gestational age is predictive of moderate to severe fetal anemia and is an indication for percutaneous umbilical blood sampling for precise determination of fetal hemoglobin concentration. Intrauterine fetal transfusion should follow if indicated. **After 35 weeks' gestation, this test may produce a higher false-positive rate (Figures 15-2 and 15-3).**

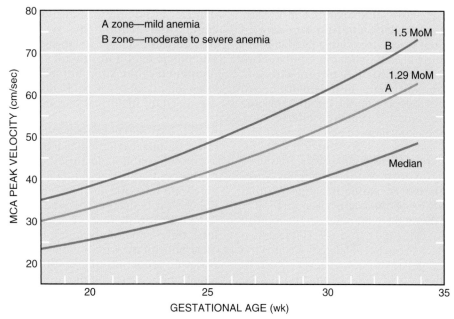

FIGURE 15-2 Middle cerebral artery (MCA) Doppler peak velocities based on gestational age. *MoM,* Multiples of the median. (Data from Moise KJ Jr: Management of rhesus alloimmunization in pregnancy. *Obstet Gynecol* 100:600–611, 2002.)

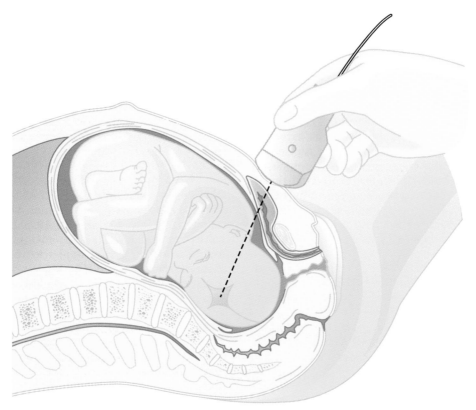

FIGURE 15-3 Obtaining a middle cerebral artery Doppler peak systolic velocity.

The ultrasonic examination should include a detailed fetal assessment for anatomy, growth, estimated fetal weight, and (if viable) biophysical profile, plus a determination of placental size and thickness and hepatic size. **Both the placenta and the fetal liver are enlarged with hydrops fetalis. Fetal hydrops is easily diagnosed on ultrasound by the characteristic appearance of two or more of the following: ascites, pleural effusion, pericardial effusion, skin edema, or polyhydramnios.** Appearance of any of these factors during an ultrasonic examination necessitates therapeutic intervention, depending on the fetal gestational age.

AMNIOTIC FLUID SPECTROPHOTOMETRY

Before widespread use of MCA Doppler studies, spectrophotometric analysis of amniotic fluid bilirubin concentration was the most frequently used method of gauging the severity of fetal hemolysis. The optical density deviation (ΔOD) at 450 μ from a baseline drawn between the OD values at 365 and 550 μ measures the amniotic fluid unconjugated bilirubin level, which in turn correlates with the cord blood hemoglobin of the newborn at birth.

Liley devised a graph based on the correlation of cord blood hemoglobin concentrations at birth and the amniotic fluid ΔOD at 450 μ. Using this method, he was able to establish the Liley graph or curve with predictive zones for mild, moderate, and severe disease. **The great drawback of using amniotic fluid spectrophotometry to determine the severity of fetal hemolytic disease is that amniocentesis, especially if transplacental, can increase the severity of fetomaternal transfusion and worsen the severity of the disease. For this reason and others, amniotic fluid spectrophotometry has been replaced by serial Doppler assessments of MCA peak systolic velocities and is discussed for historical purposes only.**

PERCUTANEOUS UMBILICAL BLOOD SAMPLING

If there is ultrasonic evidence of fetal hydrops, or if the MCA peak systolic velocity is greater than 1.5 multiples of the median for gestational age (see Figure 15-2), moderate to severe fetal anemia may be present and there is an indication for fetal blood sampling if the fetus is at less than 35 weeks' gestation. Advances in fetal interventional techniques and high-resolution ultrasonography have made direct fetal blood sampling the most accurate method for the diagnosis of fetal hemolytic disease. **Percutaneous umbilical blood sampling (PUBS) can allow measurement of fetal hemoglobin, hematocrit, blood gases, pH, and bilirubin levels.** If the fetal hematocrit is less than 30, or more than two standard deviations below the mean for gestational age, intrauterine transfusion is indicated.

The technique for fetal blood sampling is similar to that described for fetal intravenous transfusion. One drawback is that it requires expertise above and beyond that required for amniocentesis. **The major risk is fetal exsanguination from tears in placental vessels,** so in most cases blood will have been ordered before the procedure and will be on hand in case an intrauterine transfusion is needed (see below). If the procedure is performed by an experienced practitioner, the risk of this complication and fetal death is no more than 1-2%. **However, there is a greater risk of fetomaternal hemorrhage.** Percutaneous umbilical blood sampling should not be a first-line method of assessing fetal status unless clearly indicated.

Management of the At-Risk Pregnancy

INTRAUTERINE TRANSFUSION

Intrauterine transfusion, initially introduced in 1963 as an intraperitoneal transfusion and currently usually administered as an intravascular transfusion, has markedly changed the prognosis for severely affected fetuses. **The goal is to transfuse fresh group O, Rh-negative packed red blood cells.** In addition to routine blood bank screening for viruses such as hepatitis and HIV, the blood for transfusion is irradiated, washed, processed through a leukocyte-poor filter, and screened for cytomegalovirus. Transfusions are done under ultrasonic guidance using sterile technique, either in or near the operating room if the fetus is potentially viable so that delivery can be accomplished expeditiously should the fetal status deteriorate irreversibly.

Transfusions usually cannot be done until 18 to 20 weeks' gestation, because fetal size limits vascular access. Repeat transfusions are generally scheduled at 1- to 3-week intervals, and the final transfusion is typically performed at 32 to 35 weeks' gestation. In general, the fetus is delivered when the lungs are mature, when it reaches 37 weeks, or if antepartum testing indicates severe fetal compromise.

The overall survival rate following intrauterine transfusion is about 90%, but it is significantly lower for fetuses with hydrops before the transfusion. Approximately 90% of survivors are reported to have normal neurologic outcomes.

Fetal Intraperitoneal Transfusion

Red blood cells are absorbed via the subdiaphragmatic lymphatics and proceed via the right lymphatic duct into the fetal intravascular compartment. After transfusion, the absorption of blood may be monitored with serial transverse ultrasonic scans of the fetal abdomen. **In nonhydropic fetuses, the blood should be absorbed within 7 to 9 days.** In the presence of hydrops, absorption is variable and the survival rate of hydropic fetuses is lower than after intravascular transfusion. Because of this, intravascular transfusion is the method of choice for correcting fetal anemia, and intraperitoneal transfusion is reserved for cases in which intravascular transfusion is not possible, such as gestational age less than 20 weeks.

Intravascular Transfusion

In most cases, intravascular transfusion is the preferred method. Fetal survival is better with this technique than after intraperitoneal transfusions, especially if there is ascites or other evidence of hydrops. In addition, transfusion into the peritoneal cavity can result in fetal bradycardia or a pseudosinusoidal fetal heart rate pattern following the procedure because of compression at the site of insertion of the umbilical cord.

Under ultrasonic guidance, and using sterile technique, a 22-gauge spinal needle is inserted into the umbilical vein near the placental insertion. An initial fetal hematocrit is determined, and a paralyzing agent is injected. The volume of blood to be transfused is based on the estimated fetal body weight, as determined by ultrasonography, the initial fetal hematocrit, the target fetal hematocrit, and the hematocrit of the packed red cells to be transfused.

OTHER MODES OF THERAPY

Maternal plasmapheresis combined with administration of intravenous immunoglobulin may be helpful in cases of severe erythroblastosis when intrauterine transfusions have not been successful, but further research must be done before this can be recommended. **Phenobarbital** has been used to induce fetal hepatic enzyme maturation, thereby increasing uptake and excretion of bilirubin by the liver. Treatment with phenobarbital is initiated at least 1 week before delivery.

TIMING OF DELIVERY IN THE RH-SENSITIZED FETUS

In addition to serial MCA Doppler studies and detection of hydrops, these fetuses should be evaluated twice weekly from at least 32 weeks until delivery for fetal well-being (nonstress tests, modified biophysical profile) and every 3 weeks for fetal growth. **Although the goal is a term delivery, the risks of intrauterine demise, including that caused by procedure-related losses, must be balanced against the risks of prematurity.** There is no absolute gestational age cutoff for intrauterine transfusions, but after 35 weeks the risk of an intrauterine loss may be greater than the risk of a neonatal death. It may be prudent in this setting to deliver the fetus and transfuse the neonate, if necessary. **If delivery is expected to occur before 34 weeks' gestation (or if amniocentesis suggests an immature lung profile), betamethasone should be given at least 48 hours before delivery to enhance fetal pulmonary maturation.**

Prevention of RhD Alloimmunization

Because RhD immunization occurs in response to exposure of an RhD-negative mother to the RhD antigen, the mainstay for prevention is the avoidance of maternal exposure to the antigen. Rh immune globulin diminishes the availability of the RhD antigen to the maternal immune system, although the exact mechanism by which it prevents RhD alloimmunization is not well understood.

Rh immune globulin is prepared from fractionated human plasma obtained from hyperreactive sensitized donors. The plasma is screened for hepatitis B surface antigen and anti-HIV-1. The globulin is available in several dosages for intramuscular injection. **Since the advent of its use in 1967, Rh immune globulin has dramatically reduced the incidence of Rh isoimmunization. Three hundred micrograms (or 1 U) of Rh immune globulin can neutralize 30 mL of fetal RhD-positive blood in the maternal circulation.**

Because the greatest risk for fetomaternal hemorrhage occurs during labor and delivery, Rh immune globulin was initially administered only during the immediate postpartum period. This resulted in a 1-2% failure rate, which is thought to be caused by exposure of the mother to fetal red blood cells during the antepartum period. **The indications for the use of Rh immune globulin have therefore been broadened to include any antepartum event (such as amniocentesis) that may increase the risk of transplacental hemorrhage. The routine prophylactic administration of Rh immune globulin at 28 weeks' gestation is now the standard of care.** Despite adherence to this suggested Rh immune globulin protocol, 0.27% of primiparous RhD-negative patients still become sensitized. Although this is a low rate, it is still unacceptable, given that it is preventable.

It is the responsibility of every health care practitioner who is involved in the care of pregnant women to prevent RhD alloimmunization by the appropriate administration of Rh immune globulin. Box 15-1 lists the indications and dosing for Rh immune globulin.

IRREGULAR ANTIBODIES

Although RhD alloimmunization is the most common cause of hemolytic disease in the newborn, **other antigens in the Rh system (C, c, E, e) and other blood group systems, such as Kell, Duffy, or Kidd, can also cause fetal hemolytic disease.** Kell antigen can elicit a strong IgG response similar to RhD alloimmunization.

BOX 15-1

INDICATIONS AND DOSING FOR RH IMMUNE GLOBULIN

- Blood type and antibody screen are performed for all pregnant women at their first prenatal visit.
- Women who are RhD-negative with a negative initial screen should have a repeat screen at 28 weeks.
- Those women with a negative screen at 28 weeks should receive 300 µg of Rh immune globulin (prophylactically).
- Those women with a positive screen should have their antibodies identified. If RhD-negative, they should also receive 300 µg of Rh immune globulin.
- All pregnant women who are RhD-negative and who are not sensitized (anti-D–negative) and who experience (1) spontaneous or induced abortion, (2) ectopic pregnancy, (3) significant vaginal bleeding, (4) amniocentesis, (5) abdominal trauma, or (6) cephalic version should receive 50-100 µg of Rh immune globulin before 12 weeks' gestation and be administered 300 µg if later than 12 weeks.
- Rh immune globulin is not necessary for complete molar pregnancies, but it is necessary for partial molar pregnancies, where fetal tissue may be present. Because this is not always clear at the time of evacuation, 300 µg of the immune globulin should be given.
- The greatest risk of fetomaternal hemorrhage is at the time of delivery. Rh immune globulin (300 µg) should be given routinely within 72 hours of delivery to all Rh-negative, anti-D–negative women who deliver an Rh-positive child.
- Additional Rh immune globulin is indicated if the delivery is complicated by excessive hemorrhage (>30 mL of fetal blood suspected or documented by Kleihauer-Betke testing).

For this reason, any positive antibody screen in pregnancy, even in an RhD-positive woman, should be followed up with an antibody identification and titer. If the antibody screen is positive for one or more antibodies associated with hemolytic disease of the newborn, the pregnancy should be followed in a fashion similar to that advised for the RhD-sensitized pregnancy.

A potential exception to this is Kell sensitization. Antibody titers are not as reliable for the detection of fetal anemia in this situation, probably because the anemia is due more to suppression of hematopoiesis than to hemolysis. The MCA peak systolic velocity remains an excellent predictor of anemia in this setting. It is extremely important to test the Kell antigen status of the father before any invasive testing, because 90% of the population is Kell-negative.

Common Medical and Surgical Conditions Complicating Pregnancy

LONY C. CASTRO • JOSEPH C. GAMBONE

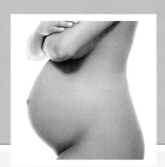

CLINICAL KEYS FOR THIS CHAPTER

- Diabetes and thyroid disorders are among the most common and consequential medical conditions that occur during pregnancy, labor, and the postpartum period. Diabetes may precede pregnancy or may occur because of pregnancy, with a return to the prepregnancy state after delivery. *Gestational diabetes mellitus* (GDM) is defined as glucose intolerance with onset or first recognition during pregnancy. Pregestational diabetes mellitus may be type 1 (insulin-dependent) or type 2. Thyroid abnormalities occur in about 2% of pregnancies, and the presentation and course of the disease may be affected by the pregnancy.

- Other important medical conditions include heart, autoimmune, renal, gastrointestinal (GI), lung, and thromboembolic disorders. Preexisting cardiovascular disease and conditions such as asthma and cystic fibrosis are encountered more commonly because of modern medical management that has allowed more women than in the past to consider pregnancy. As a general rule, most pregnancies complicated by these medical conditions are considered "high risk" for maternal and fetal morbidity and mortality. Good outcomes often require frequent maternal and fetal assessment and the ability to respond in a timely fashion to changes in the clinical status of either the mother or her fetus.

- Elective delivery for medical and surgical conditions is indicated when deteriorating maternal or fetal status occurs in the presence of a term fetus or when there is evidence of fetal lung maturity. When a preterm delivery before 34 weeks' gestation is necessary, steroids (betamethasone) should be given to enhance fetal lung maturity and improve fetal outcomes. In some cases, cesarean delivery is indicated.

- Obstetricians and other providers should focus on the mitigation of the effects and prevention of medical conditions that may complicate pregnancy. The increased prevalence of obesity in pregnant women in the United States and elsewhere has resulted in metabolic dysregulation (metabolic syndrome) that increases inflammation and insulin resistance. The risk of some medical disorders, such as diabetes, hypertension, and heart disease, is increased due to excessive body weight during pregnancy. Women should be encouraged to lose weight before pregnancy and to limit weight gain during pregnancy. Physical activity and a healthy diet are very important before, during, and after pregnancy.

- Surgical conditions that may complicate pregnancy include appendicitis, cholecystitis and cholelithiasis, acute pancreatitis, bowel obstruction, abdominal trauma, or torsion of an adnexal structure such as an ovarian tumor. When trauma is evaluated during pregnancy, the possibility of intimate partner abuse must be ruled out, as in women who are not pregnant. Strongly indicated but nonemergent surgery is most safely performed in the second trimester. Laparoscopy is becoming more common during pregnancy, and guidelines have been published that should increase the safety for both the pregnant woman and her fetus.

Most of the conditions discussed in this chapter are not unique to pregnancy and understanding the causes, diagnosis, and management of them is based on the same principles that would apply in the nonpregnant woman. **Important issues** for the management of medical and surgical problems during pregnancy include **how the physiologic changes of pregnancy may affect the diagnosis and clinical course** of the disease, as well as **how the disease may affect the pregnancy,** with particular attention to the fetus.

The most common medical and surgical disorders that may complicate pregnancy are covered in this chapter. Common and important infectious diseases of both nonpregnant and pregnant women are covered in Chapter 22, including perinatal infections (toxoplasmosis, others [syphilis, varicella zoster, parvovirus B19], rubella, cytomegalovirus [CMV], and herpes, referred to together as *TORCH infections*), human immunodeficiency virus (HIV) infection, and acquired immunodeficiency syndrome (AIDS).

Endocrine Disorders

Diabetes mellitus and thyroid disease are the two most common endocrine disorders complicating pregnancy.

DIABETES MELLITUS

Incidence and Classification

The prevalence of diabetes mellitus has greatly increased in the last 20 years. In the United States, rates appear to range from 6-12%, depending on the population studied and the diagnostic criteria used. **Overall, 80-90% of diabetes in pregnant women is gestational, and about 10% is pregestational.**

Gestational diabetes mellitus (GDM) is defined as glucose intolerance with onset or first recognition during pregnancy. Rising levels of **human placental lactogen, progesterone, prolactin, and cortisol in pregnancy are some of the primary factors associated with progressive insulin resistance during pregnancy.** Studies suggest that women who develop GDM have chronic insulin resistance and that GDM is a "stress test" for the development of diabetes later in life.

Pregestational diabetes mellitus refers to diabetes present before pregnancy and may be either type 1 or type 2 diabetes. Most obstetricians use the **White classification of diabetes during pregnancy to further refine the categories for GDM and pregestational diabetes.** This classification is helpful for assessing disease severity and the likelihood of complications (Table 16-1).

TABLE 16-1

WHITE CLASSIFICATION OF DIABETES IN PREGNANCY

Class	Description
A_1	Gestational diabetes; diagnosed in pregnancy and controlled with diet alone
A_2	Gestational diabetes; diagnosed in pregnancy and controlled with diet and glyburide or insulin
B	Pregestational diabetes developing after age 20 yr and duration <10 yr; controlled with diet and insulin
C	Pregestational diabetes developing between ages 10 and 19 yr or duration 10-19 yr and controlled with diet and insulin
D	Pregestational diabetes developing before age 10 yr or duration 20 yr or more or background retinopathy; controlled with diet and insulin
F	Pregestational diabetes at any age or duration with nephropathy; controlled with diet and insulin
R	Pregestational diabetes at any age or duration with proliferative retinopathy; controlled with diet and insulin
H	Pregestational diabetes at any age or duration with arteriosclerotic heart disease; controlled with diet and insulin

Complications

Maternal and fetal complications of diabetes are listed in Table 16-2. **Diabetes often coexists with the metabolic syndrome.** This syndrome consists of a group of risk factors for diabetes, coronary heart disease, and stroke that occur together (central obesity, insulin resistance, and hyperlipidemia). Most fetal and neonatal effects are attributed to the consequences of maternal hyperglycemia or, in the more advanced classes, to maternal vascular disease. **Glucose crosses the placenta easily by facilitated diffusion, causing fetal hyperglycemia that stimulates pancreatic β-cells, and results in fetal hyperinsulinism. Fetal hyperglycemia during the period of embryogenesis is teratogenic.** There is a direct correlation between birth defects in diabetic pregnancies and increasing glycosylated hemoglobin A1C (HbA1C) levels in the first trimester. **Fetal hyperglycemia and hyperinsulinemia later in pregnancy, especially in the third trimester, cause fetal overgrowth and macrosomia that predispose to birth trauma, including shoulder dystocia and Erb palsy. Fetal demise is most likely due to acidosis, hypotension from osmotic diuresis, or hypoxia from increased metabolism, coupled with inadequate placental oxygen transfer.**

Pregestational diabetes is generally associated with a higher rate of maternal and fetal complications due to the greater difficulty in achieving glycemic control, the higher rate of congenital malformations, and the higher likelihood of vascular disease. Maternal complications include worsening nephropathy and retinopathy, a greater incidence of preterm preeclampsia, and a higher likelihood of diabetic ketoacidosis. **Hypoglycemia is also much more common** because of the need for insulin therapy and stricter glycemic control attempted during pregnancy. **Fetal complications include an increased rate of abortions, anatomic birth defects, fetal growth restriction, and prematurity.**

Diagnosis of Gestational Diabetes Mellitus

The American College of Obstetricians and Gynecologists (ACOG) recommends a two-step method to test for GDM. The first step involves universal screening for gestational diabetes between 24 and 28 weeks' gestation with a 50-g, 1-hour oral glucose challenge test (OGCT), given without regard to most recent oral intake. This timing recognizes the progressive nature of insulin resistance in pregnancy due to rising levels of hormones such as human placental lactogen, and the test will identify most women with gestational diabetes while allowing for several weeks of therapy to reduce potentially adverse consequences. **Screening is advised at the first prenatal visit in women with risk factors** such as a previous pregnancy with GDM, a history of polycystic ovarian disease, or obesity. If overt signs and symptoms of diabetes are present, the

TABLE 16-2

MATERNAL AND FETAL COMPLICATIONS OF DIABETES MELLITUS

Entity	Monitoring
Maternal Complications	
Obstetric Complications	
Polyhydramnios	Close prenatal surveillance: blood glucose monitoring, ultrasonography
Preeclampsia	Evaluation for signs and symptoms
Infections (e.g., UTI and candidiasis)	Urine culture, wet mount, and appropriate therapy
Cesarean delivery	Blood glucose monitoring, insulin and dietary adjustment to prevent fetal overgrowth
Genital trauma	Ultrasonography to detect macrosomia, cesarean delivery for macrosomia
Diabetic Emergencies	
Hypoglycemia	Teach signs and symptoms; blood glucose monitoring; insulin and dietary adjustment
Diabetic coma	Urgent medical management required
Ketoacidosis	Check for ketones if glucose >200 mg/dL
Vascular and End-Organ Involvement or Deterioration (in patients with pregestational diabetes mellitus)	
Cardiac	Electrocardiogram, first visit and as needed
Renal	Renal function studies, first visit and as needed
Ophthalmic	Funduscopic evaluation, first visit and as needed
Peripheral vascular	Check for ulcers, foot sores; noninvasive Doppler studies as needed
Gastrointestinal disturbance	Symptomatic treatment as needed
Neurologic	
Peripheral neuropathy	Neurologic and gastrointestinal consultations as needed
After Pregnancy	
Type 2 diabetes	Postpartum glucose testing of GDM, lifestyle changes (diet and exercise)
Metabolic syndrome	Lifestyle changes (diet and exercise)
Obesity	Lifestyle changes (diet and exercise)
Cardiovascular disease	Annual check-up by physician, lifestyle changes (diet and exercise)
Fetal and Neonatal Complications*	
Macrosomia with traumatic delivery	Ultrasonography for estimated fetal weight before delivery (shoulder dystocia, Erb palsy), offer cesarean delivery if EFW >4500 g
Delayed organ maturity (pulmonary, hepatic, neurologic)	Avoid delivery before 39 weeks in GDM in the absence of maternal-fetal respiratory distress syndrome indications, unless amniocentesis indicates lung maturity
Neonatal hypocalcemia, neonatal hypoglycemia	Maintain maternal euglycemia especially intrapartum
Congenital Defects	
Cardiovascular anomalies	Preconception counseling and glucose control
Neural tube defects	Maternal serum α-fetoprotein screening; fetal ultrasonography and fetal echocardiogram
Caudal regression syndrome	
Other defects (e.g., renal)	
Fetal Compromise	
Intrauterine growth restriction	Serial ultrasonography for fetal growth and estimated fetal weight, serial fetal antepartum surveillance; avoid postterm pregnancy
Intrauterine fetal death	Doppler
Abnormal FHR patterns	NST

EFW, Estimated fetal weight; *FHR,* fetal heart rate; *GDM,* gestational diabetes mellitus; *NST,* nonstress test; *UTI,* urinary tract infection.
*Maintenance of maternal euglycemia (normal glucose levels) will decrease most of these complications.

TABLE 16-3

THREE-HOUR ORAL GLUCOSE TOLERANCE TEST	
Test	Maximal Normal Blood Glucose (mg/dL)
Fasting	95
1 hr	180
2 hr	155
3 hr	140

From Berggren EK, Boggess KA, Stuebe AM, et al: National Diabetes Data Group vs Carpenter-Coustan criteria to diagnose gestational diabetes. *Am J Obstet Gynecol* 205:253.e1-e7, 2011.

BOX 16-1

METHOD FOR CALCULATING THE STARTING DOSE OF INSULIN

Insulin Units = Body Weight (kg)
×0.6 (first trimester)
×0.7 (second trimester)
×0.8 (third trimester)

Dosage Schedule: Give Two-Thirds in AM and One-Third in PM

Before breakfast: two-thirds NPH, one-third regular or lispro
Before dinner: one-half NPH, one-half regular or lispro (if on lispro, administer additional dose before bedtime snack)

NPH, Neutral protamine Hagedorn.

patient's fasting blood sugar should be checked first. **If a first-trimester screen is done and is found to be negative, it should be repeated at 24 to 28 weeks. Glucose values above 130 to 140 mg/dL on an OGCT are considered abnormal** and have an 80-90% sensitivity in detecting GDM.

The second step involves performing a diagnostic 3-hour, 100-g oral glucose tolerance test (OGTT) if the screening test is abnormal. This involves checking the patient's fasting blood glucose after an overnight fast, having the patient consume a 100-g glucose drink, and checking her glucose levels hourly for 3 hours. **If there are two or more abnormal values on the 3-hour OGTT, the patient is diagnosed with GDM (Table 16-3). If the 1-hour screening (50 g of oral glucose) plasma glucose exceeds 200 mg/dL, an OGTT is not required and may dangerously elevate blood glucose values.**

Management

TEAM APPROACH. Management of gestational and pregestational diabetes requires a team approach involving patient education and counseling, medical-nursing assessments and interventions, strategies to achieve maternal euglycemia, and avoidance of fetal-neonatal compromise. Ideally, this team should include the patient, obstetrician, maternal-fetal medicine specialist, clinical nurse specialist, nutritionist, social worker, and neonatologist. The patient is included as an active participant in formulating management strategies.

ACHIEVING EUGLYCEMIA. The importance of strict metabolic control before and during pregnancy to decrease the incidence of congenital anomalies, perinatal morbidity, and perinatal mortality has been established. To achieve an optimal outcome, the patient's fasting blood glucose level should be less than 95 mg/dL, with the 1-hour postprandial glucose level less than 140 mg/dL and the 2-hour postprandial glucose level less than 120 mg/dL.

DIET. Caloric requirements are calculated on the basis of ideal body weight: 30 kcal/kg for those patients 80-120% of ideal body weight, 35 to 40 kcal/kg for those patients less than 80% of ideal body weight, and 24 kcal/kg for gravidas who are 120-150% of ideal body weight. The diet is composed of about 45-50% carbohydrate, 20-25% protein, and 20-25% fat. The diet should also contain a generous amount of fiber. Caloric intake is divided into 20% at breakfast, 30% at lunch, 30% at dinner, and 20% at a bedtime snack.

EXERCISE. Patients with diabetes should be encouraged to engage in mild to moderate aerobic exercise (e.g., brisk walking) for about half an hour after meals.

PHARMACOLOGIC THERAPY. Patients with GDM are usually managed with diet and exercise alone, but if euglycemia cannot be achieved, an oral hypoglycemic agent (glyburide) or insulin should be added. Glyburide does not appear to enter the fetal circulation in appreciable quantities, and it has been used successfully to treat gestational diabetes after the first trimester.

Insulin is the medication of choice to maintain euglycemia in pregnancy and is the recommended therapy in women with pregestational diabetes. The peak action of insulin lispro occurs between 30 and 90 minutes after injection, that of regular insulin occurs between 2 and 3 hours after injection, and that of neutral protamine Hagedorn (NPH) insulin occurs between 6 and 10 hours after injection. A combination of rapid- or short-acting (lispro or regular) and intermediate-acting (NPH) insulin is usually given in split morning and evening doses or more frequently to achieve euglycemia. A method for calculating insulin dosage is shown in Box 16-1.

Antepartum Obstetric Management

Aside from achieving euglycemia, adequate surveillance should be maintained during pregnancy to detect and possibly mitigate maternal and fetal complications. In addition to routine prenatal screening tests for women with pregestational diabetes, **a detailed obstetric ultrasonic study, fetal echocardiogram, and maternal serum α-fetoprotein should be obtained in the second trimester to check for congenital malformations.** This is **especially important if the first trimester HbA1C is significantly elevated (>8.5%).** Maternal renal, cardiac, and ocular function must be closely monitored. **In women with GDM as well as those with class B or C pregestational diabetes, fetal macrosomia is common and should be investigated,** whereas for women with classes D, F, or R pregestational diabetes, fetal growth restriction occurs more commonly. Abnormalities of fetal growth are most likely to be present in the third trimester and can be confirmed by ultrasound.

Serial antepartum testing should be performed in the third trimester. This testing can usually be delayed until at or after 36 weeks, or later in women with well-controlled GDM. In patients with pregestational diabetes, fetal testing should be initiated between 32 and 34 weeks, or sooner if complications develop.

The timing of delivery depends on fetal and maternal status and the degree of glucose control. In general, in the setting of well-controlled GDM without other complications, spontaneous onset of labor at term may be awaited. Earlier intervention is indicated if these conditions are not met. For macrosomic babies, increased birth trauma to both mother and fetus should be avoided. **Cesarean delivery may be elected for large fetuses (>4500 g).**

Intrapartum Management

Intrapartum management of a patient with diabetes requires the establishment of maternal euglycemia during labor. Plasma glucose levels are measured frequently, and, if elevated, a continuous infusion of regular insulin is given. **Insulin dosage is adjusted as needed to maintain a plasma glucose level between 80 and 120 mg/dL.** Many insulin-dependent patients will not require exogenous insulin during labor. Continuous electronic **fetal heart rate monitoring is recommended for all patients with diabetes.**

Postpartum Period

After delivery of the fetus and placenta, insulin requirements drop sharply because the placenta, which is the source of many insulin antagonists, has been removed. Many patients with insulin-dependent diabetes may not require exogenous insulin for the first 48 to 72 hours after delivery. **Plasma glucose levels should be monitored and lispro or regular insulin given when plasma glucose levels are elevated.** Women with pregestational diabetes can be restarted on two-thirds of the prepregnancy insulin dosage, with adjustments made as necessary. Women with GDM treated with insulin or oral hypoglycemic agents during pregnancy frequently do not need treatment postpartum.

Women with GDM should undergo a 75-g OGTT at 6 to 12 weeks postpartum.

Patients should be counseled about changes in diet. The American Diabetes Association diet with the same distribution of carbohydrates, proteins, and fat should be maintained. If the mother is breastfeeding, 500 calories/day should be added to the prepregnancy diet.

Contraception counseling should involve advising the patient that estrogen-containing oral contraceptives are not recommended for women with advanced-stage diabetes with vascular disease.

THYROID DISEASES

Thyroid diseases are relatively common disorders in pregnancy, complicating up to 2% of pregnancies. Pregnancy can alter the presentation, diagnosis, and course of thyroid disease. If inadequately treated, these disorders can lead to major maternal, fetal, and neonatal morbidity.

Normal Thyroid Physiology during Pregnancy

With the increase in glomerular filtration rate that occurs during pregnancy, the renal excretion of iodine increases and plasma inorganic iodine levels are nearly halved. Goiters caused by iodine deficiency are not likely if plasma inorganic iodine levels are greater than 0.08 μg/dL but they do occur (Figure 16-1). An inorganic iodine intake of 250 μg/day is sufficient to prevent goiter formation during pregnancy. Prenatal vitamins typically contain 150 μg of iodine.

THYROID FUNCTION TESTS. The estrogen-mediated increase in thyroid-binding globulin during pregnancy results in a pronounced rise in serum total thyroxine (T_4) and total triiodothyronine (T_3) levels. Total T_4 levels in a pregnant woman can be up to 50% greater than the

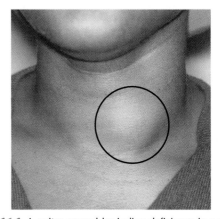

FIGURE 16-1 A goiter caused by iodine deficiency in a pregnant woman *(circle)*. Although iodine deficiency is rare during pregnancy, it can occur in areas where preconception and prenatal care are inadequate. (From Lemmi FO, Lemmi CAE: *Physical assessment findings* [CD-ROM], Philadelphia, 2009, Saunders.)

TABLE 16-4

MEDIAN VALUES OF THYROID-STIMULATING HORMONE

Pregnancy Stage	Median Value*
Nonpregnant	0.3-4.2 U/mL
First trimester	0.5-5.0 U/mL
Second trimester	0.5-3.5 U/mL
Third trimester	0.5-4.0 U/mL

*Rounded to the nearest 0.5.

upper limit of normal for nonpregnant women. **Serum free thyroxine (free T$_4$) and free triiodothyronine (free T$_3$) levels usually remain in the normal range. Human chorionic gonadotropin (hCG) levels peak in the first trimester and can cause transient, subclinical hyperthyroidism. In the setting of a molar pregnancy, the extremely high hCG levels can result in thyrotoxicosis.** When interpreting serum levels of thyroid-stimulating hormone (TSH) and free T$_4$ and T$_3$, it is best to use a laboratory that has trimester-specific values. Generally accepted TSH ranges for nonpregnant and pregnant women by trimester are shown in Table 16-4.

FETAL THYROID FUNCTION. Before 10 weeks' gestation, no organic iodine is present in the fetal thyroid. By the end of the first trimester (11 to 12 weeks), the fetal thyroid is able to produce iodothyronines and T$_4$, and by 12 to 14 weeks, it is able to concentrate iodine. Levels of these hormones remain low even at term, but they increase rapidly in the neonate within 48 hours of birth.

PLACENTAL TRANSFER OF THYROID HORMONE. Iodide freely crosses the placenta, but TSH does not. Limited transfer of T$_4$ occurs across the placenta and appears to be important for fetal neural development in the first trimester before fetal thyroid function begins. **Thyroid hormone analogues such as methimazole and propylthiouracil (PTU), with smaller molecular weights, cross the placental barrier and can potentially cause fetal hypothyroidism.** Thyroid-releasing hormone can cross the placental barrier, but there is no significant placental transfer because of circulating low levels. Thyroid-stimulating antibodies (TSH receptor antibodies) also cross the placenta and can potentially cause fetal and neonatal thyroid dysfunction.

Maternal Hyperthyroidism

The incidence of maternal thyrotoxicosis is about 1 per 500 pregnancies. It is accompanied by an increased incidence of prematurity, intrauterine growth restriction (IUGR), superimposed preeclampsia, stillbirth, and neonatal morbidity and mortality. Graves disease is an autoimmune disorder caused by thyroid-stimulating antibodies. It is the most common cause of hyperthyroidism. Other causes of hyperthyroidism in pregnancy include hCG-mediated hyperthyroidism, such as that seen in association with a hydatidiform mole, and toxic nodular goiter. Patients with Graves disease tend to have a remission during the third trimester of pregnancy and an exacerbation during the postpartum period. The increased immunologic tolerance during pregnancy may lead to a decrease in thyroid antibodies, which may account for the remission.

CLINICAL FEATURES. The clinical diagnosis of hyperthyroidism in pregnancy is difficult, because many of the signs and symptoms of the hyperdynamic circulation associated with hyperthyroidism are present in a normal euthyroid pregnant woman. A resting pulse rate greater than 100 beats per minute, a wide pulse pressure, tremor, eye changes (exophthalmos), failure to gain weight despite normal or increased food intake, and heat intolerance, when present, are all helpful in making the clinical diagnosis.

INVESTIGATIONS. An **elevated serum free T$_4$ level** and a **suppressed TSH level establish the diagnosis** of hyperthyroidism. Infrequently, a free T$_3$ determination might be needed to diagnose T$_3$ thyrotoxicosis. In cases where there is significant discordance between the clinical findings and TSH and free thyroid hormone levels, it is appropriate to measure the total T$_4$ level, accepting as normal up to 1.5 times the upper range in nonpregnant women.

THERAPY. Because radioactive iodine treatment is contraindicated during pregnancy, medical treatment is generally given. When there is significant maternal tachycardia, β-blockers such as atenolol or propranolol may be used for short-term treatment, with longer-term treatment increasing the risk of fetal growth restriction. **Thioamides are the mainstay of antithyroid therapy.** They block the synthesis, but not the release, of thyroid hormone. **PTU and methimazole (Tapazole)** are both effective, but they have different safety profiles. Both cross the placenta, and **methimazole** has been associated with aplasia cutis congenita (absence of a portion of skin at birth) and fetal gastrointestinal (GI) defects to a greater degree than PTU. For the mother, **methimazole** appears safer because there is less risk of liver toxicity. **These drugs readily cross the placenta, and a concern during maternal treatment is the development of fetal goiter and hypothyroidism.** Although there is no conclusive evidence that PTU treatment leads to cretinism or abnormalities in physical or intellectual development, 1-5% of children exposed in utero will develop a goiter (Figure 16-2). For these reasons, **PTU should be used to treat overt hyperthyroidism in the first trimester, and methimazole should be used in the second and**

A case of fetal goiter

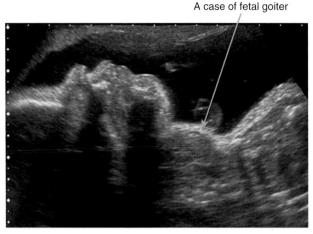

FIGURE 16-2 Ultrasonic study of a fetus with a goiter caused by maternal treatment with propylthiouracil for hyperthyroidism. (From Polak M, Luton D: Fetal thyroïdology. *Best Pract Res Clin Endocrinol Metab* 28:161-173, 2014.)

third trimesters. Importantly, antithyroid drugs should be reduced to the lowest dose that results in free T_4 levels within the upper range of normal. Free T_4 levels should be checked at least every 4 weeks. Antithyroid therapy can often be discontinued after 30 weeks' gestation, but the patient should be followed for recurrent disease postpartum.

Methimazole and PTU are excreted in breast milk, but no changes occur in the thyroid function tests of breastfed neonates. Methimazole is preferred over PTU in breastfeeding mothers because of the lower risk of liver toxicity.

Surgical management of a pregnant patient with hyperthyroidism during the second trimester is recommended only when medical treatment fails.

Thyroid Storm

The major risk for a pregnant patient with thyrotoxicosis is the development of a thyroid storm. Precipitating factors include infection, labor, cesarean delivery, or noncompliance with the medication regimen. It is not uncommon to mistakenly attribute the signs and symptoms of severe hyperthyroidism to preeclampsia. In the former, significant proteinuria is usually absent, but both may be present in the same patient. **Thyroid storm in a pregnant woman is a life-threatening medical emergency and should be treated in an intensive care setting. The signs and symptoms associated with a thyroid storm include hyperthermia, marked maternal tachycardia, perspiration, and high-output renal failure or severe dehydration.** Fetal tachycardia can also be present.

Specific treatment involves (1) blocking β-adrenergic activity and controlling maternal heart rate with propranolol, (2) blocking synthesis of thyroid hormone and conversion of T_4 to T_3 with PTU, (3) administering potassium iodide 1 to 2 hours after starting PTU to block secretion of thyroid hormone, (4) additional blocking of the deamination of T_4 to T_3 with glucocorticoids (dexamethasone), (5) replacing fluid losses, and (6) rapidly lowering the patient's body temperature with hypothermic techniques. Management also involves intensive maternal and fetal monitoring and correction of precipitating factors. It is important to stabilize the patient before attempting delivery if that is being considered. Once the patient is stabilized and no longer acutely ill, methimazole should be substituted for PTU to avoid hepatotoxicity.

Neonatal Thyrotoxicosis

About 5% of pregnant women with a history of Graves disease give birth to children with thyrotoxicosis due to transplacental transfer of TSH receptor antibodies. It is transient and lasts less than 2 to 3 months, but if clinically significant and untreated, it is associated with neonatal morbidity and mortality. Fetal thyrotoxicosis can be suspected if the baseline fetal heart rate consistently exceeds 160 beats per minute. A fetal goiter can often be identified by ultrasonography in such cases, and fetal growth restriction may be present. This situation is associated with an increase in perinatal morbidity and mortality and should be treated pre- and postnatally.

Hypothyroidism

Hypothyroidism (overt or subclinical) complicates up to 3% of pregnancies. The value of universal screening is still being debated, and ACOG is currently not recommending routine screening. However, pregnant women with symptoms consistent with low thyroid hormone levels (fatigue, intolerance to cold, excessive weight gain) or with risk factors (e.g., obesity, type 1 diabetes or history of thyroid disease) should be screened.

The most important laboratory finding of hypothyroidism is an elevated TSH level. If the TSH level is elevated, the diagnosis of overt vs. subclinical hypothyroidism can be made based on whether free T_4 levels are decreased. Once diagnosed, therapy such as levothyroxine should be started, and serum TSH levels should be measured monthly with appropriate adjustments in levothyroxine dosage. Pregnant women on appropriate thyroid replacement therapy can expect a normal pregnancy outcome, but **untreated maternal hypothyroidism has been associated with an increased risk of spontaneous abortion, preeclampsia, abruption, low-birth-weight or stillborn infants, and lower cognitive function in offspring.**

CONGENITAL HYPOTHYROIDISM. Thyroid hormone deficiency during the fetal and early neonatal periods leads to generalized cognitive impairment. The severity of symptoms depends on the time of onset and the severity of the deprivation. **The incidence of congenital hypothyroidism is about 1 in 2000 to 4000 births.** The etiologic factors include thyroid dysgenesis, inborn errors of thyroid function, and iodine deficiency. Maternal and neonatal exposure to excess iodine (e.g., amiodorone, iodine-containing contrast dyes or disinfectants, and supplements) is another potentially preventable cause. **Newborn screening programs can identify many cases of congenital hypothyroidism, and with early administration of thyroid hormone replacement, the impairment can be minimized.**

Heart Disease

Less than 5% of pregnancies in the United States are complicated by maternal cardiac disease, but it is an important cause of maternal mortality. The cardiovascular adaptations to pregnancy, delivery, and the early puerperium can trigger acute cardiovascular decompensation in women with high-risk lesions. The physiologic changes discussed in Chapter 6, including the rise in preload, decrease in afterload, and increase in cardiac output, begin in the first trimester and peak toward the end of the second or early third trimester. The corresponding physical findings of a new systolic flow murmur, an S_3 gallop, an increase in resting heart rate, a decline in diastolic blood pressure, and dependent edema can further complicate the clinical diagnosis and management of these pregnancies.

The categories of heart disease in pregnancy include **rheumatic and congenital cardiac disease** as well as **arrhythmias, cardiomyopathies,** and other forms of **acquired heart disease, such as coronary artery disease.** Better treatment of rheumatic fever and improvements in medical and surgical management of congenital heart disease have meant that in a modern tertiary referral center, **about 80% of patients with cardiac disease in pregnancy now have congenital heart disease.**

RHEUMATIC HEART DISEASE

The most common lesion associated with rheumatic heart disease is mitral stenosis, followed by mitral regurgitation. Patients with mitral stenosis, especially those with a valve area less than 1.5 cm^2, **are at high risk of developing heart failure, subacute bacterial endocarditis, and thromboembolic disease.** They also have a higher rate of fetal wastage.

During pregnancy, the mechanical obstruction associated with mitral stenosis worsens as cardiac output increases. **Asymptomatic patients may develop symptoms of cardiac decompensation or pulmonary edema as pregnancy progresses.** Atrial fibrillation is more common in patients with severe mitral stenosis, and **nearly all women who develop atrial fibrillation during pregnancy experience congestive heart failure.** Tachycardia can result in decompensation because

cardiac output in patients with mitral stenosis depends on an adequate diastolic filling time.

CONGENITAL HEART DISEASE

Congenital heart disease includes atrial or ventricular septal defects, valvular defects, primary pulmonary hypertension (Eisenmenger syndrome), and cyanotic heart diseases such as tetralogy of Fallot and transposition of the great arteries. If the anatomic defect has been corrected during childhood with no residual damage, the patient is expected to go through pregnancy without complications. Patients with persistent atrial or ventricular septal defects and those with tetralogy of Fallot with complete surgical correction generally tolerate pregnancy well. However, **patients with primary pulmonary hypertension or cyanotic heart disease with residual pulmonary hypertension are in danger of experiencing decompensation during pregnancy.** Pulmonary hypertension from any cause is associated with an increased risk of maternal mortality during pregnancy or in the immediate postpartum period. In all of these patients, care should be taken to avoid overloading the circulation and precipitating pulmonary congestion, heart failure, or hypotension, all of which may lead to hypoxia and sudden death. **In general, significant pulmonary hypertension with Eisenmenger syndrome is a contraindication to pregnancy due to the high maternal mortality that accompanies this condition.**

CARDIAC ARRHYTHMIAS

Palpitations are common in pregnancy and are a frequent indication for an electrocardiogram (ECG). **If an arrhythmia is detected, an echocardiogram should be obtained to determine if there is underlying structural heart disease. Atrial premature beats are common, but usually benign and do not require therapy** other than elimination of exogenous stimulants such as caffeine and cigarettes. **The management of supraventricular tachyarrhythmias (SVTs) with carotid massage or the Valsalva maneuver, antiarrhythmic therapy, or direct current cardioversion is based on the patient's hemodynamic status. Atrial fibrillation and atrial flutter, though much less common than SVTs, are more serious and are usually associated with underlying maternal cardiac disease.** Tests of thyroid function should also be done. Treatment is similar to that in nonpregnant adults, although antiarrhythmic agents cross the placenta and the fetal risks are largely unknown. Heparin (or low-molecular-weight heparin) should be used instead of warfarin when anticoagulation is indicated.

ISCHEMIC HEART DISEASE

It is anticipated that the number of pregnant women with coronary artery disease or other causes of ischemic heart disease will increase as the number of pregnant women with comorbidities, such as age over 40 years, obesity, chronic hypertension, and diabetes, continues to rise. Stress testing and angiography should be done before pregnancy. Use of lipid-lowering agents or angiotensin-converting enzyme (ACE) inhibitors should be avoided during pregnancy because these drugs are currently labeled class X because of concerns regarding fetal toxicity. Certain antiplatelet agents may be safe for the fetus, but they should be stopped before delivery to avoid bleeding complications.

PERIPARTUM CARDIOMYOPATHY

The occurrence of peripartum cardiomyopathy is reported to have wide regional variation. Patients with this condition have no underlying cardiac disease, and symptoms of cardiac decompensation appear during the last weeks of pregnancy or within 6 months postpartum. **Pregnant women particularly at risk of developing cardiomyopathy are those with a history of preeclampsia or hypertension and those who are poorly nourished.** It appears to be a dilatational cardiomyopathy with a decreased left ventricular ejection fraction (LVEF < 45%). Hypertensive or drug-induced cardiomyopathy, ischemic heart disease, viral myocarditis, and valvular heart disease must be excluded in these patients before the diagnosis can be made. With prompt diagnosis and skilled management (including delivery if the disease presents antepartum), maternal mortality rates have been declining but are still at least 10%. These women have a 30-50% risk of persistent cardiac dysfunction and a 20-50% recurrence rate in subsequent pregnancies.

MANAGEMENT OF CARDIAC DISEASE DURING PREGNANCY

The New York Heart Association functional classification of heart disease is of value in assessing the risk of pregnancy for a patient with acquired cardiac disease and in determining the optimal management during pregnancy, labor, and delivery (Table 16-5). In general, **the maternal and fetal risks** for patients with class I or II disease are small, whereas they **are greatly increased in patients with class III or IV disease or if they have cyanosis.** However, the type and severity of the defect is important as well. In general, mitral (valve area <2 cm^2) and aortic stenosis (valve area <1.5 cm^2) carry a much higher risk of decompensation than do mitral or aortic regurgitation, because the pregnancy-induced decrease in systemic vascular resistance improves cardiac output in the setting of lesions causing regurgitation. **Other patients at high risk of morbidity and mortality include those with significant pulmonary hypertension, a LVEF less than 40%, Marfan syndrome, a mechanical valve, a previous history of a cardiac event or arrhythmia, or significant comorbidities.**

Prenatal Management

As a general principle, **all pregnant cardiac patients should be managed with the help of a cardiologist, a maternal-fetal medicine specialist, and an anesthesiologist.** A careful history and physical examination should be performed, and an ECG and echocardiogram should be obtained. This evaluation will assist in counseling the patient about risks associated with pregnancy, and all available options (including pregnancy termination) should be presented. Frequent prenatal visits are indicated, and frequent hospital admissions may be needed, especially for patients with class III or IV cardiac disease.

AVOIDANCE OF EXCESSIVE WEIGHT GAIN AND EDEMA. There is no strong evidence to support sodium restriction in the absence of heart failure, but excessive salt intake should be avoided. Women should be encouraged to rest in the left lateral decubitus position (which avoids compression of the vena cava) for at least 1 hour every day. Adequate sleep should be encouraged. If there is evidence of chronic left ventricular failure not adequately treated with sodium restriction, a loop diuretic and β-blockers should be added. **Aldosterone antagonists should be avoided because of their potential antiandrogenic effects on the fetus.**

AVOIDANCE OF STRENUOUS ACTIVITY. Individuals with significant heart disease have decreased cardiac reserve and are unable to increase their cardiac output to meet the metabolic needs of exercise to the same extent that healthy individuals are.

AVOIDANCE OF ANEMIA. With anemia, the oxygen-carrying capacity of the blood decreases. Oxygen delivery to tissues is generally maintained by increased cardiac output. An increase in heart rate, especially with mitral stenosis, leads to a decrease in left ventricular filling time, resulting in pulmonary congestion and edema.

TABLE 16-5

NEW YORK HEART ASSOCIATION FUNCTIONAL CLASSIFICATION OF HEART DISEASE	
Class	Description
Class I	No signs or symptoms of cardiac decompensation
Class II	No symptoms at rest, but minor limitation of physical activity
Class III	No symptoms at rest, but marked limitation of physical activity
Class IV	Symptoms present at rest, discomfort increased with any kind of physical activity

AVOIDANCE OF INFECTION. This is accomplished by routine screening for sexually transmitted infections and urinary tract infections, the timely administration of appropriate immunizations, and vigilance in the evaluation and treatment of any concerning symptoms or signs of infection. Cesarean delivery should only be performed for clear obstetrical indications, in part because of the increased risk of endometritis and wound infections.

ANTICOAGULATION. Women with mechanical valves and those with atrial fibrillation require full anticoagulation with heparin or low-molecular-weight heparin in pregnancy. Warfarin may be restarted postpartum.

FETAL ECHOCARDIOGRAPHY. Women with congenital heart disease have an increased risk of having children with heart disease. Early detection with fetal echocardiography can help with plans for neonatal management.

Management of Delivery and the Immediate Postpartum Period

Cardiac patients should be delivered vaginally unless obstetric indications for cesarean delivery are present. They should be allowed to **labor in the lateral decubitus position** with frequent assessment of vital signs, urine output, and pulse oximetry. Adequate pain relief is important. **Pushing should be avoided during the second stage of labor** because the associated increase in intraabdominal pressure can lead to cardiac decompensation. The second stage of labor can be assisted by performing an **outlet forceps** delivery or by the use of a **vacuum extractor.**

The immediate postpartum period presents special risks to the cardiac patient. After delivery of the placenta, the uterus contracts and about 500 mL of blood are added to the effective blood volume. **Cardiac output increases up to 80% above prelabor values in the first few hours after a vaginal delivery and up to 50% after cesarean delivery.** To minimize the risks of volume overload or depletion, careful attention should be paid to fluid balance (avoiding overload) and **prevention of uterine atony (avoiding depletion from blood loss) with oxytocin and uterine massage. When these measures are unsuccessful, prostaglandin F2α can be administered if pulmonary hypertension and reactive airway disease are not concerns. Methergine should be avoided** due to its pronounced vasoconstrictor effects.

A particular concern is the risk of endocarditis. The 2008 American Heart Association guidelines state that, in most cases, delivery does not increase the risk of infectious endocarditis. **Antibiotic prophylaxis is recommended only for high-risk patients,** such as those with prosthetic valves, unrepaired or incom-

pletely repaired congenital heart disease, or a previous history of bacterial endocarditis.

Acute cardiac decompensation with congestive heart failure should be managed as a medical emergency, and the immediate postpartum period poses the greatest risk. Medical management is directed at correcting the precipitating factors and may include administration of morphine sulfate, supplemental oxygen with ventilatory support if needed, and an intravenous loop diuretic (e.g., furosemide) to reduce fluid retention and preload. β-Blockers should not be used in the setting of acute heart failure. Vasodilators such as hydralazine, nitroglycerin, and, rarely, nitroprusside are used to improve cardiac output by decreasing afterload. **Some patients may require inotropic support** with dopamine or dobutamine. The use of digitalis is controversial. **ACE inhibitors and similar drugs should be avoided.** Very frequent monitoring of vital signs, urine output, and pulse oximetry, along with continuous electrocardiographic monitoring, is advised. Routine use of pulmonary artery catheterization is discouraged, and it may even be contraindicated if the patient has cyanotic heart disease.

Autoimmune Disease in Pregnancy

An autoimmune disease is one in which antibodies are developed against the host's own tissues. A summary of the interactions of primary immunologic disorders and pregnancy is provided in Table 16-6.

IMMUNE THROMBOCYTOPENIA

With immune thrombocytopenia (ITP), the low platelet count occurs when peripheral platelet destruction exceeds bone marrow production. ITP is considered to be an autoantibody disorder in which immunoglobulins attach to maternal platelets, leading to platelet sequestration in the reticuloendothelial system. ITP maybe be confused with gestational thrombocytopenia. **Gestational thrombocytopenia** is unlikely to present with a platelet count less than 70,000/μL, **is not associated with bleeding complications,** does not require therapy, occurs late in pregnancy, and resolves after delivery.

Treatment

In the absence of bleeding, therapy for ITP is usually not initiated unless platelet counts are less than 50,000/μL. Oral **prednisone** at a dose of 1 mg/kg per day is given initially, and once platelet counts improve, it is tapered off over several weeks. Severe ITP can be more rapidly treated with intravenous immunoglobulin (IVIG). **In patients with life-threatening hemorrhage, platelet transfusions combined with high-dose steroids and IVIG may be required. Splenectomy is a last resort** for patients who do not respond to medical therapy. Maternal hemorrhage is unlikely if the platelet

TABLE 16-6

AUTOIMMUNE DISEASE IN PREGNANCY

Disease	Effect of Disease on Pregnancy		Effect of Pregnancy on Disease	Antibodies That Cross Placenta
	Mother	Fetus		
Rheumatoid arthritis	No significant effect	No significant effect Teratogenic effects of medication	Usually improved	None
Idiopathic thrombocytopenic purpura	Antepartum, intrapartum, and postpartum hemorrhage	None (causes neonatal intracranial bleeding)	None	Platelet antibodies
Graves disease	No significant effect (avoid magnesium sulfate)	Intrauterine growth restriction (IUGR) Neonatal thyrotoxicosis	Improved during pregnancy Exacerbation postpartum	Thyroid-stimulating immunoglobulins
Myasthenia gravis	No significant effect	Transient neonatal myasthenia gravis	Variable during pregnancy Moderate exacerbation postpartum	Antiacetylcholinesterase
Systemic lupus erythematosus	Increased incidence of uterine infection Increased incidence of preeclampsia	Abortion (spontaneous) Preterm preeclampsia IUGR Stillbirth Congenital heart block Endomyocardial fibrosis	Exacerbation of disease Deterioration of renal condition Anemia, leukopenia, and thrombocytopenia	Anti-Ro/SSA, anti-La/SSB

count is greater than 40,000/μL at the time of delivery, but concerns about the possibility of an epidural hematoma may preclude the use of epidural anesthesia. Advanced consultation with anesthesia staff is advised. **The neonate should be monitored for thrombocytopenia, because placental transfer of maternal antiplatelet antibodies can occur.** Rarely, neonatal intracranial hemorrhage may occur once the neonatal platelet count has reached its nadir after the first 2 to 3 days of life. There is no correlation between fetal platelet counts and neonatal outcome; thus, monitoring fetal platelet counts is not done in pregnancy. **Vaginal delivery is generally preferred,** because there is little evidence that the fetal outcome is improved by cesarean delivery and surgery carries additional maternal risks.

SYSTEMIC LUPUS ERYTHEMATOSUS

Systemic lupus erythematosus (SLE) is a chronic autoimmune disease with multiple organ system involvement in which patients are subject to acute exacerbations or flares. Associated antibodies include antinuclear, anti-ribonucleoprotein (anti-RNP), and anti-Smith (anti-Sm) antibodies. Anti-double-stranded DNA (anti-dsDNA) antibody is associated with nephritis and lupus activity. Anti-Ro/SSA and anti-La/SSB are present in Sjögren syndrome and neonatal lupus with heart block. Antihistone antibody is common in drug-induced SLE. The diagnosis of SLE is based on a com-

bination of clinical and laboratory criteria. The criteria proposed by the American College of Rheumatology are given in Table 16-7. The diagnosis of SLE can be made if four or more of the 11 criteria listed in Table 16-7 are present, serially or simultaneously.

SLE can flare up during any trimester or in the postpartum period. There is good evidence that the best pregnancy outcomes occur if the disease has been quiescent or under good control for at least 6 months before conception and there is no evidence of active lupus nephritis. A lupus flare, if it occurs, can be life-threatening, but it is often difficult to differentiate from superimposed preeclampsia, and both may coexist. Complement component 3 levels are usually low in a flare, but they are often elevated in patients with preeclampsia. Often only a trial of therapy will enable the two to be distinguished. Flares and active disease are generally managed with steroids and hydroxychloroquine, drugs that have less fetal toxicity than other immunosuppressive agents. The addition of heparin or low-molecular-weight heparin in prophylactic or therapeutic doses is dependent on the patient's medical and obstetric history and risk factors.

In addition to flares, worsening nephritis, and preeclampsia, SLE is associated with a relatively high rate of other pregnancy complications. **These include an increased rate of miscarriage and intrauterine fetal death, especially when associated with antiphospholipid antibodies, as well as preterm delivery and fetal**

TABLE 16-7

1997 REVISED CRITERIA OF THE AMERICAN RHEUMATISM ASSOCIATION FOR THE DIAGNOSIS OF SYSTEMIC LUPUS ERYTHEMATOSUS

Criteria*	Comments
Malar rash	Malar erythema
Discoid rash	Erythematous patches, scaling, follicular plugging
Photosensitivity	
Oral ulcers	Usually painless
Arthritis	Nonerosive involving two or more peripheral joints
Serositis	Pleuritis or pericarditis
Renal disorder	Proteinuria greater than 0.5 g/day or >3+ dipstick, or cellular casts
Neurological disorders	Seizures or psychosis without other cause
Hematological disorders	Hemolytic anemia, leukopenia, lymphopenia, or thrombocytopenia
Immunological disorders	Anti-dsDNA or anti-Sm antibodies, or false-positive VDRL, IgM or IgG anticardiolipin antibodies, or lupus anticoagulant
Antinuclear antibodies	Abnormal titer of ANAs

From Hochberg MC: Updating the American College of Rheumatology revised criteria for the classification of systemic lupus erythematosus. *Arthritis Rheum* 40:1725, 1997. Copyright 1997 American College of Rheumatology. Reprinted with permission of John Wiley & Sons, Inc.
ANA, Antinuclear antibody; *dsDNA*, double-stranded DNA; *Ig*, immunoglobulin; *Sm*, Smith; *VDRL*, Venereal Disease Research Laboratory.
*If four criteria are present at any time during the course of the disease, systemic lupus erythematosus can be diagnosed with 98% specificity and 97% sensitivity.

growth restriction. These pregnancies require close monitoring with serial assessment of renal function, blood counts, and immune markers of disease activity (complement levels and anti-dsDNA). In the third trimester, weekly maternal visits may be indicated, along with serial ultrasonic monitoring of fetal growth and twice-weekly antepartum testing. **Neonatal lupus is associated with passive transmission of anti-Ro/SSA or anti-La/SSB antibodies** and is one of the main causes of congenital heart block.

ANTIPHOSPHOLIPID SYNDROME

Antiphospholipid antibodies are circulating antibodies to negatively charged phospholipids. They include lupus anticoagulant, anticardiolipin immunoglobulin G (IgG) or IgM antibodies, and β_2-glycoprotein-1 antibodies. They **may occur alone or in association with SLE. The *antiphospholipid syndrome* is defined as the presence of at least one of these antibodies in association with arterial or venous thrombosis and/or one or more obstetric complications.** These complications

include an unexplained fetal demise after 10 weeks' gestation, a history of preterm delivery before 34 weeks' gestation due to severe preeclampsia or placental insufficiency, or three or more unexplained miscarriages before 10 weeks' gestation. Lupus anticoagulant can be screened for with an activated partial prothrombin time (aPTT) or with the dilute Russell viper venom test, a sensitive and specific radioimmunoassay that is available for the detection of anticardiolipin. In pregnancy, **a history of antiphospholipid syndrome is treated with prophylactic low-molecular-weight heparin and low-dose aspirin (81 mg), unless there is a history of thrombosis, in which case a full dosage of anticoagulants is indicated.**

Renal Disorders

ACUTE RENAL FAILURE

Acute renal failure during pregnancy or in the postpartum period may be caused by deterioration of renal function secondary to a preexisting renal disease or by a pregnancy-associated disorder. The causes can be classified as prerenal, renal, or postrenal. **With prerenal causes, a history of blood or fluid loss, such as that which occurs with obstetric hemorrhage or severe hyperemesis gravidarum, is usually apparent or can be elicited.** Treatment is aimed at correcting the hypovolemia and underlying disease process.

Renal causes are usually suspected in patients with a history of preexisting renal disease, such as lupus nephritis. Acute tubular necrosis (ATN) can complicate a septic abortion and pyelonephritis in pregnancy. **ATN can also be due to thrombotic microangiopathies** such as thrombotic thrombocytopenic purpura and hemolytic uremic syndrome, preeclampsia with hemolysis, elevated liver enzymes, and low platelet count (HELLP) syndrome (see Chapter 14), or acute fatty liver of pregnancy with disseminated intravascular coagulopathy (DIC). **Prolonged hypotension with DIC, such as that which occurs in the setting of massive abruption, retained dead fetus, or amniotic fluid embolus, can lead to acute cortical necrosis, which may present with the triad of anuria, gross hematuria, and flank pain. Treatment is directed at the underlying causes and delivery of the fetus if the patient is still pregnant.** Whereas the majority of patients with ATN recover, acute cortical necrosis has a much poorer prognosis and many of these patients will require dialysis.

Postrenal causes of acute renal failure are less common, but they should be suspected in situations in which urologic obstructive lesions are present or in which there is a history of kidney stones. In many instances, simple measures, such as turning the patient on the left side to displace the gravid uterus away from the ureters or inserting a Foley catheter into the bladder to overcome urethral obstruction, will resolve the problem. In situations in which a ureteral or renal pelvic obstruction is present (e.g., stones), surgical intervention may be indicated to relieve the obstruction.

CHRONIC RENAL DISEASE

The outcome of pregnancies complicated by chronic renal disease is less favorable than that associated with acute renal failure. Good pregnancy outcomes may be expected in mild renal disease. The risk of adverse fetal outcomes and loss of maternal renal function increases with the severity of the renal insufficiency. **In general, a serum creatinine greater than 1.5 to 2.0 mg/dL, especially if accompanied by hypertension and/or nephrotic syndrome, greatly worsens the prognosis for the mother and fetus.** Management principles include serial monitoring of renal function by 24-hour urinary creatinine clearance and protein excretion, as well as screening and treating the patient for asymptomatic bacteriuria. Diastolic pressure should be maintained at 90 mm Hg or less to prevent further renal damage. **Superimposed preeclampsia is more difficult to diagnose because hypertension and proteinuria are already present.** Fetal surveillance is important for assessing fetal growth and well-being.

PREGNANCY FOLLOWING RENAL TRANSPLANTATION

Pregnancy after renal transplantation should not be considered before thorough counseling about maternal, fetal, and neonatal risks takes place. Maternal complications of pregnancy include high rates of hypertension and preeclampsia and a significant risk of graft rejection and failure. **Fetal complications include steroid-induced adrenal and hepatic insufficiency, prematurity, and IUGR.** In addition, the infant may inherit the primary disease of the mother or other family members. The mother and fetus or neonate are both at increased risk of infection because of immunosuppressive therapy. Before a patient attempts to conceive, fetotoxic medications such as sirolimus should be replaced with immunosuppressants that are safer for the fetus, and fetotoxic infections such as CMV must be ruled out.

Patients who are good candidates for pregnancy are those who are 1 to 2 years posttransplant, have stable renal function (serum creatinine <1.5 mg/dL and proteinuria <500 mg/day), are not significantly hypertensive, and are taking low doses of prednisone and stable doses of cyclosporine. These medications do not appear to have significant teratogenic effects, but long-term consequences on growth, immune function, and neurocognitive development are unknown. Cyclosporin may have adverse maternal consequences, including a blood pressure increase, renal function decline, hyperkalemia, hyperuricemia, and, less frequently, a hemolytic uremic syndrome.

Gastrointestinal Disorders

NAUSEA AND VOMITING DURING PREGNANCY

About 50-80% of pregnant women complain of nausea and vomiting during the first trimester. The symptoms are usually mild and disappear during the early part of the second trimester. **The underlying causes of nausea and vomiting during pregnancy are not well understood.**

Treatment is usually symptomatic. Patients are instructed to avoid known triggers of nausea (e.g., coffee, strong odors, fatty foods); to eat frequent, small, protein-rich meals or snacks; to avoid the recumbent position, especially after meals; and to use an extra pillow to elevate the head when sleeping. Many patients respond to pyridoxine (vitamin B_6), whereas others may require ginger, acupressure, or first-line antiemetics such as doxylamine.

HYPEREMESIS GRAVIDARUM

Hyperemesis gravidarum is generally defined as persistent nausea and vomiting in pregnancy that is associated with ketosis and loss of more than 5% of prepregnancy body weight. Even though the exact cause is unknown, proposed theories include psychological abnormalities, hormonal changes such as high hCG and estradiol levels, gastric dysrhythmias, hyperacuity of the olfactory system, subclinical vestibular disorders, and impairment of mitochondrial fatty acid oxidation. **The overall incidence is about 1-2%. The disorder appears more frequently with first pregnancies, multiple pregnancies, and those with trophoblastic disease,** but it tends to recur with subsequent pregnancies. **Pregnancy outcome is usually good if the disorder is treated and there is catch-up weight gain.**

A history of intractable vomiting, beginning in the first trimester, is usually elicited. Physical findings of weight loss, dry and coated tongue, and decreased skin turgor are very suggestive. **Significant abdominal pain and tenderness are generally absent.** Laboratory workup includes urine tests for ketonuria and blood tests for electrolytes and acetone, blood urea nitrogen (BUN), creatinine, amylase, lipase, and liver function. Electrolyte disturbances may include hypokalemia, hyponatremia, and hypochloremic alkalosis. Liver function tests and amylase and lipase levels may be elevated. Many of these women have laboratory evidence of mild hyperthyroidism, which resolves without therapy as the pregnancy progresses.

Treatment is symptomatic and includes the interventions advised for the more benign nausea and vomiting of pregnancy noted above. **If outpatient management fails, patients must be admitted for intravenous administration of fluids, electrolytes, glucose, vitamins, and medical therapy.** Medical management involves a stepwise approach beginning with vitamin B_6 (pyridoxine) and antihistamines such as doxylamine or diphenhydramine. If vomiting persists, antiemetics of the phenothiazine class and promotility agents such as metoclopramide may be needed. Phenothiazines such as promethazine and metoclopramide should be stopped immediately if they induce any signs of tardive dyskinesia (involuntary movements, usually of the face). The addition of antacids or H_2 receptor antagonists (see "Gastroesophageal Reflux Disease" section below) may also prove beneficial. **The few patients who do not respond to medical therapy may require nasogastric feeding or parenteral nutrition.**

GASTROESOPHAGEAL REFLUX DISEASE

Some amount of gastroesophageal reflux disease (GERD) occurs in about 70% of pregnant women. The main symptoms include substernal discomfort aggravated by meals and the recumbent position. Hematemesis occasionally occurs. An unusual symptom peculiar to reflux esophagitis is water brash, which is best described as the sudden filling of the mouth with clear, watery material that has a salty taste and produces nausea.

Treatment

Treatment is usually symptomatic. Upper GI endoscopy is usually not necessary, unless there is significant GI bleeding. Patients are instructed to eliminate dietary triggers; refrain from eating large and late meals; avoid the recumbent position, especially after meals; and use an extra pillow to elevate the head when sleeping. Antacids can be helpful and should be taken 1 to 3 hours after meals and at bedtime. Those containing bismuth or bicarbonate should be avoided because of possible fetal toxicity. Sucralfate (aluminum sucrose sulfate) is a surface-binding agent useful in pregnancy for symptom relief because it is poorly absorbed and has no apparent fetal toxicity. An H_2 receptor antagonist **(cimetidine) or a proton pump inhibitor (omeprazole) is indicated if there is no response to the above-described measures. Both appear to be safe for the fetus, but proton pump inhibitors are not advised in breastfeeding women, because of lack of safety data.**

PEPTIC ULCER

Pregnancy conveys relative protection against the development of peptic ulceration and may ameliorate an already-present ulcer. Gastric acid secretion is probably not altered during pregnancy, although some studies suggest modest suppression. **The diagnosis of peptic ulcer disease is based mainly on symptomatic improvement in response to conservative treatment. Endoscopy is reserved for those patients who do not respond to treatment, have more severe GI symptoms, or manifest significant GI hemorrhage.** Treatment involves avoiding caffeine, alcohol, tobacco, and spicy foods and administering antacids (see safety issues under "Gastroesophageal Reflux Disease" above), H_2 receptor antagonists, or proton pump inhibitors. Any nonsteroidal antiinflammatory drugs should be discontinued. Antibiotic therapy should be considered for patients with *Helicobacter pylori* infection, but it is generally not given until the patient is postpartum.

ACID ASPIRATION SYNDROME (MENDELSON SYNDROME)

The pregnant patient in labor is at an increased risk of regurgitation and acid aspiration of gastric contents because of delayed gastric emptying and increased intraabdominal and intragastric pressures. This is made worse when associated with the use of sedatives, narcotics, or general anesthesia. Damage to the pulmonary tissue is greatest when the pH of the aspirated fluid is less than 2.5 or the volume of the aspirate is greater than 25 mL. **Acute gastric aspiration is a cause of acute respiratory distress syndrome (ARDS) in adults.** Treatment consists of supplemental oxygen, measures to maintain the airway, provision of ventilatory support if needed, and additional therapy for acute respiratory failure. Antibiotics are indicated if there is any suggestion of infectious pneumonitis.

Preventive efforts are directed at decreasing the acid secretion by the stomach and protecting the airway. Toward this end, women are usually not fed during labor. They should have no food intake for at least 6 hours before elective cesarean delivery and no liquid intake for 2 hours before surgery. If the patient is to undergo any surgical procedure that requires general anesthesia, acid secretion can be decreased with **preoperative administration of an H_2 receptor antagonist and sodium citrate.** In this setting, a "full stomach" should be presumed, and preoxygenation followed by rapid sequence intubation performed.

CHRONIC INFLAMMATORY BOWEL DISEASE

The two entities described under chronic inflammatory bowel disease (IBD) are **Crohn disease (regional enteritis)** and **ulcerative colitis.** In general, pregnancy appears to be associated with greater disease activity in patients with ulcerative colitis than in those with Crohn disease.

Preconception care and counseling (see Chapter 7) that prepares a woman with IBD can improve pregnancy outcome. Patients with IBD should be counseled on inheritance risks, and nutritional status should be optimized. Use of supplemental folic acid is advised, and if deficiencies are present, supplemental iron and vitamin B_{12} should be prescribed. **The best pregnancy outcomes occur in those patients who are in remission at the time of conception and whose disease activity can be controlled with medication that has**

minimal fetal toxicity. Major teratogens such as methotrexate must be discontinued before conception. Overall, pregnancy in women with IBD is complicated by **higher rates of preterm birth and IUGR,** and the frequency of these complications increases if there are acute disease exacerbations during pregnancy.

Treatment

The principles of therapy for acute exacerbations of IBD are similar for pregnant and nonpregnant patients, but care must be taken to balance medication risks to the fetus against the risks of active disease. Ionizing radiation should be avoided, and magnetic resonance enterography or flexible sigmoidoscopy should be performed, when there is a clear need for diagnostic studies. The least fetotoxic antiinflammatory and immunosuppressant medications that can control disease activity should be used. **Sulfasalazine does not appear to be associated with fetal toxicity. Prednisone is metabolized by placental enzymes and relatively little crosses the placenta.** However, first trimester use has been associated with cleft lip and palate, and high doses can inhibit fetal growth and cause adrenal suppression. Use of azathioprine in pregnancy has been reported in some studies to be associated with an increased risk of fetal anomalies and preterm birth. **If diarrhea is the main complaint, dietary restriction of lactose, fruits, and vegetables is necessary.** If a lactose-free diet is used, calcium supplementation is needed. Daily **constipating agents, such as psyllium hydrophilic mucilloid (Metamucil), are quite effective.** The use of diphenoxylate-atropine (Lomotil) or loperamide (Imodium) should be restricted to patients who are past the first trimester and in whom conservative management fails. **Surgery is indicated only for very severe complications, such as bowel perforation or abscess formation.** In the absence of compelling obstetric indications, **cesarean delivery is not recommended, unless there are perineal or rectal manifestations of Crohn disease.**

Hepatic Disorders during Pregnancy

INTRAHEPATIC CHOLESTASIS OF PREGNANCY

Although the pathogenesis of intrahepatic cholestasis of pregnancy (ICP) is not known, some distinctive features are (1) **cholestasis and pruritus in the second half of pregnancy** without other major liver dysfunction, (2) **a tendency for recurrence** with each pregnancy, (3) **an association with oral contraceptives and multiple gestations,** (4) **a benign course** in that there are usually no maternal hepatic sequelae, and (5) **an increased rate of meconium-stained amniotic fluid and fetal demise.** The reported prevalence of ICP in the United States ranges from less than 1% of pregnant women in Connecticut to nearly 6% in a Latina population in Los Angeles. Rates are higher in Latin America, with the highest reported rates being in Chile in the winter months. **The etiology of ICP is most likely multifactorial. A mutation in the *MDR3* gene may be associated with up to 15% of cases.** In addition, a strong association between ICP and natural progesterone therapy for prevention of preterm birth has recently been reported.

The main symptom of ICP is itching (most intense on the palms and soles), without abdominal pain or a rash, which may occur as early as 20 weeks' gestation. Jaundice is rarely observed. **Laboratory tests show elevated levels of serum bile acids.** Serum levels of bilirubin and liver enzymes (e.g., aspartate and alanine transaminase) are usually normal, but they may be mildly elevated. If liver enzymes and bilirubin levels are significantly elevated, abdominal ultrasonography should be performed to exclude gallbladder obstruction. **A hepatitis screen to exclude viral hepatitis and an autoantibody screen for primary biliary cirrhosis should be performed.**

Treatment and Follow-up

Symptomatic treatment with cold baths, emollients, and antihistamines such as hydroxyzine may be of some help. **The best results have been obtained with ursodeoxycholic acid.** It significantly ameliorates the pruritus and reduces serum levels of bile acids, aminotransferases, and bilirubin. **The reason for the increased rate of fetal demise is unclear.** Most happen after 37 weeks' gestation and may be secondary to pathology induced by the elevated bile acids that can cross the placenta. There is no consensus regarding timing of delivery. **Serial fetal surveillance should be performed in the third trimester, with delivery at term if testing remains reassuring. Postpartum, maternal symptoms and bile acids usually normalize quickly.** Patients should be screened for hepatitis C, and liver function tests should be followed until they return to normal because a few patients may go on to develop cholecystitis, fibrosis, or other types of liver disease.

ACUTE FATTY LIVER OF PREGNANCY

Acute fatty liver of pregnancy is a rare but extremely serious complication that can occur in the third trimester of pregnancy. It is associated with diffuse microvesicular fatty infiltration of the liver, resulting in hepatic failure. The incidence is about 1 per 14,000 pregnancies. Although the cause is unknown, it may in some instances result from an inborn error of metabolism, possibly a deficiency of long-chain 3-hydroxyacyl-coenzyme A dehydrogenase (LCHAD). **Its presentation is variable, with abdominal pain, nausea and vomiting, jaundice, and increased irritability.** Extreme polydipsia or pseudodiabetes insipidus may be present.

Hypoglycemia is frequently present and can be severe. **Hypertension and proteinuria are present in approximately 50% of patients, raising the issue of coexisting preeclampsia. Patients can develop coagulopathy with intraabdominal hemorrhage, hepatic coma, and renal failure.**

Diagnosis and Investigations

Liver biopsy is diagnostic, but this is usually not done, because of the morbidity associated with the procedure. The diagnosis is usually based on the characteristic clinical findings and laboratory tests. **Other causes of liver failure should be ruled out, especially preeclampsia with HELLP syndrome.** Laboratory findings include an increase in prothrombin time and partial thromboplastin time, hyperbilirubinemia, hyperammonemia, hyperuricemia, and a moderate elevation of the transaminase levels. BUN and creatinine levels are elevated, reflecting the degree of renal failure, and hypoglycemia is present. **Hematemesis and spontaneous bleeding become manifest as DIC develops.** Liver failure is indicated by elevated blood ammonia levels.

Treatment

Prompt delivery and intensive supportive care are indicated after diagnosis. Treatment is directed mainly at providing supportive measures, such as administration of intravenous fluids with 10% glucose to prevent dehydration and severe hypoglycemia. For the coagulopathy of hepatic failure, vitamin K supplementation is not effective, and **fresh-frozen plasma or cryoprecipitate should be given** along with platelets and packed red blood cells if there is DIC.

The disease can recur in subsequent pregnancies. It is recommended that the woman and her neonate be tested for an LCHAD defect. Early detection of such a defect in the neonate could prevent life-threatening complications. With early recognition, immediate delivery, and advances in critical care management, mortality is about 7-18%, and fetal mortality about 9-23%. **In those who survive, recovery is complete, with no signs of chronic liver disease.**

Venous Thromboembolic Disorders

Pregnancy is a hypercoagulable state with up to a fivefold increased risk of deep vein thrombosis (DVT) and pulmonary embolism (PE). **The greatest risk of a venous thromboembolism (VTE) is during the first few weeks postpartum,** especially following a cesarean delivery. Pregnancy-induced changes in coagulation factors that favor clotting include a decrease in protein S and increases in fibrinogen; factors VI, VII, and X; and von Willebrand factor. Venous stasis results from compression of the pelvic veins by the gravid uterus, as well as endocrine-mediated venodilation, often aggravated by decreased mobility. Delivery, especially an operative delivery, can cause endothelial injury to uteroplacental and pelvic vessels. Thus, all three elements of the Virchow triad (stasis, endothelial injury, and hypercoagulability) are present and predispose the pregnant woman to VTE. **Additional important risk factors are previous history of a DVT or PE, acquired or inherited thrombophilias, smoking, and prolonged immobility** as a result of prescribed bed rest for certain obstetric complications.

DEEP VEIN THROMBOSIS

Clinical Features

The clinical diagnosis of DVT is difficult. **Fifty percent of cases are asymptomatic.** Pain in the calf in association with dorsiflexion of the foot **(positive Homans sign)** is a clinical sign of thrombosis in the calf veins. Dull ache, tingling, tightness, or pain in the calf or leg, especially when walking, may be present. Acute swelling and pain in the thigh area, as well as tenderness in the femoral triangle, are suggestive of iliofemoral thrombosis. **DVT in pregnancy is usually in the left leg.** In a patient complaining of left lower-extremity pain and swelling, the finding of a 2-cm difference in calf circumference is one of the more reliable clinical signs of a DVT in pregnancy.

Investigations

Compression ultrasonography is a noninvasive technique that has high sensitivity and specificity and **is currently the primary mode of diagnosis** used for **DVT. Magnetic resonance imaging** (MRI) has been used to evaluate patients suspected of having pelvic thrombosis who have a negative Doppler ultrasonic examination. **D-Dimers** are not a reliable screening tool for VTE in pregnancy.

Therapy

Treatment of proven DVT during pregnancy should be initiated with either intravenous unfractionated heparin or subcutaneous low-molecular-weight heparin (enoxaparin sodium) to achieve full anticoagulation. The unfractionated heparin dose is adjusted to 1.5 to 2.5 times the control aPTT. Intravenous anticoagulation should be maintained for at least 5 to 7 days, after which treatment is converted to subcutaneous heparin that must be continued for the duration of the pregnancy and for up to 6 weeks postpartum, with weekly monitoring of the aPTT. **Alternatively, enoxaparin can be administered at a dose of 1 mg/kg subcutaneously every 12 hours.** The dose can be adjusted to achieve anti–factor X levels of 0.6 to 1 U/mL. **Both forms of heparin are safe for the fetus and do not cross the placenta. Unfractionated heparin is associated with a higher risk of maternal thrombocytopenia and osteoporosis than is low-molecular-weight heparin.** Supplemental calcium and vitamin D_3 (2000 IU/day) should be advised, along with periodic platelet counts. Because of its longer half-life and the increased risk of spinal hematomas with neuraxial anesthesia, **low-molecular-weight heparin should be stopped about 24 hours before delivery in the case of a planned induction or cesarean delivery. Alternatively, the patient can be switched to unfractionated heparin that can be stopped 6 hours before delivery.** If the aPTT is normal, neuraxial anesthesia can safely be administered. If there are no signs of hemorrhage postpartum, low-molecular-weight or unfractionated heparin can be restarted 12 to 24 hours postdelivery and the patient can then be transitioned to warfarin, which should be continued for at least 6 weeks postpartum. **Warfarin is a vitamin K antagonist that crosses the placenta, carries risks of fetal hemorrhage and teratogenesis, and, with few exceptions, should be used only in the postpartum period.** The international normalized ratio (INR) is commonly used to measure the effects of warfarin, and the target INR is 2.5 (range: 2.0 to 3.0). **Breastfeeding is not a contraindication to the use of warfarin, low-molecular-weight heparin, or unfractionated heparin.**

PULMONARY EMBOLISM

PE is one of the most common causes of pregnancy-related death in the United States. The maternal mortality is less than 1% if treated early and greater than 80% if left untreated. In about 70% of cases, DVT is the instigating factor. Early detection and treatment of DVT and widespread recognition of conditions or circumstances requiring DVT prophylaxis are expected to decrease the incidence of PE in pregnancy.

Clinical Features

Suggestive symptoms of PE include pleuritic chest pain, shortness of breath, air hunger, palpitations, hemoptysis, and syncopal episodes. Suggestive signs of PE include tachypnea, tachycardia, low-grade fever, a pleural friction rub, chest splinting, pulmonary rales, an accentuated pulmonic valve second heart sound, and even right ventricular failure. **In most obstetric patients, the signs and symptoms of a PE are subtle.**

Investigations

An ECG can show sinus tachycardia with or without premature heartbeats or right ventricular axis deviation. On a chest film, atelectasis, pleural effusion, obliteration of arterial shadows, and elevation of the diaphragm may be present. Arterial blood gases obtained on room air may show an oxygen tension below 80 mm Hg. **PE is ultimately a radiologic diagnosis. Three algorithms may be used. (1) Bilateral compression ultrasonography of the lower extremities: If positive for DVT, a PE may be assumed in a symptomatic patient. (2) A ventilation-perfusion scan:** This method poses minimal risk to the fetus, but it cannot be used in patients with an abnormal chest X-ray or in patients with asthma or chronic obstructive pulmonary disease. **(3) Computed tomographic pulmonary angiography:** This technique has the advantage of noninvasive visualization of a thrombus. The radiation dose to the fetus is considered acceptably low, but there is concern about the radiation exposure to maternal breast tissue.

The acute treatment of PE and follow-up during pregnancy, labor, delivery, and the postpartum period are the same as for DVT.

Thrombophilia Evaluation

A thrombophilia workup should be considered for patients with a PE or DVT, especially those with recurrent thromboses, a positive family history, or an obstetric history suggestive of antiphospholipid syndrome. Tests to order include those for acquired thrombophilias (e.g., lupus anticoagulant, anticardiolipin antibody) and inherited thrombophilias (factor V Leiden and the prothrombin G20210A mutations, as well as proteins C and S and antithrombin III titers).

Prophylactic Anticoagulant Therapy

In pregnant patients with a past history of a PE or DVT, prophylactic doses of heparin or low-molecular-weight heparin should be given during pregnancy and continued for 6 weeks postpartum. **Subcutaneous injections of a prophylactic dose of heparin (5000 to 10,000 U every 12 hours) or enoxaparin sodium (40 mg once daily)** provide sufficient prophylaxis for most patients, although some pregnant women may require full anticoagulation. All pregnant women having cesarean delivery should have pneumatic compression stockings placed for thromboprophylaxis.

SUPERFICIAL THROMBOPHLEBITIS

Superficial thrombophlebitis is more common in patients with varicose veins, obesity, limited physical activity, or a previous history of superficial thrombosis. **In most patients, superficial thrombophlebitis is limited to the calf area, and symptoms include swelling and tenderness of the involved extremity.** Physical examination reveals erythema, tenderness, warmth, and a palpable cord over the course of the involved superficial veins. **Superficial thrombophlebitis usually does not progress to DVT or lead to PE,** but lower-limb ultrasound is indicated if there is concern that the thrombosis may extend into the deep veins.

Treatment

Treatment of superficial thrombophlebitis involves elevation of the leg, pain medications, and local application of heat. **There is usually no need for anticoagulants, but antiinflammatory agents may be considered.** Ambulation is encouraged, and patients should be **instructed to wear support stockings** to help avoid a repeat episode.

Pulmonary Diseases

ASTHMA

Asthma is a chronic inflammatory disorder characterized by bronchial hyperreactivity, and it is the most common pulmonary disease in pregnancy, affecting between 3% and 9% of pregnant women. Asthma in pregnancy is currently classified according to severity as (1) mild intermittent, (2) mild persistent, (3) moderate persistent, and (4) severe persistent. During pregnancy, condition improves in about one-third of patients and deteriorates in about one-third, and about one-third have no significant change. **Most exacerbations occur before the third trimester.** Status asthmaticus, the most severe form of asthma, complicates about 0.2% of pregnancies. **Severe asthma is associated with an increased rate of miscarriage, preeclampsia, intrauterine fetal death, fetal growth restriction, and preterm birth.** These complications may occur **as a result of intrauterine hypoxia.**

Obstetric Management

Pregnancy does not induce any significant changes in peak flow (PF), forced vital capacity (FVC), forced expiratory volume in 1 second (FEV_1), or the FVC/FEV_1 ratio. Most patients with asthma have been diagnosed before pregnancy, and pregnancy does not change the criteria for diagnosis (characteristic clinical symptoms combined with abnormal spirometry [decreased FVC/FEV_1 and decreased PF with improvement after acute bronchodilator therapy]).

Pregnant women with asthma should be followed closely and educated in the use of a PF meter. The avoidance of dehydration, early and aggressive treatment of respiratory infections, and the avoidance of hyperventilation, excessive physical activity, and allergens are important. Daily measurement of PF rates can provide useful information on respiratory status. The Working Group on Asthma in Pregnancy recommends the following **treatment guidelines: For those with mild intermittent asthma, a short-acting inhaled β_2-agonist (albuterol) can be used as needed. Patients with mild persistent asthma should be treated with a daily low-dose inhaled glucocorticoid (budesonide). The preferred treatment for moderate persistent asthma is either a daily medium-dose inhaled glucocorticoid or a combination of a daily low-dose inhaled glucocorticoid and a long-acting β_2-agonist (salmeterol). Those with severe persistent asthma should be treated with a daily high-dose inhaled glucocorticoid combined with a long-acting β_2-agonist. They may require the addition of a systemic glucocorticoid.** With the exception of systemic glucocorticoids, the above-described therapies have not been associated with any significant fetal complications. Systemic combination glucocorticoids have been associated with fetal and/or neonatal complications, including cleft lip and palate, IUGR, and adrenal suppression. **Alternative therapies include inhaled cromolyn sodium, leukotriene receptor antagonists, or sustained-release theophylline. Acute severe exacerbations must be treated aggressively** with oxygen therapy, intravenous fluids, systemic glucocorticoids, administration of short-acting β_2-agonists and ipratropium by nebulized aerosol, and antibiotics if there is evidence of bacterial infection. Intravenous magnesium sulfate or subcutaneous terbutaline can be added if needed. To prevent fetal hypoxia, pulse oximetry should be used and oxygen saturation should be maintained at 95% or greater. Because of the hyperventilation and compensated respiratory alkalosis present in normal pregnancy, **an arterial blood gas with a PaO_2 less than 70 mm Hg and/or a $PaCO_2$ greater than 35 mm Hg are indicative of severe respiratory compromise.** Some patients may require endotracheal intubation and mechanical ventilation to maintain an adequate oxygen supply.

Serial fetal monitoring and ultrasonic assessment of fetal growth should be implemented. The timing of delivery is dependent on the status of both the mother and the fetus. When pregnancy is progressing well, there is no need for early delivery, and it is advisable to await the spontaneous onset of labor. **Early delivery can be considered for fetal growth restriction or maternal deterioration.**

Management of Labor and Delivery

Labor and delivery are usually not triggers of acute asthma attacks. Glucocorticoid therapy, including inhaled or high-potency topical use for more than 3 weeks, may suppress the hypothalamic-pituitary-adrenal axis, and administration of stress doses of medication during labor or delivery should be considered. An epidural block during labor reduces pain, anxiety, hyperventilation, and respiratory effort, all of which are known to aggravate the disease. **Vaginal delivery should be anticipated. Cesarean delivery is performed only for obstetric reasons.** Oxytocin is the preferred drug for the initial management of postpartum hemorrhage. **Prostaglandins should not be used, because they are likely to trigger acute bronchoconstriction.**

CYSTIC FIBROSIS

Cystic fibrosis is due to mutations in the cystic fibrosis transmembrane conductance regulator gene, *CFTR*, which is the gene that regulates epithelial cell chloride channel function. Because of improvements in diagnosis and treatment, **the majority of females with cystic fibrosis now survive to adulthood. It is the most severe form of obstructive lung disease observed during pregnancy, but there is no evidence that pregnancy increases the maternal risk, unless there is severe disease with pulmonary hypertension.** Preconception care and counseling should involve optimizing nutrition and pulmonary function, as well as testing the father's carrier status and counseling about inheritance risks to the fetus. **Women with pulmonary hypertension should be counseled about the greater risk that pregnancy poses for an adverse maternal, fetal, or neonatal outcome.** Exocrine pancreatic insufficiency is present in about 90% of patients, and screening for diabetes (if not already diagnosed) should be undertaken early in pregnancy. Women with malabsorption symptoms might become more emaciated during pregnancy, and there are risks of superimposed infections. **In addition to either having cystic fibrosis or being a carrier of it, the fetus is at increased risk of IUGR and premature delivery.** Options for prenatal diagnosis should be reviewed, and antepartum testing should be instituted in the third trimester.

For labor and delivery, epidural analgesia is recommended. Outlet forceps or vacuum-assisted delivery should also be considered. The Valsalva maneuver should be avoided because of the associated increase in maternal oxygen requirements. Breastfeeding is recommended unless the mother's condition does not allow it.

Central Nervous System Disease

In the majority of cases, seizure frequency does not change in pregnancy. Some factors during pregnancy that may contribute to increased seizure frequency include nausea and vomiting leading to missed doses, decreased GI motility, expanded intravascular volume lowering serum drug levels, induction of enzymes increasing drug metabolism, and increased glomerular filtration hastening drug clearance.

Treatment

Preconception counseling and care are important. Antiepileptic drugs (AEDs) that induce cytochrome P450 and related enzymes can decrease the efficacy of hormonal contraception. **In patients who have had no seizure activity for at least 2 years, AED therapy can be discontinued before conception.** First-generation AEDs include phenytoin, phenobarbital, trimethadione, clonazepam, valproic acid, and carbamazepine. Second-generation AEDs include lamotrigine, topiramate, and levetiracetam.

There is no ideal anticonvulsant for use in women intending to become pregnant or during pregnancy, and **all AEDs should be considered potential teratogens.** In general, **monotherapy should be attempted, using the lowest dose of the AED that most effectively controls the woman's seizures.** Valproic acid is an exception. **Valproic acid should probably not be used in a woman planning a pregnancy,** unless other drugs have proven ineffective. Its teratogenicity, especially the high risk of neural tube defects and neurodevelopmental disorders, is unacceptably high compared with

other AEDs. The neural tube closes approximately 4 weeks postconception, before many women realize they are pregnant. For this reason, **women of reproductive age who are taking AEDs are advised to take at least 0.4 to 0.8 mg of folic acid daily to protect against neural tube defects should they become pregnant.** This should be continued throughout pregnancy. Those taking valproic acid or carbamazepine should be prescribed 4 mg/day of folic acid for 1 to 3 months preconception and through the first trimester.

If seizures are well controlled during pregnancy, no change in therapy should be attempted. The AED that is effective should be used, and serum levels of the unbound drug should be followed. The maternal serum AFP should be measured at 15 to 19 weeks' gestation to screen for open neural tube defects, and an obstetric ultrasound should be done at 18 to 22 weeks to look for fetal anatomic anomalies, especially neural tube defects, cardiac anomalies, cleft lip, and cleft palate. Because some AEDs increase the rate of vitamin K degradation, supplemental vitamin K (10 to 20 mg/day) is usually advised after 35 weeks' gestation to prevent neonatal hemorrhage. Antacids and antihistamines should be avoided in patients receiving phenytoin, because they lower plasma levels of phenytoin and may precipitate a seizure attack.

For the treatment of status epilepticus, immediate hospitalization is required. Management is similar to that in the nonpregnant adult. Patency of the airway and adequate oxygenation should be ensured. After blood is drawn for plasma levels of anticonvulsants, **intravenous lorazepam should be given slowly, followed by a loading dose of phenytoin with continuous cardiac monitoring.**

The management of labor and delivery follows obstetric indications. During labor and in the immediate postpartum period, anticonvulsant drugs must be continued. The dose of the anticonvulsant drug may be lowered postpartum, provided that a therapeutic level is maintained. **Although anticonvulsants are excreted in breast milk in small amounts, breastfeeding is not contraindicated.**

Complications

Pregnant patients with epilepsy have a twofold increase in maternal complications such as preeclampsia, abruption, hyperemesis, and premature labor. Fetal hypoxia is a potential consequence of maternal seizures, and there is a high incidence of intrauterine fetal demise. In the neonate, higher rates of coagulopathy, drug withdrawal symptoms, and morbidity and mortality are reported. **Congenital anomalies are more common in neonates exposed to AEDs in utero** than among offspring of untreated women with epilepsy and women without epilepsy. **The overall risk of major malformations is 4-6%.** Small retrospective studies have raised the possibility of impaired cognitive and neurologic function in the offspring that may manifest later in life. The risk of a seizure disorder is greater among the children of mothers with epilepsy.

Reducing the Morbidity of Medical Conditions during Pregnancy

Metabolic dysregulation (metabolic syndrome) begins in women who are obese and/or gain excessive weight during pregnancy. Obesity is associated with a marked increase in inflammation in fat cells, leading to insulin resistance. Because of the current, dramatic increase in the incidence of obesity in the United States and elsewhere, weight loss beginning before pregnancy and prevention of excessive weight gain during pregnancy should be strongly recommended. Increased physical activity, known to reduce the risk of obesity, should be encouraged. Coupled with physical activity, counseling for behavioral changes to reduce psychosocial stress, known to be a factor in the development of cardiovascular disease, should also be recommended for women at risk. Finally, there should be a focus on the gut-brain connection, a new theory that links gut dysregulation (by abnormal bacteria) with brain dysregulation leading to insulin resistance and inflammation. Poor diet alters the gut microbiome, leading to gut inflammation and alterations in appetite. Dietary changes such as the "Mediterranean diet" plus probiotics can alter the gut biome, resulting in improvement in metabolism and weight loss. Consuming smaller portions while avoiding calorie-dense foods, particularly sugars and other carbohydrates, is very important.

Recently, it has been shown that changes in the gut biome and supplementation with vitamin D reduces weight gain, improves insulin sensitivity, and reduces hypertension. In order to improve the health of women and their children, reducing the impact of medical disorders in pregnancy should have a high priority. Obstetricians and other health care providers must focus on the prevention and mitigation of the effects of medical conditions that may complicate pregnancy.

Surgical Conditions during Pregnancy

Pregnancy substantially enhances the problems associated with surgery. Physiologic changes and the altered immunologic responses of pregnancy change the diagnostic parameters of surgical diseases. Surgery (especially abdominal surgery) can increase the rate of fetal loss. **Reluctance to operate on a pregnant woman with an acute surgical condition or a suspicious pelvic mass may add to critical delays and increase the mor-** **bidity, and even mortality, for both the fetus and the mother.**

GENERAL PRINCIPLES

Elective surgery should be avoided in pregnancy. When surgery must be done, but not emergently (e.g., an ovarian neoplasm), **the second trimester is the safest time.** During this period, the risks of teratogenesis and miscarriage are much lower than in the first trimester, and the risk of preterm labor is lower than in the third trimester. Regional analgesia is preferred because it is associated with lower mortality and morbidity than general anesthesia. There is little evidence of teratogenicity of commonly used anesthetics. **Pulmonary aspiration is more common.** All pregnant women should be treated as if they have a full stomach and premedicated with citrate and histamine H_2 receptor blockers. **Precautions must be taken to avoid maternal hypotension and hypoxia that have adverse effects on uteroplacental blood flow.** When possible, the patient should be in the left lateral decubitus position. Pre- and postoperative fetal and uterine monitoring are indicated in the third trimester. If significant blood loss is anticipated and the patient is anemic, it is advisable to transfuse the patient preoperatively.

ACUTE CONDITIONS

The general approach to acute surgical emergencies during pregnancy is to manage the problem, regardless of the pregnancy. Acute nonobstetric surgical emergencies occur in all three trimesters of pregnancy. The overall incidence is approximately 1 in 500 pregnancies. The more common acute conditions are discussed below.

Appendicitis

Appendectomy for presumed acute appendicitis is the most common surgical emergency during pregnancy. The incidence of acute appendicitis in pregnancy is approximately 0.05-0.1%, and it is constant throughout the three trimesters. The usual symptoms of acute appendicitis, such as epigastric pain, nausea, vomiting, and lower abdominal pain, may be less apparent during pregnancy, although **right lower-quadrant pain is still the most common presentation. The differential diagnosis may be especially confusing** (Box 16-2). The enlarging uterus displaces the appendix superiorly and laterally as pregnancy progresses (as shown in Figure 16-3). **Tenderness and guarding are elicited more laterally than expected.** The increased white blood cell count seen in normal pregnancy further confuses the issue. Surgery may be delayed, resulting in an increased rate of rupture, premature labor, infant morbidity, and, rarely, maternal death.

Imaging studies can increase the accuracy of the diagnosis of appendicitis but should never replace

BOX 16-2

DIFFERENTIAL DIAGNOSIS OF ACUTE APPENDICITIS IN PREGNANCY

Ruptured corpus luteum
Torsion of an adnexal mass
Pyelonephritis
Nephrolithiasis
Ectopic pregnancy
Hyperemesis gravidarum
Acute mesenteric lymphadenitis
Inflammatory bowel disease
Tuboovarian abscess
Acute mesenteric thrombosis
Cholecystitis/cholelithiasis
Concealed abruption

TABLE 16-8

ESTIMATED FETAL EXPOSURE FROM SOME COMMON RADIOLOGIC PROCEDURES

Procedure	Fetal Exposure (Gy)
Chest radiograph (two views)	0.000002-0.00007
Abdominal film (single view)	0.001
Intravenous pyelography	>0.01*
Hip film (single view)	0.002
Mammography	0.0007-0.002
Barium enema or small bowel series	0.02-0.04
CT scan of head or chest	<0.01
CT scan of abdomen and lumbar spine	0.035
CT pelvimetry	0.0025

Data from American College of Obstetricians and Gynecologists: Guidelines for diagnostic imaging during pregnancy. American College of Obstetricians and Gynecologists Committee opinion No. 299. *Obset Gynecol* 104:649, 2004.
CT, Computed tomography.
*Exposure depends on the number of films.

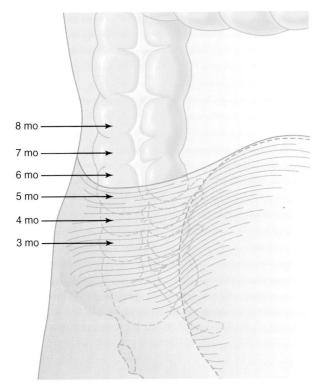

8 mo

7 mo

6 mo

5 mo

4 mo

3 mo

FIGURE 16-3 The changing position of the right colon and appendix as pregnancy progresses and the uterus enlarges upward and laterally.

initial physical evaluation. The American College of Radiology recommends nonionizing radiation techniques such as **ultrasonography** and **MRI** in pregnant women. On ultrasound, the abnormal appendix can be visualized as a noncompressible tubular structure measuring 6 mm or greater in the region of the patient's pain. Helical computed tomographic scanning has the disadvantage of radiation exposure, but appendicitis should be suspected when right lower-quadrant inflammation, an enlarged nonfilling tubular structure, and/or a fecalith are noted. The estimated fetal radiation exposure is about 0.025 Gy. Exposure to less than 0.05 Gy has not been associated with an increase in fetal anomalies or pregnancy loss. Table 16-8 shows the dose of ionizing radiation to the fetus during common diagnostic radiologic procedures. **MRI is now widely used for diagnostic assistance when appendicitis is suspected.**

When acute appendicitis is diagnosed, laparotomy with appendectomy may be carried out. A McBurney, transverse, or Rockey-Davis incision can be performed. **Laparoscopic appendectomy may also be considered.** A potential concern with laparoscopy is that **carbon dioxide used for insufflation can be absorbed across the peritoneum into the maternal blood stream and cross the placenta, leading to fetal respiratory acidosis and hypercapnia.** As gestation progresses, the likelihood increases that the pneumoperitoneum will decrease venous return, cardiac output, and uteroplacental blood flow. Guidelines to mitigate these harmful fetal effects and increase the overall safety of laparoscopy during pregnancy have been published by the Society of American Gastrointestinal and Endoscopic Surgeons. **Laparoscopic appendectomy, as well as other laparoscopic procedures, may be considered during pregnancy in accordance with the guidelines listed in Box 16-3.**

Acute Cholecystitis and Cholelithiasis

An increase in serum cholesterol and lipid levels in pregnancy, along with biliary stasis, leads to a higher

BOX 16-3

SOCIETY OF AMERICAN GASTROINTESTINAL AND ENDOSCOPIC SURGEONS GUIDELINES FOR DIAGNOSIS, TREATMENT, AND USE OF LAPAROSCOPY FOR SURGICAL PROBLEMS DURING PREGNANCY (EVIDENCE RATING)

Diagnostic laparoscopy is safe and effective when used selectively in the workup and treatment of acute abdominal processes in pregnancy (Moderate; Strong).

Laparoscopic treatment of acute abdominal diseases has the same indications in pregnant and nonpregnant patients (Moderate; Strong).

Laparoscopy can be performed safely during any trimester of pregnancy (Moderate; Strong).

Gravid patients should be placed in the left lateral decubitus position to minimize compression of the vena cava (Moderate; Strong).

Initial abdominal access can be accomplished safely with an open (Hasson) technique, Veress needle, or optical trocar if the location is adjusted according to fundal height and previous incisions (Moderate; Strong).

CO_2 insufflation of 10-15 mm Hg can be safely used for laparoscopy in the pregnant patient (Moderate; Strong).

Intraoperative CO_2 monitoring by capnography should be used during laparoscopy in the pregnant patient (Moderate; Strong).

Intraoperative and postoperative pneumatic compression devices and early postoperative ambulation are recommended as prophylaxis for deep vein thrombosis in the gravid patient (Moderate; Strong).

Laparoscopic cholecystectomy is the treatment of choice in the pregnant patient with gallbladder disease, regardless of trimester (Moderate; Strong).

Choledocholithiasis during pregnancy may be managed with preoperative endoscopic retrograde cholangiopancreatography (ERCP) with sphincterotomy, followed by laparoscopic cholecystectomy, laparoscopic common bile duct exploration, or postoperative ERCP (Moderate; Strong).

Laparoscopic appendectomy may be performed safely in pregnant patients with appendicitis (Moderate; Strong)

Laparoscopic adrenalectomy, nephrectomy, and splenectomy are safe procedures in pregnant patients (Low; Weak).

Laparoscopy is a safe and effective treatment in gravid patients with symptomatic cystic masses. Observation is acceptable for all other cystic lesions, provided ultrasound findings are not concerning for malignancy and tumor markers are normal. Initial observation is warranted for most cystic lesions.

Laparoscopy is recommended for both diagnosis and treatment of adnexal torsion, unless clinical severity warrants laparotomy (Low; Strong).

Fetal heart monitoring should occur preoperatively and postoperatively in the setting of urgent abdominal surgery during pregnancy* (Moderate; Strong).

Obstetric consultation can be obtained pre- and/or postoperatively based on the severity of the patient's disease, gestational age, and availability of the consultant (Moderate; Strong).

Tocolytics should not be used prophylactically in pregnant women undergoing surgery, but they should be considered perioperatively when signs of preterm labor are present (High; Strong).

Data from www.sages.org/publications/guidelines/guidelines-for-diagnosis-treatment-and-use-of-laparoscopy-for-surgical-problems-during-pregnancy/. Accessed May 19, 2015. An explanation of the method for the assessment of evidence along with references is provided on this website.

*The American College of Obstetricians and Gynecologists recommends continuous fetal monitoring based upon the preoperative monitoring assessment and gestational age.

incidence of cholelithiasis, biliary obstruction, and cholecystitis. High levels of estrogens in pregnancy increase the saturation of cholesterol in the bile. Virtually all of the gallstones associated with pregnancy are composed of crystallized cholesterol. Ultrasonography has revealed a fairly high incidence of cholelithiasis in pregnancy (4%). The incidence of hospitalization for cholecystitis in pregnancy is 1-2%, but only 1 in 2000 pregnant women require cholecystectomy.

Nausea and vomiting, along with right upper-quadrant tenderness and guarding, generally suggest biliary tract disease. An increasing white blood cell count with elevated alkaline phosphatase and bilirubin levels, jaundice in the presence of stones, or increased thickness of the gallbladder wall on ultrasonography serves to authenticate the diagnosis. **Viral hepatitis must be considered in the differential diagnosis.** Markedly elevated aspartate transaminase and alanine transaminase levels (>200 U/L), especially without leukocytosis, should suggest viral hepatitis.

Generally, cholecystitis can be managed medically in pregnancy. Parenteral fluids, gastric decompression, and dietary measures should comprise the primary approach. Endoscopic retrograde cholangiopancreatography (ERCP) can be performed safely in pregnancy with little ionizing radiation exposure to the fetus if the patient has cholangitis or pancreatitis caused by a common bile duct stone. If symptoms and signs persist with progressive peritonitis despite medical management or ERCP, cholecystectomy is indicated. Laparoscopic cholecystectomy has been performed in pregnancy and is considered to be both indicated and safe (see Box 16-3).

Acute Pancreatitis

Generally, pancreatitis is associated with cholecystitis, cholelithiasis, or alcoholism. It has also been associated with viral infections and drugs such as thiazide diuretics, furosemide, acetaminophen, clonidine, isoniazid, rifampin, tetracycline, propoxyphene, and steroids. It is less common in pregnancy, and the incidence in pregnancy varies from 1:1000 to 1:4000, increasing somewhat in the third trimester. However, **the mortality rate associated with pancreatitis is significantly higher in pregnancy.**

The prime symptom of pancreatitis is severe, non-colicky epigastric pain radiating to the high back, which is relieved somewhat by leaning forward. Nausea and vomiting generally are present. Upper abdominal guarding may be difficult to assess in late pregnancy. **An elevated serum amylase** (>200 U/dL) **and lipase generally confirm the diagnosis,** although cholecystitis, peptic ulcer, diabetic ketoacidosis, and hyperemesis gravidarum may also be associated with elevations of serum amylase.

Generally, the disease is self-limiting and responds within 1 to 10 days to bed rest, parenteral fluids, pain relief, and nasogastric suction. Occasionally, the disease becomes severe and protracted, with extensive pancreatic edema and autodigestion, massive ascites, hemoperitoneum, fever, and paralytic ileus. In such cases, maternal and fetal mortality are high, and peritoneal lavage, operative drainage, partial pancreatic resection, or some combination of these procedures may be required.

Bowel Obstruction

Bowel obstruction in pregnancy is usually associated with postoperative adhesions, although volvulus and intussusception are rare causes. It generally occurs in late pregnancy and is associated with traction on adhesions as the uterus enlarges. **An erect abdominal x-ray showing characteristic dilated loops of bowel and air-fluid levels serves to confirm the obstruction.**

Management does not differ from that in the nonpregnant patient. Nasogastric suction should be instituted and fluid and electrolyte balance carefully monitored. **When the obstruction does not resolve after 48 to 96 hours, an exploratory laparotomy should be carried out through an appropriate vertical incision.** If uterine contractions occur postoperatively, tocolytics may be employed.

Adnexal Torsion

Torsion of the uterine adnexa occurs somewhat more commonly in pregnancy, possibly because the supporting ligaments elongate as the gestation progresses. Ovarian tumors (e.g., cystic teratomas, corpus luteal cysts) may become ischemic if their vascular pedicles undergo torsion. Such ischemic events are usually heralded by the sudden onset of severe, intermittent abdominal pain, which may radiate to the flank and down the anterior thigh.

During the first and early second trimesters, a mass is usually felt on pelvic examination or is visualized by ultrasonography. Later in the pregnancy, it may be impossible to palpate a mass clinically. Low-grade fever and leukocytosis may be present, and serum creatine phosphokinase levels may be elevated, depending on the extent of the infarction. In the first trimester, the differential diagnosis includes ectopic pregnancy and hemorrhagic corpus luteum; later in pregnancy, a degenerating fibroid should be considered.

Although the pain may diminish somewhat after 24 hours, removal of the infarcted organ is indicated. If the excised ovary contains the corpus luteum, progesterone supplementation is generally necessary before 10 weeks' gestation.

Abdominal Trauma

By far the most common abdominal trauma in pregnancy occurs in automobile accidents. Placental abruption, uterine contusions, and fetal skull fractures may result. Placental abruptions are treated expectantly unless fetal monitoring indicates fetal distress, in which case immediate abdominal delivery is in order if the fetus is at a gestational age that is considered "viable" (23 to 24 weeks or later). Abdominal exploration may be necessary to stop bleeding and repair uterine lacerations. Lap-and-shoulder harness seat belts, rather than lap belts, are advisable for pregnant women after 12 weeks' gestation.

Gunshot wounds of the abdomen are treated the same as they are in nonpregnant patients, with measures taken to stop bleeding and repair visceral or uterine injuries. As long as the pregnancy is intact, the uterus should not be disturbed. Careful monitoring of fetal well-being should be maintained before and after the operation.

Any time that a pregnant woman is evaluated for trauma and the cause is not clearly apparent, **the possibility of domestic violence should be considered.** Chapter 29 covers the incidence of domestic violence and the approach to a patient who may be the victim of intimate partner abuse or other types of domestic violence.

Ovarian Tumors

Adnexal masses are not uncommon and are usually identified by pelvic examination or ultrasonography early in the pregnancy. Paraovarian cysts, corpus luteal cysts, and mature teratomas are the most common. Approximately 50-70% are functional cysts (e.g., corpus luteal cysts) and spontaneously resolve as the gonadotropin levels fall during the second trimester. The risk of finding a malignant ovarian tumor during pregnancy is approximately 3-7%, with germ cell and epithelial tumors both potentially occurring. Abdominal and transvaginal ultrasonography should be used for initial diagnosis, and any complex mass that persists or any simple cyst that continues to enlarge should be removed in the second trimester.

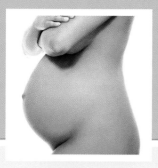

Obstetric Procedures

CALVIN J. HOBEL

CLINICAL KEYS FOR THIS CHAPTER

- Real-time (two-dimensional [2D]) ultrasonic imaging of the uterus, placenta, fetus, and cervix has become important for assessment of almost all pregnancies in the United States. Early in pregnancy, ultrasonic imaging is important for pregnancy dating and for ruling out multiple pregnancies. During mid-gestation, measurement of the biparietal diameter of the fetal head, the abdominal circumference, and the femoral length can determine normal or abnormal fetal growth, and later in pregnancy changes in these parameters can be used to assess the progress of fetal growth and well-being.

- Amniocentesis was the first invasive procedure developed to access amniotic fluid. Real-time 2D ultrasound has significantly reduced complications related to amniocentesis. Access to amniotic fluid has made biochemical testing possible for assessment of fetal genetic and metabolic parameters.

- Placental tissue and fetal cells can be obtained safely from the amnion for the assessment of fetal genetics. Amniotic fluid obtained by amniocentesis provides access to cells shed from the amnion that can be used for

genetic studies. Placental tissue obtained by either chorionic villus sampling (CVS) via the cervical route (transvaginal catheter) or by transabdominal needle aspiration may also be used for genetic analysis of the fetus.

- The cervix is an important barrier that protects the fetus from early delivery. The normal length of the cervix is 4 to 5 cm, but, in approximately 5% of pregnancies, it can silently undergo shortening. If identified after mid-pregnancy (20 to 22 weeks), a cerclage can be placed around the cervix to keep it from further shortening and dilating, which would increase the risk of early preterm delivery.

- Forceps application or the use of a vacuum extractor (VE) is sometimes warranted to safely deliver the fetus. When a woman experiences prolonged labor after complete cervical dilation and the fetus has descended to the point where the head is at a station of at least +2 (using a 0 to 5 cm scale), the second stage of labor can be reduced by the use of forceps or a VE. **When forceps or VE fails, a cesarean delivery should be performed.**

As the fetus has become more accessible for monitoring as a result of technological advances, the desire to intervene on behalf of the fetus has led to the development of a number of obstetric diagnostic and therapeutic procedures. Any procedure performed during pregnancy carries risks to both mother and fetus, so it is important to counsel the mother regarding the potential benefits and risks of all options before embarking on any obstetric intervention.

The diagnostic indications for ultrasonic imaging, amniocentesis, chorionic villus sampling (CVS), and cordocentesis are covered in this chapter, as well as the therapeutic indications for cervical cerclage, obstetric forceps, vacuum extraction, and cesarean delivery. The

techniques used in these obstetric procedures are also described.

Ultrasound

Two-dimensional (2D) ultrasound has been the standard in sonography for the past 30 years. Obstetric transvaginal and transabdominal sonography play a pivotal role in contemporary obstetric care, with ultrasonic imaging being done in approximately 90% of pregnancies in the United States today. Human data have shown no adverse fetal effects of ultrasound. Box 17-1 lists common abnormalities that may be identified prenatally with ultrasound.

BOX 17-1

EXAMPLES OF FETAL ABNORMALITIES DETECTED BY PRENATAL ULTRASOUND

Central Nervous System
- Hydrocephalus
- Anencephaly
- Arachnoid cyst
- Porencephaly
- Agenesis of corpus callosum
- Spina bifida

Face
- Cleft lip and/or palate
- Hypoplasia of the nose

Neck
- Cystic hygroma
- Goiter
- Nuchal skin thickening

Heart
- Atrial septal defect
- Ventricular septal defect
- Tetralogy of Fallot
- Transposition of the great vessels
- Arrhythmias

Lungs
- Congenital cystic adenomatoid malformation
- Lung sequestration
- Diaphragmatic hernia

Abdominal Wall
- Gastroschisis
- Omphalocele

Gastrointestinal Tract
- Bowel atresia or obstruction
- Echogenic bowel

Urinary System
- Renal agenesis
- Polycystic kidney disease
- Hydronephrosis
- Posterior urethral valves

Skeletal Dysplasia

TRANSVAGINAL ULTRASOUND

Transvaginal ultrasound is useful in the first trimester of pregnancy because the close proximity of the intravaginal ultrasonic transducer allows for high-frequency scanning and better resolution of the pelvic organs and developing pregnancy than are possible with transabdominal imaging. **Transvaginal ultrasound is commonly used in the first trimester to determine accurate dating of the pregnancy, as well as fetal location and number (see Chapter 7). The nuchal translucency measurement (first-trimester screening),** a sonographically derived assessment of the subcutaneous fluid collection at the level of the fetal neck, is a screening test for chromosomal and structural abnor-

malities. It is performed between 11 and 14 weeks' gestation, most commonly by a transabdominal approach, but also by a transvaginal approach. First-trimester vaginal ultrasound can also identify structural malformations.

Transvaginal sonographic measurement of cervical length in the mid-trimester can be used to identify patients at risk for preterm delivery. The median length of the cervix at 24 to 28 weeks is 3.5 cm. Patients with a cervical length less than 2.0 cm are at a three- to fivefold increased risk of preterm birth.

Transvaginal ultrasonic imaging of the lower uterine segment in the second or third trimester allows for very precise identification of placental location in relation to the internal cervical os. In a patient with vaginal bleeding, exclusion of placenta previa is important in overall obstetric management.

TRANSABDOMINAL ULTRASOUND

After 16 weeks' gestation, transabdominal ultrasonic machines (second-trimester screening) are used to evaluate the fetus for structural abnormalities, provide a baseline assessment of fetal growth, and obtain information regarding fetal well-being (see Chapter 7). The ability of a second-trimester scan to identify a fetus with an anomaly ranges from 17-74%. This wide-ranging variation in sensitivity is probably caused by differences in patient population and operator skill. The specificity—the ability of ultrasound to correctly identify a normal fetus—approaches 100% in all studies. Thus, **ultrasound is useful in ruling out fetal anomalies,** but it is not as reliable in detecting them.

In the third trimester, transabdominal ultrasound is useful for assessing fetal growth. Serial biometric measurements of the fetal head, abdomen, and limbs provide longitudinal information regarding the fetal growth trajectory. Software packages integral to ultrasound machines allow calculation of a fetal weight estimate from these measurements. This estimate is often used clinically. However, these estimates may have an error of ±15% (a variation of ±1 lb or 450 g in a 7-lb or 3400-g estimate), which limits the utility of ultrasonic fetal weight estimates, especially in larger fetuses (>8 lb or 4000 g).

Ultrasonic visualization of aspects of fetal behavior (e.g., body movement, fetal breathing) provide highly predictive information regarding fetal oxygenation and well-being. These aspects are combined to determine the **biophysical profile** (Box 17-2). The risk of fetal death within the week following a biophysical profile score of 8 or more is less than 1%.

THREE-DIMENSIONAL SONOGRAPHY

Three-dimensional (3D) ultrasonography provides the ability to acquire an entire volume of ultrasound-based information and then display any plane. It offers a huge number of display possibilities compared

BIOPHYSICAL PROFILE*

Fetal breathing—30 seconds of rhythmic movement of the fetal thorax

Fetal movement—At least three movements of the fetal body or limb

Fetal tone—One extension and flexion of a limb joint

Amniotic fluid—Single deepest vertical pocket of amniotic fluid >2 cm

*Two points for each time these events are documented on a real-time ultrasound during a 30-minute nonstress test, and two points for a reactive nonstress test.

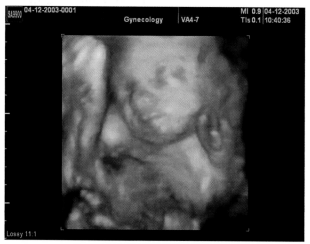

FIGURE 17-1 Three-dimensional ultrasonic image of a fetal face showing normal facial anatomy.

with 2D ultrasound. 3D volume imaging is not new, because computed tomographic and magnetic resonance imaging have been developed for subsequent 2D reconstruction. The main advantage of 3D over 2D ultrasound is the **improved imaging of the fetus with malformations.** The types of anomalies in which 3D imaging is helpful include facial defects (Figure 17-1), limb abnormalities, and neural tube defects. The most important advantage of 3D ultrasound is that more data can be gathered and reviewed over a shorter period of time than is possible with 2D ultrasound.

DOPPLER SONOGRAPHY

Pulse color flow Doppler can precisely measure the velocity profile of blood flowing through fetal vessels, which then **allows for characterization of vascular impedance (resistance).** The umbilical artery, which normally has high-velocity flow during cardiac diastole, may have low, absent, or even reversed diastolic flow in a compromised fetus with high-resistance placental vasculature. Similarly, because the peak flow velocity through a blood vessel is inversely proportional to the viscosity of the liquid flowing through it,

Doppler studies of the fetal middle cerebral artery are used as a noninvasive estimate of fetal hematocrit. This is useful in the management of severe fetal anemia in pregnancies complicated by isoimmunization (see Chapter 15).

Finally, **ultrasound is used to assist in performing invasive obstetric procedures.** Amniocentesis, CVS, and percutaneous umbilical blood sampling (cordocentesis) are examples of procedures that require continuous ultrasonic guidance.

Amniocentesis

Amniocentesis, which involves removing a sample of fluid from the amniotic cavity, is the most common invasive prenatal diagnostic procedure. With direct ultrasonic guidance, a 22-gauge needle is advanced into a clear pocket of amniotic fluid under sterile conditions, with care taken to avoid maternal bowel and blood vessels, as well as the placenta if possible. Approximately 20 mL of amniotic fluid is withdrawn for genetic studies. **Rh immune globulin (RhoGAM) must be given to the Rh-negative gravida** because of the small risk of procedure-related isoimmunization.

GENETIC DIAGNOSIS

Amniocentesis for prenatal diagnosis of chromosomal anomalies is performed at **16 to 20 weeks' gestation.** The procedure-related **risks are an approximately 0.3% pregnancy loss rate and a 1% postprocedure measurable amniotic fluid leakage rate.** Early amniocentesis done before the 15th week of gestation is associated with a higher miscarriage rate (3-4%), a higher postprocedure leakage rate (3%), and an additional risk of limb deformities, including clubfoot (1%). **Amniotic cells require 1 to 2 weeks of culture before final chromosomal analysis is possible,** although fluorescence in situ hybridization can be used with chromosome-specific probes to diagnose certain chromosomal disorders (e.g., trisomy 21, 18, and 13). This gives preliminary results in 3 days.

Single gene defects that have been characterized at the molecular level are amenable to prenatal diagnosis via amniocentesis. **By polymerase chain reaction, fetal DNA in the amniocytes can be amplified rapidly to allow for direct or indirect molecular analysis of genetic disorders.** Examples of common prenatally diagnosed genetic disorders include cystic fibrosis, Tay-Sachs disease, sickle cell disease, and fragile X syndrome (see Chapter 7).

BIOCHEMICAL TESTING

An example of biochemical testing that can be performed on amniotic fluid is the **determination of the level of α-fetoprotein (AFP).** AFP is a fetal serum protein that should, under normal circumstances, be detectable in the amniotic fluid in only trace amounts.

If the fetal dorsal or ventral wall is open (e.g., neural tube defect or gastroschisis), amniotic fluid AFP will be elevated, allowing detection of these defects even if ultrasonic imaging in both two and three dimensions is equivocal or not diagnostic.

DIAGNOSIS OF PERINATAL INFECTIONS

In the United States, the most commonly encountered prenatal infections with potential sequelae for the fetus include cytomegalovirus, parvovirus B19, varicella zoster virus, and toxoplasmosis. Often these are accompanied by findings on mid-trimester ultrasonography, including abdominal, liver, and intracranial calcifications; fetal hydrops; echogenic bowel; ventriculomegaly; and intrauterine growth restriction. These findings can prompt amniotic fluid analysis via culture or polymerase chain reaction to identify the pathogen. In addition, amniotic fluid Gram stain, white blood cell count, glucose level, interleukin-6 level, and culture have been used to diagnose preterm chorioamnionitis, which is associated with premature labor (see Chapter 22).

OTHER DIAGNOSTIC TESTING

Amniocentesis is commonly used in the third trimester to determine the risk of neonatal lung immaturity in the case of impending premature birth or before elective delivery. This is performed by measuring the pulmonary phospholipids or lamellar bodies, which enter the amniotic fluid from the fetal lungs. The presence of phosphatidylglycerol and a lecithin-to-sphingomyelin ratio greater than 2.0 are associated with minimal risk of respiratory distress in the neonate. In a case of suspected premature rupture of the membranes, when the diagnosis is unclear using standard tests, infusion of 2 to 3 mL of dye into the amniotic fluid may be performed. If the dye is then noted on a vaginally placed tampon, rupture of the membranes is confirmed.

THERAPEUTIC AMNIOCENTESIS

The primary role of a therapeutic amniocentesis has been in the management of polyhydramnios and twin-twin transfusion syndrome. *Polyhydramnios,* typically defined as a single deepest vertical pocket of amniotic fluid greater than 8 cm on ultrasound, can cause maternal respiratory embarrassment or premature labor. Excessive amniotic fluid volume may arise from lack of fetal swallowing or from excessive fetal urination. The latter condition occurs in the twin-twin transfusion syndrome (see Chapter 13). Serial amniocenteses to remove large volumes of excessive amniotic fluid from the sac of the recipient twin have been associated with improved perinatal outcome; however, recent data suggest that laser ablation of placental vascular connections between the twin placentas with twin-twin transfusion syndrome is significantly better.

Chorionic Villus Sampling

Another method used to access fetal cells for prenatal genetic diagnosis is CVS of the placenta. The indications for CVS are similar to amniocentesis. The advantage of CVS is that it can be performed earlier than amniocentesis (typically between the 10th and 12th weeks of gestation), allowing for earlier prenatal diagnosis. Although technically feasible, CVS is not performed before the 9th week, as it has been associated with an increased risk of oromandibular/limb dystrophy, presumably from a vascular insult.

CVS must be performed under sterile conditions either transcervically or transabdominally. In transcervical CVS, the distal 3 to 5 cm of a catheter is inserted through the cervix and into the placenta under sonographic guidance. A 20-mL syringe with nutrient medium is attached, and negative pressure is applied to obtain fragments of placental villi. In transabdominal CVS, an 18- to 20-gauge needle is inserted into the placenta transabdominally. With either approach, RhoGAM should be administered to Rh-negative patients. The procedure-related fetal loss is less than 1%.

Direct visual inspection of dividing villous cells obtained by CVS allows for detection of chromosomal abnormalities within 3 days, and tissue culture yields cytogenetic results in 6 to 8 days. The diagnostic precision of CVS is somewhat less than that achieved with amniocentesis because of a 1% risk of chromosomal mosaicism, which is often due to confined placental mosaicism. A disadvantage of CVS is that amniotic fluid AFP levels cannot be assessed, and thus patients at risk for neural tube defects must wait until amniocentesis can be performed in the second trimester.

Cordocentesis

Cordocentesis (percutaneous umbilical blood sampling) is a procedure in which fetal blood is obtained directly from the umbilical vein at the placental cord insertion site under direct ultrasonic guidance. Confirmation of the fetal origin of the blood is obtained by measuring the fetal mean corpuscular volume (MCV), which is typically greater than 120 fL (maternal MCV is usually <100 fL).

Historically, the most common indication for cordocentesis has been to determine fetal hematocrit in the hemolytic disease known as Rh isoimmunization. With the recent advent of assessment of fetal anemia by Doppler of the fetal middle cerebral artery, cordocentesis is becoming less frequent. Today, cordocentesis is often performed for rapid evaluation of the fetal karyotype. Unlike amniocytes, fetal leukocytes may be cultured rapidly, and results are typically available in 3 days.

The fetal loss rate is about 1% per procedure. In the case of a hydropic fetus, the risk of fetal loss may approach 7%. The cause of pregnancy loss may be chorioamnionitis, rupture of membranes, bleeding from the puncture site, bradycardia, or thrombosis of the umbilical vessel.

Cervical Cerclage

Cervical insufficiency or incompetence **is defined as the inability of the uterine cervix to retain a pregnancy in the absence of contractions or labor** (see Chapter 12). Cervical cerclage, a circumferential suture placed into the cervix, has been proposed as a surgical treatment for this condition. More recently, it has been used in combination with vaginal progesterone for the prevention of preterm birth. **The cerclage is usually placed at 13 to 16 weeks' gestation,** but it can be placed at 22 to 24 weeks when cervical shortening is observed by physical examination or by vaginal ultrasonography.

The most common procedure, the **McDonald cerclage,** involves placement of a simple purse-string monofilament suture near the cervicovaginal junction (Figure 17-2). The **Shirodkar cerclage** differs in that the stitch is placed as close to the internal os as possible. The bladder and rectum are dissected off the cervix, and the woven, tapelike suture is tied and placed under the vaginal epithelium. Transabdominal cervicoisthmic cerclage is rarely indicated; it is reserved for select patients with previously failed vaginal cerclage, cervical hypoplasia, or a cervix severely scarred from prior lacerations or surgery. This type of cerclage entails dissection of the bladder from the lower uterine segment through an abdominal incision.

For transvaginal cerclage, the suture is typically removed before the onset of labor. For abdominal cerclage, cesarean delivery is performed. Patients must be counseled thoroughly regarding the risks associated with cerclage, which include bleeding, infection, iatrogenic rupture of amniotic membranes, and damage to adjacent organs (bladder and bowel).

Operative Delivery

The incidence of operative obstetric delivery in the United States today is approximately 35-40%, of which 10-15% are operative vaginal deliveries using either a forceps or a vacuum device. **Approximately 25-30% of all deliveries are cesarean deliveries.** Each operative procedure has inherent benefits and risks.

OBSTETRIC FORCEPS

Forceps are instruments designed to provide traction and/or rotation of the fetal head when the expulsive efforts of the mother are insufficient to accomplish safe delivery of the fetus. Commonly used forceps are shown in Figure 17-3. There are two classes of obstetric forceps: classical forceps and specialized forceps. Forceps selection depends on the obstetric indication.

Classic or standard forceps are used to facilitate delivery by applying traction to the fetal skull. The components of each blade are illustrated in Figure 17-4. The blades have a **cephalic curve** designed to conform to the curvature of the fetal head. Simpson forceps (an example of classic or standard forceps) have a tapered cephalic curve that is designed to fit on a molded fetal head. The **pelvic curve** of classic forceps approximates the shape of the birth canal.

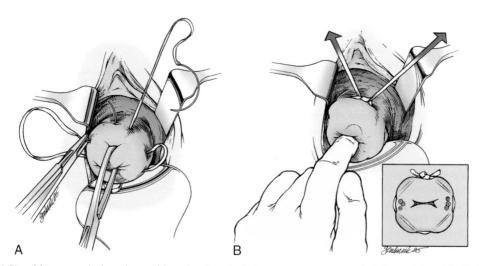

A   B

FIGURE 17-2 McDonald-type cervical cerclage. Although suture techniques may vary somewhat, four stiches (10, 7, 5, and 2 o'clock) are usually placed high into the cervix, using a nonabsorbable material such as Mersilene **(A)** and then tied (12 o'clock), providing additional support at the level of the internal cervical os **(B)**. This suture is cut for labor. (From Gabbe SG, Simpson JL, Niebyl JR, et al: *Obstetrics: normal and problem pregnancies,* ed 5, Philadelphia, 2007, Churchill Livingstone.)

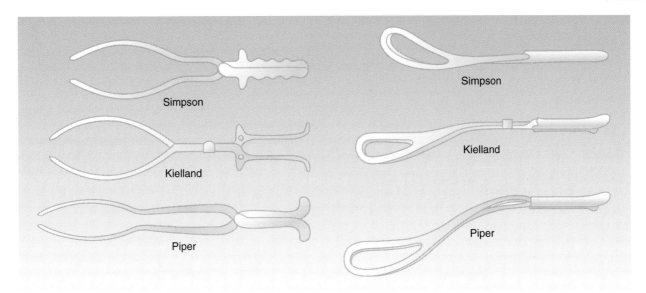

FIGURE 17-3 Types of obstetric forceps in use. Simpson forceps are an example of classic or standard forceps. Kielland forceps (for mid forceps rotation) are an example of specialized forceps and are used infrequently.

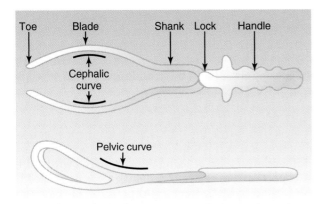

FIGURE 17-4 Components of classic forceps.

Indications

In general, there are four indications for an operative vaginal delivery:

1. **Prolonged second stage of labor.** In nulliparous women, this is defined as lack of continuing progress for 2 hours without regional anesthesia or 3 hours with regional anesthesia. In multiparous women, it is defined as lack of continuing progress for 1 hour without regional anesthesia or 2 hours with regional anesthesia.
2. **Suspicion of immediate or impending fetal compromise as defined by Category III fetal heart rate patterns.**
3. **To stabilize the after-coming head during a breech delivery** (Figure 17-5).

4. **To shorten the second stage of labor for maternal benefit.** Maternal conditions such as hypertension, cardiac disorders, or pulmonary disease, in which strenuous pushing in the second stage of labor is considered hazardous, may be indications for forceps delivery. Epidural analgesia, which also decreases strenuous pushing during the second stage of labor, may also be recommended for this purpose.

Types of Forceps Operations

Forceps application is classified according to the station and position of the presenting part at the time the forceps are applied. The American College of Obstetricians and Gynecologists has proposed the following classifications:

1. **Outlet forceps:** The scalp is visible at the introitus without separating the labia, fetal head at perineum, fetal skull at pelvic floor, sagittal suture in anteroposterior or right/left occipitoanterior or posterior position, and rotation of the fetal head not exceeding 45 degrees.
2. **Low forceps:** The leading part of the fetal skull is at station +2 cm or more (using the 5-point scale of 0 cm, +1, +2, +3, +4, and +5. Low forceps have two subdivisions: rotation of 45 degrees or less and rotation of more than 45 degrees.
3. **Mid forceps:** The fetal head is engaged, but the leading point of the skull is above station +2 cm.

Before performing a forceps-assisted vaginal delivery, appropriate consent from the patient regarding potential risks and benefits should be obtained. The indication for the procedure should be clearly outlined to the patient and in the medical record. **The cervix**

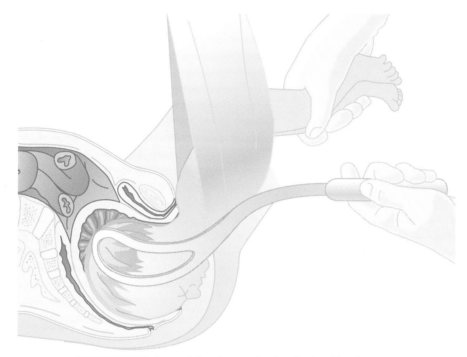

FIGURE 17-5 Delivery of the after-coming head using Piper forceps.

must be fully dilated, membranes ruptured, and the fetal head engaged into the pelvis (0 station). Clinical assessment to determine the level of the presenting part, an estimate of the fetal size, and the adequacy of the maternal pelvis is mandatory. **There must be no doubt regarding the position of the fetal head.** This evaluation is performed by palpation of the sutures and fontanels in comparison to the maternal pelvis. **Anesthesia must be adequate** via either pudendal nerve block with local infiltration (for outlet forceps only) or regional anesthesia. **The bladder should be emptied** to prevent damage to that structure and to provide more room to facilitate delivery.

Forceps Technique

The forceps blades are inserted sequentially into the vagina such that the sagittal suture of the fetal head is directly between and perpendicular to the shanks. Damage to maternal tissues may be avoided by the operator placing one hand into the vagina to guide the toe of the blade along the natural pelvic curve of the birth canal. With the next maternal pushing effort, the forceps are locked and traction is applied. The direction of pull should be parallel to the axis of the birth canal at that level, such that typically there is downward traction initially, followed by ever-increasing upward traction as delivery of the fetal head occurs. With complete delivery of the head, the shanks are nearly perpendicular to the floor. **If progress of the fetal head is not obtained with appropriate traction,** **the procedure should be abandoned (failed forceps) in favor of a cesarean delivery.**

VACUUM EXTRACTION

The vacuum extractor (VE) is an instrument that uses a suction cup that is applied to the fetal head. **Because of the relative ease of using VEs compared with using forceps, the frequency of VE delivery has increased in the United States.** After confirming that no maternal tissue is trapped between the cup and the fetal head, the vacuum seal is obtained using a suction pump. Traction is then applied using principles similar to those described above for a forceps delivery. **Flexion of the fetal head must be maintained to provide the smallest diameter to the maternal pelvis by placing the posterior edge of the suction cup 3 cm from the anterior fontanel squarely over the sagittal suture.** This is illustrated in Figure 17-6. With the aid of maternal pushing efforts, traction is applied parallel to the axis of the birth canal. Detachment of the suction cup from the fetal head during traction is termed a "pop-off." If progress down the birth canal is not obtained with appropriate traction, or if two "pop-offs" occur, the procedure should be discontinued in favor of a cesarean delivery. **The indications for vacuum delivery are the same as for forceps delivery.**

The prerequisites for use of the VE are also the same as for forceps, with a few exceptions. **The VE is contraindicated in preterm delivery** because the preterm fetal head and scalp are more prone to injury from the

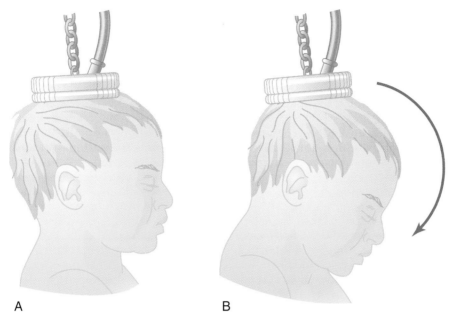

FIGURE 17-6 Application of the vacuum extractor. **A,** Incorrect application, which deflexes the fetal head, thereby increasing the presenting diameter. **B,** Correct application over the posterior fontanel, which flexes the fetal head when traction is applied.

suction cup. The VE is suitable for all vertex presentations, but unlike forceps, **it must never be used for delivery of fetuses presenting by the face or breech.**

COMPARISON OF FORCEPS AND VACUUM DELIVERY

Understanding the potential advantages and disadvantages of each operative vaginal delivery instrument allows the operator to counsel the mother appropriately and to choose the device that is best suited for the particular clinical situation.

Forceps have a higher overall success rate for vaginal delivery. **The failure rate for forceps is 7%, whereas the failure rate for vacuum extraction is 12%. In general, forceps deliveries cause higher rates of maternal injury, and vacuum extraction causes higher rates of fetal morbidity.** Forceps have an increased risk of trauma to vaginal and perineal tissues and damage to the maternal anal sphincter. In contrast, neonates delivered by vacuum have more **cephalohematomas** (accumulation of blood beneath the periosteum) and exclusively have **subgaleal hematomas** (blood in the space above the periosteum that has a large potential space and can allow significant blood loss) and retinal hemorrhages. **Sequential use of one instrument followed by the other has been associated with a disproportionately high fetal morbidity rate** and should be approached with extreme caution. Long-term retrospective studies of adolescents who were delivered by normal vaginal delivery, forceps, vacuum extractions, and cesarean delivery have shown little difference in physical or cognitive outcomes.

CESAREAN DELIVERY

Cesarean delivery is delivery of the fetus through an incision in the maternal abdomen and uterus. Hospitals offering obstetric services must have the personnel and equipment needed to perform an emergent cesarean delivery within 30 minutes. This is especially true for vaginal births after a prior cesarean delivery (VBAC), where the risk of uterine rupture is higher than in those women who have not had a prior cesarean delivery.

Cesarean delivery is the most common major operation performed in the United States today. **The rate of cesarean deliveries has increased over fivefold, from 5% of births in 1970 to at least 25-30% of births currently.** The dramatic increase in the cesarean delivery rate has been attributed to many factors, including assumed benefit for the fetus; the fact that women are postponing childbirth until a later age, when the risk is higher; relatively low maternal risk in general; societal preference; and fear of litigation.

The perinatal benefits of cesarean delivery are largely based on unquantified and scanty evidence. **There has been over a 10-fold decrease in perinatal mortality in the United States over the last 40 years** concurrent with advances in prenatal, intrapartum, and neonatal care. How much of this improvement has been due to the increased use of cesarean delivery is debatable, with the exception of management of the term breech delivery. With the latter delivery method, **perinatal and neonatal mortality and significant neonatal morbidity have been shown to improve from 5.0% for those delivered vaginally to 1.6% for those delivered by cesarean.**

The overall maternal mortality rate from cesarean delivery is currently less than 1 in 1000, but this is about five times greater than the rate for vaginal delivery. However, **recent studies have shown that the maternal mortality rate for an elective cesarean delivery approximates that of vaginal delivery.** This is due to advances in surgical techniques, anesthetic care, blood transfusions, and antibiotics.

The maternal morbidity associated with cesarean delivery is increased compared with vaginal delivery because of increased postpartum infections, hemorrhage, and thromboembolism.

Indications

Four indications account for 90% of the marked increase in cesarean deliveries over the past 40 years: dystocia (30%), repeat cesarean (25-30%), breech presentation (10-15%), and fetal distress (10-15%). **An absolute indication for a cesarean delivery is a previous full-thickness, nontransverse incision through the myometrium.** This occurs in all classical cesarean deliveries and some myomectomy surgeries. **All pregnancies complicated by placenta previa should also be delivered by cesarean delivery.**

Types of Cesarean Delivery

Cesarean deliveries are classified by the uterine incision (Figure 17-7), not by the skin incision. **In the low transverse cesarean delivery (LTCD), the uterine incision is made transversely in the lower uterine segment after a bladder flap is established.** The advantages of this approach include decreased rate of rupture

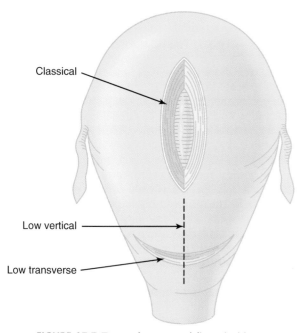

FIGURE 17-7 Types of cesarean delivery incisions.

Classical

Low vertical

Low transverse

of the scar in a subsequent pregnancy and a reduced risk of bleeding, peritonitis, paralytic ileus, and bowel adhesions.

For the classical cesarean delivery, a vertical incision is made in the upper segment of the uterus through the myometrium. A vertical incision may also be made in the lower segment, in which case the procedure is referred to as a **low vertical cesarean,** although the incision invariably extends into the upper segment. **The common indications for a classical cesarean delivery include preterm breech in a woman with an undeveloped lower uterine segment, transverse backdown fetal position, poor access to the lower segment because of myomas or adhesions, or a planned cesarean hysterectomy. The presence of cervical cancer is a rare indication.**

The type of uterine incision has important implications regarding risk of uterine rupture in future pregnancies. *Uterine rupture,* defined as separation of the uterine incision, may cause significant maternal complications caused by massive hemorrhage and fetal damage or death. **A LTCD incision is associated with a less than 1% risk of symptomatic uterine rupture in the subsequent pregnancy,** although this risk may be higher if labor induction or augmentation is carried out. **A classic cesarean delivery carries a 4-7% risk of uterine rupture.** Patients with a classical uterine incision are thus destined to have repeat cesareans for all subsequent deliveries.

Prevention

Two clinical interventions have been shown to reduce cesarean delivery rates: external cephalic version (ECV) and VBAC.

EXTERNAL CEPHALIC VERSION. ECV converts a breech fetus to the vertex position to avoid a cesarean delivery for breech presentation. This procedure is performed under ultrasonic guidance in the labor and delivery suite after the 36th or 37th week of gestation. A tocolytic may be given to decrease uterine tone. Using external manipulation, the fetus is gently guided to the vertex presentation. **Fetal risk due to umbilical cord entanglement and placental abruption is low (<1%).**

The success rate of ECV is about 60%. Parity, gestational age, placental location, cervical dilation, and fetal station affect the success rate. An ECV program can decrease the rate of cesarean delivery in this group of patients by more than half, and an obstetric service's overall cesarean delivery rate by approximately 2%.

VAGINAL BIRTH AFTER CESAREAN DELIVERY. A prior cesarean is the second most common overall cause of cesarean delivery (25-30%). In fact, about 10-15% of pregnant women have had a previous cesarean delivery.

A trial of labor may be offered if one or two previous LTCDs have been performed, the uterine incision did not extend into the cervix or upper segment, and there is no history of prior uterine rupture. Adequate maternal pelvic dimensions should be noted by clinical examination. Personnel and equipment should be immediately available in case an emergent cesarean delivery is required within 30 minutes.

The overall success rate of VBAC is approximately 70%, although it ranges from 60% (dystocia) to 90% (malpresentation), depending on the indication for the previous cesarean delivery. Compared with repeat cesarean delivery, a successful vaginal delivery is associated with less maternal morbidity without any increase in perinatal morbidity. If uterine rupture does occur, there may be a 10-fold increase in perinatal mortality and substantial maternal morbidity as well.

PART 3

Gynecology

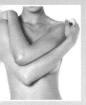
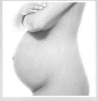
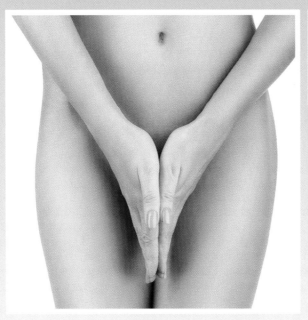
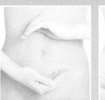

18

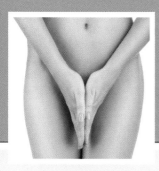

Benign Conditions and Congenital Anomalies of the Vulva and Vagina

ANITA L. NELSON • JOSEPH C. GAMBONE

CLINICAL KEYS FOR THIS CHAPTER

- Benign vulvovaginal problems are among the ten leading disorders encountered by primary care clinicians in the United States. Women with these disorders commonly present with irritation and pruritus (itching), but many conditions are asymptomatic and just visually troubling.
- There is significant variation in the normal appearance of the female vulva, with clitoral and labial size differences. Epithelial lesions in this area are often described on the basis of their appearance as white, red, or pigmented; other lesions include ulcerations, fissures, as well as solid and cystic masses.
- Biopsy may be needed in some cases to confirm a diagnosis and rule out premalignancy or malignancy before

treatment. Corticosteroid and sex-steroid creams are frequently used, but surgery is indicated in some cases.
- Benign vaginal problems include ulcerations and fistulas as well as solid or cystic masses. Traumatic injury to the vagina can occur at the time of obstetric delivery, surgical procedures, or sexual assault.
- Congenital abnormalities of the vulva frequently involve ambiguous genitalia that can present a problem with gender assignment at birth. Agenesis is the most extreme and significant congenital anomaly of the vagina. Other structural anomalies include canalization defects such as imperforate hymen, longitudinal and transverse vaginal septa, partial vaginal development, and double vagina.

Vulvovaginal problems are quite common in gynecologic practice. Definitive diagnosis may require time because complaints of pruritus (itching) and irritation are nonspecific and can be caused by a wide range of conditions.

This chapter describes a wide array of benign lesions of the vulva and vagina. Infectious conditions of the vulva and vagina are discussed in Chapter 22 and premalignant/malignant conditions are covered in Chapter 40. Although the diagnosis of many conditions can be made clinically, biopsy and other tests may be needed to establish an accurate diagnosis. The differential diagnosis for many of these conditions can be extensive. **It is important to establish an accurate diagnosis before initiating therapy.** Congenital anomalies of the vulva and vagina are also covered in this chapter.

Vulva

There is considerable variation in the appearance of normal external female genitalia. In particular, the

distance between the clitoral base and the urethra and the distance between the posterior fourchette and the anus (perineal body) vary greatly from woman to woman. Labia minora may be so small that they are completely covered by the labia majora or they may protrude by over a centimeter beyond the limits of the labia majora. The labia minora may not be symmetrical—at times, one may be considerably larger than the other. Clitoral size also differs greatly from woman to woman.

BENIGN CONDITIONS OF THE VULVA

Epithelial Changes

The epithelium of the vulva is susceptible to the same skin pathologies seen on other parts of the body. Often the appearance of those processes may be altered by the moisture and warmth of the genital tissue. In addition, there are epithelial problems that are unique to the vulva or more commonly detected in this area. Other changes reflect the impact that systemic or other diseases can have on the vulvar tissue. Most vulvar epithelial lesions present with symptoms of pruritus or pain, but a significant minority of lesions are detected only on examination. Conservative management is often appropriate, but frequently topical corticosteroids and systemic pain medications may be needed. Although the appearance of superficial vulvar lesions varies with the pigment of the woman's skin, they are generally categorized by the color most commonly associated with them—white, red or pigmented. Table 18-1 lists benign conditions of the vulva along with their clinical features and treatment.

WHITE LESIONS. Conditions that cause whitening of the vulvar epithelium range from processes that result from simple loss of pigment (vitiligo) to those that can profoundly change the architecture of the vulva (lichen sclerosus).

Vitiligo affects 1-2% of the population and is often associated with autoimmune conditions. Its initial presentation can be on the vulva, but it often involves pigment loss on other parts of the body. The diagnosis is made clinically; rarely is biopsy needed. A notable

TABLE 18-1

BENIGN CONDITIONS OF THE VULVA

Epithelial Changes	Clinical Features and Comments	Treatment
White Lesions		
Vitiligo	Loss of pigment; associated with autoimmune conditions; clinical diagnosis with biopsy rarely needed	Observation
Lichen sclerosus	Intense pruritus and dyspareunia; anogenital area of midlife women; biopsy shows loss of rete ridges with thin epidermis; recurrence is common; future squamous cell carcinoma risk increased	High potency topical corticosteroids
Lichen planus	Inflammatory autoimmune process; intense epithelial changes in the vulva, vagina, and mouth; white "Wickham striae"; scarring possible; may appear as a red lesion initially	Topical corticosteroids
Lichen simplex chronicus	Histology shows squamous hyperplasia; thickening of the epithelium; itching results in rubbing and scratching; can mimic psoriasis so biopsy is indicated	Intermediate potency topical corticosteroids
Vulvovaginal atrophy	Occurs in many postmenopausal women; underlying fat of the labia decreased with thinning of the epithelium; appears white and vaginal opening may constrict	Estrogen creams or moisturizers; lubricants may be needed for coitus
Red Lesions		
Eczema	Term that defines a dermatitis with itching, swelling, and crusting; most common on the vulva is an allergic contact dermatitis	Depends on etiology; for contact dermatitis, identify irritant(s) and discontinue use
Seborrheic dermatitis	Affects skin folds of genital area; skin has red-glazed shiny appearance; may also find dry, greasy areas of the scalp too	Topical corticosteroids
Psoriasis	Immune-mediated skin disease; red plaques with clear borders; biopsy; itching common; pustular form confused with candida	Topical corticosteroid is initial therapy
Pigmented Lesions		
Genital melanosis	Occurs in 10-15% of women; dark pigment on mucous membranes; smaller area may be lentigo; biopsy of dark, changing areas mandatory	Expectant management
Acanthosis nigricans	Increasingly common; pigmented areas on vulva, axilla, and neck; related to obesity and insulin resistance	None except weight loss and glucose control
Ulcerations and Fissures		
Aphthous ulcers	Painful lesions similar to "canker sores" in the mouth; may be small or as large as 2 cm wide and 1 cm deep	Usually symptomatic therapies
Behçet disease	Genital and oral ulceration with uveitis; may be associated with other disease processes such as inflammatory bowel disease or antiviral therapy	Depends on etiology and underlying cause
Crohn disease	Vulvar involvement of granulomatous intestinal tract inflammatory process due to fistulization	Treatment of underlying bowel disease
Traumatic ulceration	Iatrogenic or self-inflicted trauma due to scratching, overcleaning, or neglect	Counseling; suspect underlying psychiatric disorder

Continued

TABLE 18-1

BENIGN CONDITIONS OF THE VULVA—cont'd

Epithelial Changes	Clinical Features and Comments	Treatment
Solid or Cystic Masses		
Epidermal cysts	Most common type of genital cyst; may form in obstructed hair follicles; usually asymptomatic but can be visually troubling	Counseling about body hair care and/or deflation by expressing contents
Vulvar vestibular papillomatosis	Soft, slightly elongated papules	Reassurance
Genital warts	Caused by human papillomavirus	See Chapter 22
Fox-Fordyce disease	Chronic inflammation of apocrine glands causing intense itching; affects axillary area in addition to vulva	Systemic antipruritic therapy
Hidradenitis suppurativa	Painful, recurrent condition of the apocrine glands; results in red papules that have chronic purulent drainage; increased risk with obesity and smoking	Corticosteroid injection in the lesions; antibiotics only if cellulitis present; incision and drainage for comfort only; suppression with oral contraceptives reduces recurrences
Vascular lesions	Tortuous varicosities; cherry angiomas and hematomas	Evaluation, compression; possible evacuation of expanding hematoma
Urethral caruncle	Solitary red papule at the urethral meatus; usually <1 cm diameter; appears as a collar around urethral opening	Observation and biopsy as needed; estrogen creams; surgery rarely indicated

characteristic is the brightness of the depigmented areas amplified by increased pigment in the adjacent unaffected areas.

Lichen sclerosus may affect men and women of any age, and may involve the skin on any part of the body, but is most commonly found in the anogenital area of midlife women. It often presents with intense pruritus, dyspareunia and burning pain, but can also be an asymptomatic finding. Anal involvement can cause constipation. The skin is white, thin, and inelastic, with a crinkled cigarette-paper appearance on gentle stretch. Widespread excoriation is common. It starts with isolated pearly white papules and plaques that coalesce over time and form scars. The result is a "figure of 8" field of scarring from the area encircling the labia, constricting down around the perineal body and ballooning out again around the perineal area into the gluteal cleft. The clitoral hood scars, burying the clitoris (Figure 18-1). There is shrinkage or loss of the labia minora, contraction of the tissue in the vestibule and introitus, and scarring around the anus. Painful, bleeding fissures are common, especially in areas where the inelastic epithelium is put under tension, such as with attempted coitus (introital trauma) or defecation (perianal trauma). Biopsy demonstrates characteristic loss of rete ridges, a thin epidermis, and a mixed lymphocytic infiltrate lining the basement membrane. The process can be arrested by treatment with higher potency corticosteroids, but recurrence is not uncom-

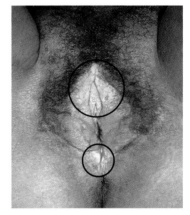

FIGURE 18-1 Vulva with lichen sclerosus *(circles)*. (From Moreland A, Kohl P: Genital and dermatologic examination. In Morse SA, Ballard RC, Holmes KK, et al, editors: *Atlas of sexually transmitted diseases and AIDS,* ed 4, Philadelphia, 2010, Elsevier, pp 1–23.)

mon and up to 10% of untreated and 3% of treated women eventually develop squamous cell carcinoma of the vulva. The histologic features of lichen sclerosus are illustrated in Figure 18-2, *A.*

Lichen planus is an inflammatory, autoimmune process that involves epithelial changes on the vulva, or in the vagina and the mouth. Symptoms include severe burning, irritation, and dyspareunia. It induces

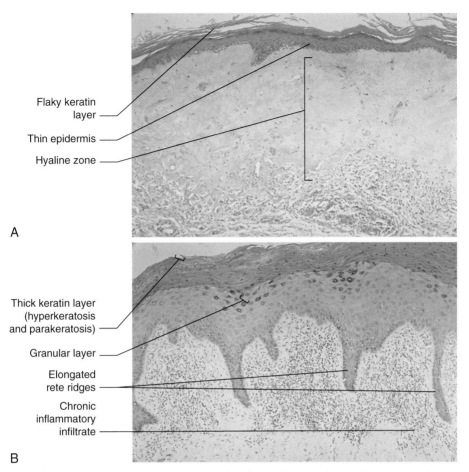

Flaky keratin layer

Thin epidermis

Hyaline zone

A

Thick keratin layer (hyperkeratosis and parakeratosis)

Granular layer

Elongated rete ridges

Chronic inflammatory infiltrate

B

FIGURE 18-2 A, Lichen sclerosus. Histology shows hyperkeratosis but the epidermis is thinner than normal. The most striking feature of lichen sclerosus is the presence of a hyaline zone in the superficial dermis. This is the result of edema and degeneration of the collagen and elastic fibers of the dermis. **B,** Squamous cell hyperplasia. Microscopy shows marked hyperkeratosis and parakeratosis with a prominent granular layer. Acanthosis, with prolongation of rete ridges, is also seen and there is a dense infiltrate of chronic inflammatory cells, mainly lymphocytes, in the superficial dermis.

an intense erythema and erosions on the vulva, which is often surrounded by reticulate white striae (Wickham striae) that appear as classic fernlike or lacy patterns. These same findings are commonly found on the mucous membranes of the mouth. Scarring, especially in the vaginal vault, is common.

Lichen simplex chronicus (referred to as squamous hyperplasia histologically), represents thickening of the epithelium, which usually results from rubbing or scratching in the absence of an underlying dermatosis. It generally appears on keratinized skin as white plaques or darker red areas; the surface is often marked with excoriations. It can often mimic other processes, such as psoriasis, lichen planus or lichen sclerosus, so biopsy is indicated. Histologically, the rete ridges deepen with hyperkeratosis of the superficial layer of the epidermis (see Figure 18-2, *B*). Intermediate potency topical corticosteroids are the cornerstone of treatment.

Vulvovaginal atrophy occurs in many postmenopausal women with the loss of ovarian production of estradiol (E2). The subcutaneous fat in the labia majora is diminished and the labia minora also shrink. The epithelium thins, appears white, and is less elastic. The vaginal introitus can constrict, creating an almost prepubertal caliber, which may make coitus uncomfortable. Estrogen creams are usually effective. Moisturizers can help women who are not candidates for hormonal therapies. Lubricants can be used for intercourse, if needed.

RED LESIONS. Many of the epithelial lesions on the vulva can be accompanied by erythema, and many infectious processes, such as **candidal infections,** can appear red. However, the lesions included in this category represent benign underlying dermatologic changes that present primarily as red lesions. These include **eczema, seborrheic dermatitis, and psoriasis.**

In the genitalia, the characteristics of many of these processes are altered by the moisture and heat in the area, friction from clothing or scratching, and secondary infection or irritation from sweat, urine, stool, or overcleansing. Fecal or urinary incontinence may cause irritation and can accelerate skin breakdown due to other etiologies.

Eczema is a term that is broadly applied to a wide range of chronic skin conditions characterized by rashes with dryness, swelling, itching, as well as crusting, flaking, cracking, blistering, oozing, or frank bleeding. The reddish appearance of eczema in the vulva is profoundly influenced by rubbing and scratching, which produce thickening and excoriation, respectively. The history of pruritus, relieved by scratching, and the shape of the lesions help with the diagnosis, but other etiologies must be ruled out first. One of the most common subtypes of eczema on the vulva is contact dermatitis. **Contact dermatitis** (either irritant or allergic) is increasing in frequency on the vulva with the use of a wide range of products on the genital tissue. Common irritants include overwashing, female hygiene products, and topical medications. These same medications, as well as chemicals found in sanitary protection products, can induce allergic reactions on the vulva with widespread erythema and even edema.

Seborrheic dermatitis causes a dry or greasy peeling, reminiscent of dandruff in the scalp, face, or eyebrows. In the genital area, the lesions tend to concentrate in the skin folds, with less prominent lesion borders or scaling. The skin has a red glazed, shiny texture, occasionally with scaling plaques, in the absence of candida or psoriasis. A diagnosis of seborrheic dermatitis is strongly supported by finding characteristic lesions elsewhere.

Psoriasis is a common chronic relapsing immune-mediated skin disease affecting 2-3% of the population. Psoriasis may involve the entire genital area, including the gluteal cleft, but there may be less extensive involvement. Both the skin fold and hair-bearing areas may be involved. Red plaques with clear borders are the hallmark of classic genital psoriasis, but the silvery-white scales are generally less prominent on the genitalia. Itching is a frequent complaint. Involvement of knees, elbows, and nails helps to make the diagnosis. Pustular psoriasis can be confused with candidal infection.

PIGMENTED LESIONS. Pigmented lesions raise the greatest concerns for malignancy, but there are several benign lesions that are darkened. The concentration of melanocytes is higher in the vulva than other body tissue, but their distribution may not be even, which can result in **physiologic hyperpigmentation.**

Genital melanosis is a relatively common finding; it occurs in 10-15% of women. It consists of flat patches and macules (0.5 to 2 cm) of dark pigment on mucous membrane (labia minora) as well as keratinized skin (labia majora). The smaller lesions may be lentigo (freckles) if they meet criteria on biopsy. There can be concerning variation of color within the lesion and the borders can be irregular, which raises differential diagnosis of melanoma, unless the lesion has been stable over time. Pigmentation can also increase following tissue trauma or inflammation.

Acanthosis nigricans is increasingly common with the rising prevalence of obesity and insulin resistance in the general population. It presents with poorly demarcated, brown, thickened, ridged lesions in the superficial layers of the skin on the vulva, axilla, and neck. The histology of acanthosis is shown in Figure 18-2, *B,* and the clinical features of acanthosis nigricans are shown in Figure 33-4.

Recent social trends have created new appearances of the vulva in some women, and made treatment of medical conditions potentially challenging. Tattooing and body piercing practices, as well as all techniques used to remove pubic hair, are examples of such trends.

Ulcerations and Fissures

Vulvar ulcerations may be the presenting complaint for many infectious conditions (herpes simplex, syphilis, chancroid, Epstein-Barr) and malignancies (squamous cell carcinoma); these conditions must always be ruled out before a benign diagnosis is made. The most common noninfectious, benign conditions causing ulcerations and fissures are **aphthous ulcers, Behçet disease and Crohn disease.**

Aphthous ulcers are extremely painful lesions, similar to the "canker sores" found in the mouth. They can be small (<1 cm) and eventually heal without scarring, or they can be larger (>2 cm diameter and 1 cm deep) and cause permanent scarring. Recurrence rates are as high as 35%. Often genital aphthous ulcers are associated with similar lesions elsewhere, as in Behçet disease, which has genital and oral ulcerations as well as uveitis. Genital ulceration can be associated with other disease processes, such as inflammatory bowel disease, or induced by medications (e.g., antiretroviral therapy).

Decubitus ulcers are most likely to develop when chronic pressure is applied to tissue over bony prominences. Tissue made moist by urinary incontinence may be more susceptible to breakdown.

Other ulceration may also be iatrogenic, such as from caustic or destructive treatments for external genital warts or vulvar intraepithelial neoplasia. Women can traumatize the area mechanically (direct scratching, overcleansing, or neglect), either as a result of a deeply held perception that the area is dirty or as part of a deeper psychiatric illness.

Crohn disease is a granulomatous inflammatory process in the intestinal tract that can extend via fistulization to or separately appear on the genital area, resulting in widespread, painful deep linear "knifelike" ulceration or fissuring in the skin folds. These fissures may be accompanied by perianal tags, edema, or abscesses. More superficial fissures can result from stretching of skin affected by lichen sclerosus.

Another more intense chronic inflammatory condition of the apocrine glands is **hidradenitis suppurativa.** This is a painful, recurrent, progressive, and disfiguring condition in which painful red papules from beneath the skin expand and eventually rupture and create ulceration and chronic, purulent draining sinuses. The ulcers heal with thick contracting scarring. Hidradenitis suppurativa can involve all genital areas. The extragenital areas most affected include the axilla and breast, along the "milk line." Obesity and smoking are risk factors. Medical and even surgical treatment is often suboptimal.

Solid or Cystic Masses of the Vulva

Epidermal cysts are the most common type of genital cyst, peaking in incidence in women in their 40s and 50s and located primarily in the labia majora, labia minora, and inguinal areas. Epidermal cysts develop when the hair follicles become obstructed; the deeper portion of the follicle swells to accommodate the desquamated cells. These cysts are generally dome-shaped, clear white to skin colored lesions rising above the surrounding epithelium. Epidermal cysts are usually asymptomatic, but can trouble the woman from a cosmetic perspective.

Vulvar vestibular papillomatosis is a normal variant very analogous to pearly penile papules in men. The papillae are the same color as the surrounding tissue from which they protrude. They are soft, slightly elongated papules generally measuring 1 to 2 mm in height and diameter arranged in a linear pattern, with one single protrusion emanating from each base, as opposed to external **genital warts** that usually have multiple protrusions from the base.

Fordyce spots are sebaceous glands that appear as small, slightly raised dome-shaped papules along the Hart line on the labia minora. On the other hand, **Fox-Fordyce disease** represents a chronic inflammation of apocrine glands that causes intense pruritus, mainly in the axilla and labia majora and minora.

Vascular lesions can be prominent on the vulva. Tortuous **varicosities** can involve the labia majora, especially in pregnancy. Large varicose veins are usually a characteristic blue color, but smaller veins appear darker red. The lesions disappear temporarily with compression. **Cherry angiomas** and **angiokeratomas** are clustered/superficial capillaries or small blood vessels that appear as dark red to purple dots on the vulva. **Hematomas** are loculated collections of blood that collect following trauma such as accidental injuries (bike accidents), incidental injuries (birth trauma), or sexual assault. The soft tissues of the labia can accommodate substantial amounts of blood, but dissection into the perivaginal and retroperitoneal space occurs commonly; significant blood loss can occur into these spaces. Complete evaluation of all the affected tissues, including periurethral and perivaginal areas, must be done to insure that there is no continued active bleeding or tissue injury requiring urgent surgery.

Other Vulvar Masses

Nevi can be flat or elevated pigmented lesions that must be distinguished from melanoma. **Acrochordons** are called **skin tags** when they are larger. Skin tags are more commonly found in obese people and those with insulin resistance. They are mainly found in the axilla, neck, and skin folds of the genital area. **Lipomas, neurofibromas,** and **endometriomas** can also be found on the vulva. **Femoral hernias** can dissect into the labia majora. Swelling of the labia can be generalized or focal, depending on the etiology. **Galactoceles** in the vulva are rare, but are milk-filled cysts that may form in the milk line.

Two particular masses involve the urethral meatus. A **urethral caruncle** is a solitary red papule at the meatus. It generally measures less than 1 cm in diameter and is pedunculated or dome-shaped (Figure 18-3, *A*). It must be distinguished from an **overt urethral prolapse,** which occurs at the two age extremes. It appears as a swollen red cuff that surrounds the meatus circumferentially, much as a collar around the opening. The histology of a urethral caruncle is shown in Figure 18-3, *B*.

CONGENITAL ANOMALIES OF THE VULVA

The most significant of the vulvar anomalies are those that pose challenges to the assignment of gender at birth. Caution, sensitivity, complete evidence collection, and clear communication with often anxious family members are all required. A thorough evaluation may include careful physical examination, pelvic ultrasonography or magnetic resonance imaging (MRI), hormonal assays, karyotyping, and often consultation with specialists before a recommendation is made to the family about which gender would be better for rearing the newborn. In general, if there is suboptimal development of penile or scrotal structures, the infant should be assigned the female gender, because reconstructive surgery for females is much more likely to be successful.

Ambiguous genitalia can present with clitoromegaly, bifid clitoris, or midline fusion of the labioscrotal folds. **Clitoromegaly** in adult women is defined as being present when the product of the length of the clitoris and the width of its base exceeds 35 mm^2, or when the clitoral base exceeds 1 cm in diameter. At birth, clitoromegaly is determined by the relative size of the clitoris in relation to the other vulvar structures. **Clitoral agenesis** may result from the failure of the

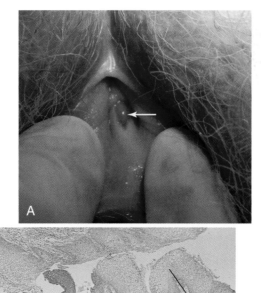

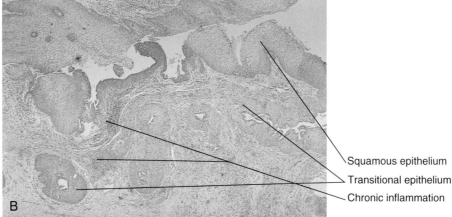

Squamous epithelium

Transitional epithelium

Chronic inflammation

FIGURE 18-3 Urethral caruncle *(arrow)*. **A,** This lesion usually presents as a small, painful, red lump at the urethral meatus. **B,** In this histologic example, transitional epithelium can be recognized and there is a papillomatous pattern involving small, neighboring glands. A little chronic inflammation is seen. (**A,** From Lemmi FO, Lemmi CAE: *Physical assessment findings* [CD-ROM], Philadelphia, 2009, Saunders.)

genital tubercle to develop. Incomplete development of the genitalia can result in a cloaca with no separation of the bladder and the vagina. Many of these defects are associated with other problems, such as bladder exstrophy.

Female pseudohermaphroditism is caused by in utero masculinization due to androgens from maternal or fetal congenital adrenal hyperplasia, androgen-producing tumors of the mother's ovary or adrenal glands, or the mother's use of exogenous androgens. Often the infant will present with ambiguous genitalia. The enlarged clitoris is the most conspicuous abnormality. Fusion of the labioscrotal folds can produce a hypospadiac urethral meatus and a malpositioned introitus, but the internal genital organs will be normal. **Male pseudohermaphroditism,** which most commonly results from mosaicism, may occur with varying degrees of virilization and müllerian development.

Androgen insensitivity syndrome (a form of male pseudohermaphroditism and formerly called testicular feminization) is a genetic deficiency of androgen receptors that results in a 46,XY infant developing female external genitalia and, later in life, secondary sexual characteristics. The syndrome may be complete or partial (Figure 18-4). In utero, müllerian-inhibiting hormone (MIH) is produced, which results in absence of the uterus and fallopian tubes. The vaginal depth is variable but seldom normal. The testes are usually located in the inguinal canals, labia, or abdomen (usually along the pelvic sidewalls) and should be removed after the young woman has experienced breast development, but before any malignant transformation of her gonads takes place. The higher body temperature in the areas where the male gonads are located is thought to play a role in this transformation. Surgical removal of gonadal tissue is recommended just after puberty in these women.

True hermaphroditism is rare. The affected child has some degree of both female and male development externally and internally; dual gonadal development occurs with either a combined ovotestes or separate gonads. The extent of masculinization depends on the relative amount of functioning testicular tissue and testosterone levels.

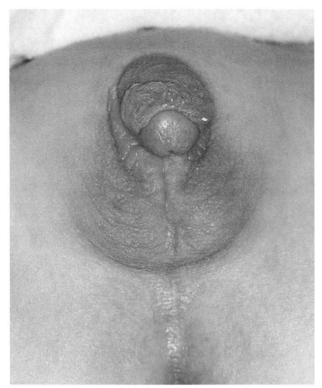

FIGURE 18-4 Ambiguous genitalia in a child with an XY karyotype and partial androgen insensitivity. (From McKay M: Vulvar manifestations of skin disorders. In Black M, McKay M, Braude P, et al, editors: *Obstetric and gynecologic dermatology,* ed 2, Edinburgh, 2003, Mosby, p 121.)

IATROGENIC ANATOMICAL CHANGES

Anatomical changes due to medical procedures are frequently encountered on the vulva. The most common relate to childbearing scars from episiotomies or obstetric lacerations, which can radiate posteriorly from the introitus to the rectum, anteriorly to the urethral meatus, or laterally into the labia. Other iatrogenic changes may be culturally dependent. **Female genital mutilation** (previously called female circumcision) has been performed on more than 130 million women worldwide and continues to be a common practice in many societies where the role of women is limited and an explicit demonstration of virginity is required for marriage. This practice is generally condemned in Western societies. Box 18-1 contains the World Health Organization (WHO) classification of the different types of female genital mutilation, in increasing severity.

Vagina

BENIGN CONDITIONS OF THE VAGINA

Epithelial Changes

The appearance of the vaginal walls varies greatly from one woman to another. In part, this is because the epi-

---

BOX 18-1

WORLD HEALTH ORGANIZATION (WHO) CLASSIFICATION OF FEMALE GENITAL MUTILATION

Type I—Partial or total removal of the clitoris and/or prepuce (clitoridectomy)

Type II—Partial or total removal of the clitoris and labia minora, with or without the excision of the labia majora (excision)

Type III—Narrowing of the vaginal orifice with creation of a covering seal by cutting and appositioning the labia minora and/or the labia majora, with or without excision of the clitoris (infibulation)

Type IV—All other harmful procedures to the female genitalia for nonmedical purposes; for example, pricking, piercing, incising, scraping, and cauterizing

---

thelium is very sensitive to estrogen. In well-estrogenized women, the epithelium is pink, moist, thickened, and folded into distensible rugae. Occasionally **papillomatosis** may occur in the vagina, appearing much like an extensive human papillomavirus (HPV) infection. In prepubescent girls, postmenopausal women, and estrogen-deficient reproductive aged women, the epithelium of the vagina is pale, flat, smooth, dry, and fragile. Such atrophy can be uncomfortable for women who attempt coitus, as well as for those who are not sexually active; for the latter, the thin, raw, dry characteristics of the atrophic epithelium can cause symptoms of burning or irritation. It can be particularly painful when a woman recommences sexual intercourse after a long period of abstinence. Lack of sexual intercourse will have altered the lining of the vagina and constricted its diameter. Acute traumatic injury can ensue. Such a woman will benefit greatly from prior topical estrogen therapy and use of a water-based lubricant during intercourse.

The epithelium of the vagina is also subject to **chemical irritants and contact dermatitis** with the use of various solutions for douching, allergic reactions to vaginal antibiotic or antimycotic creams, spermicides, or latex contraceptives. Table 18-2 lists the important vaginal conditions, along with clinical features and treatment options for them.

Ulceration and Fistulas

Most ulceration in the vagina is associated with acute infections, such as **herpes simplex** or **cytomegalovirus.** Vaginal **lichen planus** initially presents with small ulcerations and generalized, intense erythema, with densely packed leukocytes in the vaginal discharge. If left untreated, the vault can agglutinate and literally scar the vagina closed. The vaginal secretions irritate the vulva and cause an intense burning irritation in that area also.

Fistulas from the bladder into the vagina can form as a result of surgical complications, prolonged

TABLE 18-2

BENIGN CONDITIONS OF THE VAGINA

Epithelial Changes	Clinical Features and Comments	Treatment
Papillomatosis	Appears like human papillomavirus infection	Reassurance
Contact dermatitis	Chemical irritation due to the use of douching solutions; allergic reactions to antimicrobial creams, spermicides, or latex condoms	Identify irritant and discontinue
Ulcerations and Fistulas		
Ulcers	Most ulceration of the vagina is associated with acute infection due to herpes simplex or cytomegalovirus; vaginal lichen planus may present as ulcers	See Chapter 22 for diagnosis and treatment of infectious causes; topical steroids
Fistulas	Fistulas from the bladder or rectum into the vagina may occur due to surgical complication, infection, or malignancy	Surgical repair if conservative management unsuccessful unless due to advanced cancer
Cystic Masses		
Bartholin cyst	Cystic mass below hymenal ring at 4 or 8 o'clock; must rule out underlying malignancy in older women	If asymptomatic, no treatment; if symptomatic, consider drainage with Word catheter placement or marsupialization
Gartner duct cyst	Thick walled, soft cystic structures formed from remnants of the Wolffian duct; usually asymptomatic	Treatment is usually not needed; surgical removal if symptomatic or increasing in size
Other		
Traumatic injury	Vaginal injury during obstetric delivery, surgery, or sexual assault; attention to any hematoma progression	Surgical repair; sexual assault reporting protocol (see Chapter 29)
Dermatologic	Vaginal atrophy secondary to lower estrogen effect during pregnancy or after menopause; condyloma due to the papillomavirus; herpes simplex infection	Vaginal estrogen cream or systemic estrogen patch (menopause); removal or destruction of condyloma; antivirals for herpes simplex (see Chapters 22 and 35)
Vaginismus	Involuntary contraction of the muscles surrounding the vaginal introitus	Psychological cause takes extensive counseling; treat any underlying physical cause
Foreign objects	Objects placed and forgotten in the vagina; most common in young girls and older women who may have forgotten a pessary; vaginal bleeding and/or odor usually present	Removal; awareness of possible toxic shock syndrome (see Chapter 22)

pressure applied during labor, or malignancies. Fistulas from the bowel into the vagina can result from incomplete healing of fourth degree lacerations, surgical complications, malignancies, or granulomatous processes, such as tuberculosis or Crohn disease.

One unique lesion involves an acute and chronic inflammation of the vestibular glands found near the introitus, scattered around the hymen or hymenal tags. The lesion appears as a 1- to 3-mm red dot, which is extremely tender. This lesion is found in women with focal provoked **vulvodynia** (vestibulodynia). Careful inspection is often needed to locate these lesions. Gentle touch with a cotton tip swab will elicit significant pain, which confirms the diagnosis. The tenderness of this lesion may prevent not only intromission and any sexual intercourse, but also any speculum or digital examination.

Cystic Masses

As a thin epithelial structure, the vagina only infrequently develops significant benign masses. Thick-walled, soft cysts resulting from embryonic remnants can present in the vagina. **Gartner duct cysts** are the most common of these. They arise from the remnant of the Wolffian duct (mesonephros). They vary in size from 1 to 5 cm and are found on the anterolateral walls in the upper half of the vagina and more laterally in the lower half. Most are asymptomatic and require no treatment. They may be surgically removed when symptomatic.

Bartholin cysts start with occlusion of the Bartholin duct at the 4 and 8 o'clock positions of the vaginal introitus. The trapped mucinous secretions from the Bartholin gland accumulate and develop into a smooth, skin colored cystic structure ranging from 1 to 5 cm in diameter. Often they represent remnants of old Bartholin abscesses. Occasionally they may develop bilaterally. Digital examination of the duct underlying the cystic structure is important to rule out a malignant mass, particularly in an older woman who presents with a new Bartholin cyst. Treatment of these benign cysts is needed only if the woman is symptomatic (experiences pressure-like discomfort) or if there is a rapid change in the size or character of the cyst. Treatment can be with a Word catheter or by marsupialization (Figure 18-5). Cystectomy is rarely indicated.

Trauma

Injury to the vagina can occur at the time of delivery, during surgery, or more generally as a result of sexual assault. Large hematomas that dissect into the broad ligament or retroperitoneal space can contain liters of blood and cause profound anemia and even shock. Thorough examination is needed to rule out ongoing bleeding. Red, raised, friable granulation tissue can sometimes be seen along recent surgical scars, particularly at the apex of the vault following hysterectomy or along episiotomy scars postpartum.

Other Benign Abnormalities of the Vagina

Some dermatologic changes may occur due to the effect of lower estrogen levels on the vaginal epithelium during pregnancy or after the menopause. The resulting **atrophic vaginitis** may be treated with estrogen cream. Infectious lesions such as **vaginal warts** from HPV or **herpes simplex blisters** can affect the vaginal epithelium.

Vaginismus is an involuntary contraction of the muscles surrounding the introitus. It may have psychological and/or physical causes, but the contraction makes any vaginal penetration either extremely painful or impossible. Many women with vaginismus report prior sexual abuse, but others may deny any such

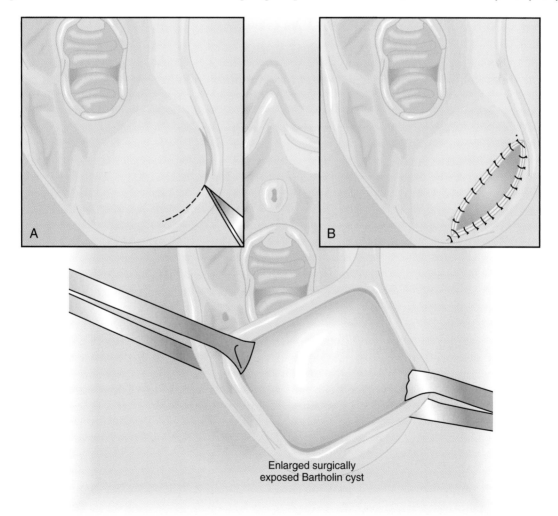

Enlarged surgically
exposed Bartholin cyst

FIGURE 18-5 Bartholin cysts are rarely removed, because of excessive bleeding that may occur. More commonly, they are drained by inserting a Word catheter or by marsupialization by first incising over the cyst **(A)** and then externalizing an opening to allow for drainage **(B)**. The cyst lining is sutured to the vaginal epithelium to create a drainage opening for cyst fluid.

trauma. It is important that the health care professional understands that vaginismus is an involuntary reaction much like the reflex to shut the eyelid when a foreign object is seen to be approaching. Voluntary control can be learned, but it takes much counseling and patience.

Foreign bodies can be forgotten in the vagina. Little girls may place small beads or paper into that pocket when they discover it. Older women may neglect to remove tampons, contraceptive devices, or pessaries. Generally, a strong odor and copious vaginal discharge compels them to seek professional help. Toxic shock syndrome must be ruled out. Removal of the foreign body, if necessary under general anesthesia, is the first step in therapy. Examination of the tissue for any abrasions, then vaginal irrigation can help shorten the recovery time.

Implants of **endometriosis** can occasionally be found arising from the vaginal walls. They may cause pain or they may be asymptomatic. These implants may respond to cyclic hormones (see Chapter 25). The anatomic changes associated with pelvic relaxation, including anterior vaginal wall prolapse **(cystocele)**, posterior vaginal prolapse **(rectocele)**, and herniation of bowel **(enterocele)**, are discussed in detail in Chapter 23.

CONGENITAL ABNORMALITIES OF THE VAGINA

Vaginal agenesis represents the most extreme instance of a vaginal anomaly, with total absence of the vagina except for the most distal portion that is derived from the urogenital sinus, which may appear as a dimple on the vulva. If the uterus is absent but the fallopian tubes are spared, the defect is **müllerian agenesis** or **Rokitansky-Küster-Hauser syndrome.** Isolated vaginal agenesis with normal uterine and fallopian tube development is rare, and is thought to be the end result of isolated vaginal plate malformation. The more common structural anomalies of the vagina include canalization defects such as **imperforate hymen, transverse and longitudinal vaginal septa, partial vaginal development, and double vagina.**

Imperforate hymen represents the mildest form of these canalization abnormalities. It occurs at the site where the vaginal plate contacts the urogenital sinus. After birth, a bulging, membrane-like structure may be noticed in the vestibule, usually blocking egress of mucus. If not detected until after menarche, an imperforate hymen may be seen as a thin, dark bluish or thicker, clear membrane blocking menstrual flow at the introitus (Figure 18-6, *A* and *B*). A similar anomaly, the **transverse vaginal septum,** is most commonly found

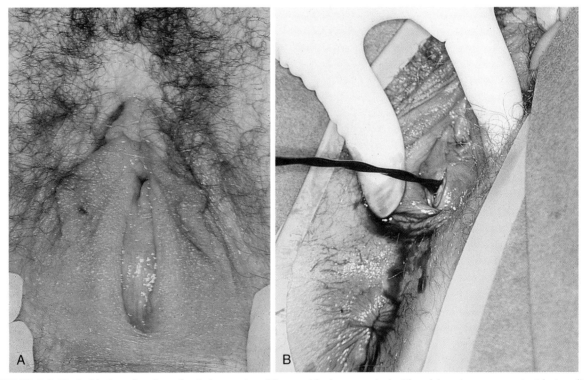

FIGURE 18-6 **A,** Vaginal bulge of an imperforate hymen in a 13-year-old who presented with pelvic pain, now constant but cyclical in the past. **B,** Old blood (hematocolpos) and some mucous (mucocolpos) is released after a stab incision is made through the hymen. (From McKay M: Vulvar manifestations of skin disorders. In Black M, McKay M, Braude P, et al, editors: *Obstetric and gynecologic dermatology,* ed 2, Edinburgh, 2003, Mosby, p 122.)

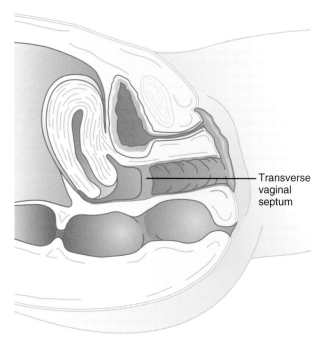

FIGURE 18-7 Illustration of a transverse vaginal septum.

at the junction of the upper and middle thirds of the vagina (Figure 18-7). Patients with an imperforate hymen or transverse vaginal septum usually have normal development of the upper reproductive tract.

A **midline longitudinal septum** may be present, creating a double vagina. The longitudinal septum may be only partially present at various levels in the upper and middle vagina, either in the midline or deviated to one side. In addition, a longitudinal septum may attach to the lateral vaginal wall, creating a blind vaginal pouch, with or without a communicating sinus tract. These septa are usually associated with a **double cervix** and one of the various duplication anomalies of the uterine fundus, although the upper tract is often entirely normal.

Adenosis of the vaginal wall consists of islands of columnar epithelium in the normal squamous epithelium. It is often located in the upper third of the vagina. The incidence of this finding is much higher in women exposed to diethylstilbestrol in utero.

Urethral diverticula are small (0.3 to 3 cm), sac-like projections that can be found along the posterior urethra in the midline of the anterior vaginal wall. They may or may not communicate with the urethra, and they may cause dyspareunia. Urethral diverticula can cause recurrent urinary tract infections (see Chapter 22).

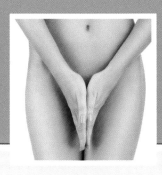

CHAPTER 19

Benign Conditions and Congenital Anomalies of the Uterine Corpus and Cervix

WILLIAM H. PARKER • JOSEPH C. GAMBONE

CLINICAL KEYS FOR THIS CHAPTER

- Uterine fibroids (also called leiomyomas) are benign smooth muscle tumors, and about 80% are asymptomatic. They are very common, with an estimated prevalence of 70% by the sixth decade of life. Uterine tumors presenting as fibroids are rarely malignant, with less than 1 in 1000 leiomyosarcomas found at the time of surgical removal. Fibroids may cause abnormal uterine bleeding, pelvic discomfort, and pressure when they enlarge. They can cause pain (sometimes severe) if degeneration and infarction occur.

- Fibroids arise within the myometrium (intramural) but may grow near the serosal surface (subserosal) or near the endometrium (submucosal). Some fibroids are pedunculated. About 40% of fibroids enlarge during the first trimester of pregnancy, but rarely thereafter.

- Medical treatment with progestins, gonadotropin-releasing hormone (GnRH) analogues, or other hormones may be indicated initially for uterine bleeding and

fibroid enlargement. Uterine artery embolization (UAE) and magnetic resonance directed ultrasound may be used as alternatives to surgery. Surgical treatment ranges from myomectomy (removal of one or several fibroids) for women who desire fertility or uterine preservation to hysterectomy when less invasive treatments fail.

- Endometrial and cervical polyps may cause uterine bleeding and must be biopsied to rule out cancer. Complex atypical endometrial hyperplasia progresses to endometrial cancer in about 20-30% of cases. Simple hyperplasia may be treated medically.

- Congenital anomalies of the uterus and cervix are most often due to incomplete fusion of the paramesonephric (müllerian) ducts, incomplete dissolution of the midline fusion of those ducts, or formation failures. Diagnosis of uterine defects can be made by hysterosalpingogram or magnetic resonance imaging. Some defects may be diagnosed and treated by hysteroscopy.

Congenital anomalies of the uterus and cervix are most often caused by incomplete fusion of the paramesonephric (müllerian) ducts, incomplete dissolution of the midline fusion of those ducts, or formation failures. Diagnosis of uterine defects can be made by hysterosalpingogram (HSG) or magnetic resonance imaging (MRI). Some defects may be diagnosed and treated by hysteroscopy.

Benign conditions of the uterine corpus and cervix are commonly encountered in gynecologic practice, because they may adversely affect a woman's fertility, cause abnormal uterine bleeding, or cause pelvic pain. In this chapter, benign neoplasms, epithelial changes, functional disorders of the uterus (corpus and cervix), and congenital anomalies are discussed along with both conventional and emerging therapies. Cervical dysplasia along with cervical cancer is covered in Chapter 38.

Benign Neoplastic Conditions

UTERINE FIBROIDS (LEIOMYOMAS)

Uterine fibroids are benign tumors derived from the smooth muscle cells of the myometrium. They are also referred to as leiomyomas or myomas, but "fibroid" is most often used today. Fibroids are the most common neoplasm of the uterus. Estimates are that more than 70% of women have fibroids by the age of fifty, but most are asymptomatic. However, **fibroids may be associated with heavy menstrual bleeding or infertility, pelvic pressure related to uterine bulk and, rarely, pain secondary to degeneration.** Fibroids are the primary indication for as many as one-third of the 500,000 hysterectomies performed in the United States each year. Although fibroids have the potential to grow to be large, **they rarely become malignant.** Leiomyosarcomas occur in less than 1 per 1000 women operated on for presumed fibroids. Rapid growth is not always a reliable sign of leiomyosarcoma.

Risk factors associated with developing fibroids include increasing age during the reproductive years, ethnicity, nulliparity, and family history. African American women have a 2- to 3-fold increased risk of developing fibroids compared with white women, and they may develop more numerous fibroids and at a younger age. Some studies have suggested that higher body mass index (BMI) may be associated with a greater risk of developing fibroids. In other studies, oral contraceptive pills have been associated with a reduced risk.

Pathogenesis of Fibroids

Factors that initiate fibroids are not known. **These benign growths are monoclonal, and about 40% are chromosomally abnormal.** The remaining 60% may have as yet undetected mutations or epigenetic changes. Genetic differences between fibroids and leiomyosarcomas indicate that leiomyosarcomas do not result from malignant degeneration of fibroids. Ovarian sex steroids, both estrogen and progesterone, are important for the growth of fibroids. Fibroids rarely develop before menarche and seldom develop or enlarge after menopause, unless stimulated by exogenous hormones. **Approximately 40% of fibroids enlarge during pregnancy.** Most of the growth occurs in the first trimester and they seldom interfere with the course of the pregnancy.

Fibroids have increased levels of estrogen and progesterone receptors compared with other smooth muscle cells. Estrogen stimulates the proliferation of smooth muscle cells, whereas progesterone increases the production of proteins that interfere with programmed cell death (apoptosis). Many growth factors are over-expressed in fibroids, including those that stimulate the production of fibronectin and collagen, both of which are major components of the extracellular matrix that characterizes fibroids. Other growth factors include those that increase smooth muscle proliferation and DNA synthesis, as well as those that promote mitogenesis and angiogenesis.

Characteristics of Fibroids

Fibroids are usually elliptical or spherical, well-circumscribed, white, firm lesions with a whorled appearance on cut section. Although the fibroid appears discrete, it does not have a true cellular capsule. Compressed smooth muscle cells on the tumor's periphery provide the false impression of a true capsule. **This pseudocapsule contains a rich network of blood vessels, but few blood vessels and lymphatics actually traverse the pseudocapsule into the fibroid.**

Fibroids can undergo degenerative changes, **most commonly hyaline acellularity,** in which the fibrous and muscular tissues are replaced with hyaline tissue. If the hyaline substance breaks down from a further reduction in blood supply, **cystic (fluid) degeneration may occur. Calcification may occur in degenerated fibroids,** particularly after the menopause. **Fatty degeneration may also occur** but is rare. **During pregnancy, 5-10% of women with fibroids undergo a painful red or carneous degeneration** caused by hemorrhage into the tumor.

Fibroids always arise within the myometrium **(intramural)** but may develop near the serosal surface **(subserosal)** or the endometrium **(submucosal),** as depicted in Figure 19-1. Fibroids very near the serosal or endometrial surfaces may develop pedicles. The submucosal fibroids can be propelled by uterine contractions until they extend through the endocervical canal and deliver through the cervical os. This process can be associated with significant bleeding and cramping pain. A subserosal fibroid on a long

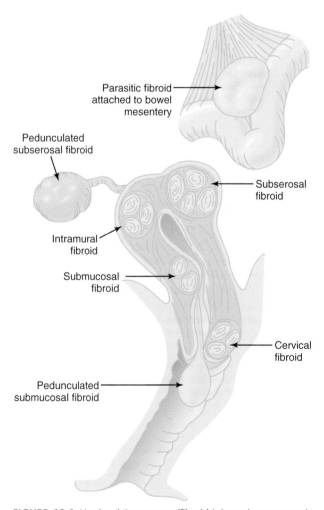

FIGURE 19-1 Uterine leiomyomas (fibroids) in various anatomic locations.

pedicle can present as a mass that feels separate from the uterus. MRI is often helpful to differentiate a pedunculated fibroid from other types of pelvic masses. Very rarely, pedunculated subserosal fibroids attach to the blood supply of the omentum or bowel mesentery and lose their uterine connections to become **parasitic growths.** Fibroids can also arise in the cervix, between the leaves of the broad ligament (intraligamentous), and very rarely in the various supporting ligaments (round or uterosacral) of the uterus.

Symptoms of Fibroids

The majority of uterine fibroids (approximately 80%) cause no symptoms. Occasionally, a woman may be able to feel a lower abdominal mass when the fibroid protrudes above the pelvis. For women with fibroids that are asymptomatic or mildly to moderately symptomatic, "watchful waiting" may allow treatment to be deferred, perhaps indefinitely. Symptomatic women **may complain of pelvic pressure, congestion, bloating, or a feeling of heaviness in the lower abdomen. Rarely, lower back pain may be associated with fibroids.** If the fibroid presses upon the bladder, it may cause frequency of urination or nocturia. A large fibroid in the lower uterine segment or near the cervix may compress the vesicourethral junction and lead to urinary retention. Compression of the ureters with resultant hydronephrosis is very rare and, if suspected, can be ruled out with a renal ultrasound.

Prolonged or heavy menstrual bleeding may be associated with submucosal fibroids. Growth factors secreted by fibroids interfere with the blood-clotting cascade. Intermenstrual bleeding is not characteristic of these tumors but may occasionally occur with submucosal fibroids ulcerating through the endometrial lining. Excessive bleeding may result in anemia, weakness, and even dyspnea.

Fibroids do not usually cause pain, but **severe pain may occur when degeneration (acute infarction) occurs within a fibroid.** Dyspareunia can occur with posterior fibroids near the vaginal cul-de-sac. There is an increased incidence of secondary dysmenorrhea in women with uterine fibroids, generally caused by heavy menstrual bleeding. Although many women with uterine fibroids become pregnant and carry their pregnancies to term, **submucosal fibroids may be associated with an increased incidence of infertility,** possibly due to growth factor secretion by the fibroid that may interfere with implantation.

Signs of Fibroids

Fibroids smaller than a 12- to 14-week gestation are usually confined to the pelvis, but larger fibroids can be palpated abdominally. Before examination, the bladder should be emptied because a full bladder will alter the examiner's impression of uterine size. **On bimanual pelvic examination, a firm, irregularly**

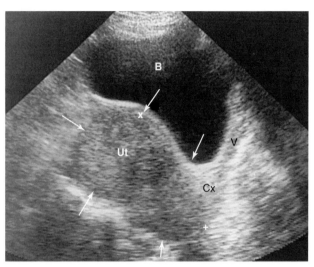

FIGURE 19-2 Ultrasonic image of a uterus enlarged and irregularly distorted by multiple fibroids *(arrows)*. Such studies are useful to help rule out ovarian enlargement too. *B*, Bladder; *Cx*, cervix; *Ut*, uterus; *V*, vagina. (From Mettler FA: *Essentials of radiology,* ed 2, Philadelphia, 2005, Saunders.)

enlarged uterus with smoothly rounded or bosselated protrusions may be felt if the fibroids are subserosal or intramural. The tumors are usually nontender, although degenerating fibroids can be tender to palpation. Their consistency may vary from rock hard, as in the case of a calcified postmenopausal leiomyoma, to soft or even cystic, as in the case of cystic degeneration. In general, the fibroid uterus is in the midline, but sometimes a large portion of the fibroid lies in the lateral aspect of the pelvis and may be indistinguishable from an adnexal mass. **If the mass moves with the cervix, it is suggestive of a fibroid.** Often the presence of a fibroid precludes a proper evaluation of the adnexa, but ultrasonic imaging, as seen in Figure 19-2, can help to distinguish adnexal masses from laterally placed fibroids.

Differential Diagnosis for Fibroids

Fibroids present as pelvic masses and thus the differential diagnosis is extensive and includes other uterine pathology. This includes adenomyosis (see Chapter 25), uterine sarcoma (rarely), and other pelvic processes, such as **an ovarian neoplasm, a tubo-ovarian inflammatory mass, a pelvic kidney, a diverticular or inflammatory bowel mass, or cancer of the colon.** Ultrasonography may be helpful to visualize the fibroids and identify normal ovaries apart from the fibroids. MRI is the most accurate way to diagnose uterine fibroids if the diagnosis is uncertain. Figure 19-3 shows the gross appearance of an irregularly enlarged uterus with multiple fibroids and Figure 19-4 is an MRI of a similarly deformed uterus preoperatively.

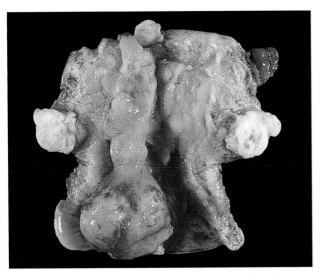

FIGURE 19-3 Gross appearance of an irregularly enlarged uterus with multiple fibroids. (From Voet RL: *Color atlas of obstetric and gynecologic pathology,* St Louis, 1997, Mosby.)

Management of Fibroids

In general, when asymptomatic fibroids are detected, treatment is not necessary. If the fibroid uterus is causing bothersome symptoms or is implicated as a cause of infertility in a woman seeking pregnancy, then some treatment is indicated. Traditionally, rapid growth has been listed as an indication for removal but recent studies show that rapid growth is not a reliable predictor of uterine sarcoma.

Medical Management

Heavy or prolonged menstruation presumed to be caused by fibroids can initially be managed hormonally in some cases. Many women with symptomatic fibroids are in the age group of women who may also have anovulation as the cause of the bleeding. **Progestin-only therapies** (oral or injected medroxyprogesterone acetate, progestin-only oral contraceptive pills, or levonorgestrel-releasing intrauterine devices) **or combination hormonal contraceptive methods** (oral contraceptive pills, vaginal rings, or patches) **are usually the first therapeutic option.** The goal is to reduce monthly menstrual blood loss with cyclic hormonal methods or to eliminate menses with extended or continuous use of these methods. Dysmenorrhea is also markedly reduced by these measures.

Gonadotropin-releasing hormone (GnRH) analogues (agonists and antagonists) block ovarian steroidogenesis, which reduces the volume of the myometrium and fibroids and stops menstrual bleeding. However, because of the intense vasomotor symptoms and the deleterious effect the GnRH-analogues may have on bone mineral density, only short courses

of these agents can be administered. Usually their use is confined to decreasing uterine size and/or increasing hemoglobin levels for women preparing for surgical treatments, such as endometrial ablation, myomectomy, or hysterectomy.

Surgical Management Options

When uterine fibroids are not amenable to the less invasive medical therapies, surgery or embolization should be considered (Table 19-1). Even after childbearing is complete, many women desire uterine preserving treatment for symptoms of fibroids. **Myomectomy should be considered as a safe alternative to hysterectomy.** Case-controlled studies suggest that there may be less risk of intraoperative injury to the bladder, bowel, and ureters with myomectomy when compared with hysterectomy.

The surgical approach depends on the size, number, and location of the various fibroids. MRIs are the best way to localize and estimate the volume of each fibroid, and to determine its position relative to the endometrium and other anatomical structures in the pelvis. Submucosal fibroids less than 5 cm may be resected at the time of hysteroscopy. Pedunculated, subserosal, and many intramural fibroids may be removed laparoscopically or with robotic assistance. Laparotomy is generally reserved for larger or more numerous tumors. If the endometrial cavity is entered during myomectomy, future births are usually recommended to be by cesarean delivery even though the risk of rupture is reported to be very low. In skilled hands, myomectomy may often avoid hysterectomy.

Although new fibroids may form following myomectomy, only 11% of women with three or fewer fibroids and about 25% of women with four or more fibroids will require a subsequent operation because of new fibroid growth. Less invasive techniques using laparoscopy and hysteroscopy for the removal of fibroids, including morcellation, have significantly reduced the hospital stay necessary for myomectomy as well as the morbidity associated with larger incisions and longer operating times. Although this may be of great benefit to the large majority of appropriate patients, any fast growing fibroid in a premenopausal woman or enlarging fibroid in a postmenopausal woman should be removed at open operation. At least, women in these two circumstances should be warned about the possibility of a sarcoma and the potential lethal dangers of spread caused by open morcellation.

For women desiring uterine preservation but not future fertility, surgical management of excessive bleeding is possible using procedures that ablate the endometrium. **With endometrial ablation, over 70% of women have a significant and satisfactory decrease in menstrual blood loss after one treatment, while others require repeat ablation or undergo hysterectomy. Uterine artery embolization (UAE) is a**

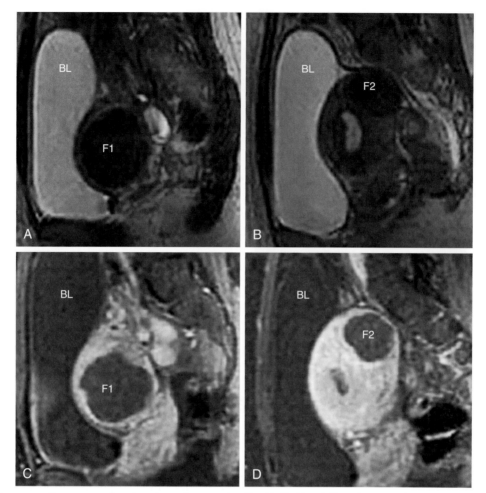

FIGURE 19-4 Two magnetic resonance imaging views of two uterine fibroids F1 (**A** and **C**) and F2 (**B** and **D**). Significant uterine deformity due to fibroids can result in symptoms such as abnormal uterine bleeding when the fibroids are submucosal (entering the uterine cavity) or pelvic pressure and a feeling of fullness. Large fibroids may put pressure on the bladder (BL) resulting in urinary frequency. Fibroids rarely cause pain except when they undergo degeneration (infarction). (From Bouwsma EV, Gorny KR, Hesley GK, et al: Magnetic resonance-guided focused ultrasound surgery for leiomyoma-associated infertility. *Fertil Steril* 96:e9-e12, 2011, Figure 1.)

TABLE 19-1

INTERVENTION FOR PATIENTS WITH FIBROIDS NOT AMENABLE TO MEDICAL THERAPY*

Clinical Presentation	Nonmedical Options	Comments
Desired fertility or uterine preservation	Myomectomy or uterine artery embolization (UAE)†	Usually used for a limited number of fibroids
Poor surgical risk	Endometrial ablation or UAE	UAE only for a limited number of fibroids
No desired fertility or uterine preservation	Endometrial ablation or hysterectomy	Hysterectomy is definitive therapy
Rapidly growing uterus (double in size in 6 months)	Exploratory laparotomy, abdominal hysterectomy	More extensive surgery if malignancy discovered

*Generally failed medical therapy or large (>12 to 14 weeks' gestational size) uterus.
†Pregnancies after UAE are at higher risk.

procedure performed under conscious sedation using microspheres or small coils introduced into the uterine artery via a transcutaneous femoral approach. These coils and/or particles occlude the artery feeding the fibroid, leading to necrosis of the myoma. Fibroids often shrink in volume, and bleeding is successfully reduced in 90% of women. After UAE is performed, pregnancy may still be possible, but there is a higher risk of placental complications (accreta), postpartum hemorrhage, premature delivery, and malpresentation.

Hysterectomy provides definitive therapy for uterine fibroids. Approximately 200,000 hysterectomies are done annually in the United States to treat fibroids. If the uterus is very large or bulky, laparotomy is generally the preferred approach. Vaginal hysterectomy or total laparoscopic hysterectomy are both excellent options for women with smaller uteri. If a woman desires a supracervical hysterectomy, the vaginal approach is not possible but laparoscopic supracervical hysterectomy may be used. Usually ovarian preservation is encouraged unless the woman is over age 60, or has risk factors for ovarian carcinoma (see Chapters 20 and 39).

Other technologies have been developed recently to offer newer treatment options. **Magnetic resonance-guided focused ultrasonography** (seldom used) produces energy that penetrates through soft tissue to produce regions of protein denaturation and necrosis, with minimal (20%) reduction of fibroid volume. **Radio frequency ablation** through a laparoscope, aided by intraoperative ultrasonic guidance, can also be used to treat individual fibroids.

ENDOMETRIAL POLYPS

Endometrial polyps (named for their shape and not their histology) form from the endometrium to create abnormal protrusions of friable tissue into the endometrial cavity. They can cause irregular menstrual bleeding during the reproductive years and postmenopausal bleeding after menopause. On ultrasound, endometrial polyps may appear as a focal thickening of the endometrial stripe. **They can be more clearly recognized on saline infusion sonography (SIS) or visualized directly by hysteroscopy** (see Figure 34-1). Endometrial polyps may evade detection by endometrial aspiration or dilation and curettage (D&C) because they are too large to be aspirated through the sampling orifice and are very flexible and can be pushed out of the path of the sharp curette. Histologic evaluation of the polyp is imperative, because although most are benign, endometrial hyperplasia, endometrial carcinoma, and carcinosarcomas may also present as polyps. Malignant or hyperplastic polyps are significantly more common in postmenopausal compared with premenopausal women (5% versus 2%), and more common in women with abnormal bleeding compared to those without bleeding (4% versus 2%).

Squamocolumnar junction

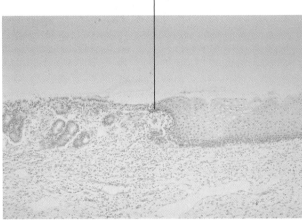

FIGURE 19-5 Squamocolumnar junction. In the "ideal" cervix, the original squamous epithelium abuts the columnar epithelium. The squamocolumnar junction thus formed may be situated at the external cervical os, but in most women of childbearing age, the original squamocolumnar junction is located on the vaginal portion of the cervix.

NORMAL CERVIX

At birth, a pale pink squamous epithelium covers the outer rim of the cervix. The inner region of the exocervix (or ectocervix) is covered with the taller columnar cells. The junction between the two is called the original squamocolumnar junction, as seen in Figure 19-5. The columnar epithelium appears redder because of the closer proximity of its underlying blood vessels to the surface. **With acidification of the vagina at menarche, the exocervix (or ectocervix) undergoes an accelerated rate of squamous metaplasia in a radial pattern, from the squamocolumnar junction inward, which produces the transformation zone.** A new squamocolumnar junction is formed that moves progressively up the endocervical canal (see Figure 38-1). Younger women are often found to have a reddish ring of tissue surrounding the os, which is sometimes called a **cervical ectropion,** but in reality, this is an area of columnar epithelium that has not yet undergone normal squamous metaplasia.

Under the influence of estrogen (birth control pills, pregnancy), the columnar epithelium of more mature women may evert and present as an ectropion that appears similar. The columnar cells produce mucus and are more vulnerable to trauma and infection with chlamydia. Therefore, **women with a cervical ectropion may notice more vaginal secretions and, occasionally, postcoital spotting.** Once other etiologies have been ruled out, no treatment is needed for the friable tissue.

Nabothian cysts on the cervix are so common that they are considered a normal variant. They result from

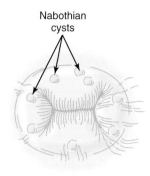

Nabothian cysts

FIGURE 19-6 Cervix of a multiparous woman with nabothian cysts.

the process of squamous metaplasia. A layer of superficial squamous epithelium entraps an invagination of columnar cells beneath its surface. The underlying columnar cells continue to secrete mucus, and a mucous retention cyst is created. Nabothian cysts are opaque, with a yellowish or bluish hue. They vary generally in size from 0.3 to 3 cm (Figure 19-6), although larger nabothian cysts have been reported.

CERVICAL POLYPS

Ectocervical and endocervical polyps are the most common benign neoplastic growths of the cervix. A polyp is a localized proliferation of cells (usually columnar) located in the endocervix. Endocervical polyps tend to the more beefy red in color and arise from the endocervical canal on a long, pedunculated stalk. Ectocervical polyps are less common, are generally pale, and arise from the exocervix (or ectocervix) to create a broad-based protrusion. Cervical polyps may be isolated or multiple and vary in diameter from a few millimeters to several centimeters. **If symptomatic, they most commonly cause coital bleeding or menorrhagia.** Narrow-based polyps are removed by twisting the polyp off at its base. Broader-based polyps may be better removed with cautery or other modalities that can control bleeding after removal. **Although the incidence of malignancy is very low (1% or less), both squamous cell carcinomas and adenocarcinomas can present as polyps.** All specimens must be sent for pathologic examination.

Trauma of the Uterine Corpus and Cervix

Most trauma to the uterus has an obstetric basis, such as uterine rupture from prolonged labor, caused by a Bandl ring, or rupture along a previous uterine scar. However, uterine perforation is also possible with operative procedures such as D&C, endometrial aspiration, or intrauterine contraceptive (IUC) placement.

Similarly, most trauma to the cervix occurs during vaginal delivery. The cervix can tear if the infant delivers through an incompletely dilated cervical os. Lacerations can also occur when instruments such as forceps are used for delivery or during gynecologic operations, such as cervical conization, hysteroscopy, or abortion. Trauma to the cervix can occur with sexual assault.

Epithelial Conditions of the Uterus

ENDOMETRIAL HYPERPLASIA

Endometrial hyperplasia represents an overabundant growth of the endometrium generally caused by persistent levels of estrogen unopposed by progesterone. **Hyperplasia is most frequently seen at the extremes of a woman's reproductive years when ovulation is infrequent.** It also occurs in association with unopposed estrogenic stimulation, such as the following:
1. **Polycystic ovarian syndrome (PCOS) and anovulation**
2. Estrogen-producing tumors such as **granulosa-theca cell tumors**
3. **Obesity** because of peripheral conversion of androgens to estrogen in adipose cells
4. Prolonged use of **exogenous estrogens** without progesterone or progestins
5. Use of **tamoxifen**

A spectrum of histologic variations exists. **There are two categories (simple hyperplasia and complex hyperplasia) and two subcategories (with and without atypia).** Complex atypical hyperplasia has the greatest malignant potential; about 20-30% of cases progress to endometrial carcinoma, if untreated. Figure 19-7 shows photomicrographs of normal proliferative endometrium, simple hyperplasia (without atypia), and complex hyperplasia with atypia.

Diagnosis

Endometrial hyperplasia should be suspected when women develop intermenstrual bleeding, or when high-risk women develop unexplained heavy or prolonged bleeding. In premenopausal women, endometrial sampling is necessary to obtain a histologic diagnosis, especially for women at high risk of hyperplasia (chronic anovulation, obesity, diabetes mellitus). Office endometrial biopsy is easy to perform, but fractional D&C or hysteroscopically directed biopsy may be needed to rule out carcinoma or other pathology. **Postmenopausal women who have bleeding can be evaluated with transvaginal ultrasound and a thin (<4 mm) endometrial stripe is reassuring. Those whose endometrial stripe is thicker should be sampled.**

Treatment

Treatment of simple hyperplasia in reproductive aged women without atypia generally consists of a thor-

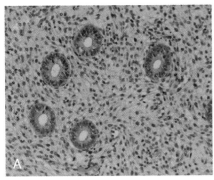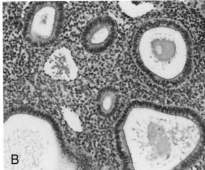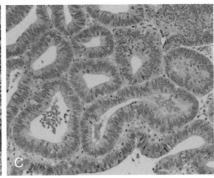

FIGURE 19-7 Endometrial biopsies of normal proliferative endometrium (A), simple endometrial hyperplasia without atypia (B), and complex endometrial hyperplasia with cellular atypia (C). (From Espindola D, Kennedy KA, Fischer EG: Management of abnormal uterine bleeding and the pathology of endometrial hyperplasia. *Obstet Gynecol Clin North Am* 34:717-737, 2007.)

ough, coordinated sloughing of the hyperplastic endometrium and therapies directed at preventing recurrence. **Simple hyperplasia without atypia should be treated initially with a progestin, such as 10 days each month for 3 months,** then biopsy should be repeated to confirm normalization of the endometrium. **Complex hyperplasia must be evaluated with a fractional D&C and should be initially treated with daily progestin therapy for 3 to 6 months. The levonorgestrel intrauterine system may also be successful in reversing hyperplasia. Test of cure with another biopsy is then needed.** In the longer run, a source of progestin must be supplied. **Complex hyperplasia with atypia is best treated by hysterectomy** once carcinoma has been excluded. **Endometrial ablation is absolutely contraindicated in any of these situations until the endometrium normalizes.**

ASHERMAN SYNDROME

Asherman syndrome is a condition where the endometrium is denuded and the endometrial cavity is filled with adhesions. Most commonly, the scarring results from curettage in high-risk settings, such as postpartum hemorrhage or septic abortion, although vigorous scraping under any circumstances can result in the loss of the endometrium and consequent adhesion of opposing myometrial surfaces. Endometrial ablation procedures are designed to deliberately destroy the endometrium and create such scarring. Subsequent bleeding disorders can range from irregular bleeding to amenorrhea depending on the amount of intrauterine scarring.

Functional Conditions of the Uterine Corpus and Cervix

Noncongenital cervical stenosis usually arises after trauma (endocervical curettage, conization) or **hypoestrogenism** (menopause, prolonged depot medroxyprogesterone acetate [MPA] use). Problems arise if blood from the endometrium cannot escape into the vagina, in which case the uterus becomes grossly distended **(hematometra).** Similarly, sperm may be less likely to enter the upper genital tract. Cervical stenosis may also compromise cervical sampling for microscopic evaluation.

Cervical incompetence is a condition in which the cervix is unable to maintain closure under the pressure of a progressively enlarging pregnant uterus and painlessly dilates, resulting in pregnancy loss, most commonly in the second trimester (see Chapter 12). **Cervical incompetence may be intrinsic** (caused by poor ground substance in the cervix), or **the result of cervical surgery** (especially loop electrosurgical excision procedure [LEEP] and cold knife conization) for cervical dysplasia.

Congenital Anomalies of the Uterine Corpus and Cervix

The upper vagina, cervix, uterine corpus, and fallopian tubes are formed from the paramesonephric (müllerian) ducts. **The absence of a Y chromosome and the resultant absence of müllerian inhibiting substance lead to the development of the paramesonephric system, with the regression of the mesonephric system.** The paramesonephric ducts first arise at 6 weeks lateral to the cranial pole of the mesonephric duct and expand caudally. By 9 to 10 weeks, they fuse in the midline at the urogenital septum to form the uterovaginal primordium. Later, dissolution of the septum between the fused paramesonephric ducts leads to the development of a single uterus and cervix.

The most common anomalies of the uterus result from either incomplete fusion of the paramesonephric ducts, incomplete dissolution of the midline

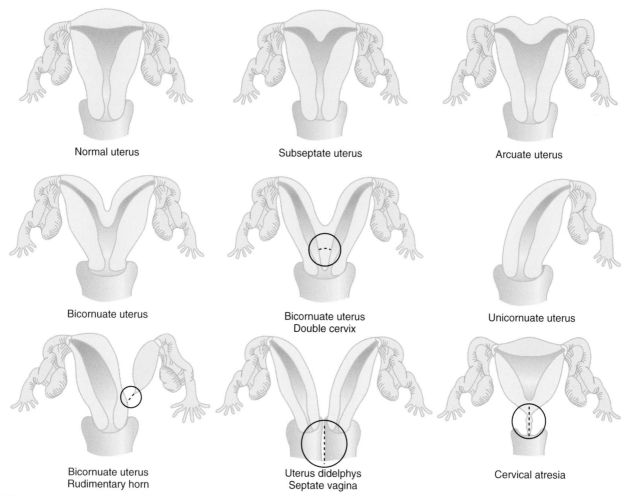

FIGURE 19-8 Variations in uterine development. The *dotted lines within circles* represent potential sites of communication or obstruction.

fusion of those ducts, or formation failures. Figure 19-8 shows variations of the uterine and cervical development and demonstrates that communication between the dual systems can exist at several levels. Failure of fusion is most evident in **uterus didelphys,** which presents with two separate uterine bodies, each with its own cervix and attached fallopian tube and vagina. **A bicornuate uterus with a rudimentary horn** also represents a fusion failure. Less complete fusion failure is seen in the **bicornuate uterus with or without double cervices.** Incomplete dissolution of the midline fusion of the paramesonephria explains the **septate uterus.** Failure of formation can be seen in the **unicornuate uterus. In müllerian agenesis, there is complete lack of development of the paramesonephric system.** The affected woman generally has an incomplete development of the fallopian tubes associated with the absence of the uterus and most of the vagina. All of these conditions occur in normal karyotypic and phenotypic females, but can be associated with important anomalies of the urinary system such as a horseshoe or pelvic kidney.

The most common congenital cervical anomalies are the result of malfusion of the paramesonephric (müllerian) ducts with varying degrees of separation, as seen in the didelphys cervix or septate cervix.

These different anatomies may have a significant effect on a woman's risk of infertility and early pregnancy loss, and may also cause dysmenorrhea and dyspareunia. Women with fusion anomalies may present with menstrual blood trapped in a noncommunicating uterine horn or vagina.

In addition to these macroscopic differences, subtle anomalies may exist within the uterine vascular system, such as an **arteriovenous malformation,** rupture of which may cause life-threatening hemorrhage.

Although all of these anomalies can occur spontaneously, they may also be caused by early maternal exposure to certain drugs. Historically, the most notable of these drugs is diethylstilbestrol (DES), which increases the risk of a small T-shaped endometrial cavity or cervical deformity.

DIAGNOSIS AND TREATMENT OF CONGENITAL ANOMALIES

Certain congenital anomalies of the uterus may need to be treated, especially if they are thought to be interfering with normal function, fertility, or causing other symptoms. The diagnosis of intrauterine defects can be made by imaging studies such as HSG or MRI, and may be suspected at the time of laparoscopy because of visualized uterine distortion. Hysteroscopy may be performed to both diagnose and treat defects such as the resection of a uterine septum. A bicornuate uterus can be repaired laparoscopically by performing a metroplasty, thereby creating one functional uterine cavity (see Chapter 31).

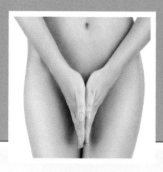

CHAPTER 20

Benign Conditions and Congenital Anomalies of the Ovaries and Fallopian Tubes

WILLIAM H. PARKER • JOSEPH C. GAMBONE

CLINICAL KEYS FOR THIS CHAPTER

- The adnexa are composed of the ovaries and fallopian tubes, along with the blood vessels, ligaments, and connective tissues located along both sides of the uterus. Benign ovarian masses may be classified as functional, inflammatory, metaplastic, or neoplastic. Functional cysts are the most common masses and almost always resolve spontaneously. Differentiating between benign and malignant ovarian masses is extremely important and can be challenging.

- A risk assessment tool, the Risk of Malignancy Index (RMI), may be used to help determine the likelihood that ovarian masses are malignant. Nonmalignant masses are generally unilateral, cystic (without solid components), mobile, and without ascites. CA-125 tumor marker levels are usually normal but false positives may occur. Benign ovarian neoplasms are divided into three cell types: epithelial, stromal, and germ-cell.

- The most common ovarian neoplasm in the premenopausal woman is the benign cystic teratoma or dermoid cyst which is a germ-cell type of tumor. In postmeno-

pausal women serous cyst adenomas are the most common. Management of ovarian masses ranges from observation and ultrasonographic follow-up for presumed functional cysts, to surgical removal. Laparoscopic cystectomy is appropriate for cystic masses that are considered very low risk for malignancy after appropriate evaluation.

- Recent evidence suggests that some ovarian cancers may actually originate in the fallopian tubes. Benign neoplasms of the tubes include epithelial adenomas and polyps, myomas from the tubal musculature, inclusion cysts, and angiomas. Paraovarian cysts are usually located within the broad ligament.

- Congenital anomalies of the ovaries are uncommon. Absence, duplication, and ectopic location of ovarian tissue, as well as supernumerary ovaries may occur. Rarely, an ovatestis (ovarian and testicular tissue) may be present, resulting in intersex problems. Turner syndrome (45 XO) is characterized by rudimentary streak gonads.

The ovaries and fallopian tubes, along with the blood vessels, ligaments, and connective tissues located along both sides of the uterus, are referred to as the adnexa. In this chapter, after presenting the recommended workup and management of benign adnexal masses, the abnormal development and congenital anomalies of the ovaries and fallopian tubes are discussed.

Benign Conditions of the Ovaries

The human ovary is prone to develop a wide variety of tumors, the majority of which are benign. **Ovarian cysts are common, with a reported clinical prevalence of 15% in premenopausal and 8% in postmenopausal women.** Most of these cysts resolve over time without treatment. As indicated in Table 20-1, ovarian masses

may be functional, inflammatory, metaplastic, or neoplastic. **During the childbearing years, 70% of noninflammatory benign ovarian tumors are functional.** The remainder are either neoplastic (20%) or metaplastic (endometriomas, accounting for 10%).

The management of ovarian tumors, whether functional, benign, or malignant, involves difficult decisions that may affect a woman's hormonal status or her future fertility. Although only functional cysts and benign ovarian neoplasms are considered in detail in this chapter, diagnostic methods to differentiate benign masses from malignant ones are discussed.

FUNCTIONAL OVARIAN CYSTS AND TUMORS

Dozens of ovarian follicles form the "cohort of follicles" of each menstrual cycle. It is from this cohort that usually only one dominant follicle will fully develop to

TABLE 20-1

DIFFERENTIAL DIAGNOSIS OF OVARIAN MASSES

Pathogenesis	Specific Type
Functional	Follicular cysts Corpus luteal cysts Theca-luteal cysts Polycystic ovaries (multiple follicular cysts)
Inflammatory	Salpingo-oophoritis Pyogenic oophoritis—puerperal, abortal, or intrauterine device–related Granulomatous oophoritis
Metaplastic	Endometriomas
Neoplastic	Premenarchal years—10% are malignant Menstruating years—15% are malignant Postmenopausal years—50% are malignant

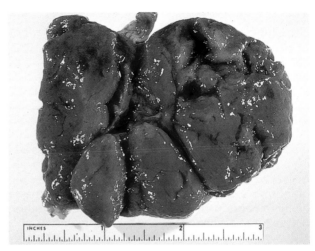

FIGURE 20-1 Gross appearance of a luteoma of pregnancy. Note the multiple brown nodules. (From Voet RL: *Color atlas of obstetric and gynecologic pathology*, St Louis, 1997, Mosby.)

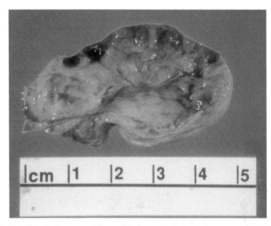

FIGURE 20-2 Ovary with multiple cysts lining the capsule consistent with polycystic ovarian syndrome. (Courtesy Dr. Sathima Natarajan, Ronald Reagan—UCLA Medical Center.)

about 2 cm in size in each cycle (see Chapter 4). If ovulation occurs, the remaining follicle becomes the corpus luteum. Functional cysts, including follicular and corpus luteal cysts, may appear from time to time as part of the normal function of the ovary. **To be classified a "functional cyst," the follicle must reach a diameter of at least 3 cm.** Functional cysts may cause a dull sensation or heaviness in the pelvis or, occasionally, pelvic pain.

A **follicular cyst,** lined by one or more layers of granulosa cells, develops when an ovarian follicle fails to rupture. Similarly, **a corpus luteal cyst** may develop if the corpus luteum grows to over 3 cm and fails to regress normally after 14 days. **Hemorrhagic cysts** form when invasion of ovarian vessels into the corpus luteal cyst 2 to 3 days after ovulation causes bleeding within the cyst. Hemorrhagic corpus luteal cysts are more likely to cause symptoms and, on occasion, rupture.

Other specific types of lutein cysts may occur in association with abnormally high serum levels of human chorionic gonadotropin (hCG) or increased ovarian sensitivity to gonadotropins. **Theca-luteal cysts may develop in association with the high levels of hCG present in patients with a hydatidiform mole or choriocarcinoma. Patients undergoing ovulation induction with gonadotropins, clomiphene, or letrozole may also develop theca-lutein cysts.** Theca-lutein cysts are usually bilateral, may become quite large (>30 cm), and characteristically regress slowly after the gonadotropin level falls. Rarely, when follicles are stimulated with gonadotropins, theca-lutein cysts can become so extensive as to cause massive ascites and dangerous problems with systemic fluid imbalance. This condition is referred to as **ovarian hyperstimulation syndrome** or OHSS (see Chapter 34).

A **luteoma of pregnancy** is a related condition in which there is a hyperplasic reaction of ovarian theca cells, presumably from prolonged hCG stimulation during pregnancy. The luteomas characteristically appear as brown to reddish-brown nodules that may be cystic or solid. A luteoma of pregnancy (Figure 20-1) may be associated with multifetal pregnancies or hydramnios. **They can cause maternal virilization in 30% of women** and, less often, ambiguous genitalia in a female fetus. Although ovarian enlargement may be impressive, surgical resection is not indicated, because **luteomas regress spontaneously postpartum.**

Polycystic ovarian syndrome, a functional disorder generally associated with chronic anovulation, hyperandrogenism, and insulin resistance, can also produce enlarged ovaries with multiple simple follicles (Figure 20-2). The hormonal aspects and treatment of this syndrome are discussed further in Chapter 33.

Clinical Features

An ovarian follicular cyst is usually asymptomatic, but a patient may present with delayed menses, abnormal uterine bleeding, or pelvic pain. Occasionally, a functional cyst may undergo **torsion** (see below) or it may **rupture,** which may produce acute lower abdominal pain and tenderness and the differential diagnosis must include ectopic pregnancy, pelvic abscess, or adnexal torsion of an ovarian neoplasm. Occasionally, a significant **hemoperitoneum** may be present.

Most follicular cysts are unilocular ("simple"), and rarely can be as large as 15 cm in diameter. Regression usually occurs during the subsequent menstrual cycles. In general, **a corpus luteal cyst** is apt to be smaller but more firm or even solid in consistency, and **is more likely to cause pain or signs of peritoneal irritation.** Because it may continue to produce progesterone, it is also more likely to cause delayed menses.

Diagnosis

The presumptive diagnosis of a functional ovarian cyst is usually made when a 5- to 8-cm cystic adnexal mass is noted on bimanual examination and imaged with transvaginal ultrasonography; it is confirmed when the lesion regresses over the course of the next several cycles. **In general, a functional cyst is mobile, unilateral, and not associated with ascites.** On rare occasions, the mass may exceed 8 cm and be quite tender to palpation. Occasionally, hemorrhagic corpus luteal cysts may have a solid rather than a cystic consistency, and can be confused with ovarian cancer.

Masses that are suspicious for malignancy are more solid, fixed, and irregular, and they may be bilateral. Any adnexal mass found in the presence of ascites or an upper abdominal mass should be considered malignant until proven otherwise, unless the patient has hyperstimulation syndrome.

Table 20-2 lists the current modalities that are available to evaluate adnexal masses along with the sensitivity and specificity as calculated by the U.S. Agency for Healthcare Research and Quality (AHRQ). None of these modalities is accurate enough to be used alone for diagnosis.

A pelvic ultrasound will confirm the cystic nature of the mass, but it cannot differentiate with certainty between a functional and a neoplastic tumor. Table 20-3 contains a risk assessment tool that can be useful for evaluating suspicious adnexal masses in pre- and postmenopausal women. It is called the **Risk of Malignancy Index** or **RMI.** CA-125 levels may be "falsely" elevated in some premenopausal women with endometriosis or fibroids as well as other benign conditions, and assay numbers for CA-125 may vary among laboratories. For these reasons **the RMI should be interpreted carefully, particularly in premenopausal patients.**

A follow-up ultrasound should be performed 6 weeks after the initial ultrasound. A cyst that enlarges and increases in complexity should be considered suspicious. Based upon a recent large study of over 30,000 women, cysts that do not enlarge or increase in complexity may be followed with ultrasound every few months until stability is documented, and then frequent follow-up imaging may be safely discontinued. According to the study findings, care for clinical judgment must occur because the adverse consequences of delayed diagnosis of ovarian cancer is significant.

Management

If the RMI is low and the cyst is considered to be functional, it is appropriate to **wait and reexamine the patient after her next menses.** Low-dose contraceptive agents may be given to suppress gonadotropin

TABLE 20-2

MODALITIES FOR THE EVALUATION OF ADNEXAL MASSES		
Modality	Sensitivity (%)	Specificity (%)
Gray-scale transvaginal ultrasonography (UTX)	0.82-0.91	0.68-0.81
Doppler UTX	0.86	0.91
Computed tomography	0.90	0.75
Magnetic resonance imaging	0.91	0.88
Positron emission tomography	0.67	0.79
CA-125 level measurement	0.78	0.78

Data from Agency for Healthcare Research and Quality (AHRQ): *Management of adnexal mass,* AHRQ Publication No. 06-E004, Rockville, MD, 2006, AHRQ.

TABLE 20-3

CALCULATION OF THE RISK OF MALIGNANCY INDEX FOR AN OVARIAN MASS	
Criteria	Scoring System
A. Menopausal Status	
Premenopausal	1
Postmenopausal	3
B. Ultrasonic Features	
Multiloculated	1 feature = 1
Solid areas Bilaterality Ascites	2 or more features = 3
C. Serum CA-125 titer	Absolute value (normal = <35 U/mL)

Data from Jacobs I, Oram D, Fairbanks J, et al: A risk of malignancy index incorporating CA 125, ultrasound and menopausal status for the accurate preoperative diagnosis of ovarian cancer. *Br J Obstet Gynaecol* 97:922, 1990.
Risk of Malignancy Index = A × B × C.
A Risk of Malignancy Index (RMI) score of >200 will discriminate a benign from a malignant mass with a sensitivity of 87% and a specificity of 97%.

levels and to prevent development of another cyst which may confuse the evaluation.

If the lesion does not fulfill the requirements for observation because it is solid, painful, fixed, or has an elevated RMI, surgical exploration and/or referral to a gynecologic oncologist is indicated. In a premenopausal woman laparoscopic cystectomy to allow histologic evaluation may be needed to differentiate between a functional and a neoplastic ovarian cyst. **Aspiration of the fluid as a diagnostic tool is inappropriate because the false-negative rate for the cytologic examination is high and slow leakage of the fluid will disseminate cancer if the cyst is malignant.**

BENIGN NEOPLASTIC OVARIAN TUMORS

Ovarian neoplasms may be divided generally by cell type of origin into three main groups: epithelial, stromal, and germ-cell. Taken as a group, the epithelial tumors are by far the most common, although **the single most common benign ovarian neoplasm in a premenopausal woman is the benign cystic teratoma (dermoid cyst),** which is a germ-cell tumor. Interestingly, the aggressive form of serous "ovarian" cancer has been shown to originate frequently from the fallopian tubes (see Chapter 39).

Epithelial Ovarian Neoplasms

These tumors are believed to be derived from the mesothelial cells lining the surface of the ovary and also lining the peritoneal cavity. A mucinous ovarian neoplasm cytologically resembles the endocervical epithelium, an endometrioid neoplasm resembles the endometrium, and serous tumors resemble the lining of the fallopian tubes. The most common epithelial ovarian tumors are serous cystadenomas. Figure 20-3, *A* and *B* shows the gross appearance of a mucinous (A) and serous (B) cystadenoma.

Each of the epithelial ovarian neoplasms has characteristic clinical and histologic features. The serous tumors are bilateral in about 10% of cases. **Of all serous tumors, about 70% are benign, 5-10% have borderline malignant potential, and 20-25% are malignant,** depending largely on the patient's age. Larger serous cystadenomas tend to be multilocular, although small unilocular serous cystomas also occur. Histologically, serous tumors characteristically form **psammoma bodies** (from the Greek *psammos*, meaning sand), which are calcific, concentric concretions. Psammoma bodies occur occasionally in benign serous neoplasms and frequently in serous cystadenocarcinomas. Papillary patterns are also common.

The mucinous neoplasms of the ovary can attain a huge size, often filling the entire pelvis and abdomen. They are often multilocular, and benign mucinous tumors are bilateral in less than 10% of cases. **About 85% of mucinous tumors are benign.** Mucinous tumors are often associated with a mucocele of the appendix. **Rarely, a benign mucinous tumor may be complicated by pseudomyxoma peritonei,** a condition in which a great many benign implants are seeded onto the surface of the bowel and other peritoneal surfaces and produce large quantities of mucus.

The **Brenner tumor** is a small, smooth solid ovarian neoplasm, usually benign, with a large fibrotic component that encases epithelioid cells that resemble transitional cells of the bladder (Figure 20-4). In about 33% of cases, Brenner tumors are associated with mucinous epithelial elements.

Sex Cord–Stromal Ovarian Neoplasms

These tumors include thecomas, granulosa-theca cell tumors, Sertoli-Leydig cell tumors, and fibromas. Combinations of granulosa-theca cell and Sertoli-Leydig cell tumors are termed gynandroblastomas.

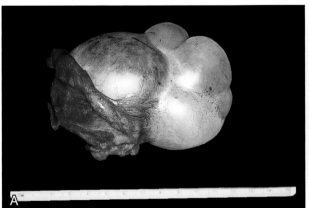
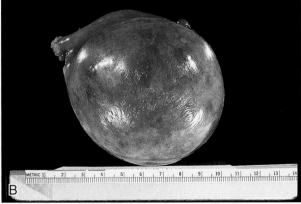

FIGURE 20-3 Gross appearance of a mucinous (**A**) and serous (**B**) cystadenoma of the ovary. The mucinous type is generally multiloculated and can be quite large. (**A,** From Voet RL: *Color atlas of obstetric and gynecologic pathology,* St Louis, 1997, Mosby, Figure 6-31; **B,** from Voet RL: *Color atlas of obstetric and gynecologic pathology,* St Louis, 1997, Mosby, Figure 6-20.)

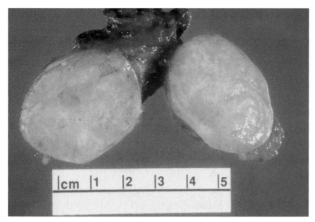

FIGURE 20-4 Gross appearance of a cut-open Brenner tumor. (Courtesy Dr. Sathima Natarajan, Ronald Reagan—UCLA Medical Center.)

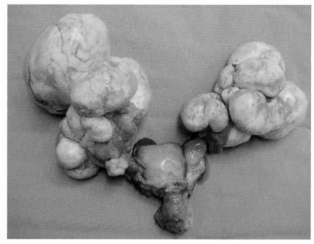

FIGURE 20-5 Bilateral ovarian fibromas in a surgical specimen with the uterus (corpus and cervix) in the middle. (Courtesy Dr. Neville Hacker.)

The tumors in this category derive from the sex cords and specialized stroma of the developing gonad. The embryologic origins of granulosa and theca cells as well as their counterparts in the testes, the Sertoli and Leydig cells, arise from cells that make up this specialized gonadal stroma. If the ultimate differentiation of cell types occurring in the tumor is feminine, the neoplasm becomes a **granulosa-cell tumor,** a **theca-cell tumor,** or in many instances, a **mixed granulosa-theca cell tumor.** Neoplasms containing cells that take on a masculine differentiation become **Sertoli-Leydig cell tumors.** This is far less common.

The **granulosa-theca cell neoplasms as well as their androgenic counterparts are generally referred to as functioning (not functional) ovarian tumors.** They occur in any age group, from birth on, but more commonly in the postmenopausal years. Their functioning characteristics are responsible for a variety of associated presenting signs and symptoms. **The granulosa-theca cell tumors promote feminizing signs and symptoms,** such as precocious menarche, precocious thelarche, or premenarchal uterine bleeding during infancy and childhood. In the reproductive years, menorrhagia (with alternating amenorrhea), endometrial hyperplasia, and, not infrequently, endometrial cancer, breast tenderness, and fluid retention occur. Postmenopausal bleeding may occur in older women with granulosa theca cell tumors.

In contrast, **the less frequent Sertoli-Leydig cell tumors are responsible for virilizing effects,** such as hirsutism, temporal baldness, deepening of the voice, clitoromegaly, and a defeminizing change in body habitus to a muscular build. Fifteen percent of these tumors produce no obvious endocrinologic effects. **Except for the pure thecoma or fibroma, all of these tumors have low malignant potential** and are discussed further in Chapter 39.

The **ovarian fibroma,** another ovarian stromal tumor, forms a solid, encapsulated smooth-surfaced tumor made up of interlacing bundles of fibrocytes. It is not hormonally active. The **fibroma** represents a stromal cell neoplasm developing from mature fibroblasts in the ovarian stroma. Figure 20-5 illustrates a gross surgical specimen of bilateral ovarian fibromas. On occasion, this tumor is associated with ascites caused by the transudation of fluid from the ovarian tissue. The flow of this ascitic fluid through the transdiaphragmatic lymphatics into the right pleural cavity may result in **Meigs syndrome** (ascites and hydrothorax in association with an ovarian fibroma). These effusions will spontaneously resolve when the fibroma has been removed. The ovarian fibroma may be associated with theca-cell elements called a fibrothecoma.

Germ-Cell Tumors

Germ-cell neoplasms can occur at any age. They make up about 60% of ovarian neoplasms occurring in infants and children.

The most common ovarian neoplasm in the premenopausal woman is the benign cystic teratoma, a germ-cell tumor that can take on a great variety of forms with virtually all adult tissues being represented within the mass (Figure 20-6). Ten to 15% of teratomas are bilateral. The benign cystic teratoma, commonly referred to as a dermoid cyst, is composed primarily of ectodermal tissue (such as sweat and sebaceous glands, hair follicles, and teeth), with some mesodermal and rarely endodermal elements.

These are slow-growing tumors and half the tumors are diagnosed in women between 25 and 50 years of age. Most are less than 10 cm in diameter. Because of the oily secretion of the sebaceous glands, the desquamated squamous cells, the presence of hair, and the

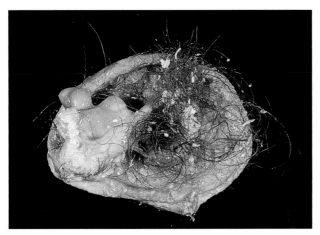

FIGURE 20-6 Gross appearance of a cut-open dermoid cyst. Note the presence of hair-bearing skin. (From Voet RL: *Color atlas of obstetric and gynecologic pathology,* St Louis, 1997, Mosby.)

presence of a dermoid tubercle (of Rokitansky), which often contains a hard, well-formed tooth, the dermoid cyst has a characteristic gross and histologic appearance (see Figure 20-6). **These tissues also have a characteristic appearance on ultrasonography,** usually allowing a preoperative diagnosis. Other tissue components commonly found in benign cystic teratomas include mature brain, bronchus, thyroid, cartilage, intestine, bone, and carcinoid cells. As opposed to similar tissues found in a malignant immature teratoma, the tissues making up the benign (mature) teratoma are all of an adult, well-differentiated form.

Mixed Ovarian Neoplasms

The most common ovarian tumor in which the neoplastic elements are composed of more than one cell type is the **cystadenofibroma,** or the fibrocystadenoma. These tumors generally take their characteristics from the epithelial component, although they tend to be more solid than the epithelial ovarian neoplasms.

The **gonadoblastoma** is a tumor composed of cells resembling those of a dysgerminoma and others resembling granulosa and Sertoli cells. Characteristically, calcific concretions are a prominent feature of this neoplasm. **Almost all patients with a gonadoblastoma have dysgenetic gonads, and a Y chromosome has been detected in more than 90% of cases.** Although the gonadoblastoma is initially benign, about half of these tumors may predispose to the development of dysgerminomas or other malignant germ-cell tumors.

Diagnosis of Benign Ovarian Tumors

The clinical features of benign ovarian tumors are often nonspecific. Except for the functioning ovarian neoplasms, **most benign ovarian tumors are asymptomatic unless they are larger than 6 to 8 cm.** They usually enlarge very slowly, so that an increase in abdominal girth or pressure on surrounding organs is not perceived until the later stages of growth.

Any pelvic pain is generally mild and intermittent, unless the tumor twists on its pedicle (torsion), when infarction may induce severe pain and tenderness. On rare occasions, **an ovarian cyst may rupture spontaneously from internal hemorrhage or intracystic pressure,** resulting in pain and peritoneal irritation. A cyst may also rupture occasionally during or following a bimanual pelvic examination or with intercourse. Depending on the cystic contents, pain of varying degrees of severity can result. The escape of thin serous fluid without hemorrhage may evoke some pain or tenderness, but the oily contents of a dermoid cyst or the thick mucinous fluid of a mucinous cystadenoma are irritating to both the parietal and the visceral peritoneum, and can lead to chemical peritonitis and severe pain. Without surgical treatment and irrigation and suctioning of the fluid, the peritonitis can lead to the subsequent formation of pelvic adhesions.

Bimanual pelvic examination generally indicates the presence of the mass in the pelvis, but it may be too small to be palpated. On the other hand, if the mass is large enough, it may be detected by abdominal palpation. Examination may suggest a cystic mass or a solid tumor. Movement of the mass separate from the uterus supports the suspicion of an adnexal mass instead of a uterine fibroid. Percussion of the abdomen in a patient with a large ovarian cyst may reveal dullness anteriorly with tympany in the flanks as the bowel is displaced laterally by the tumor.

If the tumor has undergone torsion and infarction or rupture, signs of peritoneal irritation may be present. If complete infarction has occurred, there may be abdominal rigidity. Paralytic ileus may also be present.

Pelvic ultrasonography, particularly **transvaginal ultrasonography,** with or without color Doppler, may help to identify the size, consistency, and location of the mass. It is particularly helpful in the diagnosis of a dermoid cyst.

In postmenopausal patients in particular, tumor markers, such as **serum CA 125,** as part of the **RMI** (see above and Table 20-2) may help to distinguish between a benign and a malignant mass. When clinical evaluation, pelvic ultrasonography, and tumor markers all indicate malignancy, the patient should be referred to a gynecologic oncologist for evaluation and treatment.

MANAGEMENT OF OVARIAN NEOPLASMS

Most benign-appearing ovarian cysts may be observed and followed with ultrasonography. If they are symptomatic or enlarging, laparoscopic management is usually appropriate. If the patient is premenopausal, the ovarian neoplasm is unilocular, and there are no excrescences within the cyst, an ovarian cystectomy with preservation of the ovary can be performed. **In postmenopausal women, at least unilateral salpingo-oophorectomy would be appropriate.** The contralateral ovary should be carefully inspected to exclude a bilateral lesion. Because of the possible coexistence of an appendiceal mucocele with a mucinous cystadenoma, appendectomy should also be performed.

Laparotomy is usually indicated if the mass is suspicious for malignancy. Any ascitic fluid should be collected on opening the peritoneal cavity and sent for cytologic examination. **A frozen-section histologic diagnosis should be obtained intraoperatively** to exclude malignancy. The definitive treatment will depend on the type of neoplasm, the patient's age, and her desire for future childbearing.

Stromal-cell neoplasms of the ovary are generally treated by unilateral salpingo-oophorectomy when future pregnancies are a consideration.

Cystic teratomas ("dermoids") can be treated by ovarian cystectomy. Because 15-20% are bilateral, the contralateral ovary should be carefully evaluated and any cysts resected.

In a patient with a gonadoblastoma, dysgenetic ovaries are usually present, necessitating bilateral salpingo-oophorectomy, particularly in the presence of a Y chromosome. With embryo transfer now available to these patients, the uterus should be left in situ if future fertility is desired.

OVARIAN REMNANT SYNDROME

Ovarian remnant syndrome may be the cause of cyclic pelvic pain and deep dyspareunia in women who have previously undergone hysterectomy with salpingo-oophorectomy. A residual part of the ovary may be left inadvertently and adhere to the vaginal cuff or the retroperitoneal space near a ureter. Surgical excision of the small mass is required to relieve the pain.

The ovarian remnant syndrome must be distinguished from the **residual ovary syndrome.** In the latter, an ovary is intentionally left at the time of hysterectomy but subsequently causes deep dyspareunia if it becomes adherent to the vaginal cuff.

Congenital Anomalies of the Ovaries

Abnormal embryologic development of the ovaries is uncommon. Congenital duplication or absence of ovarian tissue may occur, as may ectopic ovarian tissue and supernumerary ovaries. Although rare, the sexual bipotentiality noted in embryologic development can progress without the usual regression of one system, producing an ovotestis and subsequent intersex problems.

Genetic chromosomal disorders, such as **Turner syndrome (45 XO),** are associated with a lack of normal gonadal development, as evidenced by the rudimentary streaked ovaries that are a hallmark of the disorder. **Women with Turner syndrome usually progress through puberty and develop secondary sexual characteristics, but enter menopause shortly thereafter.** This provides evidence that two X chromosomes are required for normal ovarian development. Testicular predominance occurs with the addition of a single Y chromosome, even in the face of multiple X chromosomes. Such predominance is seen in **Klinefelter syndrome (47 XXY),** in which testicular development occurs embryologically. In **complete androgen insensitivity syndrome (46 XY), which is also known as testicular feminization,** the lack of androgen receptors produces a phenotypic female in the face of a Y chromosome. The gonads in these women (functioning testes) should be removed (usually after puberty) because of their significant malignant potential.

Benign Conditions of the Fallopian Tubes

Most benign "tumors" of the fallopian tubes are inflammatory/infectious enlargements such as a fluid-filled tube from previous infection (hydrosalpinx) and a pyosalpinx (pus-filled tube) from a more recent and active infection (Figure 20-7). When the fallopian tube and ovary are involved the infectious mass is called a tubo-ovarian abscess or TOA (see Chapter 22).

Benign neoplasms of the oviducts are rare. Although the tubes, uterine corpus, and uterine cervix are from the same müllerian anlage (primordial tissue),

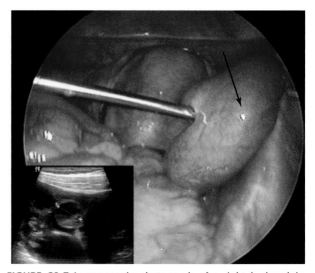

FIGURE 20-7 Laparoscopic photograph of a right hydrosalpinx *(arrow)* with the ultrasonic image *(inset)* of this clear fluid-filled fallopian tube that represents previous infection and inflammation. (From Hornemann A, von Koschitzky H, Bohlman MK, et al: Isolated pyosalpinx in a 13-year-old virgin. *Fertil Steril* 91:2732.e9–e10, 2009, Figure 1.)

the tubes have been thought to have less of a tendency toward neoplastic transformation. **Recent evidence, however, suggests that some serous "ovarian" cancers may actually arise in the fallopian tubes** (see Chapter 39).

Benign tubal neoplasms that do occur are **epithelial adenomas and polyps, myomas** from the tubal musculature, **inclusion cysts** from the mesothelium, or **angiomas** from the tubal vasculature. It is usually difficult to differentiate a tubal neoplasm from other adnexal masses on examination, although ultrasonography may identify the ovary separate from the mass and determine its tubal origin. Salpingectomy represents the definitive treatment.

As the name paraovarian (beside the ovary) implies, **paraovarian neoplasms are generally located within the broad ligament** between the tube and the ovary. These tumors are generally small compared with ovarian cysts, measuring less than 8 cm in diameter. Histologically, most appear to be derived from paramesonephric (müllerian) structures or occasionally from mesonephric (wolffian) remnants. Although the malignancy rate is less than 10%, it is necessary to resect the cystic mass to obtain a pathologic assessment.

Torsion either of the ovary alone or of both the ovary and fallopian tube (adnexal torsion) represents an acute surgical emergency. Torsion is a complication of benign ovarian tumors, paraovarian cysts, and tubal ligation remnants. Adnexal torsion causes severe acute, unilateral lower abdominal pain, which starts often as less severe pain alternating with a dull soreness. This pattern results from intermittent twisting and untwisting of the mass. With torsion, the venous blood supply is occluded, which increases pressure in the mass and can cause hemorrhage into the mass. With more prolonged and extensive torsion, the arterial supply is occluded and the mass necroses.

The diagnosis may be confusing because the patient may also have fever, nausea, vomiting, and leukocytosis suggestive of appendicitis. Ultrasonic studies, including Doppler color flow studies, can help pinpoint the diagnosis preoperatively, but prompt surgical intervention is required. If the mass has not undergone significant necrosis, it may be untwisted. In some cases, the ovary may be sutured to the pelvic side wall to make recurrence less likely. If the tube has undergone significant necrosis, a unilateral salpingectomy or salpingo-oophorectomy may be necessary.

Congenital Anomalies of the Fallopian Tubes

Isolated anomalies of the fallopian tubes, the end result of abnormal development of the proximal unfused portions of the paramesonephric ducts, are rare. **Aplasia or atresia,** usually of the distal ampullary segment of the fallopian tube, is most commonly unilateral in the presence of otherwise normal development. Bilateral aplasia is noted in some cases of uterine and vaginal agenesis. **Complete duplication** of the fallopian tubes is rarely seen, but distal duplication and accessory ostia are relatively common.

In addition, women exposed in utero to certain drugs, such as diethylstilbestrol (DES), may have abnormalities in the architecture of the fallopian tubes; **with DES exposure, the tubes may be shortened, distorted, or clubbed.**

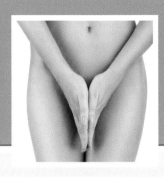

CHAPTER 21

Pelvic Pain
Acute, Cyclic (Dysmenorrhea), and Chronic

ANDREA J. RAPKIN • JOSEPH C. GAMBONE

CLINICAL KEYS FOR THIS CHAPTER

- Acute pelvic pain of sudden onset can be caused by both gynecologic and nongynecologic disorders. Adnexal accidents such as rupture or torsion of ovarian cysts, pelvic infections, tubal rupture of ectopic pregnancies, and aborting intrauterine pregnancies are the more common gynecologic causes. Gastrointestinal conditions, such as appendicitis and bowel obstruction, and genitourinary problems, such as cystitis and ureteral stones are the significant nongynecologic causes. Early diagnosis and expeditious treatment, often surgical, are important for safe and effective clinical management of acute pelvic pain.

- The most common type of cyclic pelvic pain is recurrent painful menstruation or dysmenorrhea. Dysmenorrhea may be primary, when caused by excessive production of prostaglandins (PGs), mainly $PGF_{2\alpha}$, or secondary, when an underlying condition for the pain such as adenomyosis or endometriosis is diagnosed. Primary dysmenorrhea occurs in ovulatory cycles and in younger women (17 to 22 years). Other causes of secondary menstrual and perimenstrual recurrent pain include chronic pelvic infection, degenerating fibroids, and pelvic congestion. Secondary dysmenorrhea is not limited to pain only during menses and typically occurs in older women (>30 years of age).

- Treatment of primary dysmenorrhea involves provision of an explanation for the cause of the pain, and reassurance, along with nonsteroidal antiinflammatory drugs (NSAIDs), hormonal contraceptives to block ovulation, and other nonpharmaceutical interventions such as transcutaneous nerve stimulation and acupuncture. Treatment of secondary dysmenorrhea depends on the underlying cause of the pain, with NSAIDs the preferred initial choice.

- Chronic pelvic pain (CPP) is noncyclic pain that lasts for more than 6 months. Like other forms of pelvic pain, CPP has both gynecologic and nongynecologic causes. Chronic pain, including CPP, differs from acute pain in several important and measurable ways. With acute pain, the pain perception, suffering, and behavior are usually commensurate with the degree of sensory input. With chronic pain, such as CPP, the suffering and behavioral responses may be quite exaggerated, and may persist even after the pain stimulus has remitted.

- The appropriate evaluation and treatment of CPP is challenging. The most effective treatment occurs when a multidisciplinary team manages the patient with ongoing, as opposed to episodic care. Psychiatric referral for psychopharmacologic therapy may be needed. This aspect of therapy is crucial, because many of these patients may be severely depressed and they may be withdrawn interpersonally, sexually, and occupationally.

Pelvic pain is a frequent complaint in gynecology. It may be acute, cyclic, and associated with menstruation, or chronic, lasting for more than 6 months. **Acute pelvic pain** is sudden in onset and is usually associated with significant neuroautonomic reflexes such as nausea and vomiting, diaphoresis, and apprehension. There are several important gynecologic and nongynecologic causes of acute pain.

Half of all menstruating women are affected by painful menstruation or dysmenorrhea making it the most common type of pelvic pain. Ten percent of these women have severe symptoms necessitating time off from work or school. **Chronic pelvic pain (CPP) includes reproductive and nonreproductive organ–related pelvic pain** that is primarily acyclic and that lasts for 6 months or more.

Acute Pelvic Pain

It is important for the gynecologist to be aware of both the gynecologic and nongynecologic causes of acute pelvic pain (Box 21-1). Delayed diagnosis and treatment of acute pelvic pain may increase the morbidity and even the mortality.

Adnexal accidents, including **torsion or rupture of an ovarian or fallopian tube cyst** (Figure 21-1), can cause severe lower abdominal pain. Normal ovaries and fallopian tubes rarely undergo torsion, but cystic

---

BOX 21-1

CAUSES OF ACUTE PELVIC PAIN

Gynecologic

Adnexal accidents, e.g., ovarian cyst torsion, rupture, or hemorrhage

Acute infections, e.g., endometritis or pelvic inflammatory disease

Pregnancy complications, e.g., ectopic gestation or abortion

Nongynecologic

Gastrointestinal, e.g., appendicitis, enteritis, or intestinal obstruction

Genitourinary, e.g., cystitis, ureteral stones, or urethral syndrome

Other, e.g., pelvic thrombophlebitis, vascular aneurysm, or porphyria

---

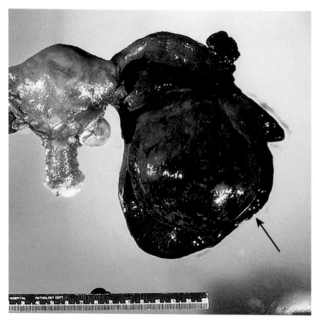

FIGURE 21-1 Torsion of an ovarian cyst and adnexal blood vessels. Note the large clot that has formed in the adnexal area *(arrow)* due to obstruction of venous outflow from a left ovarian cyst. (From Clement PB, Young RH: *Atlas of gynecologic surgical pathology,* Philadelphia, 2000, Saunders.)

or inflammatory enlargement predisposes to these adnexal accidents. The pain of adnexal torsion can be intermittent or constant, is often associated with nausea, and has been described as reverse renal colic because it originates in the pelvis and radiates to the loin. An enlarging pelvic mass is found on examination and ultrasound, with decreased or absent blood flow to the adnexa on Doppler-ultrasonic studies. The need for surgical intervention is common and urgent.

Functional ovarian cysts (e.g., corpus luteum or follicular cysts) **may rupture** causing leakage of fluid or blood that causes acute pain from peritoneal irritation. When there is significant associated bleeding, the pain may be followed by a hemoperitoneum and hypovolemia. Surgical intervention is mandatory in this setting, after adequate resuscitation with packed red cells and intravenous fluids.

Reproductive organ infections such as endometritis or salpingo-oophoritis (commonly referred to as pelvic inflammatory disease or PID) **can present acutely.** Rupture of a tubo-ovarian abscess is a surgical emergency that can progress to hypotension and oliguria after initially presenting with diffuse lower abdominal pain. Pelvic infection is covered in greater detail in Chapter 22.

Several complications of early pregnancy, such as ectopic gestation (see Chapter 24) **and threatened or incomplete abortion, can cause acute pelvic pain** and are generally associated with abnormal bleeding. Ectopic tubal pregnancies produce pain as the fallopian tube dilates and ruptures into the abdominal cavity, and can be life-threatening when not diagnosed expeditiously.

Nongynecologic causes of acute lower abdominal pain (see Box 21-1) are frequently in the differential diagnosis when a woman presents with pelvic pain. **Appendicitis** is a common gastrointestinal cause of acute lower abdominal pain that eventually localizes to the right lower quadrant of the abdomen (McBurney point). The unilateral intensity of the pain usually differentiates it from salpingo-oophoritis. Rupture of an infected appendix into the pelvic cavity can have a significant adverse effect on female fertility and may be a diagnostic challenge during pregnancy (see Chapter 16). **Diverticular abscess** is also not uncommon but usually occurs in postmenopausal women.

Acute cystitis (see Chapter 22) and **ureteral stone formation** (lithiasis) and passage are both frequently painful. **Urethral syndrome** can present acutely and become chronic over time when not recognized and treated. Painful pelvic floor disorders are covered in more detail in Chapter 23.

Cyclic Pelvic Pain: Dysmenorrhea

Dysmenorrhea is painful menstruation with absence of pain, generally, between menstrual periods. It may be **primary** when there is no readily identifiable cause, or **secondary** to organic pelvic disease. The typical age range of occurrence for primary dysmenorrhea is between 17 and 22 years, whereas secondary dysmenorrhea is more common in older women (>30 years of age).

PRIMARY DYSMENORRHEA

Pathophysiology

Primary dysmenorrhea occurs during ovulatory cycles and usually appears within 6 to 12 months of the menarche. The etiology of primary dysmenorrhea has been attributed to uterine contractions with ischemia and production of prostaglandins. Women with dysmenorrhea have increased uterine activity, which results in increased resting tone, increased contractility, and increased frequency of contractions. During menstruation, prostaglandins are released as a consequence of endometrial cell lysis, with instability of lysosomes and release of enzymes which break down cell membranes.

The evidence that prostaglandins are involved in primary dysmenorrhea is convincing. Menstrual fluid from women with this disorder has higher than normal levels of prostaglandins (especially $PGF_{2\alpha}$ and PGE_2), and these levels can be reduced to below normal with nonsteroidal antiinflammatory drugs (NSAIDs), which are effective treatments. Infusions of $PGF_{2\alpha}$ or PGE_2 reproduce the discomfort and many of the associated symptoms such as nausea, vomiting, and headache. Secretory endometrium contains much more prostaglandin than proliferative endometrium. Women with primary dysmenorrhea have upregulated cyclooxygenase (COX) enzyme activity as a major cause of their pain. **Anovulatory endometrium (without progesterone) contains little prostaglandin, and these menses are usually painless. The thin endometrium in women using hormonal contraceptives also exhibits decreased prostaglandin synthesis.**

Figure 21-2 summarizes the relationships among endometrial cell wall breakdown, prostaglandin synthesis, uterine contractions, ischemia, and pain.

Clinical Features

The clinical features of primary dysmenorrhea are summarized in Box 21-2. Cramping usually begins a few hours before the onset of bleeding and may persist for hours or days. It is localized to the lower abdomen

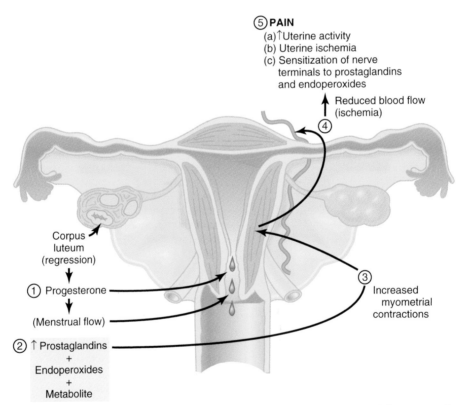

⑤ **PAIN**
(a) ↑Uterine activity
(b) Uterine ischemia
(c) Sensitization of nerve
  terminals to prostaglandins
  and endoperoxides

Reduced blood flow
(ischemia)
④

Corpus
luteum
(regression)

① Progesterone

(Menstrual flow)

② ↑ Prostaglandins
+
Endoperoxides
+
Metabolite

③
Increased
myometrial
contractions

FIGURE 21-2 Postulated mechanism of pain generation in primary dysmenorrhea. Nonsteroidal antiinflammatory drugs inhibit cyclooxygenase, the enzyme that catalyzes the formation of prostaglandins from arachidonic acid. Hormonal contraceptives that block ovulation significantly reduce the formation of prostaglandins. Both drugs can mitigate this mechanism of pain and are effective treatment for primary dysmenorrhea. (Modified from Dawood MY: Hormones, prostaglandins and dysmenorrhea. In Dawood MY, editor: *Dysmenorrhea,* Baltimore, 1981, Williams & Wilkins.)

BOX 21-2
FEATURES OF PRIMARY DYSMENORRHEA

Initial Onset
90% experience symptoms within 2 years of menarche (i.e., when ovulation begins).

Duration and Type of Pain
Dysmenorrhea begins a few hours before or just after the onset of menstruation and usually lasts 48-72 hours.
Pain is described as cramp-like and is usually strongest over the lower abdomen, but may radiate to the back or inner thighs.

Associated Symptoms
Nausea and vomiting
Fatigue
Diarrhea
Lower backache
Headache

Pelvic Examination
Normal findings

BOX 21-3
TREATMENT OF PRIMARY DYSMENORRHEA

General Measures
Reassurance and explanation

Medical Measures
Nonsteroidal antiinflammatory drugs
Hormonal contraceptives (including hormone-releasing intrauterine devices and vaginal rings)
Progestins
Analgesics

Other Measures
Transcutaneous nerve stimulation
Acupuncture
Psychotherapy
Hypnotherapy

and may radiate to the thighs and lower back. The pain may be associated with altered bowel habits, nausea, fatigue, dizziness, and headache.

Treatment

NSAIDs, which act as COX inhibitors, are highly effective in the treatment of primary dysmenorrhea (Box 21-3). Typical examples include **ibuprofen** (400 to 600 mg every 6 to 8 hours), **naproxen sodium** (250 to 500 mg every 8 hours), and **mefenamic acid** (500 mg every 8 hours). Decreasing prostaglandin production by enzyme inhibition is the basis of all NSAIDs. Pain relief is better if NSAIDs are started 2 to 3 days before menstrual flow. Hormonal contraceptives, such as **oral contraceptive pills (OCs), patches, or transvaginal rings, reduce menstrual flow and inhibit ovulation**

and are also effective therapy for primary dysmenorrhea. Extended cycle use of OCs or the use of long-acting injectable or implantable hormonal contraceptives or progestin-containing intrauterine devices minimizes the number of withdrawal bleeding episodes that users have. Some patients may benefit from using both hormonal contraception and NSAIDs.

Resistant cases may respond to high dose continuous daily progestogens (especially **medroxyprogesterone acetate** or **dydrogesterone**). Nonpharmacologic pain management, particularly **acupuncture or transcutaneous electrical stimulation (TENS) may be useful, as is psychotherapy, hypnosis, and heat patches.** Surgical procedures such as **presacral neurectomy and uterosacral ligament section have been largely abandoned.**

If a patient fails to respond to hormonal contraception and NSAID therapy, the diagnosis of primary dysmenorrhea should be questioned, and consideration given to a secondary cause. Ultrasonic imaging, laparoscopy, and possibly hysteroscopy should be performed to exclude pelvic disease.

SECONDARY DYSMENORRHEA
Pathophysiology
The mechanism of pain in secondary dysmenorrhea depends on the underlying (secondary) cause and in most cases is not well understood. Prostaglandins may also be involved in this type of dysmenorrhea, although NSAIDs and hormonal contraceptives that do not suppress menses altogether are less likely to provide satisfactory pain relief.

Clinical Features
The clinical features of some of the underlying causes of secondary dysmenorrhea are summarized in Box 21-4. In general, secondary dysmenorrhea is not limited to the menses, and can occur up to 2 weeks before as well as up to a week after the menses. In addition, secondary dysmenorrhea is less related to the first day of flow, develops in older women (in their 30s or 40s), and is usually associated with other symptoms such as dyspareunia, infertility, or abnormal uterine bleeding.

Treatment
Management consists of the treatment of the underlying disease. The treatments used for primary dysmenorrhea are often helpful. Other specific treatments are discussed in the chapters dealing with the underlying causes.

Chronic Pelvic Pain

CPP refers to pelvic pain of more than 6 months' duration that has a significant effect on daily function and quality of life. CPP includes reproductive and nonreproductive organ–related pain. Although CPP is an enigmatic disorder, it is one of the most common presenting complaints in a gynecologic practice. **As a public health problem, it results in great cost to society in terms of hospital services, loss of productivity, and human misery.**

BOX 21-4

CHARACTERISTICS OF SOME CAUSES OF SECONDARY DYSMENORRHEA

Endometriosis

Pain extends to premenstrual or postmenstrual phase or may be continuous; may also have deep dyspareunia, premenstrual spotting, a fixed retroverted uterus, and tender pelvic nodules (especially on the uterosacral ligaments); onset is usually in the 20s and 30s but may start in the teens.

Pelvic Inflammation

Initially pain may be menstrual, but often with each cycle it extends into the premenstrual phase; may have intermenstrual bleeding, dyspareunia, and pelvic tenderness.

Adenomyosis, Fibroid Tumors

Uterus is generally symmetrically enlarged and may be mildly tender; dysmenorrhea is associated with a dull pelvic dragging sensation; hypermenorrhea and dyspareunia may be present.

Ovarian Cysts (Especially Endometriosis and Luteal Cysts)

Should be clinically evident.

Pelvic Congestion

A dull, ill-defined pelvic ache, usually worse premenstrually, relieved by menses; not all investigators agree that this is a cause of chronic pelvic pain.

Obviously, not all lower abdominal and low back pains are of gynecologic origin. **Careful evaluation is needed to distinguish gynecologic pain from that of orthopedic, gastrointestinal, urologic, neurologic, and psychosomatic origin.** The relationship between pelvic pain and the underlying gynecologic pathology is often inexplicable, and frequently the pain is thought to be psychosomatic.

Anatomy and Physiology

The innervations of the pelvic organs that convey information related to pain are shown in Table 21-1. Painful impulses that originate in the skin, muscles, bones, joints, and parietal peritoneum travel in somatic nerve fibers, whereas those originating in the internal organs travel in visceral nerves.

Visceral pain is more diffusely spread than somatic pain because of a phenomenon called *viscerosomatic convergence*, and the lack of a well-defined projection area in the sensory cortex for its identification. Viscerosomatic convergence occurs in all second-order neurons in the dorsal horn of the spinal cord that receive visceral input. No second-order neurons in the dorsal horn receive only visceral input. The viscerosomatic neurons have larger receptive fields than do the somatic second-order neurons. Visceral pain is therefore usually referred to the skin, which is supplied by the corresponding spinal cord segment **(referred pain).** For example, the initial pain of appendicitis is referred to the epigastric area because the affected structures are innervated by the thoracic cord segments T8, T9, and T10.

The structures of the female genital tract vary in their sensitivity to pain. The skin of the external

TABLE 21-1

NERVES CARRYING PAINFUL IMPULSES FROM THE PELVIC ORGANS

Organ	Spinal Segments	Nerves
Perineum, vulva, lower vagina	S2-4	Pudendal, inguinal, genitofemoral, posterofemoral cutaneous
Upper vagina, cervix, lower uterine segment, posterior urethra, bladder trigone, uterosacral and cardinal ligaments, rectosigmoid, lower ureters	S2-4	Pelvic parasympathetics
Uterine fundus, proximal fallopian tubes, broad ligament, upper bladder, cecum, appendix, terminal large bowel	T11-12, L1	Sympathetics via hypogastric plexus
Outer two-thirds of fallopian tubes, upper ureter	T9-10	Sympathetics via aortic and superior mesenteric plexus
Ovaries	T9-10	Sympathetics via renal and aortic plexus and celiac and mesenteric ganglia
Abdominal wall	T12-L1	Sympathetics via renal and aortic plexus and celiac and mesenteric ganglia
	T12-L1	Iliohypogastric
	T12-L1	Ilioinguinal
	L1-2	Genitofemoral

genitalia is exquisitely sensitive. Pain sensation is variable in the vagina, and the upper vagina is somewhat less sensitive than the lower. **The cervix is relatively insensitive to small biopsies but is sensitive to deep incision or to dilation.** The uterus is quite sensitive. The ovaries are insensitive to many stimuli, but they are sensitive to rapid distention of the ovarian capsule or compression during physical examination.

Patient Evaluation

HISTORY

A pain history should be obtained during the first visit. Characteristics of the pain should be determined, including its location, radiation, severity, alleviating and aggravating factors, as well as the effects of menstruation, level of stress, work, exercise, and intercourse. Symptoms related to the gastrointestinal, genitourinary, musculoskeletal, and neurologic systems should be ascertained. This process can be guided by the Pain History Mnemonic outlined in Box 21-5.

PHYSICAL EXAMINATION

The abdomen should be examined initially, and the patient should be asked to point to the exact location of the pain and its radiation. An attempt should be made to duplicate the pain by palpating each abdominal quadrant. The severity of the pain should be quantified on a 0 to 10 scale (0 = no pain, 10 = hitting thumb with a hammer).

BOX 21-5

PAIN HISTORY MNEMONIC (OLD CAARTS)

Onset: When and how did the pain start? Does it change over time?
Location: Localize specifically—can the woman put a finger on it?
Duration: How long does it last?
Characteristics: e.g., cramping, aching, stabbing, itching
Alleviating/aggravating factors: What makes it better (e.g., change of position, medication, stress reduction) or worse (e.g., menstrual cycle, stress, specific activity)?
Associated symptoms:
  Gynecologic (e.g., dyspareunia, dysmenorrhea, abnormal bleeding, discharge)
  Gastrointestinal (e.g., constipation, diarrhea, bloating, gas, rectal bleeding)
  Genitourinary (e.g., urinary frequency, dysuria, urgency, incontinence)
  Neurological (specific nerve distribution of the pain)
Radiation: Does the pain move to other areas of the body?
Temporal: Time of day and relationship to daily activities
Severity: On a scale of 0 to 10 (from no pain to the most severe imaginable)

Modified from Rapkin AJ, Howe CN: Chronic pelvic pain: a review. In *Family practice recertification,* Monroe Township, NJ, 2006, Medical World Communications, 28:59-67.

The abdominal wall should be examined for evidence of myofascial trigger points and for iliohypogastric (T12, L1), ilioinguinal (T12, L1), or genitofemoral (L1, L2) nerve entrapment. Each dermatome of the abdominal wall and back should be palpated with a fingertip and points of severe tenderness or "jump signs" should be marked with a pen. The patient should be asked to tense the abdominal muscles by performing a straight-leg raising maneuver (both legs raised at least 6 inches with both knees straight) or a partial sit-up. Points that are more tender or that reproduce the patient's pain suggest nerve entrapment, impingement, or a muscular trigger point pain. These points should be injected with 2 to 3 mL of 0.25% bupivacaine. Chronic abdominal wall pain is confirmed if the pain level is reduced by at least 50% and outlasts the duration of the local anesthetic.

A thorough pelvic examination should be performed, with an attempt made to reproduce and localize the patient's pain. The examination should be performed gently so as to prevent involuntary guarding, which may obstruct the findings. The examination may be suggestive of specific pelvic pathology. For example, patients with endometriosis may have a fixed retroverted uterus with tender uterosacral nodularity. An adnexal mass may suggest ovarian pathology. Bilateral, tender, irregularly enlarged adnexal structures may suggest prior salpingitis with subsequent formation of adhesions and bilateral hydrosalpinges. A prolapsed uterus may account for pelvic pressure, pain, or low backache.

FURTHER INVESTIGATIONS

Psychological evaluation should be requested if an obviously traumatic event has occurred with the onset of pain; if there is obvious depression, anxiety, catastrophizing, psychosis, or secondary gain; or to aid in the planning of pain management sessions. The latter may involve cognitive behavioral and stress reduction therapy.

Laboratory studies are of limited value in the diagnosis of CPP, although a complete blood count, erythrocyte sedimentation rate (ESR), and urinalysis are indicated. The ESR is nonspecific and will be increased in any type of inflammatory condition, such as subacute salpingo-oophoritis, tuberculosis, or inflammatory bowel disease. Patients who are engaging in sexual intercourse should have a pregnancy test if they have a uterus and are not postmenopausal. **Pelvic ultrasonography** should be performed because the pelvic examination may miss an adnexal mass, particularly in obese patients or in those who are unable to relax. Routine urine analysis and studies to rule out sexually transmitted infections are indicated depending on the patient's symptoms and risk factors. If bowel or urinary symptoms are present, an abdominal and pelvic computed tomographic (CT) scan, endoscopy, cystoscopy, or CT urogram may be useful. Similarly, if there is clinical evidence of musculoskeletal disease, a lumbosacral x-ray film, CT scan, magnetic resonance imaging (MRI) scan, or orthopedic consultation may be in order.

Diagnostic laparoscopy is the ultimate method of diagnosis for patients with CPP of undetermined etiology. Laparoscopic examination and bimanual examination may differ in 20-30% of cases. Laparoscopy should only be performed if no etiology for the pain can be identified, or when indicated to treat specific pathology.

Differential Diagnosis

CAUSES OF CHRONIC PELVIC PAIN

Of women with CPP who are subjected to diagnostic laparoscopy, approximately a third have no apparent pathology, a third have endometriosis, somewhat less than the remaining third have adhesions or stigmata of past pelvic inflammatory disease (PID), and the small remainder have other causes (Box 21-6).

Endometriosis

Endometriosis may be missed visually at the time of diagnostic laparoscopy in as many as 20-30% of women who have histologically proven disease, so it is justifiable to initiate hormonal treatment based on a presumptive diagnosis of the disease once other etiologies have been ruled out. Current hormonal therapies are often very effective and may preclude the need to undergo a costly surgical procedure that is not without risk.

The size and location of the endometriotic implants do not appear to correlate with the presence of pain, and the reasons for the pain are not fully understood, although prostaglandins, cytokines, and innervation of lesions have been hypothesized. Endometriosis is covered more extensively in Chapter 25.

Chronic Pelvic Inflammatory Disease

Chronic PID may cause pain because of anatomic distortions (hydrosalpinges and adhesions between the tubes, ovaries, and intestinal structures) that result

---

BOX 21-6

GYNECOLOGIC CAUSES OF CHRONIC PELVIC PAIN

Endometriosis
Salpingo-oophoritis (pelvic inflammatory disease)
Ovarian remnant syndrome
Pelvic congestion syndrome
Cyclic pelvic (uterine) pain
Myomata uteri (degenerating)
Adenomyosis
Adhesions

---

from the acute infection. It is also thought that prior PID may lead to "upregulation" of sensory processing from the previously inflamed tissue. Persistent active infection is called acute PID, even if fever and peritoneal signs are absent. Recurrent active infections that require antibiotic therapy must be ruled out. PID is also discussed in Chapter 22.

Before ascribing symptoms to adhesions, one must have specifically noted adhesions in the area of pain localization, because most patients with extensive pelvic adhesions discovered incidentally during surgery for other reasons are asymptomatic.

Ovarian Pain

Ovarian cysts are usually asymptomatic, but episodic pain may occur secondary to rapid distention of the ovarian capsule or rupture or leakage of irritating fluid into the peritoneal cavity. **An ovary or an ovarian remnant may occasionally become retroperitoneal secondary to inflammation or previous surgery, and cyst formation in these circumstances may be painful.** Some women, for unknown reasons, may develop multiple recurrent functional hemorrhagic ovarian cysts that seem to cause pelvic pain and dyspareunia on an intermittent basis.

Hormonal suppression of ovulation is usually an effective treatment for painful functional cysts. The differential diagnosis of ovarian masses is covered in Chapter 20. An ovarian cyst may also be an endometrioma, and if an endometrioma is suspected based on history, physical examination, and ultrasonography, surgical excision is usually indicated. Other benign and malignant ovarian neoplasms can contribute to CPP, but are often asymptomatic. A benign cystic teratoma (dermoid) for example can intermittently twist and untwist, causing repeated episodes of subacute pain.

Uterine Pain

Adenomyosis (or endometriosis interna) can cause dysmenorrhea, dyspareunia, and menorrhagia, but rarely does it cause chronic daily intermenstrual pain. **Uterine myomas usually do not cause pelvic pain unless they are degenerating, undergoing torsion (twisting on their pedicles), or compressing pelvic nerves. A completely submucous leiomyoma can attempt to deliver via the cervix, which may cause considerable crampy uterine pain akin to childbirth.** This is generally associated with heavy vaginal bleeding. During pregnancy, uterine myomas can cause pain from rapid growth or infarction.

Pelvic pain is not likely to be caused by variations in uterine position, but **deep dyspareunia may occasionally be associated with uterine retroversion,** especially when the uterus is fixed in place by adhesions or endometriosis. The pain has been ascribed to irritation of pelvic nerves by the stretching of the uterosacral ligaments as well as to congestion of pelvic veins secondary to retroversion. The dyspareunia is typically worse during intercourse in the missionary position and is improved in the female superior position. A tender uterus that is in a fixed retroverted position usually signifies other intraperitoneal pathology, such as endometriosis or PID, and diagnosis rests on laparoscopic findings.

Pelvic Congestion Syndrome

The concept of a pelvic congestion syndrome still has many proponents. **This entity has been described in multiparous women who have pelvic vein varicosities and congested pelvic organs.** The pelvic pain is worse premenstrually and is increased by fatigue, standing, and sexual intercourse. Many women with this condition are noted to have a mobile, retroverted, soft, boggy, and slightly enlarged uterus. **There may be associated menorrhagia and urinary frequency.** Dilated veins may be seen on pelvic MRI with contrast. Factors other than venous congestion may be involved in the genesis of pain, because most women with pelvic varicosities have no pain. Surgery for this condition, consisting of **hysterectomy and oophorectomy, may be beneficial for women who have completed their families,** as is ovarian hormonal suppression (decreased blood flow to the pelvic organs) and cognitive behavioral therapy. A few uncontrolled studies have suggested that embolization of involved veins by an interventional radiologist may be helpful.

Genitourinary Pelvic Pain

A variety of genitourinary problems may result in CPP. **Urethral syndrome, trigonitis, and interstitial cystitis/painful bladder syndrome are prime examples. Urinary urgency, frequency, nocturia, and midline pelvic pain may suggest interstitial cystitis/painful bladder syndrome.** A thorough genitourinary evaluation is an important part of the workup for CPP when the above symptoms are reported. As many as one in five women have interstitial cystitis/painful bladder syndrome (see Chapter 23).

Gastrointestinal Pain

Gastrointestinal sources of CPP include penetrating neoplasms of the gastrointestinal tract, irritable bowel syndrome, functional abdominal pain syndrome (FAPS), celiac disease, partial bowel obstruction, inflammatory bowel disease, diverticulitis, and hernia formation. Because the innervation of the lower intestinal tract is the same as that of the uterus and fallopian tubes, pelvic pain may be confused with pain of gynecologic origin. Irritable bowel syndrome is the most common gastrointestinal cause of pelvic pain. Pain that is present at times of alteration of form or frequency of bowel movements, increased before and improved after a bowel movement, and especially if worse with stress and eating, may be irritable bowel syndrome. Red flags for a possible gastrointestinal malignancy include onset of pain over age 50, family history of bowel cancer, blood in the stool, nocturnal pain, and alteration of stool caliber.

Neuromuscular Pain

Pain of neuromuscular origin, which is experienced as low back pain or abdominal wall pain, usually increases with activity and stress. Trigger points and myalgia of the abdominal wall and pelvic floor muscles can cause pelvic pain, vulvodynia, and dyspareunia. **Chronic low back pain without lower abdominal pain is seldom of gynecologic origin.** Fibromyalgia, or generalized myofascial pain syndrome can also cause pelvic pain. Occasionally, neuromuscular symptoms are accompanied by a pelvic mass on examination or diagnostic imaging, and surgical exploration may reveal a neuroma, sarcoma, or bony tumor. Entrapped or compressed nerves in the abdominal wall (iliohypogastric and ilioinguinal nerves most commonly) or pelvic floor (pudendal nerve) are often unrecognized sources of pain. The nerves may become entrapped after surgery, physical trauma, pregnancy and delivery, or occupational injury.

PSYCHOLOGIC FACTORS

A pathologic diagnosis may not be made in approximately one third of patients with CPP, even after laparoscopy. This has led to the postulation that **psychological factors** may be primary. **When subjected to the Minnesota Multiphasic Personality Inventory (MMPI), these patients have shown a greater degree of anxiety, hypochondriasis, and hysteria than control subjects. The profiles are similar, however, in patients who have chronic pain with organic pathology, indicating that chronic pain per se engenders a complex, debilitating, psychological response.** Patients with chronic pain, with or without anatomic pathology, tend to feel depressed, anxious, fearful, helpless, and passive. They withdraw from social and sexual activity and are overwhelmed by pain and suffering. Many have post-traumatic stress disorder (PTSD) from emotional, physical, or sexual trauma. **Women with CPP are also at risk of developing chronic fatigue syndrome.** Women with depression, anxiety, or PTSD must be treated with psychological and/or psychopharmacological therapy as part of the multidisciplinary management of their CPP.

Pain Perception Factors

Chronic pain is characterized by neurophysiological, emotional, and behavioral responses that are different from those of acute pain. Both acute and chronic pain involve a stimulus and a psychic response; for acute pain, these responses may be adaptive and appropriate, whereas for chronic pain this may not be the case. **The response to chronic pain may be greatly affected** by operant conditioning. The patient's reaction to pain and the reaction of significant others to the patient and her pain may be so reinforcing that the behavior may persist even after the painful stimulus has resolved. With acute pain, the pain perception, suffering, and behavior are *usually* commensurate with the degree of sensory input. **In chronic pain, the suffering and behavioral responses to a given sensory input may be quite exaggerated and may persist even after the stimulus has remitted.**

Modulation of Sensation

Pain impulses are subjected to a large amount of modulation en route to, and within, the central nervous system. **The first synapse in the dorsal horn is an important focus of enhancement, inhibition, or facilitation. Modulation of sensations may also occur within the spinothalamic system, the descending inhibitory neurosystems, the frontal cortex, and other brain regions.** Various neurotransmitters and neuromodulators are present in the dorsal horn and at higher levels of the neuraxis. Some excitatory modulators include substance P, glutamate, aspartate, calcitonin gene–related peptide (CGRP), and vasoactive intestinal peptide (VIP). Inhibitory neuromediators include endogenous opioid peptides, norepinephrine, serotonin, and γ-aminobutyric acid (GABA). Nerve axons that have been compromised after inflammation, stretch, or crush injury can develop abnormal sodium channels. These changes play an important role in the development of allodynia (pain with gentle touch) and hyperalgesia (pain with stimuli that are not normally painful) in many women with CPP.

Within this context, anxiety, loss of self-efficacy, fear of pain, depression, and other psychological states are also considered to be facilitators or inhibitors of neurologic transmission. It is possible that many forms of CPP may result from modulation of afferent impulses (upregulation) or abnormality of descending inhibition in the dorsal horn, spinal cord, or brain.

Management

When treating patients with CPP, a therapeutic, supportive, and sympathetic (but structured) physician-patient relationship should be established. The patient should be given regular follow-up appointments, and should not be told to call only if the pain persists. This reinforces pain behavior as a means of procuring sympathy and medical attention.

A negative evaluation or pathological findings not amenable to therapy (e.g., dense pelvic adhesions) does not mean that the patient should be discharged from care without therapy directed toward her symptoms. **After initial reassurance that there is no serious underlying pathology and education as to the likely** mechanisms of pain production (including central nervous system factors), symptomatic therapy should be undertaken. The symptoms of pain should be approached with the seriousness and direction afforded to any other condition.

THE MULTIDISCIPLINARY TEAM

The most productive strategy for the management of patients with CPP is a multidisciplinary approach. The personnel should include a **gynecologist,** a **psychologist** who also has expertise in chronic pain, sexual and marital counseling, a **physical therapist** with pelvic floor muscle expertise, and for more complex cases requiring diagnostic or therapeutic nerve blocks, an **anesthesiologist.** An **acupuncturist** may also be a useful referral. It is the role of the psychologist to provide cognitive behavioral pain management and stress reduction, assertiveness training, and adaptive coping strategies, as well as marital and sexual counseling. Psychiatric referral for psychopharmacologic therapy may be needed. This aspect of therapy is crucial, because many of these patients have become severely depressed and often withdrawn interpersonally, sexually, and occupationally. Depression may be secondary to pain, but without treatment of the depression, the pain may persist. **Relaxation, cognitive and behavioral therapies are employed to replace the pain behavior and its secondary gain with effective behavioral responses. Multidisciplinary management has been shown to be more effective than traditional gynecologic management.**

MEDICAL AND SURGICAL MANAGEMENT

The gynecologist continues to assess progress, coordinate care, and provide periodic gynecologic examinations. **In the initial stages of therapy, a trial of ovulation and or menstrual suppression with combined hormonal contraception (pills, patches, rings; cyclic or continuous), high-dose or intrauterine progestins or a gonadotropin-releasing hormone analogue (GnRH-a) may be helpful.** Ovulation and/or menstrual suppression is especially helpful in patients who have midcycle, premenstrual, or menstrual exacerbation of pain, or in those who have ovarian pathology, such as periovarian adhesions or recurrent functional cyst formation. **NSAIDs are also useful.** Pharmacologic approaches to increase inhibitory neuromodulators such as norepinephrine, serotonin (5-HT), and GABA or sodium channel blockers are frequently used in the form of tricyclic antidepressants, selective serotonin reuptake inhibitors (SSRIs), anticonvulsants or other GABA-ergic agents, and topical or injectable local anesthetics.

Surgical procedures that have not proved to be effective for CPP without pathology include unilateral adnexectomy for unilateral pain or total abdominal hysterectomy, presacral neurectomy, or uterine

4-QUADRANT INJECTION TECHNIQUE

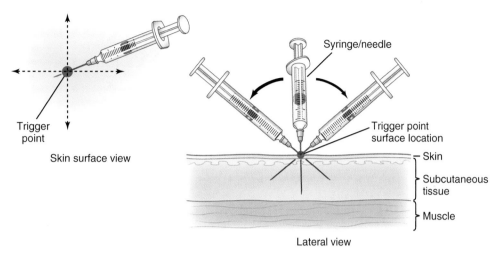

FIGURE 21-3 Trigger point injection technique for the abdominal wall for a patient with chronic pelvic pain. (From Auerbach PS: *Wilderness medicine,* ed 5, Philadelphia, 2007, Mosby.)

suspension for generalized pelvic pain. Lysis of adhesions is also usually nonproductive, with the possible exception of the situations where the site of adhesions, as visualized by the laparoscope, specifically coincides with the localization of pain. However, pelvic adhesions often recur following surgical lysis. **Without proof of organic pathology or a reasonable functional explanation for the pelvic pain, a thorough psychosomatic evaluation should be carried out before any surgical procedure is considered.**

INJECTION THERAPIES

Acupuncture, nerve blocks, and trigger-point injections of local anesthetics may provide prolonged pain relief. Acupuncture has been used successfully for dysmenorrhea, and trigger-point injections and nerve blocks with local anesthetics have been used successfully for neuropathic and musculoskeletal pain. Acupuncture probably increases spinal cord endorphins. In women with CPP, trigger points are typically found either in the lower abdominal wall, lower back, or the vagina. **A significant percentage of patients with pelvic pain have abdominal wall trigger points or nerve entrapments that respond to weekly or biweekly injections of a local anesthetic (usually up to five injections is sufficient) combined with alterations of activity or modification of behaviors that affect the area of pain.** Injection of local anesthetic into myofascial trigger points (Figure 21-3) may abolish pain by lowering the impulses from the area of referred pain, thereby diminishing the afferent impulses reaching the dorsal horn to a level below the threshold for pain transmission (but the exact mechanism is not known). Repeated local anesthetic nerve blocks of areas of nerve impingement/entrapment combined with instructions to patients about alteration in physical activity and or physical therapy can be helpful. Along with nerve threshold altering medications, these interventions can down regulate neural hypersensitivity and permanently decrease or eliminate pain.

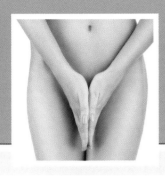

Infectious Diseases of the Female Reproductive and Urinary Tract

BASSAM H. RIMAWI • DAVID E. SOPER

CLINICAL KEYS FOR THIS CHAPTER

- Bacterial vaginosis (BV) is caused by an alteration of normal vaginal bacterial flora that results in the loss of hydrogen peroxide-producing lactobacilli, thereby allowing an overgrowth of predominantly anaerobic bacteria. Women with BV are at increased risk for pelvic inflammatory disease (PID) and postabortal and postoperative infection. Trichomonas vaginitis, caused by a flagellated parasite, is another sexually transmitted infection (STI) that often accompanies BV. Both are treated with metronidazole.

- PID is caused by microorganisms that colonize the endocervix and ascend into the uterine lining and fallopian tubes. Sexually transmitted *Neisseria gonorrhoeae* and *Chlamydia trachomatis* are the two most common causes of PID. Traditionally, the diagnosis of PID has been based on the triad of symptoms and signs: pelvic pain, cervical and adnexal tenderness, and fever. Many women have more subtle and mild symptoms that may delay the diagnosis. Treatment of PID is with broad-spectrum antibiotics on an outpatient basis. Any sexual partner(s) should be evaluated and treated. A possible end-stage development of PID is tubo-ovarian abscess(es) that requires hospitalization.

- Genital ulcer disease is usually caused by herpes simplex virus (HSV) or syphilis, with chancroid, lymphogranuloma venereum (LGV), and granuloma inguinale as rare causes. Genital warts, caused by the sexually transmitted human papillomavirus (HPV), are common and treated by removal/destruction. Infection with HPV types 6, 11, 16, and 18 can be prevented by vaccination.

- Cystitis and pyelonephritis are infections of the urinary tract, with *Escherichia coli* the causative bacteria 80% of the time. Pyelonephritis during pregnancy is associated with premature labor and delivery when not treated in a timely manner.

- Infections during pregnancy include chorioamnionitis (also called intraamniotic infection syndrome or IAIS), postpartum endometritis, and postabortal sepsis. IAIS is an ascending infection caused by highly virulent organisms such as Group-B streptococcus. IAIS can interfere with labor and should be treated before delivery. Hepatitis, human immunodeficiency virus (HIV), and perinatal infections can complicate the management of pregnancy for the fetus and mother.

Infectious diseases of the reproductive and urinary tracts are interesting and challenging disorders in gynecology. Some are difficult to treat, with frequent recurrences. Some occur during pregnancy and have an impact on its course and outcome.

Infections of the vulva, vagina, and cervix (lower reproductive tract) and the uterine corpus, fallopian tubes, and ovaries (upper reproductive tract) are the most common gynecologic problems. Many are sexually transmitted infections (STIs) that require screening, early recognition, and treatment. The diagnosis and management of common reproductive and urinary tract infections in both nonpregnant and pregnant women are discussed in this chapter. Also covered are the important perinatal infections that may impact the mother and/or her fetus.

The Normal Female Reproductive Tract

Normal vaginal secretions are composed of vulvar secretions from sebaceous, sweat, Bartholin, and Skene glands; transudate from the vaginal wall; exfoliated vaginal and cervical cells; cervical mucus; endometrial and oviductal fluids; and microorganisms and their metabolic products. **The normal vaginal flora is mostly aerobic, with an average of six different species of bacteria, the most common of which is the hydrogen peroxide–producing lactobacillus.** The microbiology of the vagina is determined by factors that affect the ability of bacteria to survive. These factors include vaginal pH and the availability of glucose for bacterial metabolism. **The pH of the normal vagina is lower** than 4.5, which is maintained by the production of lactic acid. Estrogen-stimulated vaginal epithelial cells are rich in glycogen. Vaginal epithelial cells break down glycogen to monosaccharides, which can be converted by the cells themselves, and by lactobacilli to lactic acid. Normal vaginal secretions are floccular in consistency, white in color, and usually located in the dependent portion of the vagina (posterior fornix).

Vaginal secretions can be analyzed by a wet-mount preparation. A sample of vaginal secretions is suspended in 0.5 mL of normal saline in a tube, transferred to a slide, covered with a slip, and assessed by microscopy. Microscopy of normal vaginal secretions reveals many superficial epithelial cells, few white blood cells (less than 1 per epithelial cell), and few, if any, clue cells. **Clue cells are superficial vaginal epithelial cells with adherent bacteria, usually _Gardnerella vaginalis,_** which obliterate the crisp cell border when visualized microscopically (Figure 22-1). Potassium hydroxide (KOH) 10% may be added to the slide or a separate preparation can be made to examine the secretions for evidence of fungal elements. **Gram stain reveals normal superficial epithelial cells and a predominance of gram-positive rods (lactobacilli).**

Vaginal Infections

BACTERIAL VAGINOSIS

Bacterial vaginosis (BV) is an alteration of normal vaginal bacterial flora that results in the loss of hydrogen peroxide–producing lactobacilli and an overgrowth of predominantly anaerobic bacteria. Anaerobic bacteria can be found in less than 1% of the flora of normal women. **In women with BV, the concentration of anaerobes, and _G. vaginalis_ and _Mycoplasma hominis,_ is 100 to 1000 times higher than in normal women.**

Lactobacilli are usually absent. **Women with BV are at increased risk for pelvic inflammatory disease (PID), postabortal PID, postoperative cuff infections after hysterectomy, and abnormal cervical cytology.** Pregnant women with BV are at risk for premature rupture of the membranes, preterm labor and delivery, chorioamnionitis, and postcesarean endometritis.

Office-based testing is required to diagnose BV. Figure 22-1 reveals a microscopy of a clue cell. The addition of potassium hydroxide to the vaginal secretions **(the "whiff" test)** releases a fishy, amine-like odor. Clinicians who are unable to perform microscopy can use alternative diagnostic tests such as a pH and amines test card, detection of _G. vaginalis_ ribosomal RNA, or Gram stain. Culture of _G. vaginalis_ is not recommended as a diagnostic tool because of its lack of specificity.

Ideally, treatment of BV should inhibit anaerobes but not vaginal lactobacilli. **Metronidazole,** an antibiotic with excellent activity against anaerobes but poor activity against lactobacilli, **is the drug of choice for the treatment of BV.** Clindamycin is an alternative agent. Table 22-1 illustrates the 2015 Centers for Disease Control and Prevention (CDC) guidelines for the treatment of bacterial vaginosis. Table 22-2 lists alternative regimens for the treatment of bacterial vaginosis. Many clinicians prefer intravaginal treatment to avoid systemic side effects such as mild to moderate gastrointestinal upset and an unpleasant taste. **Treatment of the male sexual partner does not improve therapeutic response and therefore is not recommended.**

TRICHOMONAS VAGINITIS

Trichomonas vaginitis is caused by the sexually transmitted, flagellated parasite, _Trichomonas vaginalis._

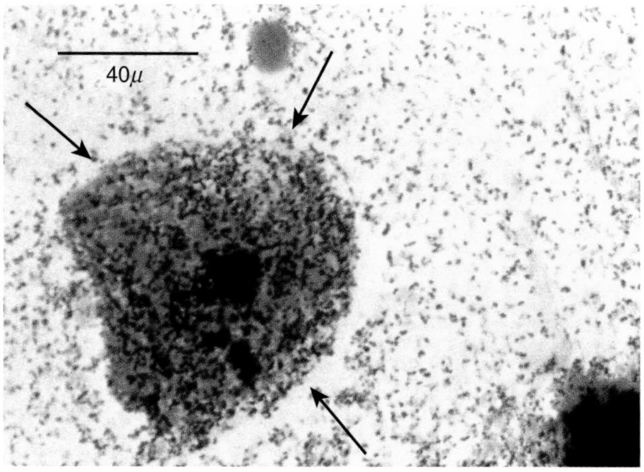

FIGURE 22-1 Wet mount microscopy of vaginal secretions from a patient with bacterial vaginosis. Note the presence of a clue cell, which is an epithelial cell with "serrated" edges caused by bacteria *(arrows).*

TABLE 22-1
2015 CENTERS FOR DISEASE CONTROL (CDC) RECOMMENDED FIRST-LINE REGIMEN FOR BACTERIAL VAGINOSIS
Metronidazole 500 mg orally twice a day for 7 days*
OR
Metronidazole gel 0.75%, one full applicator (5 g) intravaginally, once a day for 5 days
OR
Clindamycin cream 2%, one full applicator (5 g) intravaginally at bedtime for 7 days[†]

From Diseases Characterized by Vaginal Discharge: Sexually Transmitted Diseases Treatment Guidelines, 2015. www.cdc.gov.
*Consuming alcohol should be avoided during treatment and for 24 hours thereafter.
[†]Clindamycin cream is oil-based and might weaken latex condoms and diaphragms for 5 days after use (refer to clindamycin product labeling for additional information).

TABLE 22-2

2015 CENTERS FOR DISEASE CONTROL (CDC) RECOMMENDED ALTERNATIVE REGIMEN FOR BACTERIAL VAGINOSIS

Tinidazole 2 gm orally once daily for 2 days

OR

Tinidazole 1 g orally once daily for 5 days

OR

Clindamycin 300 mg orally twice daily for 7 days

OR

Clindamycin ovules 100 mg intravaginally once at bedtime for 3 days

From Diseases Characterized by Vaginal Discharge: Sexually Transmitted Diseases Treatment Guidelines, 2015. Available at http://www.cdc.gov/std/treatment/2015/vaginal-discharge.htm. Accessed February 19, 2015.

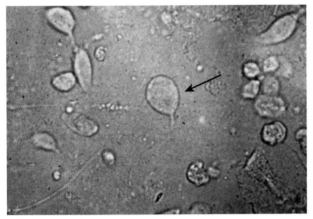

FIGURE 22-2 Microscopic view (high power) of a trichomonad *(arrow)* in a saline wet-mount preparation. The organisms are usually motile in this type of preparation.

The transmission rate is high; **70% of men contract the disease after a single exposure to an infected woman,** which suggests that the rate of male-to-female transmission is even higher. The parasite, which exists only in trophozoite form, is an anaerobe that has the ability to generate hydrogen to combine with oxygen to create an anaerobic environment. **Bacterial vaginosis** can be diagnosed in as many as 60% of patients with trichomonas vaginitis.

Trichomonas vaginitis is associated with a profuse, purulent, malodorous vaginal discharge that may be accompanied by vulvar pruritus. In patients with high concentrations of organisms, a patchy vaginal erythema and colpitis macularis (**"strawberry" cervix**) may be observed. Microscopy of the secretions may reveal **motile trichomonads** (Figure 22-2) and increased numbers of leukocytes, but the sensitivity of this test is

poor (50%). For this reason, nucleic acid amplification testing is recommended when trichomoniasis is suspected but not confirmed by microscopy.

Because of the sexually transmitted nature of trichomonas vaginitis, women with this infection should be tested for other STIs, particularly *Neisseria gonorrhoeae* and *Chlamydia trachomatis*. Serologic testing for syphilis and human immunodeficiency virus (HIV) infection should be considered.

Metronidazole is the drug of choice for treatment of vaginal trichomoniasis. Both a single-dose (2 g orally) and a multidose (500 mg twice daily for 7 days) regimen are highly effective and have cure rates of about 95%. **The sexual partner should be treated.**

Women who do not respond to initial therapy should be treated again with metronidazole, 500 mg, twice daily for 7 days. If repeated treatment is not effective, the patient should be treated with a single 2-g dose of metronidazole once daily for 5 days or tinidazole 2 g, in a single dose for 5 days. Patients who do not respond to repeated treatment with metronidazole or tinidazole and for whom the possibility of reinfection is excluded should be referred for expert consultation. In these uncommon refractory cases, an important part of management is to obtain cultures of the parasite to determine its susceptibility to metronidazole and tinidazole.

VULVOVAGINAL CANDIDIASIS

An estimated 75% of women will experience at least one episode of vulvovaginal candidiasis (VVC) during their lifetimes. Nearly 45% of women will experience two or more episodes. A few are plagued with a chronic, recurrent infection. *Candida albicans* is responsible for 85-90% of vaginal yeast infections. The extensive areas of pruritus and inflammation, often associated with minimal invasion of the lower genital tract epithelial cells, suggest that an extracellular toxin or enzyme may play a role in the pathogenesis of this disease. **A hypersensitivity phenomenon may be responsible for the irritative symptoms associated with VVC,** especially for patients with chronic, recurrent disease.

Factors that predispose women to the development of symptomatic VVC include antibiotic use, pregnancy, and diabetes. Pregnancy and diabetes are associated with a qualitative decrease in cell-mediated immunity, leading to a higher incidence of candidiasis.

The symptoms of VVC consist of vulvar pruritus associated with a discharge that can vary from watery to homogeneously thick. Vaginal soreness, dyspareunia, vulvar burning, and irritation may be present. Examination may reveal erythema and edema of the labia and vulvar skin. Discrete pustulopapular peripheral lesions may be present. **The vagina may be erythematous with an adherent, whitish discharge.** The cervix appears normal. Fungal elements, either budding

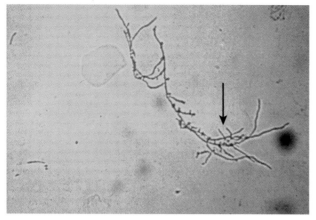

FIGURE 22-3 Mycelial tangles of yeast (arrow) pseudohyphae in potassium hydroxide wet-mount preparation.

yeast forms or mycelia, appear in as many as 80% of cases (Figure 22-3).

Treatment

The treatment of VVC involves the use of topically applied azole drugs, which are more effective than nystatin. Table 22-3 illustrates the 2010 CDC guidelines for the treatment of VVC. **Treatment with azoles results in relief of symptoms and negative cultures in 80-90% of patients.** Symptoms usually resolve in 2 to 3 days. Short-course regimens up to 3 days are recommended. **The oral antifungal agent, fluconazole, used in a single 150-mg dose, is also recommended** for the treatment of VVC. It has equal efficacy when compared with topical azoles in the treatment of mild to moderate VVC. Symptoms will persist for 2 to 3 days. Adjunctive treatment with a weak topical steroid, such as 1% hydrocortisone cream, may be helpful in relieving some of the external irritation.

RECURRENT VULVOVAGINAL CANDIDIASIS

A small number of women develop recurrent VVC (RVVC), defined as four or more episodes in a year. **The treatment of patients with RVVC consists of inducing a remission of chronic symptoms with fluconazole** (150 mg every 3 days for three doses), then **maintaining a suppressive dose of this agent** (fluconazole, 150 mg weekly) **for 6 months.** On this regimen, 90% of women with RVVC will remain in remission. After suppressive therapy, approximately half will remain asymptomatic. Recurrence will occur in the other half and should prompt reinstitution of suppressive therapy.

ATROPHIC VAGINITIS

Estrogen plays an important role in the maintenance of normal vaginal ecology. **Hypoestrogenic women having undergone natural or surgical menopause may have dyspareunia and postcoital bleeding result-**

ing from atrophy of the vaginal and vulvar epithelium. Examination reveals atrophy of the external genitalia, along with a loss of the vaginal rugae. The vaginal epithelium may be somewhat friable in areas. Microscopy of the vaginal secretions shows a predominance of parabasal epithelial cells and an increased number of leukocytes.

Atrophic vaginitis is treated with vaginal estrogen cream. Maintenance estrogen therapy, either topical or systemic, should be considered to prevent recurrence of this disorder.

TABLE 22-3
2015 CENTERS FOR DISEASE CONTROL (CDC) RECOMMENDED FIRST-LINE REGIMEN FOR VULVOVAGINAL CANDIDIASIS
Over-the-Counter Intravaginal Agents
Clotrimazole 1% cream 5 g intravaginally for 7-14 days
OR
Clotrimazole 2% cream 5 g intravaginally for 3 days
OR
Miconazole 2% cream 5 g intravaginally for 7 days
OR
Miconazole 4% cream 5 g intravaginally for 3 days
OR
Miconazole 100 mg vaginal suppository, one suppository for 7 days
OR
Miconazole 200 mg vaginal suppository, one suppository for 3 days
OR
Miconazole 1200 mg vaginal suppository, one suppository for 1 day
OR
Tioconazole 6.5% ointment 5 g intravaginally in a single application
Prescription Intravaginal Agents
Butoconazole 2% cream (single dose bioadhesive product), 5 g intravaginally for 1 day
OR
Terconazole 0.4% cream 5 g intravaginally for 7 days
OR
Terconazole 0.8% cream 5 g intravaginally for 3 days
OR
Terconazole 80 mg vaginal suppository, one suppository for 3 days
Oral Agent
Fluconazole 150 mg oral tablet, one tablet in single dose

From Diseases Characterized by Vaginal Discharge: Sexually Transmitted Diseases Treatment Guidelines, 2015. Available at http://www.cdc.gov/std/treatment/2015/vaginal-discharge.htm. Accessed February 19, 2015.

INFLAMMATORY VAGINITIS

Desquamative inflammatory vaginitis (DIV) is a fairly rare clinical syndrome characterized by diffuse exudative vaginitis, epithelial cell exfoliation, and a profuse purulent vaginal discharge. DIV presents as vaginal erythema. There may also be an associated vulvar erythema, vulvovaginal ecchymotic spots, and colpitis macularis **("strawberry cervix").** DIV can resemble atrophic vaginitis, but can also occur in women with normal estrogen levels. By the time women are diagnosed, their symptoms have usually been present for years, and they have typically been treated repeatedly for a "vaginal infection" without any long-term improvement.

Initial therapy should be with 2% clindamycin cream, one applicator full (5 g) intravaginally daily for 7 days. If this is not effective, intravaginal 10% hydrocortisone daily for 14 days may be tried.

Uterine and Adnexal Infections

ENDOCERVICITIS

N. gonorrhoeae and *C. trachomatis* are associated with mucopurulent endocervicitis 50% of the time. Other etiologies include *M. genitalium,* bacterial vaginosis, and birth control pills.

The diagnosis of cervicitis is based on the finding of a purulent endocervical discharge, generally yellow or green in color, and referred to as "mucopus" (see Figure 22-4). In addition, the zone of ectopy (glandular epithelium) is friable or easily induced to bleed. Touching the ectropion with a cotton swab or spatula can assess this characteristic sign. Tests for gonorrhea and chlamydia, preferably using nucleic acid amplification tests, should be performed. The microbial etiology of endocervicitis is unknown in about 50% of cases in which neither gonococci nor chlamydia is detected.

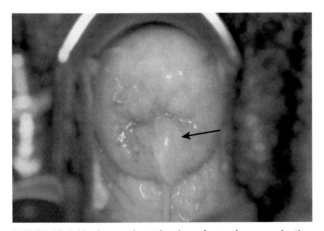

FIGURE 22-4 Uterine cervix at the time of speculum examination with yellow mucopus protruding from the os *(arrow).*

Treatment

Table 22-4 illustrates the 2015 CDC guidelines for the treatment of uncomplicated gonococcal and chlamydial infections of the cervix, urethra, and rectum. There is an ongoing problem with the emergence of strains of gonococcal isolates that are resistant to the fluoroquinolones, tetracyclines, and now the cephalosporins. For this reason, **dual therapy is recommended,** and should include an intramuscular injection of ceftriaxone 250 mg, and a single oral dose of azithromycin (1 g). The azithromycin is added not for the presumptive treatment of chlamydia, but to insure treatment of gonococci that are potentially resistant to ceftriaxone.

It is imperative that all sexual partners be treated with a similar antibiotic regimen. Cervicitis is commonly associated with BV, which, if not treated concurrently, leads to significant persistence of the symptoms and signs of cervicitis.

PELVIC INFLAMMATORY DISEASE

Microorganisms colonizing the endocervix and ascending to the endometrium and fallopian tubes cause PID. This is a clinical diagnosis implying that the patient has upper genital tract infection and

TABLE 22-4
2015 CENTERS FOR DISEASE CONTROL (CDC) RECOMMENDED FIRST-LINE REGIMEN FOR UNCOMPLICATED GONOCOCCAL AND CHLAMYDIAL INFECTIONS OF THE CERVIX, URETHRA, AND RECTUM
Recommended Regimen
Ceftriaxone 250 mg in a single intramuscular dose
PLUS
Azithromycin 1 g orally in a single dose or **doxycycline** 100 mg orally twice daily for 7 days*
Alternative Regimens
If ceftriaxone is not available: **cefixime** 400 mg in a single oral dose
PLUS
Azithromycin 1 g orally in a single dose or **doxycycline** 100 mg orally twice daily for 7 days*
PLUS
Test-of-cure in 1 week
If the patient has severe cephalosporin allergy: **azithromycin** 2 g in a single oral dose
PLUS
Test-of-cure in 1 week

From Centers for Disease Control and Prevention. Updated recommended treatment regimens for gonococcal infections and associated conditions—United States, April 2015. www.cdc.gov.
*Because of the high prevalence of tetracycline resistance among Gonococcal Isolate Surveillance Project isolates, particularly those with elevated minimum inhibitory concentrations to cefixime, the use of azithromycin as the second antimicrobial is preferred as **dual therapy.**

inflammation. The inflammation may be present at any point along a continuum that includes endometritis, salpingitis, and peritonitis. **PID is commonly caused by the sexually transmitted microorganisms *N. gonorrhoeae* and *C. trachomatis.*** Recent evidence suggests that *Mycoplasma genitalium* can cause PID and may present with mild clinical symptoms similar to chlamydial PID. Endogenous microorganisms found in the vagina, particularly the BV microorganisms, are often isolated from the upper genital tract of women with PID. The BV microorganisms include anaerobic bacteria such as *Prevotella* and peptostreptococci, as well as *G. vaginalis.* Less frequently, respiratory pathogens such as *Haemophilus influenzae,* group A streptococci, and pneumococci can colonize the lower genital tract and cause PID.

Traditionally, the diagnosis of PID has been based on a triad of symptoms and signs, including pelvic pain, cervical motion and adnexal tenderness, and the presence of fever. There is wide variation in many symptoms and signs among women with this condition, which makes the diagnosis of acute PID difficult. Many women with PID exhibit subtle or mild symptoms that are not readily recognizable as PID. The diagnosis should be considered in women with any genitourinary symptoms, including, but not limited to, lower abdominal pain, excessive vaginal discharge, heavy and irregular vaginal bleeding, fever, chills, and urinary symptoms.

Pelvic organ tenderness, either uterine tenderness alone or uterine tenderness with adnexal tenderness, is usually present in patients with PID. Cervical motion tenderness suggests the presence of peritoneal inflammation, which causes pain when the peritoneum is stretched by moving the cervix and causing traction of the adnexa on the pelvic peritoneum. Direct or rebound abdominal tenderness may be present.

Evaluation of both vaginal and endocervical secretions is an important part of the workup of a patient with PID. In women with PID, an increased number of polymorphonuclear leukocytes may be detected in a wet mount of the vaginal secretions or the cervix may have a mucopurulent discharge.

Therapeutic regimens for PID must provide empirical, broad-spectrum coverage of likely pathogens, including *N. gonorrhoeae, C. trachomatis, M. genitalium,* gram-negative facultative bacteria, anaerobes, and streptococci. Recommended first-line outpatient treatment regimens for PID, per the 2015 CDC guidelines, are listed in Table 22-5, and parenteral treatment is illustrated in Table 22-6.

An outpatient regimen of cefoxitin and doxycycline is as effective as an inpatient parenteral regimen of the same antimicrobials. Box 22-1 lists the clinical criteria for hospitalization with parenteral treatment. Hospitalized patients can be considered for discharge when their fever is less than 99.5° F for more than 24

TABLE 22-5
2015 CENTERS FOR DISEASE CONTROL (CDC) RECOMMENDED FIRST-LINE REGIMEN FOR OUTPATIENT TREATMENT OF PELVIC INFLAMMATORY DISEASE
Recommended Regimen
Ceftriaxone 250 mg intramuscularly in a single dose
PLUS
Doxycycline 100 mg orally twice a day for 14 days
WITH or WITHOUT
Metronidazole 500 mg orally twice a day for 14 days
OR
Cefoxitin 2 g intramuscularly in a single dose and probenecid, 1 g orally administered concurrently in a single dose
PLUS
Doxycycline 100 mg orally twice a day for 14 days
WITH or WITHOUT
Metronidazole 500 mg orally twice a day for 14 days
OR
Other parenteral third-generation cephalosporin (e.g., ceftizoxime or cefotaxime)
PLUS
Doxycycline 100 mg orally twice a day for 14 days
WITH or WITHOUT
Metronidazole 500 mg orally twice a day for 14 days

From Pelvic Inflammatory Disease: Sexually Transmitted Diseases Treatment Guidelines, 2015. Available at http://www.cdc.gov/std/treatment/2015/pid.htm. Accessed February 19, 2015.

hours, the white blood cell count is decreasing, rebound tenderness is absent, and repeat examination shows marked amelioration of abdominal tenderness.

Sexual partners of women with PID should be evaluated and treated for urethral infection caused by chlamydia or gonorrhea. One of these STIs is usually found in the male sexual partners of women with PID even if her diagnosis is not associated with chlamydia or gonorrhea.

TUBO-OVARIAN ABSCESS

Tubo-ovarian abscess (TOA), an endstage process of acute PID, is diagnosed when a patient with PID has a pelvic mass that is palpable during bimanual examination. The condition usually reflects an agglutination of pelvic organs (tube, ovary, and bowel) forming a palpable complex. Occasionally, an ovarian abscess can result from the entrance of microorganisms through an ovulatory site. Tubo-ovarian abscess is treated with an antibiotic regimen administered on an inpatient basis. Table 22-6 illustrates the parenteral treatment of PID, as per the 2015 CDC guidelines. **About 75% of women with a tubo-ovarian abscess respond to antimicrobial therapy alone. Failure of medical therapy suggests**

TABLE 22-6

CENTERS FOR DISEASE CONTROL (CDC) RECOMMENDED FIRST-LINE REGIMEN FOR PARENTERAL TREATMENT OF PELVIC INFLAMMATORY DISEASE
Recommended Parenteral Regimen A
Cefotetan 2 g IV every 12 hours
OR
Cefoxitin 2 g IV every 6 hours
PLUS
Doxycycline 100 mg orally or IV every 12 hours
Recommended Parenteral Regimen B
Clindamycin 900 mg IV every 8 hours
PLUS
Gentamicin loading dose IV or IM (2 mg/kg of body weight), followed by a maintenance dose (1.5 mg/kg) every 8 hours. Single daily dosing (3 to 5 mg/kg) can be substituted.
Alternative Parenteral Regimens
Ampicillin/sulbactam 3 g IV every 6 hours
PLUS
Doxycycline 100 mg orally or IV every 12 hours

From Pelvic Inflammatory Disease: Sexually Transmitted Diseases Treatment Guidelines, 2015. Available at http://www.cdc.gov/std/treatment/2015/pid.htm. Accessed February 19, 2015.
IM, Intramuscularly; *IV,* intravenously.

BOX 22-1

PELVIC INFLAMMATORY DISEASE: CLINICAL CRITERIA FOR HOSPITALIZATION AND PARENTERAL TREATMENT

1. Surgical emergencies (e.g., appendicitis) not ruled out
2. Failed oral treatment (no improvement with short-term treatment)
3. Compliance questionable (i.e., patient unable to follow or tolerate outpatient regimen)
4. Severe illness (toxicity: nausea, vomiting, high fever)
5. Tubo-ovarian abscess demonstrated on ultrasonography or suspected clinically

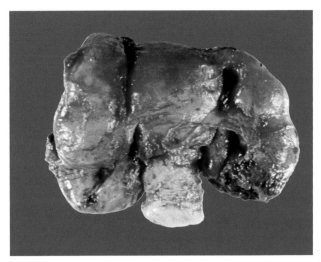

FIGURE 22-5 Gross appearance of bilateral tubo-ovarian abscesses. (From Kumar V, Fausto N, Abbas A: *Robbins and Cotran pathologic basis of disease,* ed 7, Philadelphia, 2005, Saunders.)

the need for drainage of the abscess. Although drainage may require surgical exploration, **percutaneous drainage, guided by imaging studies (ultrasonography or computed tomography) should be used as an initial option if possible.** Trocar drainage, with or without placement of a drain, is successful in up to 90% of cases in which the patient has failed to respond to antimicrobial therapy after 72 hours. Figure 22-5 depicts a surgical specimen with bilateral TOAs.

Genital Ulcer Diseases

HERPES SIMPLEX AND SYPHILIS

In the United States, most patients with genital ulcers have genital herpes simplex virus (HSV) infection or syphilis.

Chancroid, lymphogranuloma venereum (LGV), and granuloma inguinale (donovanosis) round out the infectious diagnoses. **These infections are associated with an increased risk for HIV.** Other infrequent and noninfectious causes of genital ulcers include abrasions, fixed drug eruptions, carcinoma, and Behçet disease. Genital ulcers in nonsexually active girls are usually apthmous ulcers and are not related to sexually transmitted infections.

A diagnosis based on history and physical examination alone is often inaccurate. Therefore, **all women with genital ulcers should undergo a serologic test for syphilis.** Because of the consequences of inappropriate therapy, such as tertiary disease and congenital syphilis in pregnant women, diagnostic efforts should be directed at excluding syphilis. Optimally, the evaluation of a patient with a genital ulcer should include dark-field examination or direct immunofluorescence testing for *Treponema pallidum,* culture or antigen testing for HSV, and culture for *Haemophilus ducreyi.* Dark-field or fluorescent microscopes and selective media to culture for *H. ducreyi* often are not available in most offices and clinics. **Even after complete testing, the diagnosis remains unconfirmed in one-fourth of patients with genital ulcers.** For this reason, most clinicians base their initial diagnosis and treatment recommendations on their clinical impression.

Several clinical presentations are highly suggestive of specific diagnoses. **A painless and minimally tender ulcer, not accompanied by inguinal lymphadenopathy, is likely to be syphilis,** especially if the ulcer is indurated. A nontreponemal rapid plasma reagin (RPR) test, or venereal disease research laboratory (VDRL) test, and a confirmatory treponemal test—syphilis IgG enzyme immunoassay (EIA), fluorescent treponemal antibody absorption (FTA ABS) or microhemagglutinin–*T. pallidum* (MHA TP)—should be used to diagnose syphilis presumptively. Some laboratories screen samples with treponemal EIA tests, the results of which should be confirmed with nontreponemal tests. The results of nontreponemal tests usually correlate with disease activity and should be reported quantitatively.

Grouped vesicles mixed with small ulcers, particularly if there is a history of such lesions, are usually pathognomonic of genital herpes. Nevertheless, laboratory confirmation of the findings is recommended because the diagnosis of genital herpes is traumatic for many women, alters their self-image, and affects their perceived ability to enter new sexual relationships and bear children. **A culture test is the most sensitive and specific test;** sensitivity approaches 100% in the vesicular stage and 89% in the pustular stage, but drops to as low as 33% in patients with ulcers. Nonculture tests are about 80% as sensitive as culture tests. Because false-negative results are common with HSV cultures, especially in patients with recurrent infections, type-specific glycoprotein G-based antibody assays are useful in confirming a clinical diagnosis of genital herpes.

One to three extremely painful ulcers, accompanied by tender inguinal lymphadenopathy, are unlikely to be anything except chancroid. This is especially true if the adenopathy is fluctuant. If no vulvar ulcer is present, the most likely diagnosis of an inguinal bubo is LGV. Treatment of diagnoses specific to genital ulcers is noted in Table 22-7.

GENITAL WARTS

External genital warts are a manifestation of human papillomavirus (HPV) infection (Figure 22-6). The nononcogenic HPV types 6 and 11 are usually responsible. The warts tend to occur in areas most directly affected by coitus, namely the posterior fourchette and lateral areas of the vulva. Less frequently, warts can be found throughout the vulva, in the vagina, and on the cervix. Minor trauma associated with coitus can cause breaks in the vulvar skin, allowing direct contact between the viral particles from an infected man and the basal layer of the epidermis of his susceptible sexual partner. Infection may be latent or may cause viral particles to replicate and produce a wart. **External genital warts are highly contagious; more than 75% of sexual partners develop this manifestation of HPV infection when exposed.**

The goal of treatment is removal of the warts; it is not possible to eradicate the viral infection. Treatment is most successful in patients with small warts that have been present for less than 1 year. It has not been determined whether treatment of genital warts reduces transmission of HPV. Selection of a specific treatment regimen depends on the anatomic site, size,

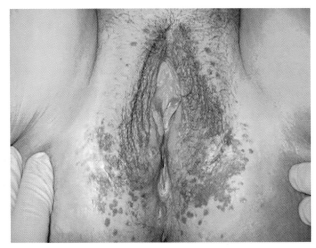

FIGURE 22-6 Venereal warts (HPV infection). (From Monk BJ, Tewari KS: The spectrum and clinical sequelae of human papillomavirus infection. *Gynecol Oncol* 107:S6–S13, 2007.)

and number of warts, and the expense, efficacy, convenience, and potential adverse effects. Treatment of genital warts is noted in Table 22-7. **Recurrences more often result from reactivation of subclinical infection than reinfection by a sexual partner;** therefore, examination of sexual partners is not absolutely necessary. However, many partners may have external genital warts and may benefit from therapy and counseling concerning transmission of warts. **HPV infection with types 6, 11, 16, 18, 31, 33, 45, 52, and 58 can be prevented with the nonavalent HPV vaccine.**

Urinary Tract Infections

ACUTE CYSTITIS

Women with acute cystitis generally have an abrupt onset of multiple, severe urinary tract symptoms including dysuria, frequency, and urgency associated with suprapubic or low-back pain. Suprapubic tenderness may be noted on physical examination. Urinalysis reveals pyuria and sometimes hematuria. **Several factors increase the risk for cystitis, including sexual intercourse, the use of a diaphragm and a spermicide, delayed postcoital micturition, and a history of a recent urinary tract infection.**

Escherichia coli **is present in the urine of 80% of young women with acute cystitis** and *Staphylococcus saprophyticus* is present in an additional 5-15% of patients. The pathophysiology of cystitis in women involves the colonization of the vagina and urethra with coliform bacteria from the rectum. For this reason, the effects of an antimicrobial agent on the vaginal flora play a role in the eradication of bacteriuria.

High concentrations of trimethoprim and fluoroquinolone in vaginal secretions can eradicate *E. coli* while minimally altering normal anaerobic and

TABLE 22-7

TREATMENT OF GENITAL (VULVAR) ULCERATIVE INFECTIONS

Disease	Microorganism(s) Involved	Preferred Treatment	Alternative Treatment
Herpes	Herpes simplex virus	**First Episode** **Acyclovir** 400 mg PO three times daily OR **Famciclovir** 250 mg PO three times daily OR **Valacyclovir** 1 g PO twice daily for 7-10 days	**Recurrent Episode** **Acyclovir** 400 mg PO twice daily OR **Famciclovir** 250 mg PO twice daily OR **Valacyclovir** 1 g PO daily
Syphilis	Treponema pallidum	**Primary, Secondary, and Early* Latent Disease** **Benzathine Penicillin G** 2.4 million units IM in a single dose	**ALL immunocompromised patients with a penicillin allergy must be desensitized and given penicillin**
		Late† Latent Syphilis **Benzathine Penicillin G** 2.4 million units IM weekly × three doses	**Doxycyline** 100 mg PO twice daily for 28 days
Chancroid	Haemophilus ducreyi	**Azithromycin** 1 g PO × 1 dose	**Ceftriaxone** 250 mg IM × 1 dose **Ciprofloxacin** 500 mg PO twice daily for 3 days **Erythromycin base** 500 mg PO four times daily for 7 days
Granuloma inguinale (donovanosis)	Klebsiella granulomatis (Calymmatobacterium granulomatis)	**Azithromycin** 1 g PO once a week for 3 weeks	**Doxycycline** 100 mg PO twice daily for 3 weeks **Ciprofloxacin** 750 mg PO twice daily for 3 weeks **Erythromycin base** 500 mg PO four times daily for 3 weeks **Sulfamethoxazole** (800 mg), **Trimethoprim** (160 mg), **Bactrim** (double strength) 1 PO twice daily for 3 weeks
Lymphogranuloma venereum (LGV)	Chlamydia trachomatis Serovars: L1, L2, L3	**Doxycycline** 100 mg PO twice daily for 21 days or until signs and symptoms have resolved	**Erythromycin base** 500 mg PO four times daily or for 21 days until signs and symptoms have resolved
Condylomata accuminata	Human papillomavirus	**Excision of warts using either:** Trichloroacetic acid Electrodessication Cautery Laser	Cryotherapy OR Imiquimod 5% cream OR Sinecatechins 15% ointment OR Popofilox 0.5%

From Centers for Disease Control and Prevention. The sexually transmitted infections treatment guidelines. *MMWR Morb Mortal Wkly Rep* 2015.
IM, Intramuscularly; *IV,* intravenously; *PO,* orally.
*Early latent syphilis—defined at the first year of latent syphilis.
†Late latent syphilis—defined as beyond 1 year of latent syphilis.

microaerophilic vaginal flora. **There has been an increasing linear trend in the prevalence of resistance of E. coli (>10%) to the fluoroquinolones (e.g., ciprofloxacin).** Despite a similar increase in *E. coli* resistance (9-18%) to trimethoprim-sulfamethoxazole, therapeutic efficacy remains stable. In contrast, no such increase in resistance has been noted with nitrofurantoin. **Nitrofurantoin** (macrocrystals, 100 mg orally twice daily for 5 days) **or trimethoprim-sulfamethoxazole** (160/800 mg orally twice daily for 3 days) **are the optimal choices for empirical therapy for uncomplicated cystitis.**

In patients with typical symptoms, an abbreviated laboratory workup followed by empirical therapy is recommended.** The diagnosis can be presumed if pyuria is detected by microscopy or leukocyte esterase testing. Urine culture is not necessary, and a short course of antimicrobial therapy should be given. No follow-up visit or culture is necessary unless symptoms persist or recur.

RECURRENT CYSTITIS

About 20% of premenopausal women have recurrent episodes of cystitis. More than 90% of these recurrences are caused by exogenous reinfection. **Recurrent cystitis should be documented by culture to rule out resistant microorganisms.** Patients may be treated by one of three strategies: (1) continuous prophylaxis, (2) postcoital prophylaxis, or (3) therapy initiated by the patient when symptoms are first noted.

Postmenopausal women may have frequent reinfections. Hormonal therapy or topically applied estrogen cream, along with antimicrobial prophylaxis, is helpful in these patients.

URETHRITIS

Women with dysuria caused by urethritis have a more gradual onset of mild symptoms, which may be associated with abnormal vaginal discharge or bleeding related to concurrent cervicitis. Patients may have a new sexual partner or experience lower abdominal pain. Physical examination may reveal the presence of mucopurulent cervicitis or vulvovaginal herpetic lesions. *C. trachomatis, N. gonorrhoeae, or genital herpes may cause acute urethritis.* Pyuria is present on urinalysis, but hematuria is rarely seen.

ACUTE PYELONEPHRITIS

The clinical spectrum of acute, uncomplicated pyelonephritis in young women ranges from gram-negative septicemia to a cystitis-like illness with mild flank pain. *E. coli* **accounts for more than 80% of these cases.** Microscopy of unspun urine reveals pyuria and gram-negative bacteria. A urine culture should be obtained in all women with suspected pyelonephritis; blood cultures should be performed in those who are hospitalized, because results are positive in 15-20% of cases. In the absence of nausea and vomiting and severe illness, outpatient oral therapy can be given safely. Patients who have nausea and vomiting, and are moderately to severely ill, should be hospitalized. **Pyelonephritis in a pregnant patient can cause premature labor and preterm delivery if not treated promptly.**

Outpatient treatment regimens include trimethoprim-sulfamethoxazole (160/800 mg every 12 hours for 14 days) or a quinolone (e.g., levofloxacin 750 mg daily for 7 days). Inpatient treatment regimens include the use of parenteral **levofloxacin** (750 mg daily), **ceftriaxone** (1 to 2 g daily), **ampicillin** (1 g every 6 hours), and **gentamicin** (especially if *Enterococcus* species are suspected) or **aztreonam** (1 g every 8 to 12 hours). Symptoms should resolve after 48 to 72 hours. **If fever and flank pain persist after 72 hours of therapy, ultrasonography or computed tomography should be considered to rule out a perinephric or intrarenal abscess or ureteral obstruction.** A follow-up culture should be obtained 2 weeks after the completion of therapy.

Infections during and after Pregnancy

CHORIOAMNIONITIS

Intraamniotic infection syndrome (IAIS), also referred to as chorioamnionitis, is a clinically detectable infection of the amniotic fluid and fetal membranes during pregnancy. **Most cases of IAIS originate when vaginal microorganisms ascend into the intrauterine cavity after rupture of the membranes.** In full-term pregnancies, IAIS is associated with dysfunctional labor. Approximately 75% of infected women require augmentation of labor with oxytocin, and approximately **35% require cesarean delivery, usually because of arrest of progress in labor.** Risk factors for IAIS include prolonged duration of labor or rupture of membranes, multiple vaginal examinations, young age, low socioeconomic class, nulliparity, and preexisting bacterial vaginosis.

Women with IAIS have a select group of high virulence microorganisms, such as Group-B streptococcus, *Escherichia coli*, genital mycoplasmas, and pathogenic anaerobes, e.g., *Prevotella bivia*, present in significantly high quantities, causing an inflammatory response and systemic signs of infection. Many of these microorganisms (especially anaerobic bacteria, the mycoplasmas, and *Gardnerella vaginalis*) are associated with bacterial vaginosis.

The clinical diagnosis of IAIS is imprecise but is based on the presence of fever (>38° C or >100.4° F) and at least two other findings: maternal and/or fetal tachycardia, maternal leukocytosis (defined as a white blood cell count >15,000), uterine tenderness, and foul-smelling amniotic fluid. The vast majority of these gravidas will have concomitant ruptured membranes. Practically, clinicians tend to base the diagnosis on the presence of intrapartum fever plus one additional criterion. Maternal and fetal tachycardia are common with fever and add little additional information. **Uterine tenderness is often obscured by conduction anesthesia, and foul-smelling amniotic fluid is rare.** Maternal white blood cell counts increase with duration of labor, but no reliable breakpoint has been established to reliably distinguish fever from infectious and noninfectious causes.

Given the imprecision of the diagnosis of IAIS, antibiotic therapy should be considered in laboring gravidas with fever (>38° C or > 100.4° F). Antimicrobial therapy for IAIS is aimed at preventing bacteremia in the mother as well as initiating intrapartum treatment of the fetus while awaiting delivery. **Improved neonatal and maternal outcome is noted when antibiotic therapy is begun intrapartum rather than immediately postpartum.** Delivery of the fetus and placenta removes the sites of infection, much like draining an abscess, making this intervention a significant part of therapy. Because group B streptococci and *E. coli* are the most common isolates from infected newborns and maternal therapy initiates fetal therapy, **a combination of ampicillin plus gentamicin is a reasonable initial regimen for IAIS.** This regimen is sufficient to treat the mother if the delivery is vaginal with only one additional dose of the antibiotic regimen needed postpartum. **If cesarean delivery is required, up to 15% of patients given only ampicillin and gentamicin will develop postpartum endometritis.** These patients require continued broad-spectrum antibiotic coverage, and a drug such as clindamycin or metronidazole should be added to the treatment regimen. This antibiotic regimen should be continued until the patient has been afebrile (temperature <38° C or <100° F) for 24 hours.

Although delivery is essential for cure, no critical diagnosis-to-delivery interval has been identified. Accordingly, labor must be managed actively, but cesarean delivery should be performed only for accepted obstetric indications.

POSTPARTUM ENDOMETRITIS

Postpartum infection of the uterus, the most common cause of puerperal fever, is designated endomyometritis. **Cesarean delivery, particularly after labor or rupture of the membranes of any duration, is the most accurate predictor of postpartum endomyometritis (PPE).** The pathogenesis of this infection involves inoculation of the amniotic fluid after membrane rupture or during labor with vaginal microorganisms. The myometrium, leaves of the broad ligament, and the peritoneal cavity are then exposed to this contaminated fluid during cesarean surgery. **The reported incidence of PPE after cesarean delivery is less than 10% in patients receiving appropriate antibiotic prophylaxis.** The diagnosis is uncommon after vaginal delivery.

Risk factors for postcesarean endomyometritis include prolonged labor or rupture of the membranes, presence of bacterial vaginosis, frequent vaginal examinations, and use of internal fetal monitoring. Antimicrobial prophylaxis is associated with a 50% reduction in infection in all populations studied. All patients undergoing cesarean delivery, either elective or emergent, are candidates for antibiotic prophylaxis. When given before the skin incision rather than after cord clamping, the incidence of postcesarean endomyometritis and total infectious morbidities are decreased, without adversely affecting neonatal outcomes. Many patients who develop postcesarean endometritis despite antibiotic prophylaxis have histologic evidence of incipient infection.

PPE is a polymicrobial infection caused by a wide variety of bacteria. Group B streptococci, enterococci, other aerobic streptococci, *G. vaginalis*, *E. coli*, *P. bivia*, *Bacteroides* spp., and peptostreptococci are the most common endometrial isolates, with group B streptococci and *G. vaginalis* the most common isolates from the blood.

Chlamydia trachomatis has been associated with a late form of PPE that occurs more than 2 days to 6 weeks after delivery in women who deliver vaginally. Group A β-hemolytic streptococcal endometritis is rare. It is characterized by early onset and rapid progression, with few localizing symptoms or physical signs.

The diagnosis of PPE is suggested by the development of fever, usually on the first or second postpartum day. Significant fever is defined as an oral temperature of 38.5° C or higher in the first 24 hours after delivery or 38° C or higher for at least four consecutive hours 24 or more hours after delivery. Other consistently associated findings are lower abdominal pain, uterine tenderness, and leukocytosis. These women may also exhibit a delayed postoperative return of bowel function due to an associated local peritonitis.

Patients with suspected PPE should have the uterus assessed for size, consistency, and tenderness. A test for *Chlamydia* should be performed in patients with mild PPE commencing more than 7 days after delivery. Adolescents in particular are at high risk of chlamydial infection.

Clindamycin plus gentamicin has proved to be the most effective regimen in treating PPE, especially if PPE occurs after cesarean delivery. Alternative regimens used for the treatment of PPE include one of the extended-spectrum penicillins or second-generation cephalosporins (e.g., ampicillin/sulbactam, ticarcillin/clavulanic acid, piperacillin/tazobactam, cefotetan, cefoxitin). Antimicrobial regimens used in the treatment of postcesarean endometritis should provide satisfactory coverage of penicillin-resistant anaerobic microorganisms (e.g., *P. bivia*).

Parenteral therapy should be continued until the temperature has remained lower than 37.8° C (100° F) for 24 hours, the patient is pain free, and the leukocyte count is normalizing. **The use of oral antibiotics after discharge has been shown to be unnecessary.** Women with late-onset PPE can be treated as outpatients with oral azithromycin or doxycycline therapy, with or without metronidazole, depending on whether or not they have coexistent bacterial vaginosis.

Early-onset PPE should respond to parenteral antimicrobial therapy within 48 hours, with the

patient becoming afebrile within 96 hours. If fever persists despite apparently appropriate antimicrobial therapy, the differential diagnosis includes a wound or pelvic abscess, refractory postpartum fever, and non-infectious fever (e.g., drug fever, breast engorgement). **Appropriate imaging studies,** usually pelvic ultrasonography or computed tomography, **may confirm the presence of a wound or pelvic hematoma or abscess. Pelvic collections** usually involve the space between the lower uterine segment and bladder. If present, percutaneous drainage by interventional radiology should be considered.

POSTABORTAL INFECTION

Infection after abortion is an ascending process that occurs most commonly in the presence of retained products of conception or operative trauma. Risk factors include greater duration of pregnancy, technical difficulties with the procedure, and the unsuspected presence of sexually transmitted pathogens or bacterial vaginosis. Symptoms include fever, chills, abdominal pain, and vaginal bleeding, often with the passage of placental tissue. Postabortal infection typically has its onset within 4 days of the procedure.

Physical findings include an elevated temperature, tachycardia, tachypnea, and abdominal tenderness. Along with bacteremia, hypotension and frank shock may occur, and the patient may be agitated and disoriented. Pelvic examination reveals a sanguinopurulent discharge and uterine tenderness, with or without adnexal and parametrial tenderness. **It is important to inspect for cervical or vaginal lacerations, especially with a suspected illegal abortion.** Transvaginal ultrasonography can assess the intrauterine cavity for the presence of retained products of conception, suggesting the need for uterine curettage.

Simple endometritis, defined as low-grade fever associated with mild uterine tenderness after uncomplicated elective abortion, can be treated with oral regimens recommended for the treatment of PID (see Table 22-6).

Laboratory evaluation of patients with more than early uncomplicated postabortal endometritis should include a complete blood count, urinalysis, culture of a specimen of the endometrial cavity taken with an endometrial suction curette, blood cultures, a computerized tomographic (CT) scan of the abdomen and pelvis, and an upright chest x-ray, looking for a foreign body or the presence of intrauterine gas. **Patients with established infection, as indicated by fever >38° C, pelvic peritonitis, or tachycardia, should be hospitalized for parenteral antibiotic therapy and prompt uterine evacuation if retained products of conception are suspected.** Table 22-8 contains the first-line antibiotic regimen for women with suspected sepsis.

TABLE 22-8

RECOMMENDED ANTIBIOTIC REGIMENS FOR POSTPARTUM/POSTABORTAL INFECTION*

Oral Regimens for Patients with Milder Disease Treated as Outpatients

Trimethoprim/sulfamethoxazole 160/800 mg by mouth every 12 hours

PLUS

Metronidazole 500 mg by mouth every 12 hours

OR

Amoxicillin-clavulanic acid 875 mg/125 mg by mouth twice daily

Parenteral Regimen for Moderate to Severe Disease in Hospitalized Patients

Triple Antibiotics

Ampicillin 2 g then 1 g IV every 6 hours

PLUS

Gentamicin 3 mg/kg of body weight IV daily

PLUS

Clindamycin 900 mg IV every 8 hours

OR

Carbapenems

Ertapenem 1 g IV daily

Meropenem 1 g IV every 8 hours

Imipenem-cilastatin 500 mg IV every 6 hours

OR

*Extended Spectrum Penicillins with β-lactamase Inhibitors**

Penicillin-tazobactam 4.5 g IV every 8 hours

From Centers for Disease Control and Prevention. The sexually transmitted infections treatment guidelines. *MMWR Morb Mortal Wkly Rep* 2015.
IV, Intravenously.
*Outpatient and inpatient regimens should include antimicrobial therapy against anaerobes.

Surgical removal of infected tissue is essential in all but the mildest of postabortal infections. Pelvic ultrasonography can be used to confirm the presence of retained tissue. In most cases, prompt curettage controls the infection. **Indications for laparotomy and possible hysterectomy include failure to respond to uterine evacuation and appropriate medical therapy, perforation and infection with suspected bowel injury, pelvic or adnexal abscess, and clostridial necrotizing myonecrosis (gas gangrene).**

Avoidance of unwanted pregnancies by making contraceptives widely available is the most important preventive measure (see Chapter 27). Screening for sexually transmitted infections and bacterial vaginosis before performance of elective abortion is optimal but often impractical. Routine use of periabortal antibiotics, such as doxycycline, may prevent up to half of all cases of postabortal infections.

Human Immunodeficiency Virus, Hepatitis B and C, and Perinatal Infections

HUMAN IMMUNODEFICIENCY VIRUS

Women who are infected with other STIs are at least two to five times more likely to acquire HIV. Without treatment, nearly all HIV-infected individuals will progress to acquired immunodeficiency disease syndrome (AIDS) and die of the illness. It is therefore recommended by the Centers for Disease Control (CDC) in the United States to **screen for HIV in those seeking care for any STIs.** Despite the predictable effect on morbidity and mortality from HIV, some women may be inadequately treated. This is often due to, or complicated by, inadequate adherence to therapy, once started.

The estimated prevalence of HIV in the United States has been reported to be 0.32% of all adults based on testing a sample of over 11,000 individuals between 1988 and 1994. Although all patients who acquire HIV should be treated, the commencement of antiretroviral (ARV) therapy should be individualized, **especially in pregnant patients, where vertical transmission is a concern and may cause a perinatal problem.**

Recommendations regarding HIV screening and treatment of pregnant women and prophylaxis for perinatal transmission of HIV have evolved considerably and continue to do so worldwide over the last 25 years, reflecting changes in the epidemiology and the science of prevention. With the implementation of recommendations for universal prenatal HIV counseling and testing, ARV prophylaxis, scheduled cesarean delivery, and avoidance of breastfeeding, **the rate of perinatal transmission of HIV has decreased to less than 2% in the United States and Europe.**

The benefits of ARV drugs for a pregnant woman must be weighed against the risks of adverse events to her, the fetus, and newborn. Combination drug regimens are considered the standard of care both for treatment of HIV infection and for prevention of perinatal transmission of HIV. After counseling and discussion about ARV drug use during pregnancy, a pregnant woman's informed choice should be respected.

The latest perinatal HIV guidelines are constantly being updated and can be accessed at http://aidsinfo.nih.gov/guidelines/html/3/perinatal-guidelines/0.

HEPATITIS B AND C

The hepatitis B virus is a DNA virus that is transmitted via blood, saliva, vaginal secretions, semen, and breast milk and across the placenta. The population at greatest risk includes intravenous drug users, homosexuals, individuals of Asian descent, and health care workers. Infection with the virus is either asymptomatic or expressed as acute hepatitis. Ten percent of individuals go on to develop chronic active or persistent hepatitis.

Impact on Pregnancy

The course of acute hepatitis is unaltered in pregnancy. Fetal infection may occur and is most likely if maternal infection occurs in the third trimester. **Chronic active hepatitis is associated with an increased risk of prematurity, low birth weight, and neonatal death.** Maternal prognosis is very poor if the disease is complicated by cirrhosis, varices, or liver failure.

If a pregnant woman is found on screening to be HBsAg-positive, liver function tests and a complete hepatitis panel should be performed. Household members and sexual contacts should be tested and offered vaccination if they are susceptible. **Transmission to the infant is believed to occur by direct contact during delivery.** Therefore the newborn should be given hepatitis immune globulin and hepatitis vaccine soon after delivery, which will reduce the risk of infection to less than 10%. **Pregnant women at high risk for becoming infected with hepatitis B who test negative for the HBsAg should be offered vaccination.** Available vaccines are produced by recombinant DNA technology and are therefore safe for use in pregnancy. The Centers for Disease Control and Prevention has also recommended that all children receive vaccination against hepatitis B.

Hepatitis C (HCV) is the most common chronic blood borne infection in the United States. Vertical transmission is reported in 3-6% of pregnant women. Co-infection with HIV has been shown to increase the risk of vertical transmission of HCV. In HIV-negative women, route of delivery does not influence vertical transmission. Amniocentesis is a potential risk for transmission. There is no evidence of an increased risk of HCV transmission in HIV-negative women who breastfeed.

Treatment for HCV has recently become available for infected individuals. Treatment during pregnancy, however, **has not been adequately studied** and all treatment (for pregnant and nonpregnant women) is evolving. The latest information regarding potential treatment should be obtained from the American College of Obstetricians and Gynecologists (ACOG) website at www.acog.org, the Centers for Disease Control at www.cdc.gov, or www.perinatology.com; search for "infections during pregnancy."

PERINATAL INFECTIONS

Perinatal infections are sometimes listed using the acronym "TORCH," the letters standing for *T*oxoplasmosis, *O*ther, *R*ubella, *C*ytomegalovirus, and *H*erpes simplex virus. The category "other" includes syphilis, hepatitis B and C, and HIV. Hepatitis and HIV have been discussed above. The potential perinatal effects from HSV, syphilis, and the other TORCH infections are covered briefly below.

Toxoplasmosis

Toxoplasmosis is caused by an obligate intracellular protozoan organism *Toxoplasma gondii.* It is uncommon and occurs most often in Europe. Household cats may play a role in contaminating soil, which is then transferred to a litter box in the house. Uncooked/undercooked food from infected beef, lamb, and other animals is another source. **The infection is usually without symptoms in the mother, but when symptoms do occur they involve fever, rash, and fatigue.** Testing of the mother is by serology, although polymerase chain reaction (PCR) testing is under development and about 7% of infected pregnant women will have neonates with congenital toxoplasmosis. This infection can result in an enlarged placenta and fetal hepatomegaly and ascites. **Fetal microcephaly occurs in 5% of affected cases.** Routine screening is not recommended because of the relatively rare occurrence with the following preventive activities encouraged: avoidance of raw or undercooked meat or eggs; washing fruits and vegetables; avoidance of cat litter when pregnant; and keeping household cats away from outside (potentially contaminated) soil.

Treatment during pregnancy for infected women is available using spiramycin. The latest dosage and duration should be obtained from the ACOG website, the Centers for Disease Control at www.cdc.gov, or www.perinatology.com; search for "infections during pregnancy."

Rubella

Rubella is caused by an RNA virus with primary infections occurring mostly in unvaccinated children and adolescents. **Vaccination has reduced the rate of infection in pregnant women with a reported incidence of <0.1% of pregnancies. The vaccine should not be given during pregnancy.** Rubella spreads by respiratory droplets, and has an incubation period of 2 to 3 weeks. The symptoms are malaise and myalgia in the presence of a nonpruritic, maculopapular, reddish rash. The highest risk to the fetus is associated with infection during the first trimester. Deafness, retinopathies, and central nervous system and cardiac malformations are the most common teratogenic manifestations. No treatment is available for rubella, but prevention using the measles, mumps and rubella (MMR) vaccine is strongly recommended.

Cytomegalovirus

Cytomegalovirus (CMV) is the most common intrauterine viral infection. Some studies show up to 2.5% of all neonates may be affected. **The transmission is via contaminated urine, blood, saliva, semen, or cervical secretions.** There are usually no symptoms, resulting in a low rate of diagnosis. **A vaccine is available but should not be administered during pregnancy.** Pregnant women who are affected are usually exposed to children with the infection. **The highest rate of transmission is in the third trimester but the severity of fetal effects is highest in the first trimester.** The infection may also be "reactivated" during pregnancy. **Perinatal fetal effects include jaundice, thrombocytopenia, intrauterine growth restriction (IUGR), and microcephaly.**

The **"blueberry muffin baby"** has been described with the appearance caused by numerous petechiae on the skin. Amniotic fluid is positive (by PCR) for CMV with active infection, and for 4 to 8 months maternal IgM antibodies for CMV may be detected and are also indicative of active infection. IgG avidity testing is recommended in those women with IgM antibodies. Avidity testing provides an estimate of the duration of a primary CMV infection.

Treatment has not been well studied during pregnancy. **Ganciclovir and valacyclovir have been used in nonpregnant women and in neonates after birth.** For the latest recommendations on vaccination, diagnosis, and treatment of CMV, consult the ACOG website at www.acog.org, the Centers for Disease Control at www.cdc.gov, or www.perinatology.com; search for "infections during pregnancy."

Herpes Simplex

It is estimated that 20-30% of pregnant women are IgG positive for HSV-2 before pregnancy and are therefore at risk for shedding virus during pregnancy. Gravidas with a history of genital herpes should receive antiviral prophylaxis during the third trimester. About 2-4% of IgG negative women acquire HSV-2 during pregnancy and are usually not diagnosed because of a lack of symptoms. Immunocompromised women and those who have another STI are at highest risk. The mother may develop disseminated HSV disease that can cause hepatitis and encephalitis. **The neonatal effects may be severe and are due to exposure to the virus in utero or during delivery.** The complications of disseminated neonatal disease are seizures, tremors, poor feeding, and bulging fontanelles. Up to 30% of newborns may die, with more than 50% having neurological damage despite antiviral therapy.

Syphilis

A perinatal infection with *Treponema pallidum* may cause stillbirth, IUGR, nonimmune hydrops, rhinitis, hepatosplenomegaly, "mulberry molars" and "saber shins," "saddle nose deformity," and interstitial keratitis. Prenatal testing for syphilis is mandated in the United States.

VERTICAL TRANSMISSION OF SYPHILIS
- Primary: 90-100%
- Secondary: 70-90%

- Early latent: 40-60%
- Late latent: 10%
- Tertiary: 5%

Pregnancy can be affected at any gestational age. As the pregnancy advances, the frequency of infection increases and the severity of fetal infection decreases. ACOG recommends that all patients be tested at their first prenatal visit. Repeat testing is recommended in the third trimester (at 28 to 32 weeks) and again at delivery in women who are at high risk for syphilis, or those who had a positive screening test in the first trimester. Any woman who delivers a stillborn infant after 20 weeks should also be tested.

The treatment for syphilis in pregnancy is benzathine penicillin. Dosage depends on the stage of the disease. In those patients with a history of penicillin-allergy, a penicillin skin test to check that a genuine allergy exists should be offered. If the penicillin skin test is negative, treatment with penicillin should proceed.

Patients who have a positive penicillin skin test should be desensitized and treated with penicillin, because the risks associated with syphilis during pregnancy outweigh the risks of inpatient treatment of a penicillin allergy. Close monitoring of nontreponemal tests (RPR or VDRL) should be followed to ensure an appropriate response to therapy. Because syphilis is a sexually transmitted infection, all the patient's partners should be tested and treated appropriately, to decrease the risk of reinfection.

Pelvic Floor Disorders
Pelvic Organ Prolapse, Urinary Incontinence, and Pelvic Floor Pain Syndromes

AMY E. ROSENMAN

CLINICAL KEYS FOR THIS CHAPTER

- Effective clinical evaluation of patients with disorders of the female pelvic floor, such as pelvic organ prolapse (POP) and stress urinary incontinence (SUI), requires a clear understanding of female pelvic anatomy. Defects of vaginal support include anterior vaginal prolapse (cystocele), posterior vaginal prolapse (rectocele and enterocele), and apical uterine prolapse. Symptoms of POP generally affect quality of life, but when complete uterine prolapse (procidentia) occurs, ureteral obstruction and kidney damage may result.

- A staging system has been developed for POP so that outcomes of surgical and nonsurgical treatment can be quantified, followed, and improved. Medical management of mild to moderate cases of POP includes pelvic muscle exercises and the use of pessaries. Surgical procedures include anterior and posterior repairs (colporrhaphy) using existing natural tissue and synthetic mesh materials, vaginal vault suspension (colpopexy) for apical vaginal prolapse, and complete vaginal closure procedures (colpocleisis) for some women who no longer desire coital function. Robot-assisted procedures are now used for some of these interventions.

- *Urinary incontinence* is defined as the involuntary loss of urine that is a social or hygienic problem. It is estimated that as many as 50% of women have some urinary incontinence at some time during their lives. SUI occurs in response to physical exertion, coughing, or sneezing. After appropriate testing to document SUI, surgical procedures include retropubic urethropexy, suburethral sling placement, or bulking injections.

- *Overactive bladder* (OAB) and *urge urinary incontinence* (UUI) are used interchangeably to describe incontinence that occurs when there is a strong urge to pass urine with a decreased ability to prevent passage. Treatments include behavior modification (bladder training), medications, electrical stimulation, or injections.

- Overflow incontinence and urinary fistulas may also be causes of involuntary passing of urine. Neuropathies account for most of the cases of overflow incontinence, whereas pelvic surgery and radiation damage cause 95% of fistulas. Surgical repair of fistulas is almost always needed. Pelvic pain disorders include painful bladder and myofascial pelvic pain syndrome.

An accurate knowledge of the anatomy of the female pelvic floor enables the student to understand pelvic organ prolapse and its management. Female pelvic medicine and reconstructive surgery (FPMRS) is the newest board-certified subspecialty within the specialties of obstetrics and gynecology as well as urology. This new certification process recognizes the importance of disorders of the female pelvic floor and the increased knowledge and skills necessary to evaluate and treat these disorders.

Normal Pelvic Anatomy and Supports

The bony pelvis acts like a basket, supporting the muscular attachments, pelvic organs, vessels, and nerves contained within it. The pelvic organs, including the vagina, uterus, bladder, urethra, and rectum, are supported within the pelvis by the bilaterally paired and posteriorly fused levator ani muscles. **The anterior separation between the levator ani is called the** *levator hiatus.* Inferiorly, the levator hiatus is covered by the urogenital diaphragm. **The urethra, vagina, and rectum pass through the levator hiatus and urogenital diaphragm as they exit the pelvis. The endopelvic fascia is a visceral pelvic fascia that invests the pelvic organs and forms bilateral condensations referred to as *ligaments* (i.e., pubourethral, cardinal, and uterosacral ligaments).** These ligaments attach the organs to the fascia of the pelvic side walls and bony pelvis. Damage to the vagina and its support system allows the urethra, bladder, rectum, and small bowel to herniate and protrude into the vaginal canal.

The **perineal body** is a central point for the attachment of the perineal musculature. **Although the contents of the abdominal cavity bear down on the pelvic organs, they remain suspended in relation to each other and to the underlying levator sling and perineal body.**

Pelvic Organ Prolapse

Pelvic organ prolapse (POP) refers to the protrusion of the pelvic organs into the vaginal canal or beyond the vaginal opening. It occurs because of a weakness in the endopelvic fascia investing the vagina, along with its ligamentous supports. **Defects in vaginal support may occur in isolation** (e.g., anterior vaginal wall only), **but they are more commonly combined.** The nomenclature of POP has evolved such that older terms such as *cystocele, rectocele,* and *enterocele* have been replaced by more anatomically precise terms (Figure 23-1).

ANTERIOR VAGINAL PROLAPSE (CYSTOCELE)

The anterior vagina is the most common site of vaginal prolapse. Women with this type of defect will describe symptoms of vaginal fullness, heaviness, pressure, and/or discomfort that often progress over the

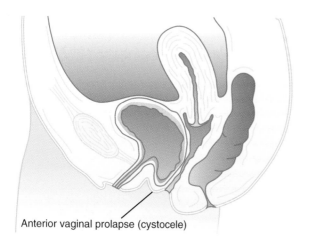

Anterior vaginal prolapse (cystocele)

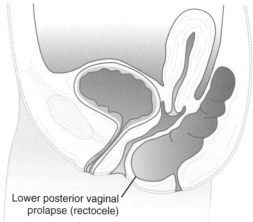

Lower posterior vaginal prolapse (rectocele)

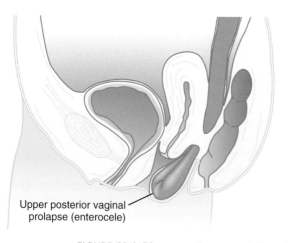

Upper posterior vaginal prolapse (enterocele)

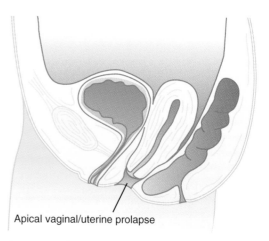

Apical vaginal/uterine prolapse

FIGURE 23-1 Diagrammatic representation of the four types of vaginal uterine prolapse.

course of the day and are most noticeable after prolonged standing or straining. Women may have to apply manual pressure to empty their bladder completely. Other symptoms include stress urinary incontinence (SUI), urinary urgency, and frequency. Significant anterior vaginal wall prolapse that protrudes beyond the vaginal opening (hymen) can cause urethral obstruction caused by kinking, resulting in urinary retention or incomplete bladder emptying.

POSTERIOR VAGINAL PROLAPSE (RECTOCELE AND ENTEROCELE)

Posterior vaginal defects occur when there is weakness in the rectovaginal septum. Symptoms can be indistinguishable from other types of prolapse because the discomfort, pressure, and the sense of a vaginal bulge are nonspecific. **When difficulties with bowel function and defecation occur, lower posterior vaginal prolapse is likely.** Straining or the need to manually splint for complete bowel elimination may occur. Upper posterior vaginal wall prolapse is nearly always associated with herniation of the pouch of Douglas, and because this is likely to contain loops of bowel, it is called an *enterocele.*

APICAL VAGINAL UTERINE PROLAPSE

Although vaginal prolapse can occur without uterine prolapse, the uterus cannot descend without carrying the upper or apical portion of the vagina with it.

Complete procidentia (uterine prolapse through the vaginal hymen) represents failure of all the vaginal supports (Figure 23-2). Hypertrophy, elongation, congestion, and edema of the cervix may sometimes cause a large protrusion of tissue beyond the hymen that may be mistaken for a complete procidentia. **Vaginal vault prolapse or eversion of the vagina may be seen after vaginal or abdominal hysterectomy** and represents failure of the supports around the upper vagina.

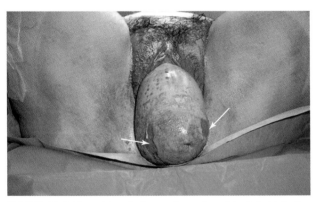

FIGURE 23-2 Complete uterine prolapse (procidentia). Note the lesions on either side of cervical dimple *(arrows),* representing pressure ulcerations from clothing/undergarments. (Courtesy C.M. Tarnay, MD, Ronald Reagan—UCLA Medical Center.)

Symptoms of POP mainly affect a woman's quality of life. However, significant sequelae of POP can occur in neglected cases of procidentia, which may be complicated by excessive purulent discharge, decubitus ulceration, and bleeding. **Ureteral obstruction with hydronephrosis is also a possible result of complete procidentia.**

ETIOLOGY OF PROLAPSE

The pelvic fascia, ligaments, and muscles may become attenuated from excessive stretching during pregnancy, labor, and difficult vaginal delivery, especially with forceps or vacuum assistance. Asian and black women appear less likely than white women to develop prolapse.

Increased intraabdominal pressure resulting from a chronic cough, ascites, repeated lifting of heavy weights, or habitual straining as a result of constipation may predispose women to prolapse. Atrophy of the supporting tissues with aging, especially after menopause, also plays an important role in the initiation or worsening of pelvic relaxation. **Iatrogenic factors include failure to adequately correct all pelvic support defects at the time of pelvic surgery, such as hysterectomy.**

DIAGNOSIS

Vaginal examination is facilitated by using a single-blade speculum. While the posterior vaginal wall is being depressed, the patient is asked to strain down. This demonstrates the descent of the anterior vaginal wall consistent with prolapse and urethral displacement. Similarly, retraction of the anterior vaginal wall during straining will accentuate posterior vaginal defects and uncover an enterocele and rectocele if present. **Rectal and vaginal examinations are often useful to demonstrate a rectocele and to distinguish it from an enterocele.**

QUANTIFYING AND STAGING PELVIC ORGAN PROLAPSE

The preferred method for describing and documenting the severity of POP is the **Pelvic Organ Prolapse Quantification (POP-Q) system.** The extent of prolapse is evaluated and measured relative to the hymen, which is a fixed anatomic landmark. The anatomic positions of the six defined points for measurement are denoted in centimeters above the hymen (negative number) or centimeters below the hymen (positive number). The plane at the level of the hymen is defined as zero (Figure 23-3).

Stages of POP can be assigned according to the most severe portion of the prolapse after the full extent of the protrusion has been determined. An ordinal system is used for measurements of different points along the vaginal canal, which allows for better communication

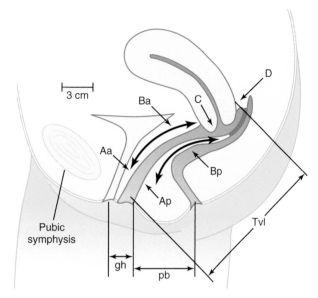

FIGURE 23-3 Illustration showing a side view of the female pelvis. Six sites (points Aa, Ba, C, D, Bp, and Ap), genital hiatus (gh), perineal body (pb), and total vaginal length (Tvl) used for pelvic organ support quantitation. (Reproduced with permission from Bump RC, Mattiasson A, Bø K, et al: The standardization of terminology of female pelvic organ prolapse and pelvic floor dysfunction. *Am J Obstet Gynecol* 175:10–17, 1996.)

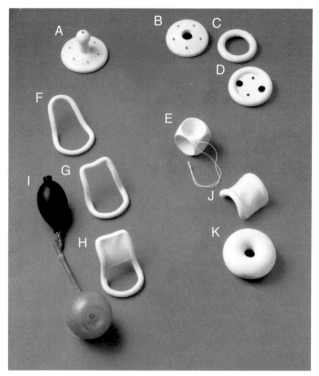

FIGURE 23-4 Some types of vaginal pessaries used for prolapse. **A,** Gellhorn; **B,** Shaatz; **C,** ring; **D,** ring with support; **E,** cube; **F,** Smith; **G,** Hodge; **H,** Hodge with support for cystocele; **I,** Inflatoball; **J,** Gehrung; **K,** donut.

between clinicians. This staging system enables more objective tracking of surgical outcomes.

MANAGEMENT

Prophylactic measures to mitigate the symptoms of POP include identifying and treating chronic respiratory and metabolic disorders, correction of constipation and intraabdominal disorders that may cause repetitive increases in intraabdominal pressure, and, for menopausal women, administration of estrogen. **Failure to recognize and treat significant support defects at the time of concomitant gynecologic surgery may lead to progression of existing prolapse** and the development of urinary incontinence or retention and urinary tract infections (UTIs).

Nonsurgical Treatment

When only a mild degree of pelvic relaxation is present, pelvic floor muscle exercises may improve the tone of the pelvic floor musculature. Pessaries (Figure 23-4), which provide intravaginal support, **may be used to correct prolapse by internally supporting the vagina. They can be considered when the patient is medically unfit** or refuses surgery or during pregnancy and the postpartum period. They are also useful to promote healing of a decubitus ulcer before surgery. In many patients, pessaries are the treatment of choice, as they are almost risk-free, immediately available, and

useful for interim treatment in those wishing to delay surgery.

Pessaries require proper fitting and must be selected in the appropriate type and size. They should be removed, cleaned, and reinserted every 6 to 12 weeks. They may cause vaginal irritation and ulceration. **Neglect may result in serious consequences,** including fistula formation, impaction, bleeding, and infection. Many patients are capable of caring for their pessaries themselves. In those cases, the patient inserts, removes, and cleans her pessary several times each week, if not daily. It is similar to the care and use of a contraceptive diaphragm.

Surgical Treatment

The main objectives of surgery are to relieve symptoms and restore normal anatomic relationships and visceral function. Preservation or restoration of satisfactory coital function, when desired, and a lasting operative result are also important goals.

REPAIR OF VAGINAL PROLAPSE. Anterior colporrhaphy corrects anterior vaginal wall prolapse and helps support the urethra. It involves **plication of the pubocervical fascia** to support the bladder and urethra. When the anterior prolapse involves a direct detachment of lateral vaginal support, it is considered a

paravaginal defect. Paravaginal defect repairs involve exposure of the retropubic space. **Interrupted permanent sutures are used to reattach bilaterally the anterior superior vaginal sulci to the arcus tendineus fasciae ("white line"),** extending from the ischial spine to the lower edge of the pubic ramus. When the defect is more central, a midline plication of endopelvic fascia is effective in adding support to the anterior vaginal wall. **Polypropylene mesh** may be used in appropriate patients to augment the weakened native tissue repair. In the presence of SUI, additional supportive measures are taken to achieve suspension of the bladder neck and proximal urethra.

Posterior colporrhaphy corrects a posterior vaginal wall prolapse and is similar in principle to anterior colporrhaphy. Site-specific posterior vaginal repairs can be performed after identification of the discrete endopelvic fascial breaks and reapproximation of this thicker tissue identified during rectal examination. Perineorrhaphy repairs a deficient perineal body. The outcomes of the site-specific repair are similar to the results of midline plication of the endopelvic fascia.

Recent modifications of these procedures involve the use of permanent suture or the addition of graft materials to augment the durability of the repair. These modifications can be accomplished using minimally invasive techniques such as endoscopic repair. **Permanent mesh grafts are not recommended in the posterior compartment,** because the incidence of complications is higher and outcomes are not as good as those achieved with repairs performed using native tissues.

REPAIR OF APICAL PROLAPSE. When the uterus is present, hysterectomy may be performed to facilitate exposure of the apical support structures. Hysterectomy, however, is not an absolute requirement in settings where uterine removal is not otherwise indicated or desired. The repair of apical defects may require peritoneal entry for the **repair of an enterocele.** After identification of the enterocele, the contents are reduced, the neck of the peritoneal sac is ligated, and the defect is repaired by approximating the uterosacral ligaments and levator ani muscles to restore continuity in the endopelvic fascia. **The uterosacral ligaments can be reattached to the cervix by either the vaginal or abdominal route.**

Vaginal vault suspension (colpopexy) for apical prolapse is performed to secure a durable fixation point for the top of the vagina. This can be accomplished vaginally or abdominally by suspending the vaginal vault to the sacrum, the sacrospinous ligaments, the uterosacral ligaments, or other firm points of fixation. This can be done with natural existing tissues or with polypropylene mesh.

Robot-assisted surgery for POP may be performed when a stronger attachment is needed in a very active or relatively young patient or for a woman with a prior failed prolapse repair. Abdominal sacrocolpopexy with polypropylene mesh has been performed for over 30 years using an open incision, and more recently laparoscopically assisted procedures have been used. Since 2008, sacrocolpopexy has been performed with the aid of a surgical robot. This is a minimally invasive abdominal operation in which mesh is placed between the bladder and vagina, the rectum and the vagina, and over the apex of the vagina or the cervical stump. The mesh is supported by attaching it to the sacral promontory. **The robot-assisted procedure is now considered to give the longest-lasting results for POP.**

VAGINAL CLOSURE PROCEDURES. For women with advanced vaginal prolapse who no longer desire coital function, there are less invasive surgical options. A LeFort colpocleisis involves suturing the partially denuded anterior and posterior vaginal walls together in such a way that the uterus remains in situ and is supported above the partially occluded vagina. **In women with posthysterectomy prolapse, a complete colpocleisis** involves total obliteration of the vagina. These "obliterative" procedures have traditionally been reserved for elderly women who are not likely to tolerate more invasive reparative operations. Most of these women will get complete resolution of their symptoms with a repair that is much less invasive and is associated with fewer risks and complications.

Urinary Incontinence

Urinary incontinence **is defined as the involuntary loss of urine that is a social or hygienic problem.** Urinary incontinence has been reported to affect 15-50% of women. The problem increases in prevalence with age, rising above 50% in elderly persons in nursing homes. **It is estimated that the direct financial cost of urinary incontinence in the United States is between $10 billion and $15 billion per year.**

ANATOMY AND PHYSIOLOGY OF THE LOWER URINARY TRACT

In the adult woman, the urethra is a muscular tube, 3 to 4 cm in length, lined proximally with transitional epithelium and distally with stratified squamous epithelium. It is surrounded mainly by smooth muscle. **The striated muscular urethral sphincter, which surrounds the distal two-thirds of the urethra, contributes about 50% of the total urethral resistance and serves as a secondary defense against incontinence.** It is also responsible for the interruption of urinary flow at the end of micturition.

The two posterior pubourethral ligaments provide a strong suspensory mechanism for the urethra and serve to hold it forward and in close proximity to the

pubis under conditions of stress. They extend from the lower part of the pubic bone to the urethra at the junction of its middle and distal thirds.

INNERVATION

The lower urinary tract is under the control of both parasympathetic and sympathetic nerves. **The parasympathetic fibers originate in the sacral spinal cord segments S2 through S4.** Stimulation of the pelvic parasympathetic nerves and administration of cholinergic drugs cause the detrusor muscle to contract. Anticholinergic drugs reduce vesical pressure and increase bladder capacity.

The sympathetic fibers originate from thoracolumbar segments (T10-L2) of the spinal cord. The sympathetic system has α- and β-adrenergic components. The β-fibers terminate primarily in the detrusor muscle, whereas the α-fibers terminate primarily in the urethra. α-Adrenergic stimulation contracts the bladder neck and the urethra and relaxes the detrusor muscle. β-Adrenergic stimulation relaxes the urethra and the detrusor muscle. **The pudendal nerve (S2-S4) provides motor innervation to the striated urethral sphincter.**

FACTORS INFLUENCING BLADDER BEHAVIOR

Sensory Innervation

Afferent impulses from the bladder, trigone, and proximal urethra pass to the S2 through S4 levels of the spinal cord by means of the pelvic hypogastric nerves. The sensitivity of these nerve endings may be enhanced by acute infection, interstitial cystitis, radiation cystitis, and increased intravesical pressure. The latter may occur in the standing or bending-forward position or in association with obesity, pregnancy, or pelvic tumors.

Inhibitory impulses, probably relayed by the pudendal nerve, also pass to S2 through S4 following mechanical stimulation of the perineum and anal canal. Their passage may explain why pain in this region can cause urinary retention or urgency and frequency.

Central Nervous System

In infancy, the storage and expulsion of urine are automatic and controlled at the level of the sacral reflex arc. Later, connections to the higher centers become established, and by training and conditioning, this spinal reflex becomes socially influenced so that voiding can be voluntarily accomplished. Although organic neurologic diseases may interrupt the influence of the higher centers on the spinal reflex arc, patterns of micturition may also be profoundly altered by mental, environmental, and sociologic disturbances.

CONTINENCE CONTROL

The bladder must store and hold urine painlessly and then, in the appropriate social setting, empty urine effectively. The normal bladder holds urine because

the intraurethral pressure exceeds the intravesical pressure. The pubourethral ligaments and surrounding endopelvic fascia support the urethra so that abrupt increases in intraabdominal pressure are transmitted equally to the bladder and proximal third of the urethra, thus maintaining a pressure gradient between the two structures. In addition, a reflex contraction of the levator ani compresses the mid-urethra, decreasing the likelihood of urine loss.

Stress Urinary Incontinence

Stress urinary incontinence **(SUI) is involuntary leakage of urine in response to physical exertion, sneezing, or coughing.**

ETIOLOGY

The most commonly accepted theory for the pathogenesis of SUI is urethral hypermobility due to vaginal wall relaxation that displaces the bladder neck and proximal urethra downward. When this occurs, increased intraabdominal pressure caused by coughing, sneezing, or physical exertion is no longer transmitted *equally* to the bladder and proximal urethra. The normal urethral resistance is overcome by this increased bladder pressure, and leakage of urine results.

The second possible mechanism is intrinsic sphincter deficiency whereby the urethra fails to close in response to increases in intraabdominal pressure. This cause of SUI is analogous to having a leaky "valve" in the urethra.

Factors that contribute to SUI include childbearing, previous urogenital surgery or trauma, pelvic radiation, estrogen deficiency (menopause), and medications, such as diuretics and α-adrenergic blockers.

PELVIC EXAMINATION

Inspection of the vaginal walls should be performed with a single-blade speculum, which allows optimal visualization of the anterior vaginal wall and urethrovesical junction. Scarring, tenderness, and rigidity of the urethra from previous vaginal surgeries or pelvic trauma may be indicated by a scarred anterior vaginal wall. Because the distal urethra is estrogen-dependent, the patient with urogenital atrophy also has atrophic urethritis.

DIAGNOSTIC TESTS AND PROCEDURES

Cough Stress Test

The patient is examined with a full bladder in the lithotomy position. While the physician observes the urethral meatus, the patient is asked to cough. SUI is present if short spurts of urine escape simultaneously with each cough. A delayed leakage, or loss of large volumes of urine, suggests uninhibited bladder contractions. If loss of urine is not demonstrated in the lithotomy position, the test should be repeated with the patient in a standing position.

Cotton Swab (Q-Tip) Test

This test determines the mobility and descent of the urethrovesical junction on straining and allows differentiation from anterior vaginal laxity alone. With the patient in the lithotomy position, the examiner inserts a lubricated cotton swab into the urethra to the level of the urethrovesical junction and measures the angle between the cotton swab and the horizontal. The patient then strains maximally, which produces descent of the urethrovesical junction. Along with the descent, the cotton swab moves, producing a new angle with the horizontal. **The normal change in angle is up to 30 degrees. In patients with pelvic relaxation and SUI, the change in cotton swab angle ranges from 50 to 60 degrees or more** (Figure 23-5).

Postvoid Residual (PVR) Test

This test determines how well the patient empties her bladder. Within 10 minutes of voiding into the toilet, a catheter is introduced into the bladder to see how much urine is left behind. This can also be determined noninvasively by ultrasound. Less than 50 mL is con-sidered normal. This determination of PVR is helpful in diagnosing the cause of the incontinence and in assisting with the formulation of a treatment plan. If a woman has a high PVR, it is important to avoid treatments that interfere further with emptying or that increase bladder outlet resistance or obstruction.

Urethrocystoscopy

Urethrocystoscopy allows the physician to examine inside the urethra, urethrovesical junction, bladder walls, and ureteral orifices. This procedure is useful to detect bladder stones, tumors, diverticula, or sutures or mesh from prior surgeries.

Cystometry

Cystometry consists of distending the bladder with known volumes of water and observing pressure changes in bladder function during filling. **The most important observation is the presence of a detrusor reflex and the patient's ability to control or inhibit this reflex.**

The first sensation of bladder filling should occur at volumes of 150 to 200 mL. The critical volume (400 to 500 mL) is the capacity that the bladder musculature tolerates before the patient experiences a strong

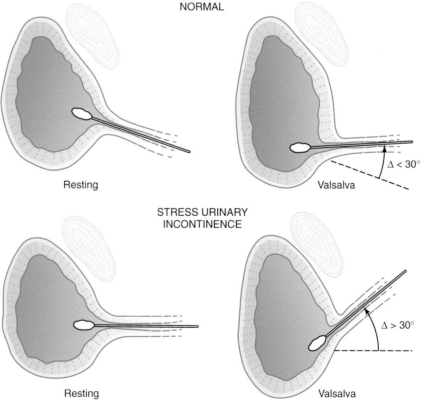

FIGURE 23-5 Diagrammatic representation of the Q-tip (cotton swab) test showing mobility of the urethrovesical junction in a continent patient and in a patient with stress urinary incontinence.

desire to urinate. At this point, if the patient is asked to void, a terminal contraction may appear and is seen as a sudden rise in intravesical pressure. At the peak of the contraction, the patient is instructed to inhibit this reflex (indicated by *arrows* in Figure 23-6, *A* and *B*). A healthy person should be able to inhibit this detrusor reflex and thereby bring down intravesical pressure

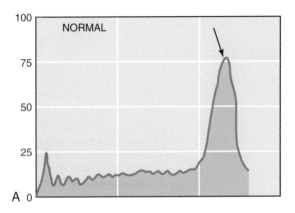

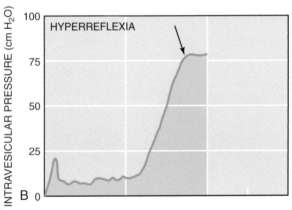

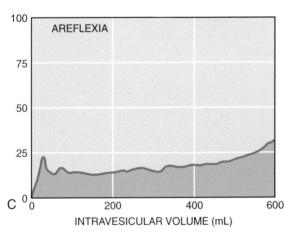

FIGURE 23-6 Water cystometry in a healthy patient **(A)**, a patient with detrusor hyperreflexia **(B)**, and a patient with detrusor are-flexia (hypotonic bladder) **(C)**. *Arrows* in **A** and **B** indicate peak of bladder contraction.

(see Figure 23-6, *A*). In patients with urologic or neurologic abnormalities, the detrusor reflex may appear without the specific instruction to void, and the patient cannot inhibit it (see Figure 23-6, *B*). This observation is referred to as an **uninhibited detrusor contraction.** Other terms for this disorder include *overactive bladder, detrusor hyperreflexia, irritable bladder, unstable bladder,* and *uninhibited neurogenic bladder.*

These cystometric procedures allow differentiation between patients who are incontinent as a result of uninhibited detrusor contraction and those who have SUI. Conversely, the hypotonic bladder accommodates excessive amounts of gas or water with little increase in intravesical pressure, and the terminal detrusor contraction is absent when the patient is asked to void (see Figure 23-6, *C*). The hypertonic bladder is a result of either neurologic disorders or fibrosis of the bladder secondary to inflammation or radiation.

Urethral Pressure Measurements

A low urethral pressure may be found in patients with SUI, whereas an abnormally high urethral closing pressure may be associated with voiding difficulties, hesitancy, and urinary retention.

Urethral function can be evaluated with cystometric testing. The urethral closing pressure profile is a graphic record of pressure along the length of the urethra. The urethral closing pressure normally varies between 50 and 100 cm H_2O. A Valsalva maneuver and/or an abdominal leak point pressure less than 60 cm H_2O or a urethral closure pressure of less than 20 cm H_2O are suggestive of the diagnosis of **intrinsic sphincteric deficiency (ISD).**

Uroflowmetry

Uroflowmetry is performed to record rate of urine flow through the urethra when the patient is asked to void spontaneously.

Voiding Cystourethrography

In this radiologic investigation, fluoroscopy is used to observe bladder filling, the mobility of the urethra and bladder base, and the anatomic changes during voiding. The procedure provides valuable information regarding bladder size and the competence of the bladder neck during coughing. It may detect any bladder trabeculation; vesicoureteral reflux during voiding; funneling of the bladder neck, bladder, or urethral diverticula; and outflow obstruction.

Complex Urodynamics

This combination of tests includes a cystometrogram, urethral pressure profile and flow study, a Valsalva leak point pressure reading, and an electromyogram. Complex urodynamics should be reserved for patients with severe incontinence, those who have had prior surgery for incontinence, or patients whose condition has been refractory to all conservative treatment. Patients with simple stress incontinence do not usually benefit from extra testing, unless their prior surgery has failed.

Other Imaging

By performing real-time or sector ultrasonography, information can be obtained about the inclination of the urethra, flatness of the bladder base, and mobility and funneling of the urethrovesical junction, both at rest and with a Valsalva maneuver. In addition, bladder or urethral diverticula may be identified.

Video urodynamics incorporate fluoroscopy with concurrent measurement of bladder and urethral pressures. Dynamic **magnetic resonance imaging (MRI)** studies are used to detect pelvic floor and relaxation defects in patients with incontinence.

SUMMARY

For a significant percentage of patients with SUI, a good history and physical examination, the cotton swab test, and the cough stress test are adequate investigations. The addition of uroflowmetry, cysto-urethroscopy, and cystometry are appropriate when more detailed information is needed for diagnosis and treatment. Additional urodynamic, electromyographic, electrophysiologic, and radiologic studies may be necessary in patients with a history of multiple previous surgeries for urinary incontinence and for patients with associated neurologic disease.

TREATMENT

Medical Therapy

In postmenopausal women with incontinence, **estrogens improve urethral closing pressure, vaginal epithelial thickness and vascularity, and reflex urethral function although paradoxically, estrogen has not been shown to reduce loss of urine.** α-Adrenergic stimulants, such as phenylpropanolamine or pseudoephedrine, may enhance urethral closure and improve continence, but they are unproven in placebo-controlled trials. The search for an effective medication to treat SUI is ongoing.

Physical Therapy

Pelvic floor muscle exercises, also known as Kegel exercises, constitute a proven first-line therapy to improve or cure mild to moderate forms of SUI. These exercises involve instructing a woman with SUI to tighten her pelvic muscles repeatedly over time. When performed correctly, the Kegel technique leads to stronger pelvic floor muscles and decreased urethral hypermobility. The exercises require diligence and a willingness to practice at home and/or at work. Some women find them difficult, fatiguing, or time-consuming, but when they are performed diligently, about 80% of women report decreased episodes of incontinence. **Kegel exercises before and after delivery may help patients with postpartum urinary incontinence.**

Intravaginal Devices

Larger sizes of pessaries (see Figure 23-5) have been used to elevate and support the bladder neck and urethra. They have been shown to be effective for SUI. Some are designed to give added support to the urethra.

Surgical Therapy

Surgery is the most successful and expeditious treatment for SUI. The aim of all surgical procedures is to correct the pelvic relaxation defect and to stabilize and restore the normal supports of the urethra. The approach may be vaginal or abdominal, or a combined abdominovaginal approach may be used.

ABDOMINAL APPROACH. Abdominal retropubic urethropexy has a long-term success rate of 80%. **The retropubic urethropexy is performed extraperitoneally (in the space of Retzius) by placing sutures in the fascia lateral to and on each side of the bladder neck and proximal urethra and elevating the vesicourethral junction by attaching the sutures to the symphysis pubis (Marshall-Marchetti-Krantz procedure) or to the Cooper ligament (Burch procedure).**

Postoperatively, a transurethral or suprapubic catheter is left in the bladder for continuous bladder drainage for 48 to 72 hours before instituting spontaneous voiding. Some patients (20-30%) may need prolonged postoperative bladder drainage (more than 7 days). Occasionally, a patient may develop osteitis pubis after the Marshall-Marchetti-Krantz procedure.

The recent popularity of operative laparoscopy for many gynecologic procedures has resulted in the **use of the laparoscope for bladder neck suspension procedures. When the laparoscopic procedure is performed by placing two sutures on each side of the bladder neck, the long-term success is similar to that achieved with the open abdominal approach for retropubic urethropexy.** Figure 23-7 illustrates the suture placement for a typical retropubic urethropexy.

VAGINAL APPROACH. Suburethral sling procedures have long been used to treat patients whose condition has been refractory to therapy or patients with severe SUI. Conventional slings often required harvesting a patient's own fascial tissue to be placed under the bladder neck, but their effectiveness has been plagued by high rates of urinary retention.

The tension-free synthetic (polypropylene) mesh placed at the level of the mid-urethra was introduced into the United States from Sweden in the late 1990s. The tension-free vaginal tape was developed as a minimally invasive technique, and **traditionally a mid-urethral sling has been placed retropubically. A**

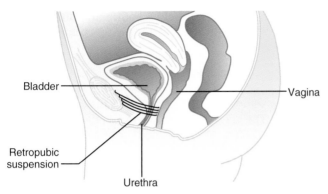

FIGURE 23-7 Illustration of a typical retropubic urethropexy with suture placement.

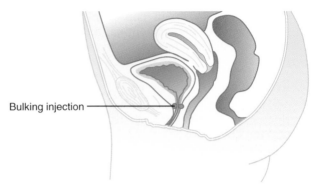

FIGURE 23-9 Illustration of the bulking injection procedure for urethral hypermobility.

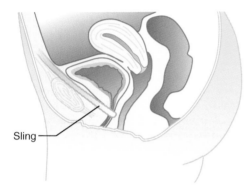

FIGURE 23-8 Illustration of a mid-urethral sling procedure.

variation is the transobturator approach. Rather than using a retropubic passage, in this approach the sling is passed through the obturator foramen laterally. The potential advantage of this approach is a reduction in bladder, bowel, or vascular injury. **The retropubic mid-urethral sling has better success rates than the transobturator sling when there is sphincter compromise as well.** The success rate of both approaches is about 85-90%. **Another variant of the mid-urethral sling is the one-incision sling or minisling.** These small lengths of polypropylene mesh are attached to the obturator fascia with small tissue hooks. Although there are fewer complications with this approach, it is somewhat less effective.

The mid-urethral sling is now considered a gold standard for the treatment of SUI. It is the most studied procedure in the history of randomized controlled surgical trials. Figure 23-8 is an illustration of a mid-urethral sling procedure for patients with SUI.

Bulking Injections

Conventional surgical procedures for incontinence sometimes fail in patients with a diagnosis of **urethral ISD.** ISD is a subtype of SUI marked by a very poorly functioning urethral sphincter. These patients are

treated with a suburethral sling procedure or **peri- or transurethral bulking injections** to improve urethral function. A commonly used bulking material is **nonabsorbable calcium hydroxylapatite,** which is nontoxic, nonantigenic, and unlikely to degrade. Figure 23-9 illustrates the bulking injection procedure for the ISD form of SUI.

Overactive Bladder/Urge Urinary Incontinence

The terms *overactive bladder* (OAB) and *urge urinary incontinence* (UUI) are often used interchangeably to describe a problem with bladder control that is associated with a strong desire to pass urine with a decreased ability to control it. UUI is defined as the involuntary leakage of urine accompanied by or immediately preceded by urgency. UUI can be associated with small losses of urine between normal micturitions or large volume losses with complete bladder emptying. **OAB,** previously described as UUI associated with detrusor muscle instability, is a more descriptive, symptom-based term that more accurately encompasses the common clinical presentation. **OAB is defined as "urgency, usually with but sometimes without urge incontinence and with frequency and nocturia."** OAB has become the preferred term as it comprises symptoms of urgency, UUI, frequency, and nocturia.

The incidence of OAB increases with age and is approximately 30% in the geriatric patient population. **In most patients, the exact etiology of OAB remains unknown,** but a number of risk factors (Box 23-1) are associated with its development.

Classically, women with OAB describe a sudden, strong urge to urinate with an inability to suppress the feeling, rushing to the bathroom, and experiencing leaking before making it to the toilet. Awakening several times a night to urinate is also a prominent feature (nocturia).

BOX 23-1

TYPES OF URINARY INCONTINENCE

Stress Urinary Incontinence (SUI)

- Involuntary leakage of urine in response to physical exertion, sneezing, or coughing
- Etiology: Urethral hypermobility due to vaginal wall relaxation displacing the bladder neck and proximal urethra downward; intrinsic sphincter deficiency (leaky valve)
- Contributing factors include childbearing, previous urogenital surgery, trauma, pelvic radiation, estrogen deficiency, and medications (e.g., diuretics and α-adrenergic blockers)
- Diagnosis: Cotton swab (Q-tip) and cough stress tests; additional urodynamic testing in appropriate women
- Treatments: Retropubic urethropexy, urethral sling procedure, and bulking injection procedures (see Figures 23-8 through 23-10)

Overactive Bladder (OAB)/Urge Urinary Incontinence (UUI)

- Both terms (OAB and UUI) are used interchangeably; both describe problems with bladder control associated with a strong desire to urinate with decreased ability to control flow
- Etiology: Poorly understood; risk factors include older age, chronic disorders, pregnancy, menopause (estrogen deficiency), operative trauma, medications (e.g., diuretics and psychotropic agents), and smoking
- Diagnosis: Unstable bladder as demonstrated during urodynamic testing

- Treatments: Behavior modification first, then add medications, Botox injections, or neuromodulation

Overflow Urinary Incontinence (OUI)

- Urinary retention and OUI may result from detrusor areflexia or a hypotonic bladder
- Etiology: Lower motor neuron disease, spinal cord injury, neuropathy due to diabetes mellitus, or outflow obstruction
- Diagnosis: Symptoms of bladder fullness, pressure, and frequent urination
- Treat the underlying causes if possible; intermittent or continuous bladder drainage (suprapubic catheter)

Mixed and Other Urinary Incontinence

- Some women may have signs and symptoms of both SUI and OAB; fistulas are an uncommon cause of incontinence in countries where modern obstetric care is available
- Etiology: For mixed incontinence, the causes are the same as for SUI and OAB; in developed countries, fistulas usually result from surgical injuries
- Diagnosis: The diagnosis of mixed incontinence can be challenging and inconsistent; incontinence from fistulas presents as painless leakage of urine from the vagina
- Treatment: A combination of treatments for SUI and OAB is usually initiated; fistulas may heal spontaneously or with estrogen cream, but surgical repair is usually necessary (e.g., muscle flap or diversion procedure)

TREATMENT

The optimal treatment of OAB starts with behavior modification (see below). Pharmacologic and physical interventions, such as electrical stimulation, can be added as needed. Identification of any dietary triggers, such as caffeine, alcohol, acidic or spicy foods, or carbonated beverages, is important. The use of a self-report bladder diary can be helpful for obtaining this information.

Behavior Modification

Reducing fluid intake and avoiding liquids during the evening hours are good initial behavior changes. Gradually **increasing the intervals between voidings,** as well as pelvic floor muscle strengthening exercises, such as **Kegel exercises,** are effective for attaining better bladder control.

Pharmacologic Treatment

Antimuscarinics, or anticholinergics, have become the mainstay of drug treatment for OAB. They work by suppressing uninhibited bladder contractions.

Current drug therapies include **oxybutynin chloride (Ditropan) and tolterodine (Detrol).** Oxybutynin chloride has been shown to improve symptoms of urinary urgency in approximately 70% of patients. **Tolterodine** also has anticholinergic activity. Because of its bladder specificity, tolterodine has a more favorable side effect profile than oxybutynin. It is also dosed less frequently, which improves patient compliance. Both are available in immediate-release and long-acting formulations. Oxybutynin is also available for delivery in a transdermal patch.

Trospium chloride, solifenacin, and **darifenacin** are newer agents used in the treatment of OAB. All significantly improve OAB symptoms compared with placebo. Evidence suggests that side effect profiles will be similar to or lower than those of the less specific antimuscarinics.

Mirabegron, the most recent agent, is a β_3-adrenergic agonist that aids in the storage of urine by assisting relaxation of the detrusor muscle.

Imipramine hydrochloride is a tricyclic antidepressant that acts through its anticholinergic properties to increase bladder storage. The drug improves bladder compliance rather than counteracting uninhibited detrusor contractions. It is given in doses lower than those recommended for use as an antidepressant. It also blocks postsynaptic noradrenaline uptake and thereby increases bladder outlet resistance. With its dual action, **imipramine may be effective in patients with mixed incontinence (both SUI and OAB).** It should be taken in the evening, as it may be sedating, and it should be used with caution in elderly patients because of its potential to cause orthostatic hypotension.

Functional Electrical Stimulation

Functional electrical stimulation offers an alternative for treating stress or urge incontinence when other treatments fail. A vaginal or rectal probe is inserted, usually twice daily for 15 to 30 minutes, to provide electrical stimulation to the pelvic floor muscles or to the nerves to these structures. Stimulation of the afferent fibers of the pudendal nerve can produce contractions of the pelvic floor and periurethral skeletal muscles, improving their tone and function in women with SUI.

Posterior Tibial Nerve Stimulation

Posterior tibial nerve stimulation (PTNS) involves the placement of an acupuncture-like needle into the posterior tibial nerve near the ankle and the application of electrical stimulation to this site. It is a form of neuromodulation that may reduce OAB symptoms with 3 to 4 months of treatment.

Sacral Stimulation (InterStim Device)

In appropriate patients, an implantable device used to stimulate the sacral nerve directly in the spine is effective for the treatment of OAB (or fecal incontinence).

Botulinum Toxin A Injection

Botulinum toxin A (Botox) can be injected into the bladder submucosa and detrusor muscle for 6 to 9 months of relief from OAB. It is as efficacious as other medications, has far fewer side effects, and gives longer benefit. **Cost-effectiveness studies show it to be more beneficial than oral medication.**

Overflow Incontinence

Urinary retention and overflow incontinence may result from detrusor areflexia or a hypotonic bladder, as is seen with lower motor neuron disease, spinal cord injuries, or autonomic neuropathy (diabetes mellitus). These patients are best managed by intermittent self-catheterization.

Overflow incontinence may also occur when there is an outflow obstruction. Straining to void, poor stream, retention of urine, and incomplete emptying may indicate an obstructive disorder. Overdistention of the bladder because of unrecognized urinary retention may occur in the postoperative period. This is a temporary problem related to postoperative pain and may be managed by continuous bladder drainage by catheter for 24 to 48 hours.

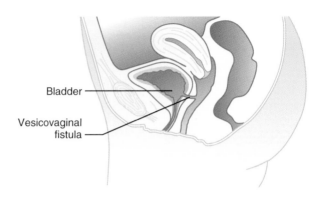

FIGURE 23-10 Illustration of a typical vesicovaginal fistula.

Urinary Fistulas

Fistulas are an uncommon cause of urinary incontinence in developed countries, because obstetric injuries, once the leading cause of urinary fistulas, have almost disappeared. When they do occur, they usually result from operative deliveries (e.g., forceps) rather than from neglected labor and pressure necrosis. **Obstetric fistulas remain a tremendous source of social and physical distress in developing countries.**

Pelvic surgery, irradiation, or both now account for 95% of the vesicovaginal fistulas in the United States. More than 50% occur following simple abdominal or vaginal hysterectomy (Figure 23-10). Approximately 1-2% of radical hysterectomies are followed in 10 to 21 days by a urinary fistula that is usually **ureterovaginal.** These fistulas are usually caused by devascularization of the ureter rather than by direct injury. Of all approaches to hysterectomy, vaginal hysterectomy has the lowest incidence of urinary tract injury.

Urethrovaginal fistulas generally occur as complications of surgery for urethral diverticula, anterior vaginal wall prolapse, or SUI. Urethral diverticula are rare, can cause incontinence, and are best diagnosed by MRI.

DIAGNOSIS OF A FISTULA

The usual history of painless and continuous vaginal leakage of urine soon after pelvic surgery is strongly suggestive of a fistula. **Instillation of methylene blue dye into the bladder will discolor a vaginal tampon or pack if a vesicovaginal fistula is present. Intravenous indigo carmine is excreted in the urine and will discolor a vaginal tampon or pack in the presence of a vesicovaginal or ureterovaginal fistula.** In addition, cystourethroscopy should be performed to determine the site and number of vesical fistulas. The majority of posthysterectomy vesicovaginal fistulas are located just anterior to the vaginal vault. **A computed tomographic (CT) scan with contrast dye or a retrograde pyelogram should be obtained to localize a ureterovaginal fistula.**

FISTULA REPAIR

Most obstetric fistulas can be repaired immediately on detection. For postsurgical fistulas, it is usual to wait some weeks to allow the inflammation to resolve. During this waiting period, UTIs should be treated and estrogen therapy instituted in postmenopausal women. **Steroids have been advocated to hasten resolution of inflammatory changes and allow early surgical intervention. Their use in this circumstance is controversial. Bladder rest with a Foley catheter, with or without tissue glue, may be effective in resolving isolated, small vesicovaginal fistulas. The majority of cases require surgical repair.**

Vesicovaginal Fistula

The vaginal approach **(Latzko operation)** is the procedure of choice. **A bulbocavernosus muscle flap or fat pad (Martius graft) may be interposed between the bladder and vagina to provide support, vascularity, and strength to the suture line, especially in patients who have had multiple previous attempted repairs and in those with a postradiation fistula.** Large radiation-induced fistulas may necessitate urinary diversion.

Ureterovaginal Fistula

Treatment of a ureterovaginal fistula depends on its size and location. **Small fistulas usually close spontaneously after placement of a ureteric stent (double J), provided the tissues have not been irradiated.**

If the fistula is close to the ureterovesical junction, the ureter proximal to the fistula can be reimplanted into the bladder **(ureteroneocystostomy).** If the fistula is several centimeters from the bladder, a **Boari flap** may be useful, a **segment of ileum may be interposed** between the proximal ureter and the bladder, or, rarely, a **transureteroureterostomy** may be employed.

Pelvic Floor Pain Syndromes

PAINFUL BLADDER SYNDROME

Painful bladder syndrome (PBS) refers to the continuum of lower urinary tract symptoms of discomfort that begin with mild OAB and end with interstitial cystitis. **PBS includes the following symptoms and signs: bladder pain, frequency, urgency, nocturia, dysuria, dyspareunia, and a feeling of incomplete bladder emptying, all in the absence of detectable infection or anatomical abnormality.**

Diagnosis is based on a careful history and physical examination to localize the pain in the bladder and urethra, negative urine cultures, and otherwise nondiagnostic cystourethroscopic and urodynamic studies. One theory of causation is a defect in the waterproof mucopolysaccharide lining of the bladder that allows caustic urine to seep into the submucosal tissue, causing inflammation and pain.

Treatment of PBS, starting with bladder training and behavior management, **includes pentosan polysulfate sodium (Elmiron),** an oral form of heparin; **hydroxyzine,** an oral antihistamine and anti-inflammatory agent; **and amitriptyline (Elavil),** a potent agent for treating neuropathy. When women are not responding, an intravesical combination of heparin, lidocaine, and sodium bicarbonate may be instilled weekly for relief, in addition to the oral agents listed above. Urethritis, which is usually caused by an infection with *Mycoplasma* or *Ureaplasma* species, may contribute to pelvic floor pain. This infection can be treated with 2 weeks of tetracycline or erythromycin after cultures have been obtained.

MYOFASCIAL PELVIC PAIN SYNDROME

Myofascial pelvic pain syndrome (MFPPS) is most likely a reaction of pelvic floor tissues to the other causes of pelvic floor pain mentioned above. The muscles of the pelvis that form the basket containing the pelvic organs react with chronic contraction and spasm to pain from other causes, resulting in more pain. MFPPS is diagnosed on the basis of physical examination by identifying a painful reaction when the levator and lateral obturator muscles, along with the anterior retropubic attachments of the pubourethral ligaments, are palpated. This condition can cause severe pain at trigger points. The pain and spasm can interfere with defecation or voiding. **The treatment includes medications such as amitriptyline, gabapentin, duloxetine, or specialized transvaginal physical therapy. Intramuscular injection of botulinum toxin A is also effective** in stopping the spasm in some cases. The prognosis for relief of pain is good with appropriate treatment.

24

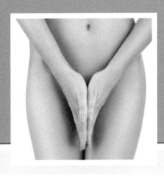

Ectopic Pregnancy

ANITA L. NELSON • JOSEPH C. GAMBONE

CLINICAL KEYS FOR THIS CHAPTER

- *Ectopic pregnancy* refers to those pregnancies that implant outside the uterine cavity. Although more than 95% of ectopic pregnancies implant in the fallopian tube, occasionally they may implant in other sites, such as the ovary, the uterine cervix, or, very rarely, in the abdominal cavity or a cesarean uterine scar. Following the use of assisted reproductive technologies (ARTs), the incidence of ectopic pregnancy has more than doubled to 2-3%, and the likelihood of implantation in more unusual sites has increased.

- The trophoblast of an early ectopic pregnancy that implants in the fallopian tube erodes through the tubal mucosal layer and into the tubal vessels. As the fetus grows, the blood from the eroded vessels dissects along the tubal wall, resulting in any of the following: (1) tubal rupture and intraperitoneal hemorrhage, (2) resorption of the pregnancy because of restricted blood supply, or (3) tubal abortion into the peritoneal cavity, where it may rarely result in an abdominal pregnancy.

- Clinical presentation of ectopic pregnancies may vary, but the classic triad of symptoms is (1) missed menses, (2) vaginal bleeding (usually spotting), and (3) lower abdominal pain. For individual women, there are three possible clinical presentations: (1) an acutely ruptured ectopic pregnancy, (2) a probable ectopic pregnancy with significant pelvic pain and vaginal spotting or bleeding, or (3) a possible ectopic pregnancy.

- Most often, the workup begins with testing to locate a "pregnancy of unknown location" (PUL). Other kinds of abnormal early pregnancies and other illnesses in early pregnancy may account for the signs and symptoms of ectopic pregnancy. The two most important diagnostic tests performed to diagnose an ectopic pregnancy are serial serum human chorionic gonadotropin (hCG) levels in maternal serum and sequential ultrasonic imaging.

- The key to proper management of ectopic pregnancy is early diagnosis. Treatment options depend on the clinical situation and, where possible, patient preferences. Surgery is necessary when rupture has occurred or is threatened or if the diagnosis remains uncertain. Medical therapy with methotrexate (MTX) is now widely used for probable and possible ectopic pregnancies. Irrespective of the type of treatment, most patients should be informed that they are at an increased risk of a future ectopic pregnancy.

An ectopic pregnancy is one that implants outside the endometrial cavity. The most common site for an ectopic pregnancy is in the fallopian tube, but a wide range of implantation sites is possible. Some treatments for infertility significantly increase the risk. They may also affect where the implantation occurs (Table 24-1). Although early diagnosis has enabled more effective intervention and lowered maternal mortality caused by ectopic pregnancies, the disorder is still a leading cause of maternal death in the first trimester of pregnancy.

Etiology and Risk Factors

Ectopic pregnancies generally result from abnormalities in the structure or function of the fallopian tube. The role that the conceptus itself may play is not known, but it is clear that chromosomal abnormalities do not cause ectopic pregnancies.

The most common cause of tubal abnormality associated with ectopic pregnancy is internal inflammation (salpingitis). Other causes include external tubal scarring secondary to endometriosis, ruptured

TABLE 24-1

INCIDENCE AND SITES OF ECTOPIC PREGNANCY

	Natural Conception	Assisted Reproductive Technologies
Overall incidence	About 1%	2-3%
Fallopian tube	>95%	<90%
Ovarian and abdominal	1-2%	5%
Cervical	0.15%	1.5%
Cesarean scar	1 in 1800	Unknown
Heterotopic*	1 in 30,000	1 in 100

*More than one site.

appendicitis, or previous surgery. Classically, **gonococcal salpingitis** causes significant symptoms of fever and pelvic pain and results in visible tubal damage. The fallopian tubes become distended with purulent material; the fimbriae can be clubbed; and the passage through the tube becomes tortuous with blind pouches (diverticuli) that physically block the progress of the fertilized egg into the endometrial cavity. **Chlamydial salpingitis** is usually associated with milder symptoms, and the tubal damage is more subtle. The heat shock protein released by *Chlamydia trachomatis* destroys the cilia lining the tubal mucosa, which are responsible for sweeping the conceptus through the tube.

Salpingitis isthmica nodosa is another inflammatory process that distorts the portion of the fallopian tube closest to the tubal ostia (opening into the uterine cavity). Thirty percent of all pregnancies that follow **tubal ligation** are ectopic. Other tubal surgeries (e.g., anastomosis, lysis of adhesions) also increase the risk of ectopic pregnancy. **One of the greatest risk factors is a history of a previous ectopic pregnancy. Recurrence rates are about 30%.** Uterine fibroids located near the ostia can distort or block tubal patency and increase the risk of ectopic pregnancy.

Tubal peristalsis is slowed by progestins, such as those that are released by the hormonal contraceptive intrauterine devices (IUDs), contraceptive implants, injections, and oral contraceptives. Although all of these methods of birth control significantly reduce the absolute risk of any pregnancy, when a failure (pregnancy) occurs during their use, the relative risk of an ectopic pregnancy is greatly increased. For example, it is estimated that 40-60% of pregnancies that occur during use of the levonorgestrel IUDs are ectopic (see Chapter 27).

The higher levels of progesterone induced by ovarian hyperstimulation during use of assisted reproductive technologies (ARTs) can also slow tubal motility. When multiple embryos are transferred during in vitro fertilization (IVF), the risk of ectopic pregnancy and the risk of heterotopic pregnancy (simultaneous intrauterine and ectopic) increase from

1:30,000 to 1:100 pregnancies. Other risk factors include a history of **infertility and smoking.**

Incidence and Classification

Now that many cases of ectopic pregnancy are managed medically in ambulatory settings, the incidence of ectopic pregnancy is not as well documented. The latest statistics from the mid-1990s indicated that 1-2% of all pregnancies in the United States were ectopic. Minority women have twice the risk of white women and a fourfold higher risk of ectopic pregnancy–related mortality. Recently, there have been counterbalancing shifts in the prevalence of risk factors for ectopic pregnancy (less pelvic infection but more advanced infertility treatment), so it is reasonable to assume that **about 1 in 80 pregnancies in the United States will be located outside the uterine cavity.**

The fallopian tubes are the site of over 95% of ectopic pregnancies. Those ectopic pregnancies are characterized by the portion of the salpinx in which the pregnancy implants: ampullary (75-80%), isthmic (12%), infundibular or fimbrial (6-10%), and interstitial or cornual (2-4%). Cornual ectopic pregnancies are particularly dangerous, because the pregnancy can continue to expand throughout the first trimester, and its rupture can lead to a sudden and rapid fatal exsanguination in less than 1 hour. Bilateral fallopian tube pregnancies occur in 1 in 200,000 pregnancies. Other sites for ectopic pregnancy include the cervix, the ovary (implantation below the ovarian cortex), the abdomen, and cesarean delivery scars. There has been a distinct increase in the numbers of cesarean scar pregnancies as cesarean delivery has become more common. Heterotopic pregnancies, in which pregnancies simultaneously implant in both the endometrium and in an extrauterine site, may occur as frequently as 1 in 100 IVF pregnancies.

Natural History

The trophoblasts of the conceptus implanted in the mucosa of the fallopian tube rapidly erode through that layer and invade into the underlying blood vessels. This induces local bleeding, some of which dissects into the tubal lumen and spills into the endometrial cavity (causing spotting), and some of it passes into the peritoneal cavity (causing a hemoperitoneum). Most of the blood generally is trapped between the serosal and mucosal layers and distends the tube with clot, which explains the common finding of cervical motion tenderness. If the bleeding is extensive enough, it can cause pressure necrosis of the overlying tubal serosa, resulting in acute rupture and causing a significant hemoperitoneum. Occasionally, the local blood supply to the pregnancy is so compromised that the pregnancy is resorbed (spontaneously resolved) or aborted into the peritoneal cavity, a process that may be asymptomatic.

Clinical Presentation

The clinical presentation of tubal ectopic pregnancies can vary from subtle lower abdominal discomfort and light uterine spotting to symptoms consistent with hypovolemic shock due to massive internal hemorrhage from tubal rupture. Ectopic pregnancies in other sites may have slightly different presentations, but the common finding of all ectopic pregnancies is that the symptoms occur in the setting of a positive pregnancy test. Clinical presentations should be evaluated in terms of three possibilities: (1) an acutely ruptured (or rupturing) ectopic pregnancy, (2) a probable ectopic pregnancy in a symptomatic woman, and (3) a possible ectopic pregnancy in a mildly symptomatic woman with a pregnancy of unknown location (PUL).

ACUTELY RUPTURED ECTOPIC PREGNANCY

Fortunately, **only a small number of women with fallopian tube pregnancies present with symptoms indicative of massive internal hemorrhage from acute tubal rupture.** This presentation is particularly likely to occur in women with poor access to care and occasionally in those whose medical therapy fails. Women may present with dizziness or loss of consciousness and sudden onset of severe pain. **Some shoulder pain may be present because of irritation of the phrenic nerve by blood and clotting in the abdominal cavity.**

During a physical examination, **hemodynamic instability is indicated by tachycardia, diaphoresis, and hypotension.** The abdomen may be distended, and both abdominal guarding and rebound tenderness may be present. There may be only minor bleeding from the cervix found by speculum examination, but noticeable cervical motion tenderness and a slightly enlarged, globular uterus may be detected by bimanual examination. A palpable adnexal mass may or may not be present.

An acute rupture of an ectopic pregnancy represents a surgical emergency. Large-bore intravenous lines must be established, and fluid resuscitation must be started immediately. Blood transfusion should follow as soon as possible, but surgery should not be delayed. **In the hemodynamically unstable patient, laparotomy is usually required.** Laparoscopy may be performed in less compromised patients. Generally, tubal damage after rupture is so extensive that salpingectomy is required.

PROBABLE ECTOPIC PREGNANCY

Hemodynamically stable women who have a positive pregnancy test and present with notable pelvic pain and vaginal spotting or bleeding should be classified as having a "probable ectopic pregnancy" after other

---

BOX 24-1

OTHER PAIN-PRODUCING PROBLEMS THAT MAY OCCUR EARLY IN PREGNANCY

Gynecologic Problems
1. Threatened or incomplete abortion
2. Ruptured corpus luteal cyst
3. Acute pelvic inflammatory disease (rare)
4. Adnexal torsion
5. Degenerating leiomyoma (especially in pregnancy)

Nongynecologic Problems
1. Acute appendicitis
2. Pyelonephritis
3. Pancreatitis

---

disease processes that may present with similar symptoms in early pregnancy have been ruled out (Box 24-1). Such patients generally have other clinical signs, such as tenderness of the abdomen with adnexal or cervical motion tenderness. On ultrasound, a variable amount of free fluid may be detected in the cul-de-sac. **Only occasionally will the ectopic pregnancy be seen on ultrasound as a "double-ring" sign in the adnexa, but a corpus luteal cyst is often present.** In such symptomatic women, even though they have stable vital signs, surgical exploration is generally recommended. Conservative surgical procedures that preserve the fallopian tube are generally performed in women desiring future fertility (see Management section below).

POSSIBLE ECTOPIC PREGNANCY

Most ectopic pregnancies fall into the category of possible ectopic pregnancy and are initially diagnosed as PUL. In the face of a positive pregnancy test, all of the differential diagnoses listed in Table 24-2 should be considered and ruled out. For women with possible ectopic pregnancies, the symptoms are more subtle than they are in the other two ectopic categories. Lower abdominal pain is present in most cases, although it is usually mild. Missed menses or an abnormal last menstrual period is seen in 75-90% of cases. More than one-half present with abnormal vaginal bleeding that can range from minor spotting to bleeding consistent with a normal menstrual flow.

A physical examination reveals most patients to be afebrile, and fewer than half are found to have a discernable adnexal mass on pelvic examination. Often, the mass is palpated on the side opposite the ectopic pregnancy and represents a corpus luteum in that ovary. The uterus is soft and is either of normal size or is slightly enlarged. On ultrasound, a thin, triple-layered endometrial stripe (lining) may be seen, or it may be thickened because of human chorionic gonadotropin (hCG) stimulation induced by placental hCG (an Arias-Stella reaction). There may be a small amount of fluid

TABLE 24-2

DIFFERENTIAL DIAGNOSIS FOR PREGNANCY OF UNKNOWN LOCATION

Diagnosis	hCG Levels	Ultrasonic Findings
Intrauterine Pregnancies		
Normal, ongoing pregnancy	Appropriately rising	Yolk sac or embryo in gestational sac in endometrial cavity
Anembryonic gestation	Variable pattern	Empty gestational sac in face of hCG > discriminatory zone or no appearance of embryo at appropriate time
Embryonic demise	Variable pattern	Embryo visualized with no cardiac activity
Incomplete abortion	Variable pattern	Retained placental tissue seen after (presumed) passage of fetus
Pregnancy Loss		
Complete abortion: intrauterine spontaneous or elective	Appropriately falling	Empty uterus, no suspicious adnexal findings
Complete abortion: ectopic	Appropriately falling	Empty uterus, no suspicious adnexal finding
Ectopic pregnancy (or persistent PUL)	Abnormally low increase, stable or abnormally decreasing	Empty uterus (without evacuation or following evacuation with no chorionic villi seen histologically) Possible visualization of extrauterine gestational sac or embryo

hCG, Human chorionic gonadotropin; *PUL,* pregnancy of unknown location.

seen in the cul-de-sac, representing some intraperitoneal blood. Rarely is the ectopic pregnancy actually visualized. A diagnosis of PUL is made until a longer-term evaluation can be conducted to determine if a more definitive diagnosis can be made. The final diagnosis may be a normal intrauterine pregnancy, an abnormal uterine pregnancy, or an ectopic pregnancy. **In the face of an early failing or failed pregnancy, the location of the implantation may never be determined and the diagnosis of PUL will thus remain.**

Diagnostic Tests for Pregnancies of Unknown Location

Because the consequences of ectopic pregnancy can be so serious, a high index of suspicion for ectopic pregnancy must be maintained until testing can establish the normalcy of the early pregnancy and its implantation site. Ectopic pregnancy must be included in the list of differential diagnoses in women who present with a positive pregnancy test, abnormal bleeding, and/or abdominopelvic pain. Generally, serial testing is needed over the course of several days during which time the patient must be reassessed clinically. **The two most important diagnostic tests are serial quantitative hCG levels in serum and sequential ultrasonic imaging.** The first test establishes the well-being of the pregnancy. The second is used to identify the implantation site and to determine a possible treatment plan. Endometrial evacuation and tissue identification procedures can also provide valuable information.

HUMAN CHORIONIC GONADOTROPIN TESTING

hCG is a glycoprotein consisting of two linked subunits: α and β. The α-subunit consists of 92 amino acids and is the same in luteinizing hormone (LH), follicle-stimulating hormone (FSH), and thyroid-stimulating hormone. The β-subunit is larger, with 145 amino acids; is different for each glycoprotein hormone; and provides for unique biologic activity. Before the development of sensitive and specific assays for the entire hCG molecule, tests for only the β-subunit of hCG were routinely used for assessment in early pregnancy, and especially to rule out ectopic pregnancies. This was because of the increased likelihood of false-positive results due to the cross-reactivity with other glycoprotein hormones (e.g., LH and FSH), which have the same α-subunits. Although the possibility of false-positive results still exists because of circulating factors in the serum that may interact with hCG antibody, **the more common laboratory test performed today is for the entire hCG molecule.** Although results of the more recent specific assay are still frequently referred to as *β-hCG,* we use the designation of *hCG* in this chapter.

The conceptus produces hCG before implantation, but the hormone does not enter the maternal circulation until after implantation. Sensitive assays for hCG can detect its presence within hours of implantation. The serum levels of hCG increase rapidly in a nonlinear fashion. The doubling time of serum hCG varies from 1.2 days shortly after implantation to 3.5 days at 2 months' gestational age. Healthy, normally developing pregnancies can be detected by a normal increase of maternal serum hCG levels. **More than 66% of normal pregnancies have a doubling time of 48 hours in the first few weeks of pregnancy.** The expected rise in 48 hours for a viable intrauterine pregnancy is generally acknowledged to be at least 50%, although researchers in one recent, large study suggested that a threshold of 35% should be used to capture all normal intrauterine pregnancies.

Approximately 60% of ectopic pregnancies show an initial increase in hCG levels, and 40% show a decrease. In fact, more than one-fourth of ectopic pregnancies initially show hCG increases consistent with a normal intrauterine pregnancy. Therefore, hCG titers need to be followed over time to document a pattern of sustained normal increase until they reach a threshold, at which time the embryo can be visualized within the endometrial cavity by ultrasound. **This *discriminatory zone* (DZ) is defined as the range of hCG values in which an ultrasonic image can first detect the signs of an intrauterine pregnancy.** Each institution sets its own DZ, depending upon the hCG assay used, the ultrasonic equipment available, and the skill of the ultrasonographers. **Most centers quote a range of 1500 to 2000 mIU/mL of hCG as the DZ.** When the hCG level exceeds the upper limit of the DZ and no signs of an intrauterine pregnancy are seen on ultrasound, suspicion of an ectopic pregnancy increases. The possibility of multiple gestations must also be considered.

In the case of declining hCG levels, the differential diagnosis includes a complete spontaneous abortion and an abnormal PUL. Two days following a complete spontaneous abortion, the hCG levels decrease by 35-52%, and by 7 days, they should be reduced by 66-87%. Levels that fail to decline appropriately are consistent with an ongoing PUL, which could be ectopic.

TRANSVAGINAL ULTRASONOGRAPHY

Ultrasound is used to determine the presence of an intrauterine pregnancy and to check for the presence of free fluid in the peritoneal cavity. **With transvaginal ultrasonography, a gestational sac is usually visible between 4.5 and 5 weeks of gestational age.** The yolk sac can be visualized between 5 and 6 weeks and a fetal pole with cardiac motion appears between 5.5 and 6 weeks.

Early in pregnancy, inaccurate dating based on the last menstrual period can be a problem, so knowing the hCG level and the DZ for the reported level can be very helpful. When the upper level of hCG for the DZ is reached, an intrauterine pregnancy should be seen.

On ultrasound, an early normal intrauterine pregnancy has an eccentrically located echolucent area with a "double-ring" sign representing the decidual lining and the chorion around the early decidual sac. **This early gestational sac can be confused with a centrally located "pseudodecidual sac" that can be seen in ectopic pregnancies.** To confirm the diagnosis of intrauterine pregnancy, the patient is generally followed until a yolk sac or a fetal pole can be seen within the gestational sac.

OTHER TESTS FOR PREGNANCIES OF UNKOWN LOCATION

If the diagnosis of an abnormal pregnancy is made on the basis of a low rate of increase in hCG titers (<35% in 48 hours) or a decrease in hCG titers that is too slow to represent a complete abortion (<30% in 48 hours), or if the pregnancy is unwanted, an endometrial curettage can be performed. The absence of chorionic villi on examination of the biopsy specimen makes the diagnosis of ectopic pregnancy much more likely.

Serum Progesterone

Serum progesterone levels can help distinguish normal from abnormal pregnancies. The levels of progesterone remain relatively constant from 5 to 10 weeks of gestation, so only a single specimen is needed. Levels less than 5 ng/mL are consistent with an abnormal pregnancy with high specificity and a 60% sensitivity. Levels greater than 20 ng/mL indicate a healthy pregnancy with 95% sensitivity and 40% specificity. Unfortunately, most ectopic pregnancies have levels of progesterone in the 6 to 19 ng/mL range, which is not useful for diagnostic purposes.

OTHER IMAGING MODALITIES AND PROCEDURES

Magnetic resonance imaging (MRI) is used to help identify cesarean scar pregnancies and cornual pregnancies, both of which are potentially dangerous. Ultrasound may not be able to identify these ectopic sites because of their proximity to the endometrium.

Culdocentesis (needle aspiration of pelvic peritoneal fluid through the posterior fornix) has largely been replaced by ultrasonic imaging of free fluid in the cul-de-sac. However, aspiration of peritoneal fluid can help distinguish nonclotting blood (hemoperitoneum) from clear fluid (ruptured ovarian cyst) and purulent material (acute infection). This information may be useful when the clinical presentation is confusing and the results would influence the choice of therapy.

Laparoscopy can be used as a diagnostic tool for PULs if questions remain about the patient's pathology. It has the advantage of providing treatment if an ectopic gestation is found (see below), but it does entail increased surgical risks and costs. Even with laparoscopy, there is a 2-5% rate of misdiagnosis, either because the ectopic pregnancy was too small to be recognized (false-negative) or because other processes were responsible for the suspicious appearance of the fallopian tube (false-positive).

Differential Diagnosis

A number of other disorders need to be considered in the differential diagnosis of ectopic pregnancy. Although pelvic pain and a positive pregnancy test should strongly suggest ectopic pregnancy, on occasion some other pain-producing disorder may occur in conjunction with an early intrauterine pregnancy and may need to be considered (see Box 24-1). Figure 24-1 presents an algorithm for the workup and

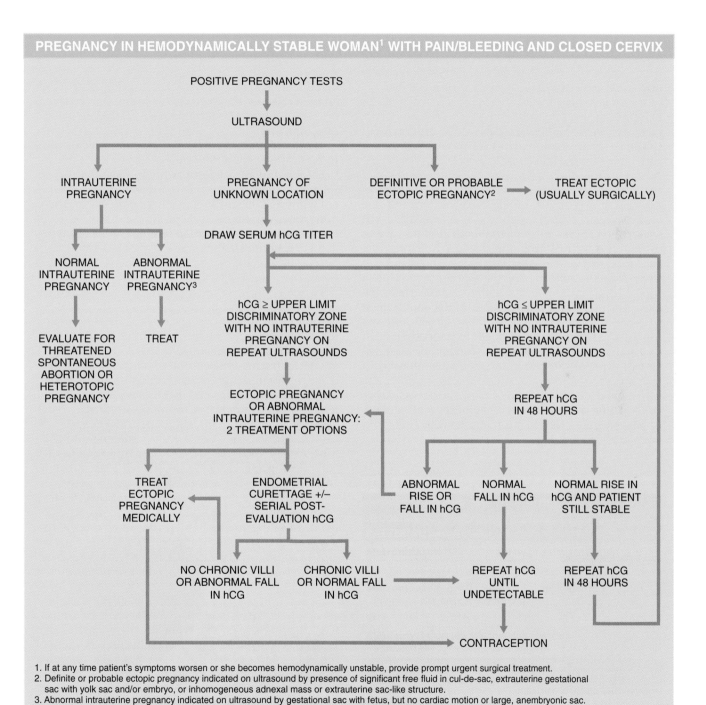

FIGURE 24-1 Algorithm for the workup and management of early pregnancy in a hemodynamically stable woman with pain, bleeding, and a closed uterine cervix. *hCG*, Human chorionic gonadotropin.

management of a hemodynamically stable woman with a positive pregnancy test, pelvic pain and bleeding, and a closed uterine cervix.

Management

The management of ectopic pregnancy in the fallopian tube depends on the stability of the patient, the availability of resources, and the patient's desire for future fertility. **In general, medical management is preferred for an early ectopic pregnancy, and surgery is reserved for unstable patients, those whose diagnosis is uncertain, and those whose medical therapy has failed.**

SURGERY

Laparotomy is the preferred surgical approach for women who are hemodynamically unstable, because rapid access to the bleeding site is critical. It is also the preferred approach whenever it is anticipated that laparoscopy would not be successful (e.g., because of extensive intraperitoneal adhesions). If it is determined intraoperatively that laparoscopy is not possible, the surgery can always be converted to laparotomy. Laparoscopy is discussed further in Chapter 31. Figure 24-2 shows a tubal ectopic pregnancy viewed through the laparoscope.

The actual surgery performed on the fallopian tube itself depends on the amount of tubal damage and the patient's wishes for future fertility. **Salpingectomy** (removal of the entire fallopian tube) is recommended when there has been significant damage to the tube, when a patient who previously has been sterilized verifies that she still does not desire future fertility, and when there is a high likelihood of retained products of conception. A laparoscopic salpingectomy is illustrated in Figure 24-3, *A*.

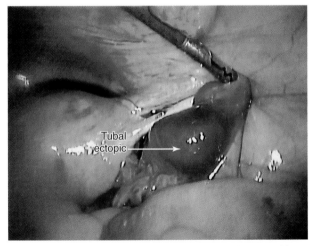

FIGURE 24-2 Tubal ectopic pregnancy as seen at the time of laparoscopy. (Courtesy B. Beller, MD, Eugene, Ore.)

Partial salpingectomy (removal of a portion of the fallopian tube) is generally performed only if the ectopic pregnancy is implanted in the mid-ampullary portion. A laparoscopic Endoloop partial salpingectomy is illustrated in Figure 24-3, *B*. **Salpingotomy** and **salpingostomy** are both procedures in which vasoconstrictive agents are injected beneath the implantation site. An incision is then made through the antimesenteric border of the fallopian tube, the products of conception are removed, and hemostasis is established. With salpingotomy, the incision is closed, whereas it is left open in a salpingostomy. A laparoscopic linear salpingostomy is illustrated in Figure 24-3, *C*. Most studies have shown that **salpingostomy** results in better long-term tubal function compared with **salpingotomy.**

If a patient's contralateral fallopian tube appears to be normal, there does not seem to be any advantage regarding future fertility if salpingectomy is performed instead of salpingostomy. In addition, there is a 10-20% risk of residual trophoblastic tissue whenever the products of conception are dissected from the fallopian tube (i.e., when salpingostomy or salpingotomy is performed). Patients who do not have resection of the affected tubal area should have repeat hCG titers 3 to 7 days postoperatively to confirm that no hCG-producing cells remain to reinvade the tube. When repeat hCG titers fail to decline appropriately, methotrexate (MTX) therapy can be started (see the following section). The risk for incomplete trophoblastic tissue removal is greatest when the ectopic products of conception are "milked" through the tube to extrude through the fimbria. This technique should never be used, even when it appears that the pregnancy is spontaneously aborting through the fimbria.

MEDICAL MANAGEMENT WITH METHOTREXATE

Ambulatory medical management of women with early, unruptured ectopic pregnancies has replaced surgical diagnosis and treatment in most cases. Randomized trials have shown no difference in overall tubal preservation, tubal patency, repeat ectopic pregnancy, or future pregnancy rates in women treated with medical management compared with tube-sparing laparoscopic surgery. The success of MTX diminishes rapidly with higher levels of hCG. Therefore, each institution should have its own criteria for offering MTX. However, in most cases, women treated with medical therapies avoid any surgical risk. The most commonly used agent is MTX, which is a folic acid antagonist that inhibits DNA synthesis and cell replication. Because of the side effects of MTX and the potential for tubal rupture, careful evaluation of the patient for possible contraindications, as shown in Box 24-2, is needed. Before MTX is considered, the woman should demonstrate a normal serum creatinine level, as well as normal liver and blood count studies.

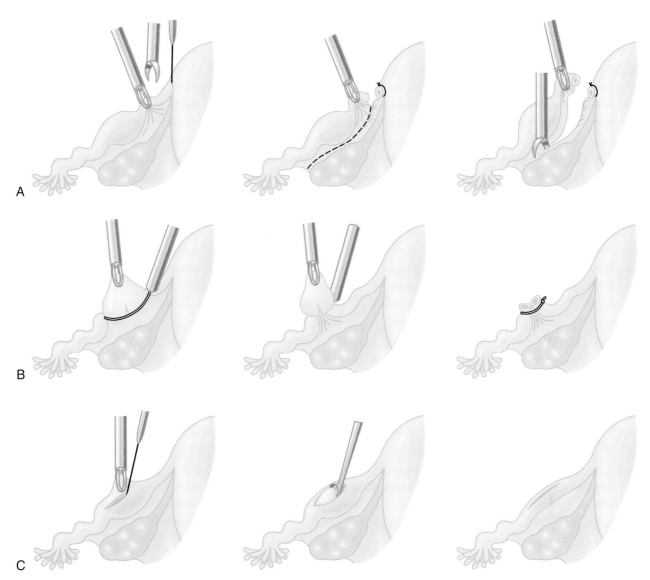

FIGURE 24-3 Methods of laparoscopic management of tubal pregnancy. **A,** Salpingectomy using Endoloop and cautery scissors for isthmic tubal pregnancy. **B,** Partial salpingectomy with Endoloop. **C,** Linear salpingostomy for an ampullary ectopic pregnancy.

There are three popular protocols used for MTX treatment: (1) the single-dose/flexible-dose protocol, (2) the two-dose protocol, and (3) the fixed multidose protocol. The most commonly used is the single-dose approach, in which the patient's response to therapy is monitored and a second dose is prescribed only if the hCG levels do not fall adequately. In this protocol, MTX is administered in a dose of 50 mg/m^2 initially. The patient returns on days 4 and 7 for repeat hCG determinations. If the hCG titers fall at least 15% between the return days, the patient can be followed at weekly intervals to verify at least a continued 15% decline every 7 days until the hCG level is undetectable (usually <5 mIU/mL). When the hCG levels plateau or fall too slowly, another dose of MTX may be given if all the

other criteria continue to be met. If the patient becomes more symptomatic or if hCG titers increase during therapy, surgical intervention is required.

Some centers prefer to routinely provide two doses of MTX—the first on day 1 and the second on day 4. If the response to these injections is suboptimal (<15% decline in hCG level), another course of therapy with MTX is given on days 7 and 11. Surgery is considered when the response is inadequate. Sometimes this protocol is followed when the baseline hCG levels approach the upper limits of the institution's threshold for MTX use.

The fixed multidose therapy today is generally reserved for cases in which the patient's hCG level is much higher than normal or embryonic cardiac motion

BOX 24-2

MEDICAL MANAGEMENT OF ECTOPIC PREGNANCY

Contraindications to the Use of Methotrexate (MTX)

Patient-Related

1. Hemodynamic instability
2. Unreliable for return visits
3. Known sensitivity to MTX
4. Overt or laboratory evidence of immunodeficiency
5. Hepatic, renal, or hematologic dysfunction
6. Active pulmonary disease
7. Peptic ulcer disease
8. Breastfeeding

Ectopic Pregnancy–Related

1. Gestational sac ≥ 3.5 cm
2. Embryonic cardiac motion seen
3. Human chorionic gonadotropin levels > institutionally predetermined value (usually between 6000 and 15,000 mIU/mL)

Modified from American College of Obstetricians and Gynecologists (ACOG): Medical management of tubal pregnancy, *Practice Bulletin No. 94*, Washington, DC, June 2008, ACOG.

is detected. In this 8-day regimen, MTX is administered intramuscularly every other day and folic acid rescue is provided on alternate days.

Patients being treated with MTX should be instructed to avoid folate supplements, nonsteroidal antiinflammatory agents, and alcohol. Pelvic rest (no sexual activity) is required, and women should also avoid sunlight exposure and vigorous physical exercise. Women should be warned about potential side effects of MTX. Gastrointestinal side effects, stomatitis, and hair loss are possible, especially with more prolonged therapy. Women may experience abdominal pain 2 to 3 days after injection, which is potentially caused by continued expansion of the pregnancy mass. They should return immediately if they have any sudden severe abdominal pain, shoulder pain, or dizziness. To avoid confusion about abdominal pain, gas-producing foods should be avoided. Women should be assured that treatment with MTX will not compromise their future fertility.

OTHER THERAPEUTIC INTERVENTIONS

When ectopic pregnancy is diagnosed at the time of laparoscopy, **MTX, prostaglandins, or hyperosmolar glucose can be injected into the amniotic sac to destroy the ectopic pregnancy without the need for any other procedure.** This technique can also be performed transvaginally using ultrasonographic guidance without laparoscopy. The potential advantage of this technique is that it is a one-time injection that reduces systemic side effects. However, the success of this approach has had mixed results, and therefore **its use should be considered experimental.**

EXPECTANT MANAGEMENT

Selected patients may qualify for expectant management (watchful waiting) if they are stable and the diagnosis of ectopic pregnancy is not yet certain or if their symptoms are resolving. **Patients managed expectantly should be reliable and relatively asymptomatic with hCG titers low enough that rupture is unlikely** (<200 mIU/mL and declining). When hCG levels are less than 200 mIU/mL, 85% of ectopic pregnancies resolve spontaneously. These women should be carefully followed with serial hCG testing and monitoring.

IMPORTANT THERAPUETIC CONSIDERATIONS

All Rh-negative, unsensitized women who have ectopic pregnancies should receive anti-Rh immunoglobulin (RhoGAM). After an ectopic gestation, pregnancy should be avoided for at least 3 months to permit the fallopian tube to normalize and to allow complete elimination of MTX if that agent has been given. Highly effective contraception should be provided as soon as the ectopic pregnancy starts to resolve.

TREATMENT OF UNCOMMON TYPES OF ECTOPIC PREGNANCIES

An **ovarian ectopic pregnancy** produces the same symptoms as a tubal pregnancy. The treatment is aimed at removing the pregnancy and preserving as much normal ovarian tissue as possible. When ovarian preservation is not possible, usually because of profuse bleeding, oophorectomy is indicated. If identified early enough, ovarian ectopic pregnancies may be treated successfully with MTX.

Cervical ectopic pregnancy usually presents with profuse vaginal bleeding, and attempts at removal of the pregnancy are often unsuccessful. MTX and arterial embolization are used to manage cervical pregnancy if the patient is not actively bleeding. An alternative is to aspirate the cervical ectopic using an oocyte aspiration needle, traversing the cervical stroma. **Hysterectomy is reserved for large cervical ectopic pregnancies not amenable to nonsurgical intervention and for actively bleeding cervical pregnancies that cannot be controlled conservatively.**

Pregnancies rarely implant in the abdominal cavity (e.g., on the omentum, bowel, or parietal or visceral peritoneum), **but when they do, the pregnancy may proceed to near or full term.** At the time of laparotomy in advanced gestations, the placenta presents a major technical difficulty. Vital organs may be entirely or partially covered by the firmly attached placenta, and any attempt at removal may cause massive bleeding. Partial bowel resection may be required if the bowel is involved. **In most cases, it is best to leave the placenta attached,** especially if the pregnancy is in the second or third trimester. Expectant management, allowing spontaneous reabsorption of placental tissue, and treatment with MTX to enhance placental reabsorption have both been reported to be successful.

The presence of an ectopic pregnancy in an old cesarean scar is reported with increasing frequency. Contrast-enhanced MRI may be needed to distinguish this from an intrauterine implantation. MTX given systemically combined with uterine artery embolization and curettage have been successful, but more extensive surgery is required in some cases.

Implications for Future Fertility

Patients who have had an ectopic pregnancy are at a 7- to 13-fold increased risk for another ectopic pregnancy and ongoing problems with infertility. In one encouraging study, researchers reported that the pregnancy rate is just over 80% after either medical or surgical treatment for ectopic pregnancy, with a mean time to conception of 9 to 12 months. Fertility rates are similar after expectant management or surgical intervention. All patients who have had an ectopic pregnancy should receive counseling about the increased risk of having another ectopic pregnancy before attempting pregnancy.

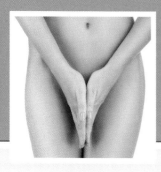

25

Endometriosis and Adenomyosis

JOSEPH C. GAMBONE

CLINICAL KEYS FOR THIS CHAPTER

- *Endometriosis* is defined as the presence of endometrial glands and stroma in extrauterine locations. An accurate prevalence for endometriosis is not known, but it is estimated that about 10% of women of reproductive age have the disease. Most women are without symptoms, but some have severe pain often manifested by dysmenorrhea, dyspareunia, and, less often, dyschezia. Infertility is often the initial sign of endometriosis.

- Retrograde menstruation, metaplastic transformation of peritoneal mesothelium, and lymphatic spread are the three most often cited hypotheses for the origins and locations of endometriosis. An immunologic factor is presumed to explain why some women who have risk factors similar to those that are affected do not develop the disease. Genetic predisposition is highly likely, based on polygenetic, multifactorial inheritance.

- The staging of endometriosis is based upon the location, extent, and appearance of the lesions. Implants of glands and stroma may be dark red, brown, bluish gray, or even white. The lesions are frequently surrounded by fibrosis, which results in puckering. Ovarian cysts filled with hemosiderin-laden, "chocolate"-colored fluid may form metaplastic endometriomas.

- The amount of endometriosis does not always correlate with the severity of symptoms. Women with minimal or no symptoms may be managed expectantly. Medical treatments consist of initial trials of nonsteroidal antiinflammatory drugs (NSAIDs) and low-dose progestins, including oral contraceptives (OCs). More advanced medical therapy includes the androgenic danazol and gonadotropin-releasing hormone (GnRH) analogues. When fertility is desired but is not occurring spontaneously and medical therapy has failed, conservative laparoscopic surgery to reduce the amount of endometriosis and reactive adhesions is indicated. More definitive extirpative surgery involves removal of all endometriosis and adhesions, along with the uterus and adnexal tissues. One or both ovaries may be preserved if they are completely free of endometriosis.

- Adenomyosis is the extension of endometrial glands and stroma into the uterine musculature more than 2.5 mm beneath the basalis layer. The uterus is homogeneously enlarged. Although many women with adenomyosis are without symptoms, some have severe dysmenorrhea, and the disorder may adversely affect fertility. Medical therapy with NSAIDs is indicated initially for the pain and uterine bleeding. Endometrial ablation may be performed for heavy bleeding, and hysterectomy is sometimes indicated when more conservative treatment has failed.

It is estimated that 5-15% of women of reproductive age have some degree of endometriosis, defined as the presence of endometrial glands and stroma in extrauterine locations. **Both endometriosis and adenomyosis** (growth of endometrial glands and stroma into the uterine muscle) **are associated with pelvic pain and infertility.** Endometriosis and adenomyosis often present difficult diagnostic and therapeutic challenges.

In the case of endometriosis, few gynecologic conditions can require such difficult surgical dissections.

Endometriosis

Endometriosis is a benign condition in which endometrial glands and stroma are present outside the uterine cavity and walls. Endometriosis is important in gynecology because of its frequency, distressing symptomatology, association with infertility, and potential for invasion of adjacent organ systems, such as the gastrointestinal and urinary tracts.

OCCURRENCE

The prevalence of endometriosis in the general population is not known, but **it is estimated that 5-15% of women have some degree of the disease.** At least one-third of women with chronic pelvic pain have visible endometriosis, as do a significant number of infertile women. Interestingly, endometriosis is noted in 5-15% of women undergoing gynecologic laparotomies, and it is an unexpected finding in approximately half of these cases.

The typical patient with endometriosis is in her 30s, nulliparous, and infertile. However, in practice, many women with endometriosis do not fit the classic picture. Occasionally, endometriosis may occur in infancy, childhood, or adolescence, but at these early ages, it is usually associated with obstructive genital anomalies such as a uterine or vaginal septum. Although endometriosis should regress following menopause unless estrogens are prescribed, 5% of new cases develop in that age group. In addition, the scarifying involution from preexisting lesions may result in obstructive problems, especially in the gastrointestinal and urinary tracts.

PATHOGENESIS

The pathogenesis of endometriosis is not completely understood. Genetic predisposition clearly plays a role. The following three hypotheses have been used to explain the various manifestations of endometriosis and the different locations in which endometriotic implants may be found:

1. **The retrograde menstruation theory** of Sampson proposes that endometrial fragments transported through the fallopian tubes at the time of menstruation implant and grow in various intraabdominal sites. Endometrial tissue, which is normally shed at the time of menstruation, is viable and capable of growth in vivo or in vitro. To explain some rare examples of endometriosis in distant sites, such as the lung, forehead, or axilla, it is necessary to postulate hematogenous spread.
2. **The müllerian metaplasia theory** of Meyer proposes that endometriosis results from the metaplastic transformation of peritoneal mesothelium into endometrium under the influence of certain generally unidentified stimuli.
3. **The lymphatic spread theory** of Halban suggests that endometrial tissues are taken up into the lymphatics draining the uterus and are transported to the various pelvic sites where the tissue grows ectopically. Endometrial tissue has been found in pelvic lymphatics in up to 20% of patients with the disease.

Most authorities believe that several factors are involved in the initiation and spread of endometriosis, including retrograde menstruation, coelomic metaplasia, immunologic changes, and genetic predisposition. A fundamental question is why all menstruating women do not develop endometriosis, given that most, if not all, women have retrograde flow into the pelvic peritoneum during menstruation. The amount of exposure to retrograde flow and the woman's immunologic response seem to be critical. Researchers have identified differences in the chemical composition and biologic pathways of endometrial cells from women with endometriosis compared with those of unaffected women. They have also found significant differences in the inflammatory and growth factors in the peritoneal fluid of affected women. A clearer understanding of the pathophysiology of endometriosis would provide insights into more effective strategies for prevention and treatment.

SITES OF OCCURRENCE

Endometriosis occurs most commonly in the dependent portions of the pelvis. Specifically, implants can be found on the ovaries, the broad ligament, the peritoneal surfaces of the cul-de-sac (including the uterosacral ligaments and posterior cervix), and the rectovaginal septum (Figure 25-1). Quite frequently, the rectosigmoid colon is involved, as is the appendix and the vesicouterine fold of peritoneum. **Endometriosis is occasionally seen in laparotomy scars,** developing especially after a cesarean delivery or myomectomy in which the endometrial cavity has been entered. It is probable that endometrial tissue is seeded into the surgical incision. **Two of three women with endometriosis have ovarian involvement.**

PATHOLOGY

Islands of endometriosis respond cyclically to ovarian steroidal hormone production. The implants proliferate under estrogenic stimulation and slough when support from estrogen and progesterone is removed with involution of the corpus luteum. The sloughed material induces a profound inflammatory response, resulting in pain immediately and fibrosis in the longer term. The macroscopic appearance of endometriosis depends on the site of the implant, the activity of the lesion, the day of the menstrual cycle, and the time since implantation.

Lesions may be raised and flat with red, black, or brown coloration; fibrotic, scarred areas that are yellow or white in hue; or vesicles that are pink, clear, or red (Figure 25-2). The color of the implant is generally determined by its vascularity, the size of the lesion, and the amount of residual sloughed material. Newer implants tend to be red, blood-filled, active lesions. Older lesions tend to be much less active hormonally, scarred, and bluish gray in color, with a puckered

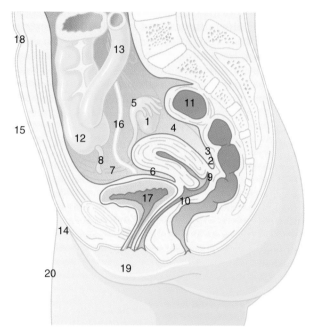

FIGURE 25-1 Common sites of endometriosis in decreasing order of frequency: (1) ovary, (2) cul-de-sac, (3) uterosacral ligaments, (4) broad ligaments, (5) fallopian tubes, (6) uterovesical fold, (7) round ligaments, (8) vermiform appendix, (9) vagina, (10) recto-vaginal septum, (11) rectosigmoid colon, (12) cecum, (13) ileum, (14) inguinal canals, (15) abdominal scars, (16) ureters, (17) urinary bladder, (18) umbilicus, (19) vulva, and (20) peripheral sites.

appearance. These older, inactive lesions have been called the tattooing of endometriosis.

Endometriomas of the ovary are cysts filled with thick, chocolate-colored fluid that sometimes has the black color and tarry consistency of crankcase oil. This characteristic fluid represents aged, hemolyzed blood and desquamated endometrium. Usually, endometrial glands and stroma are present in the cyst wall. Sometimes, however, the pressure of the enclosed fluid destroys the endometrial lining of the endometrioma, leaving only a fibrotic cyst wall infiltrated with large numbers of hemosiderin-laden macrophages. Generally, ovarian implants are associated with significant scarring of the ovary to the pelvic sidewall or broad ligament. **Histologically, two of four characteristics must be found in the endometrioma specimen to confirm the diagnosis: endometrial epithelium, endometrial glands, endometrial stroma, and hemosiderin-laden macrophages.**

Although endometriosis is a benign process, it shares many characteristics with malignancy. It is locally infiltrative, invasive, and widely disseminated. It is also curious that cyclic hormones tend to induce growth, whereas continuous hormonal exposure, especially in high doses, generally induces significant regression.

STAGING

The American Society of Reproductive Medicine employs a staging protocol in an attempt to correlate fertility potential with a quantified stage of endometriosis. This staging, which was initially based on the allocation of points depending on the sites involved and the extent of visualized disease (Figure 25-3), was modified to include a description of the color of the lesions and the percentage of surface involved in each lesion type, as well as a more detailed description of any endometrioma. The lower portion of Figure 25-3 provides sketches of normal and abnormal uterine and adnexal anatomy where mapping of implants of endometriosis and adhesions can be documented for accurate staging.

SYMPTOMS

The characteristic triad of symptoms associated with endometriosis is dysmenorrhea, dyspareunia, and, less frequently, dyschezia. The pain that women experience with endometriosis varies with the time since the onset of the disease. Early in the clinical course, women tend to have cyclic pelvic pain, which starts 1 to 2 days before the menstrual flow and resolves at the end of the menses. This secondary dysmenorrhea is thought to be related to the premenstrual swelling and extravasation of blood and menstrual debris, which induces an intense inflammatory reaction in the surrounding tissue mediated by prostaglandins and cytokines that are more directly responsible for triggering the pain sensation. Deep, infiltrating implants, especially those in the retroperitoneal space, are associated with more pain than are superficial lesions. Over time, the pain may become more chronic, with exacerbations at the time of the menses. Interestingly, **there is no clear relationship between the stage of endometriosis and the frequency and severity of pain symptoms.**

Dyspareunia is generally associated with deep-thrust penetration during intercourse and occurs mainly when the cul-de-sac, uterosacral ligaments, and portions of the posterior vaginal fornix are involved. Deep-thrust dyspareunia can also result from uterine immobility caused by significant internal scarring caused by endometriosis. Endometriomas in these circumstances may be exquisitely tender to palpation.

Dyschezia is experienced with uterosacral, cul-de-sac, and rectosigmoid colon involvement. As the stool passes between the uterosacral ligaments, the characteristic dyschezia is experienced.

Premenstrual and postmenstrual spotting is a characteristic symptom of endometriosis. Heavy menstruation is uncommon, with the amount of flow usually diminishing with endometriosis. If the ovarian capsule is involved with endometriosis, ovulatory pain and midcycle vaginal bleeding often occur. Rarely, as

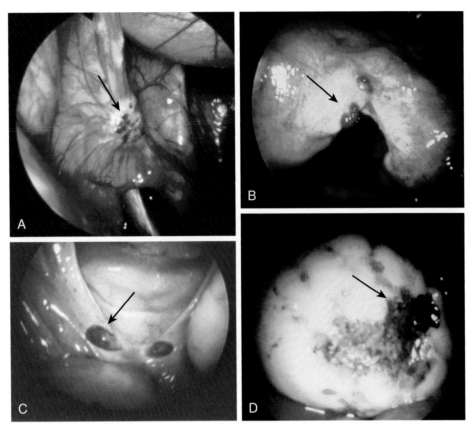

FIGURE 25-2 Appearance of red **(B)**, brown **(C)**, and black **(D)** raised lesions *(arrows)* of active endometriosis at the time of laparoscopy. The common finding of blue-gray lesions **(A)** represents less active "tatooing" of old endometriosis.

other organ systems are involved, menstrual hematochezia, hematuria, and other forms of endometriotic sloughing become evident.

The association between mild to moderate endometriosis and infertility is not clear. When more advanced stages of endometriosis distort the pelvic structures, the role of endometriosis in infertility is more predictable.

SIGNS

Endometriosis presents with a wide variety of signs, ranging from the presence of a small, exquisitely tender nodule in the cul-de-sac or on the uterosacral ligaments to a huge, relatively nontender, cystic abdominal mass. Occasionally, a small, tender, mulberry-like spot may be seen in the posterior fornix of the vagina. **Characteristically, a tender, fixed adnexal mass is appreciated on bimanual examination.** The uterus is fixed and retroverted in a substantial number of women with endometriosis. **Occasionally, no signs at all are appreciated during a physical examination.**

DIFFERENTIAL DIAGNOSIS

The main differential diagnoses in the acute phase of endometriosis are (1) chronic pelvic inflammatory disease or recurrent acute salpingitis, (2) hemorrhagic

corpus luteum, (3) benign or malignant ovarian neoplasm, and, occasionally, (4) ectopic pregnancy.

DIAGNOSIS

The diagnosis of endometriosis should be suspected in an afebrile patient with the characteristic triad of pelvic pain; a firm, fixed, tender adnexal mass; and tender nodularity in the cul-de-sac and uterosacral ligaments. The characteristic sharp, firm, exquisitely tender "barb" (so called because it is reminiscent of barbed wire) felt in the uterosacral ligament is the diagnostic sine qua non of endometriosis, but this finding is generally present only in severe cases. An ultrasonic evaluation may indicate an adnexal mass of complex echogenicity, with internal echoes consistent with old blood. Imaging studies are of limited value in most cases. Serum levels of the cancer antigen CA-125 are frequently elevated in women with endometriosis. However, the positive predictive value of CA-125 for detecting endometriosis is low (about 20%), and this test should not be used to diagnose endometriosis.

The definitive diagnosis is generally made on the basis of the characteristic gross and histologic findings obtained at laparoscopy or laparotomy. Unfortunately, even the most experienced surgeon may fail to identify endometriotic implants visually,

American Society for Reproductive Medicine
Revised Classification of Endometriosis

Patient's name _____   Date _____

Stage I (minimal)   — 1 – 5
Stage II (mild)   — 6 – 15
Stage III (moderate) — 16 – 40   Laparoscopy _____ Laparotomy _____ Photography _____
Stage IV (severe)   — > 40   Recommended treatment _____

Total _____   Prognosis _____

Peritoneum	Endometriosis	<1 cm	1-3 cm	>3 cm
	Superficial	1	2	4
	Deep	2	4	6
Ovary	R Superficial	1	2	4
	Deep	4	16	20
	L Superficial	1	2	4
	Deep	4	16	20

	Posterior cul-de-sac obliteration	Partial		Complete	
		4		40	

	Adhesions	<1/3 Enclosure	1/3–2/3 Enclosure	>2/3 Enclosure
Ovary	R Filmy	1	2	4
	Dense	4	8	16
	L Filmy	1	2	4
	Dense	4	8	16
Tube	R Filmy	1	2	4
	Dense	4*	8*	16
	L Filmy	1	2	4
	Dense	4*	8*	16

*If the fimbriated end of the fallopian tube is completely enclosed, change the point assignment to 16. Denote appearance of superficial implant types as red [(R), red, red-pink, flamelike, vesicular blobs, clear vesicles], white [(W), opacifications, peritoneal defects, yellow-brown], or black [(B), black, hemosiderin deposits, blue]. Denote percent of total described as R__%, W__%, and B__%. Total should equal 100%.

Additional endometriosis: _____   Additional pathology: _____
_____   _____
_____   _____

To be used with normal tubes and ovaries

L   R

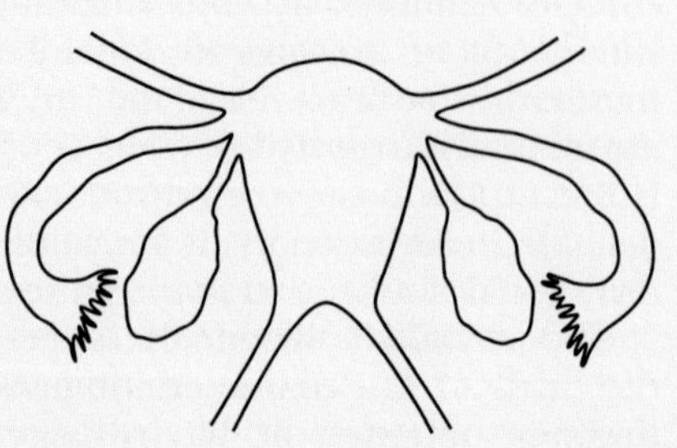

To be used with abnormal tubes and/or ovaries

L   R

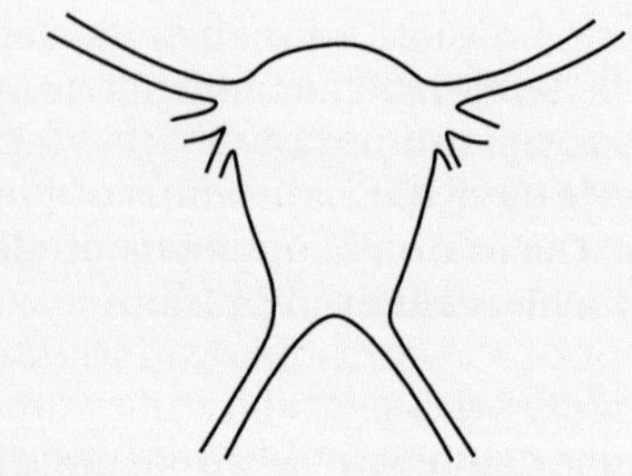

FIGURE 25-3 Modification of the revised American Society for Reproductive Medicine classification of endometriosis. (Reprinted with permission from American Society for Reproductive Medicine: Revised American Society for Reproductive Medicine classification of endometriosis: 1996. *Fertil Steril* 67:819–820, 1997.)

because the older implants may have a very subtle appearance and the deeper infiltrating lesions may not be visible at the peritoneal surface. Biopsy of any suspicious lesions improves diagnostic accuracy.

MANAGEMENT

The management of endometriosis depends on certain key considerations: (1) the certainty of the diagnosis, (2) the severity of the symptoms, (3) the extent of the disease, (4) the desire for future fertility, (5) the age of the patient, and (6) the threat to the gastrointestinal or urinary tract or both.

Treatment is indicated for endometriosis-associated pelvic pain, dysmenorrhea, dyspareunia, abnormal bleeding, ovarian cysts, and infertility caused by gross distortion of tubal and ovarian anatomy. Surgical intervention is required for an endometrioma larger than 3 cm, gross distortion of pelvic anatomy, involvement of bowel or bladder, and adhesive disease. Surgery may improve fertility for women with severe endometriosis. Medical therapy is generally the first-line treatment for other symptomatic women. **There is no convincing evidence that treatment significantly improves fertility in women with mild endometriosis.**

Asymptomatic women found incidentally to have endometriosis may not require any therapy. Some women who have minimal symptoms may choose to be managed expectantly if they are trying to conceive or if they are approaching menopause, when endometriosis generally becomes less symptomatic.

Medical Treatments

Therapy should be targeted toward relieving the patient's individual complaints and reducing the risk of disease progression. **Dysmenorrhea** that results from endometriosis **can be approached** as outlined in Chapter 21, using **nonsteroidal antiinflammatory drugs (NSAIDs) and reduction of menstrual flow with hormonal regimens such as low-dose oral contraceptives (OCs).**

For relief of noncyclic pelvic pain, short-term medical treatment may be used. **NSAIDs, OCs, and progestins (e.g., medroxyprogesterone acetate) should be considered the appropriate first-line medical treatments for symptomatic endometriosis. When an inadequate response occurs, second-line medical treatment with a gonadotropin-releasing hormone (GnRH) agonist, higher-dose progestins, or danazol appears to be equally effective.** Cost, individual patient response, and potential side effects generally guide selection of one agent or the other.

Danazol is an androgenic derivative that may be used in a "pseudomenopause" regimen to suppress symptoms of endometriosis if fertility is not a present concern. It is given over a period of 6 to 9 months, and doses of 600 to 800 mg daily are generally necessary to suppress menstruation. Through its weak androgenic properties, danazol decreases the plasma levels of sex hormone–binding globulin. The resulting increase of free testosterone may cause hirsutism and acne. **Three years after cessation of danazol, 40% of patients will have recurrence of endometriosis. After a full course of danazol therapy, use of a cyclic OC may help to delay or prevent such recurrence.**

GnRH agonists cause a temporary medical castration, thereby bringing about a marked, albeit temporary, regression of endometriosis. Treatment of women with endometriosis with GnRH agonists usually produces relief of pain and involution of implants. The disadvantages of these agonists are related to cost, hot flashes, and side effects, including vaginal dryness. They also cause calcium loss from bone and an unfavorable lipid profile. If treatment with a GnRH agonist is effective in relieving chronic pelvic pain and if surgery is not indicated, low-dose estrogen-progestin add-back therapy can permit longer-term use of GnRH agonists by mitigating the adverse impact of estrogen deficiency without reducing the efficacy of GnRH agonists.

OCs and oral medroxyprogesterone acetate are more effective than placebos in treatment of endometriosis-associated pelvic pain. The levonorgestrel-releasing intrauterine system reduces dysmenorrhea and may be helpful for inducing regression of cul-de-sac implants without diminishing circulating estrogen levels in the serum.

Surgical Treatments

The most comprehensive procedure (extirpative surgery) includes total abdominal hysterectomy, bilateral salpingo-oophorectomy with destruction of all peritoneal implants, and dissection of all adhesions. Usually, an appendectomy is also performed. A single ovary or both ovaries may be spared only if they are free of endometriosis and all other implants have been resected. Because of extensive adhesions, surgery for endometriosis is often technically very challenging. If the patient's endometriosis involves the cul-de-sac or uterosacral ligaments, the proximity to the ureter, bladder, and sigmoid colon must be considered. If the endometriosis obstructs the ureter, resection and ureteroplasty may be necessary to preserve renal function. **Nearly 25% of kidneys are lost when endometriosis blocks the ureter.** Obstruction of the rectosigmoid, and even obstruction of the small intestine, may require resection of the involved intestinal segment. The surgical risks must be explained carefully to the woman, as well as her subsequent need for treatment for loss of ovarian steroids. She also needs to understand that, postoperatively, there is a 20% recurrence rate for endometriosis, usually involving the bowel.

Often the desire for future fertility precludes this extirpative surgical option. In such circumstances, a more conservative laparoscopic or open surgical approach is designed to destroy all endometriotic implants and remove all adhesive disease. This usually involves excision (not lysis) of all adhesions and laser ablation or electrocautery of suspected implants. Endometriomas present a challenge when fertility is desired. Any surgery on the ovary, particularly in women with low ovarian reserve, could adversely affect follicular function and decrease fertility (see Chapter 34). **Large endometriomas (>3 cm) are usually amenable only to surgical resection.** Because of extensive adhesive disease that generally surrounds these cysts, cystectomy is not always possible, and an oophorectomy may be necessary. Extensive tubal disease, with or without ovarian involvement, may be treated by removal of the affected organs but with uterine preservation for in vitro fertilization when at least one ovary remains or for donor embryo transfer when both have been removed. **Preoperative treatment with medical agents such as GnRH agonists for 3 to 6 months can improve surgical success.**

The role of medical therapy postoperatively remains controversial, although it is indicated to treat women who have known residual disease diagnosed at surgery. **There is a risk of recurrence of endometriosis throughout a woman's life,** so measures should be taken to reduce the risk of retrograde menstruation or cyclic ovarian sex steroid production. Depot medroxyprogesterone acetate (DMPA), continuous OCs, and the levonorgestrel-releasing intrauterine device (IUD) are all attractive long-term options. Medical and surgical treatment options for endometriosis are summarized in Box 25-1.

PREVENTION

Whenever severe dysmenorrhea occurs in a young patient, the possibility of varying degrees of obstruction to the menstrual flow must be considered. The possibility of a blind uterine horn in a bicornuate uterus or an obstructing uterine or vaginal septum should be kept in mind. **In more than half the patients who are noted to develop endometriosis during childhood and adolescence, varying degrees of genital tract obstruction may be found.** Whenever a congenital abnormality of the urinary or intestinal tract is detected, the genital tract should be investigated for an obstructive lesion. Infants with genital tract obstruction have been noted to develop endometriosis even in the first year of life. **In all women, minimization of menstrual flow and suppression of ovarian cycling can reduce the risk of endometriosis.**

Adenomyosis

Adenomyosis **is defined as the extension of endometrial glands and stroma into the uterine musculature more than 2.5 mm beneath the basalis layer.** Often

---

BOX 25-1

OPTIONS FOR TREATING ENDOMETRIOSIS

Watchful Waiting

There is a limited role for expectant management without any medical or surgical intervention. Women who are attempting pregnancy with little or no symptoms may consider this option. In addition, women who are approaching menopause and have minimal symptoms may choose to wait for the cessation of cyclic ovarian function, at which stage endometriosis is usually far less active.

Medical Treatment

First-line therapy: Nonsteroidal antiinflammatory drugs, low-dose oral contraceptives, or progestins (e.g., medroxyprogesterone acetate). ***Note:*** This treatment should be given an adequate trial of 3 to 6 months before initiating second-line therapy.

Second-line therapy: Higher-dose progestins (e.g., medroxyprogesterone acetate or megestrol acetate [Megace]), danazol, or gonadotropin-releasing hormone analogues appear to be equally effective. ***Note:*** Laparoscopic confirmation of the diagnosis of endometriosis before initiation of second-line treatment is usually performed, but it is not required according to some guidelines. Biopsy of visualized lesions, however, is the only definitive way to diagnose endometriosis.

Surgical Treatment

Most definitive therapy: Total abdominal hysterectomy with bilateral salpingo-oophorectomy with destruction and/or removal of all peritoneal endometriotic implants and adhesions. ***Note:*** There is always a risk of recurrence, even with "definitive" treatment.

Fertility-preserving treatment: Laparoscopic or open surgery (laparotomy) with destruction and/or removal of all peritoneal endometriotic implants and adhesions. ***Note:*** Removal of endometriomas may decrease fertility potential, especially in women with already-reduced ovarian reserve (see Chapter 34). Large endometriomas >3 cm in diameter should be removed surgically. Preoperative suppressive treatment for 3 to 6 months may improve surgical success.

---

this is an incidental finding during a pathologic examination, where it is seen in up to 60% of women in their 40s. **About 15% of patients with adenomyosis have associated endometriosis.** Islands of adenomyosis do not participate in the proliferative and secretory cycles induced by the ovary.

PATHOLOGY

Generally, the gross appearance of the uterus consists of diffuse enlargement with a thickened myometrium containing characteristic glandular irregularities, with implants containing both glandular tissue and stroma (Figure 25-4). The endometrial cavity is also enlarged. Occasionally, the adenomyosis may be confined to one portion of the myometrium and take the

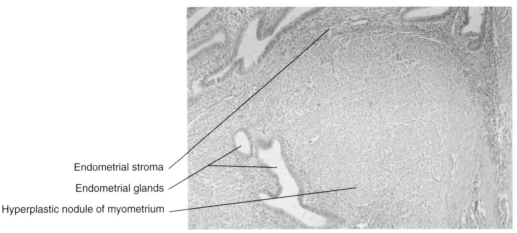

Endometrial stroma

Endometrial glands

Hyperplastic nodule of myometrium

FIGURE 25-4 Histologic illustration of adenomyosis causing enlargement of the uterus. A hyperplastic nodule of myometrium can be seen. Note the endometrial glands and stroma.

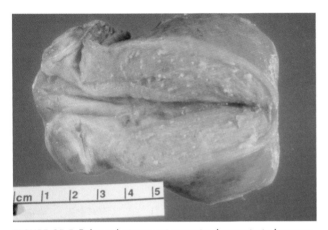

FIGURE 25-5 Enlarged uterus cut open to demonstrate homogeneous enlargement caused by adenomyosis. A diagnosis of leiomyomata may be incorrectly made at the time of pelvic examination. (Courtesy Dr. Sathima Nataratan, Ronald Reagan—UCLA Medical Center.)

form of a fairly well-circumscribed adenomyoma. Contrary to the situation with a uterine leiomyoma (fibroid), no distinct capsular margin can be detected on cut sections between the adenomyoma and the surrounding myometrium. The distinction between adenomyosis and a uterine fibroid may not always be clear on ultrasonic examination. Figure 25-5 illustrates the typical gross appearance of an enlarged uterus with extensive adenomyosis.

SYMPTOMS

Although many women with adenomyosis are asymptomatic, those who have this condition typically complain of severe secondary dysmenorrhea and heavy menstrual bleeding. Even though the islands do not cycle in response to ovarian hormonal stimulation, prostaglandin release and local inflammatory changes persist that can induce pain and tenderness and may disrupt the vasoconstriction of the arterial arcade supplying the endometrium. Deep-thrust dyspareunia, especially premenstrually, can be caused by adenomyosis.

SIGNS

Pelvic examination reveals the uterus to be generally symmetrically enlarged and somewhat boggy and tender if the examination is conducted premenstrually. Occasionally, it may enlarge asymmetrically, which makes it very difficult to distinguish adenomyosis from a myomatous uterus. The consistency of the enlarged adenomyomatous uterus is generally softer than that of a fibroid uterus.

TREATMENT

The treatment of adenomyosis depends entirely on the patient's symptoms and the possibility of other diagnoses. Any history of new onset or worsening of uterine bleeding, particularly in a woman with risk factors for endometrial cancer, should be investigated by endometrial biopsy or fractional dilation and curettage and/or hysteroscopy to rule out malignancy. **Conservative management with NSAIDs and hormonal control of the endometrium are mainstays of therapy.** Combination OCs or hormone-containing patches and vaginal rings may be used to reduce cyclic blood loss and menstrual pain. DMPA, levonorgestrel IUD, and continuous OC pills can be used to try to achieve amenorrhea. If the woman is not a candidate for any of these medical interventions or if medical treatments do not sufficiently control her symptoms, **hysterectomy may be indicated. Endometrial ablation to control the bleeding is another option.**

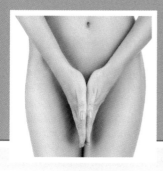

CHAPTER 26

Abnormal Uterine Bleeding

ANITA L. NELSON • JOSEPH C. GAMBONE

CLINICAL KEYS FOR THIS CHAPTER

- During the reproductive years (puberty to menopause), menstrual bleeding normally occurs every 24 to 38 days, except during the first few years of menstruation, during and for a short time after pregnancy and lactation, and in the perimenopausal period. The normal duration of bleeding is 4.5 to 8 days, and the amount of normal flow is less than 80 mL of blood. Brief deviations from normal bleeding patterns occur in many women. Once pregnancy and malignancy are ruled out, short episodes of abnormal uterine bleeding (AUB) resolve spontaneously with little or no treatment.
- Some women may experience heavy irregular AUB during their reproductive years. The causes of most cases of heavy bleeding are benign, and symptoms are often effectively managed with hormonal treatment alone. Up to 20% of women experience debilitating symptoms caused by heavy bleeding at some point during their reproductive years. Heavy menstrual bleeding may result from systemic disorders, coagulation defects, or diseases of the reproductive system.
- Traditional terminology for AUB has been replaced by more accurate descriptions of the frequency, regularity, duration, and amount of menstrual flow. A newer system for categorizing the causes of AUB (PALM-COEIN) helps to organize the evaluation and treatment of women with bleeding disorders.
- After first determining that the source of vaginal bleeding is the uterus, a series of tests is recommended to determine the cause of the AUB. Except in extreme cases, the initial therapy is medical, with a variety of hormonal and nonhormonal regimens available to control the bleeding.
- Surgical therapy is reserved for those women for whom medical management fails or for those who have obviously significant pathology (e.g., polyps) or life-threatening hemorrhage when they first present with AUB.

Abnormal uterine bleeding (AUB) patterns (unrelated to pregnancy) are common and can range from complete absence of bleeding (amenorrhea) to life-threatening hemorrhage. The etiology of the bleeding irregularities includes benign or malignant growths, systemic disease, coagulation defects, and hormonal imbalance. Bleeding pattern disruptions caused by imbalance of hormones were previously termed *dysfunctional uterine bleeding* (DUB). Newer terminology has been introduced to more accurately describe most abnormal bleeding patterns, and a new, more inclusive classification system has been adopted to categorize the various causes of AUB.

Diagnosis

Initially, abnormal vaginal bleeding is assumed to emanate from the uterus. A pelvic examination, including the insertion of a vaginal speculum, is essential to eliminate the possibility that the vulva, vagina, exocervix (or ectocervix), or even the rectum or bladder is actually the source of the bleeding. **Early pregnancy and its complications should always be ruled out as the cause of AUB in women of reproductive age.**

The newer terminology for menstrual bleeding provides information about four dimensions of a woman's cycle: (1) frequency, (2) regularity, (3) duration, and (4) blood loss. Table 26-1 outlines the normal and abnormal values for each of these dimensions and provides the newer terms to describe the abnormalities. As an example, the assessment of abnormal bleeding in a woman with complaints of "irregular menstruation" can be categorized as follows: If her cycle length (first day of menses to the first day of the next menses) is 23 days, she bleeds for 10 days during each cycle, and she loses 100 mL of blood, this would be described as "frequent, prolonged, and heavy menses." Other important traditional terms include *amenorrhea,* which refers to the absence of any menstrual bleeding or spotting for at least 3 months; *intermenstrual bleeding,* which refers to bleeding between normally spaced menses; and *postcoital bleeding,* which refers to bleeding after vaginal intercourse.

This newer, more descriptive terminology for patterns of AUB replaces the older, less precise terms listed in Box 26-1. However, it is important to become familiar with these older terms, because they have been used for decades in clinical practice and in the medical literature and are still used for diagnostic coding purposes.

The newer classification system, called *PALM-COEIN,* is depicted in Figure 26-1. Appropriate testing is needed to differentiate the various causes of AUB. The classification system takes into account that there are two different influences on AUB. On the one hand, a woman may have structural abnormalities of her uterus that are the likely causes of her bleeding, with the PALM elements standing for *p*olyps, *a*denomyosis, *l*eiomyomas (fibroids), and *m*alignancies. Rare problems such as imperforate hymen or transverse vaginal septum are more likely to present with primary amenorrhea and not with chronic bleeding problems. The COEIN portion of the classification system refers to important functional disorders such as *c*oagulation defects, *o*varian dysfunction (formerly DUB), *e*ndometrial (uterine cavity lining) causes, and *i*atrogenic. A "*n*ot yet classified" category completes the acronym and is available for a cause of bleeding that is not currently included or idiopathic.

Chapter 33 covers the causes of infrequent menses (oligomenorrhea) and both primary and secondary

TABLE 26-1

TERMINOLOGY USED TO DESCRIBE BLEEDING PATTERNS

Clinical Dimensions	Descriptive Terms	Normal Limits (5th to 95th Percentiles)
Frequency of menses (days)	Frequent Normal Infrequent Absent	<24 24-38 >38 —
Regularity of menses, cycle-to-cycle variation over 12 mo	Regular Irregular	Variation ± 2-20 days Variation >20 days
Duration of flow (days)	Prolonged Normal Shortened	>8.0 4.5-8.0 <4.5
Volume of monthly blood loss (mL)	Heavy Normal Light	>80 5-80 <5

BOX 26-1

TRADITIONAL TERMINOLOGY FOR ABNORMAL UTERINE BLEEDING*

- *Polymenorrhea:* Abnormally frequent menses at intervals of less than 24 days
- *Menorrhagia* (hypermenorrhea): Excessive and/or prolonged menses (>80 mL and >7 days) occurring at normal intervals
- *Metrorrhagia:* Irregular episodes of uterine bleeding
- *Menometrorrhagia:* Heavy and irregular uterine bleeding
- *Dysfunctional uterine bleeding:* Bleeding caused by ovulatory dysfunction

*Less descriptive terms that are no longer recommended.

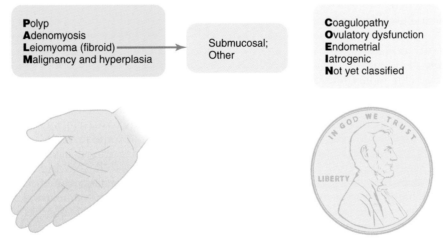

FIGURE 26-1 PALM-COEIN classification system for abnormal uterine bleeding that has been approved by the International Federation of Gynecology and Obstetrics. (Modified from Munro MG, Critchley HO, Fraser IS: The FIGO classification of causes of abnormal uterine bleeding in the reproductive years. *Fertil Steril* 95:2204–2208, 2011.)

amenorrhea. Chapters 35 and 41 address perimeno-pausal and postmenopausal bleeding. This chapter is focused on the etiology, differential diagnosis, evaluation, and treatments for both acute and chronic heavy menstrual bleeding.

Heavy menstrual bleeding occurs in 9-14% of healthy women of reproductive age and is the reason for up to 20% of outpatient clinic visits by women. Heavy menstrual bleeding can cause severe anemia, but less significant blood loss can diminish a woman's quality of life and even her income when workplace activity is adversely affected.

Acute Excessive Bleeding in Nonpregnant Women of Reproductive Age

The etiologies, workups, and therapies of excessive bleeding can differ for acute heavy bleeding compared with chronic heavy bleeding, although often there is considerable overlap. A woman who presents with heavy bleeding needs to be assessed for hemodynamic stability, anemia, and always the possibility of pregnancy. She should be asked about symptoms of dizziness, shortness of breath, or loss of consciousness. Her vital signs must be assessed for hemodynamic stability. It is helpful to get a description of her current bleeding episode as well as her recent and usual bleeding patterns, along with any previous evaluations or treatments. A complete history, including medication history, can provide insight into which of the PALM-COIEN categories is more likely, but a broad differential should be developed. It is quite possible for a woman to have more than one problem as the cause of her abnormal bleeding. Obvious causes requiring immediate surgeries should be ruled out, such as vaginal trauma or bleeding lacerations, as well as aborting fibroids (leiomyomata).

Hospitalization and transfusion are generally recommended for women who have severe anemia (hemoglobin ≤7 g/dL) and those who are hemodynamically unstable. Outpatient transfusion is an option for women with borderline presentations. Patients who decline blood transfusions or blood products in spite of severe anemia should be cared for by a team experienced with other treatment options. Before a transfusion is started, blood tests should be performed. Box 26-2 lists the tests that should be considered for the workup of AUB.

Baseline hemoglobin is mandatory, and a complete blood count (with red blood cell indices) is performed to determine the chronicity of the problem, to rule out thrombocytopenia, and to identify possible hematologic malignancies. Coagulation factors should be obtained, as well as serum iron, iron-binding capacity, and serum ferritin levels. Following these initial assess-

---

BOX 26-2

INITIAL DIAGNOSTIC TESTS FOR ACUTE EXCESSIVE BLEEDING IN WOMEN OF REPRODUCTIVE AGE

Urine tests
  Pregnancy test
Blood tests
  Blood count with reticulocyte count and differential
  Serum iron and iron-binding capacity
  Serum ferritin
  Coagulation tests (PT, PTT, and INR)
  Thyroid function tests
  Liver function tests
  Creatinine, BUN
Imaging tests, if indicated
  Pelvic ultrasonography
  Saline infusion sonography
Biopsies as necessary
  Cervical biopsy
  Endocervical biopsy
  Endometrial biopsy

BUN, Blood urea nitrogen; *INR,* international normalized ratio; *PT,* prothrombin time; *PTT,* partial thromboplastin time.

---

ments, liver, renal, and thyroid function tests may help to identify other systemic causes of excessive uterine bleeding.

Many of the test results may not be available for days, but the heavy bleeding needs to be promptly controlled. First-line therapy is generally medical. **Surgical approaches are usually reserved for women whose condition does not respond to medical therapies and for those who are bleeding so heavily that there is insufficient time to consider medical treatments.** First-line medical therapy usually involves hormonal manipulations (Box 26-3).

In the past, it was believed that high doses of estrogen were needed to induce cell proliferation over the denuded areas of endometrium that were thought to be actively bleeding. Both high-dose intravenous estrogen and high doses of combined oral contraceptive pills were recommended. **More recently, it has been recognized that high doses of estrogen may not be necessary to control the bleeding.** Furthermore, hemorrhage is known to induce a hypercoagulable state, and the addition of high-dose estrogen may increase the risk of dangerous clotting, especially in women with reactive thrombocytosis. As a result, the doses used in these estrogen-based therapies have been significantly reduced, and **high-dose progestin-only therapies have been recommended as first-line treatment for acute heavy menstrual bleeding, particularly in the outpatient setting.**

Although many hormonal regimens have been used in clinical practice, prospective clinical trials have shown that only three therapies are reliably effective for the treatment of acute excessive bleeding in

---

BOX 26-3

MEDICAL THERAPEUTIC OPTIONS FOR ACUTE HEAVY UTERINE BLEEDING

Older Estrogen-Based, High-Dose Treatments

Conjugated equine estrogen 30 mg intravenously every 3 hr for up to 24 hr

OR

50 µg of ethinyl estradiol (EE), 0.15 mg of levonorgestrel, one tablet orally every 6 hr for 5 days

Newer Therapies Prospectively Studied and Validated in Outpatient Settings

Medroxyprogesterone acetate 20 mg orally every 8 hr for 7 days, then once daily for 21 days

OR

Oral contraceptive pills with 35 µg of EE, 1.0 mg of norethindrone acetate, one tablet orally every 8 hr for 7 days, then 20 µg of EE, 1.0 mg of norethindrone acetate pills, one tablet orally once daily for 21 days

OR

Medroxyprogesterone acetate 20 mg orally every 8 hr for 3 days with intramuscular injection of depot medroxyprogesterone acetate 150 mg

Lower-Dose Oral Contraceptive Pill Treatment Proposed

Any 35-µg EE oral contraceptive pill for 1 day, then one tablet orally every 12 hr for two doses, then one tablet orally once daily for 19 days

---

BOX 26-4

MEDICAL TREATMENT OPTIONS FOR CHRONIC HEAVY MENSTRUAL BLEEDING

Normalize Prostaglandins

Ibuprofen 800 mg orally every 8 hr from start of menses through last days of heavy bleeding (<5 days)

Naproxen 500 mg orally every 12 hr from the start of menses through the last day of heavy bleeding (<5 days)

Antifibrinolytic Therapy

Tranexamic acid 650 mg, two tablets orally every 8 hr from start of menses for up to 5 days

Coordinate Endometrial Sloughing (Best for Anovulation)

MPA 10-mg tablet orally each day for last 10 days of cycle

Estrogen-containing oral contraceptive pills, transdermal patches, or vaginal rings

Endometrial Suppression (Lighter Bleeding or to Create Amenorrhea)

Progestin-only oral contraceptive or implant, MPA or NETA daily

Extended-cycle oral contraceptives, vaginal rings

DMPA 150-mg intramuscular injection every 11-13 wk

LNG-IUS 20 µg/24 hr

May be combined with hormonal therapies

Do not use with estrogen-containing products

DMPA, Depot medroxyprogesterone acetate; *LNG-IUS,* levonorgestrel intrauterine system; *MPA,* medroxyprogesterone acetate; *NETA,* norethisterone acetate.

---

women of reproductive age. This is true regardless of the underlying etiology of the heavy bleeding or the status of the endometrium (e.g., hyperplastic or atrophic).

Imaging studies can usually be delayed until the heavy bleeding is controlled. More urgent imaging may be needed if there are other symptoms, such as significant pain. In a woman with suspicious ultrasonic findings or increased risk factors for cancer, biopsy is indicated once the bleeding has been stabilized and her hemoglobin level is normal. Biopsies in women of reproductive age seldom reveal problems missed by the other tests. In fact, outpatient biopsies often miss the more common causes, such as endometrial polyps and fibroids.

When a woman with heavy uterine bleeding does not respond to the initial therapy within 12 to 24 hours, surgery is indicated. A dilation and curettage is performed to remove the remaining endometrium. When needed, **a balloon may be placed within the uterine cavity** to tamponade bleeding vessels. **Selective embolization of uterine blood vessels** can be done by an interventional radiologist if persistent active bleeding continues. **As a last resort, and only rarely, hysterectomy is indicated.**

After the initial episode has been resolved, efforts should be made to prevent a recurrence of the uterine bleeding. This usually involves correcting any specific causes identified in the workup (e.g., providing thyroxine when hypothyroidism is diagnosed) and using therapies listed in Box 26-3 for ongoing treatment of chronic heavy bleeding. Short-term treatments to suppress the endometrium may be needed after hospital discharge while awaiting test results. This can be hormonal (continuation of the initial therapy) or may involve longer-acting medications, such as gonadotropin-releasing hormone analogues.

Chronic Heavy Menstrual Bleeding

Therapies should be targeted to the underlying structural or medical problems that are detected in the workup (e.g., endometrial polypectomy, thyroid hormone replacement, desmopressin treatment). All medical therapies are intended to control bleeding from the endometrium. They can be organized as summarized in Box 26-4. The following steps should be considered: (1) normalize prostaglandins, (2) antifibrinolytic therapy, (3) coordinate endometrial sloughing, and (4) endometrial suppression. Each of these is discussed in turn in the following sections.

NORMALIZE PROSTAGLANDINS

Nonsteroidal antiinflammatory agents (NSAIDs) may be used to normalize prostaglandins. **Many women**

with heavy bleeding have an imbalance of prostaglandins. For example, levels of vasodilating prostaglandin E_2 (PGE$_2$) may exceed levels of vasoconstricting PGF$_{2\alpha}$, or there may be excessive numbers of receptors for PGE$_2$ compared with those for PGF$_{2\alpha}$. An increased PGE$_2$/PGF$_{2\alpha}$ ratio is more common among anovulatory women. NSAIDs taken in higher doses alter the prostaglandin ratios, but correct dosing and timing is needed to avoid interfering with platelet function. This therapy reduces blood loss by 20-30% and can be combined with hormonal therapies.

ANTIFIBRINOLYTIC THERAPY

Antifibrinolytic agents can be used to stabilize clots in uterine arterioles or capillaries of women who may have excessive fibrinolytic activity. Successive clots formed in the vessels feeding the endometrium are lysed in these women, and antifibrinolytic therapy can reduce blood loss by about 40%. These agents should not be combined with estrogen-containing medications.

COORDINATE ENDOMETRIAL SLOUGHING

Lack of ovulation results in very low progesterone levels. To prevent unopposed estrogenic stimulation of the endometrium that is usually seen in women with anovulatory cycles, a progestin such as oral medroxyprogesterone acetate or norethindrone can be added to emulate a luteal phase. Another approach is to prescribe additional progestin daily with conventional cycling with estrogen-progestin contraceptive pills or with patches or vaginal rings. This limits endometrial growth and provides lighter, predictable bleeding patterns. **One oral contraceptive pill has been approved by the Food and Drug Administration as treatment for heavy menstrual bleeding (a product containing estradiol valerate and dienogest),** but this benefit has been reported clinically for all combined hormonal contraceptives.

ENDOMETRIAL SUPPRESSION

Progestin-only pills and the contraceptive implant have modest but measurable impacts on blood loss, but the **levonorgestrel intrauterine system (LNG-IUS)** 20 μg/24 hours and depot medroxyprogesterone acetate injections induce complete amenorrhea in a significant percentage of women with longer use.

The higher-dose LNG-IUS is the most effective medical treatment for idiopathic heavy menstrual bleeding and **treats excessive bleeding at least as well as endometrial ablation.** It can prevent one-half of women from undergoing hysterectomy. Extended-cycle use of oral contraceptives or uninterrupted use of vaginal contraceptive rings for 3 to 12 months can also prevent scheduled bleeding for substantial periods of time.

If a woman does not respond appropriately to treatment, her evaluation must be reinitiated. Hysteroscopy can provide direct visualization of the endometrium to identify previously undetected causes of bleeding in about 25% of women whose bleeding persists despite appropriate therapy.

SURGICAL TREATMENT

Surgery is generally reserved for women whose medical therapy fails or for those in whom significant pathology has been identified in the initial evaluation. Commonly indicated procedures include polypectomy and myomectomy (see Chapter 19). After malignancy or premalignancy has been excluded, endometrial ablation is an option if the woman does not desire to become pregnant again and has not sufficiently responded to medical therapies. The endometrium can be ablated by a variety of destructive methods, such as freezing, heating, or applying ultrasonic energy. Over 70% of women who are treated with ablation have satisfactory bleeding patterns, including some with amenorrhea. Twenty percent of these women will need a second ablation, and 10% will ultimately undergo hysterectomy. Following ablation, women must be given effective contraception. Ablation causes significant damage to the endometrium, so spontaneous abortion rates are high, and there is a significant risk of abnormal placentation, such as placenta percreta.

Family Planning
Reversible Contraception, Sterilization, and Abortion

ANITA L. NELSON

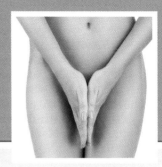

CLINICAL KEYS FOR THIS CHAPTER

■ There are three types of interventions available in family planning to prevent unwanted pregnancies. The first is contraception, which prevents fertilization by blocking the union of the gametes. The second is interception, which works after fertilization but before implantation. The third is abortion, which is defined as the interruption of an established pregnancy. The patient's perspective and preferences for family planning must always be the primary focus.

■ Ongoing contraceptive options are grouped into three tiers that are based on their efficacy in typical use. **Tier 1** methods (implants, intrauterine devices [IUDs], and permanent contraception) have the lowest failure rates. **Tier 2** methods include injections, pills, patches, and rings. **Tier 3** methods include barrier and behavioral methods.

■ Emergency contraception provides pregnancy protection after intercourse has taken place. It involves hormonal (oral contraceptives) or mechanical methods, which may be interceptive (e.g., placement of an IUD).

■ Permanent contraception (previously referred to as *sterilization*) may be performed just after childbirth, between pregnancies, or as an interval procedure at any time. Tubal interruption is the most common technique. There has been a recent recommendation that fimbriectomy or complete salpingectomy should be used because it may reduce the risk of subsequent serous ovarian or peritoneal cancer.

■ Elective termination of a pregnancy (abortion) is controversial and is unavailable in some areas of the United States. Medical and surgical abortion are as safe as other common procedures, such as tonsillectomy. Better access to effective contraception has been shown to reduce abortion rates.

Family planning plays a significant role in improving the health of women and provides a unique opportunity to optimize pregnancy outcomes by helping couples to control childbearing until conditions are favorable for them. As such, family planning contributes substantially to individual health care, to public health, and even to population control and environmental well-being.

Despite these recognized benefits, there is no other area of women's health that is as controversial and polarizing as family planning. Much of the controversy is based on a misunderstanding about reproductive facts, the safety of modern contraception, and the health risks posed by pregnancy and childbirth. Box 27-1 lists some important family planning facts and misconceptions held by many women and men.

Overview

Before going into detail about the various methods of family planning, it is important to note several facts about reproductive health. **About 85% of sexually active couples having unprotected intercourse for 1 year will experience pregnancy.** Pregnancy is not established within the uterus until about 7 days after conception, which itself may not occur for up to 5 to 7 days following intercourse. Half of all conceptions are lost before implantation, and **at least 10-15% of established pregnancies spontaneously abort.**

Although the goal of family planning is to provide couples with the ability to plan and prepare for pregnancy, efforts to date have fallen far short of that goal. **More than half of pregnancies that occur in the United**

BOX 27-1

FAMILY PLANNING FACTS

- All methods of birth control that would typically be prescribed to a woman today are far less hazardous to a woman's health than a pregnancy would be.
- In the United States, nearly half of all pregnancies are *unintended*. This has been the case for more than two decades.
- The maternal mortality rate in the United States is at its highest point in 15 years. There is currently 1 maternal mortality for every 30,000 live births.
- The mortality rate for healthy, young, nonsmoking women using oral contraceptives for 1 year is approximately 1 death in 1 million user-years.
- In spite of this, a large majority of women of reproductive age rate oral contraceptives to be more hazardous to a woman's health than pregnancy.
- A first-trimester elective pregnancy termination is safer than a tonsillectomy.
- Providing safe, affordable, and effective methods of contraception reduces the rates of abortion.

TABLE 27-1

FIRST-YEAR FAILURE RATES

Method	Percentage of Women Experiencing an Unintended Pregnancy within the First Year of Use	
	Typical Use	Perfect Use
No method	85	85
Spermicides	28	18
Fertility awareness–based methods	24	
Standard days method		5
2-Day method		4
Ovulation method		3
Symptothermal method		0.4
Withdrawal	22	4
Sponge		
Parous women	24	20
Nulliparous women	12	9
Condom		
Female (FC2)	21	5
Male	18	2
Diaphragm	12	6
Combined pill and progestin-only pills	9	0.3
ORTHO EVRA patch	9	0.3
NuvaRing	9	0.3
Depo-Provera	6	0.2
Intrauterine contraceptives		
ParaGard T 380A intrauterine copper contraceptive	0.8	0.6
Mirena LNG-IUS (20 µg/24 hr)	0.2	0.2
IMPLANON/NEXPLANON	0.05	0.05
Female sterilization	0.5	0.5
Male sterilization	0.15	0.10

LNG-IUS, Levonorgestrel intrauterine system.

States are unintended, meaning that the woman did not want to become pregnant at the time she did. More than half of these unplanned pregnancies are eventually accepted.

Most women underestimate the health risks of pregnancy and overestimate the risks of contraception. There is no method of contraception that a clinician would prescribe to a woman that is as hazardous to her health as pregnancy itself. The contraceptive needs of a couple are often given lower priority and may not be mentioned, even when clinicians prescribe drugs that may be teratogenic to women of reproductive age. The controversy that surrounds family planning makes it essential for those caring for women of reproductive age to be informed about all the available methods of birth control and to be dedicated to educating couples about their importance and safety.

Contraception

Ongoing contraceptive methods themselves may be categorized into reversible methods used before intercourse and those methods that are permanent. **The efficacy of a method is estimated by first-year failure rates measured under two different conditions: (1) correct and consistent use** (reflecting a method's full potential) **and (2) typical use** (estimates are derived from surveys of everyday, "real-world" users). Table 27-1 lists all the methods and their failure rates for both perfect and typical use. The differences in failure rates between the reversible Tier 1 methods and those in Tier 2 or 3 are so remarkable that **most authorities recommend that first-line contraceptive options for women of all ages be implants and intrauterine devices (IUDs) (Tier 1).** Any method is more effective than

unprotected intercourse, and even one of the lower-tier methods can be made quite effective if the gap between typical use and correct and consistent use is reduced. Different forms of emergency contraception are available after coitus to provide a second chance of pregnancy prevention when nonuse or method misuse occurs.

Contraceptive practice in the United States has been greatly simplified by the publication of two important documents by the Centers for Disease Control and Prevention (CDC): the United States Medical Eligibility Criteria (US MEC) for Contraceptive Use and the U.S. Selected Practice Recommendations (US SPR) for Contraceptive Use. Each of these sets of guidelines is periodically updated based on the latest available evidence, and both sets in their entirety can be accessed online:

http://www.cdc.gov/reproductivehealth/unintended pregnancy/usmec.htm and http://www.cdc.gov/reproductivehealth/unintendedpregnancy/usspr.htm. The US MEC rates the eligibility of women with a variety of medical conditions for each of the reversible Tier 1 and Tier 2 methods of birth control on a scale of 1 to 4, where 1 represents no concern and 4 represents an absolute contraindication. Added to this evaluation is a consideration of the risks that a woman would face with pregnancy and the likelihood she would experience a pregnancy if she were to use the method. For example, a woman with advanced diabetes may not experience any direct medical harm by using male condoms, but the 18% chance of pregnancy with typical use of condoms poses significant risks to her health.

Table 27-2 contains a sample of the entire US MEC to illustrate its usefulness. The complete chart can also be accessed electronically at StudentConsult.com.

The US SPR separates the elements of well-woman care from those needed for contraception, provides clear direction about the evaluations needed (beyond taking a complete medical history) before offering the method, and describes what follow-up is needed after method initiation. It also offers advice on managing potential side effects associated with each of the methods. Table 27-3 highlights the recommended testing for each method and emphasizes the importance and feasibility of initiating every method of contraception at the time a patient is seen (any time in a woman's cycle as long as she is not pregnant).

TABLE 27-2

SAMPLE CHART OF U.S. MEDICAL ELIGIBILITY CRITERIA FOR CONTRACEPTIVE USE

Condition	Sub-condition	Combined pill, patch, ring		Progestin-only pill		Injection		Implant		LNG-IUD		Copper-IUD	
		I	C	I	C	I	C	I	C	I	C	I	C
Age		Menarche to <40 = 1; ≥40 = 2		Menarche to <18 = 1; 18-45 = 1; >45 = 1		Menarche to <18 = 2; 18-45 = 1; >45 = 2		Menarche to <18 = 1; 18-45 = 1; >45 = 1		Menarche to <20 = 2; ≥20 = 1		Menarche to <20 = 2; ≥20 = 1	
Diabetes mellitus (DM)	a) History of gestational DM only	1		1		1		1		1		1	
	b) Non-vascular disease												
	i) non-insulin dependent	2		2		2		2		2		1	
	ii) insulin dependent[‡]	2		2		2		2		2		1	
	c) Nephropathy/retinopathy/neuropathy[‡]	3/4*		2		3		2		2		1	
	d) Other vascular disease or diabetes of >20 years' duration[‡]	3/4*		2		3		2		2		1	
Headaches	a) Non-migrainous	1*	2*	1*	1*	1*	1*	1*	1*	1*	1*	1*	
	b) Migraine												
	i) without aura, age <35	2*	3*	1*	2*	2*	2*	2*	2*	2*	2*	1*	
	ii) without aura, age ≥35	3*	4*	1*	2*	2*	2*	2*	2*	2*	2*	1*	
	iii) with aura, any age	4*	4*	2*	3*	2*	3*	2*	3*	2*	3*	1*	

Key:
1 No restriction (method can be used)
2 Advantages generally outweigh theoretical or proven risks
3 Theoretical or proven risks usually outweigh the advantages
4 Unacceptable health risk (method not to be used)

From Centers for Disease Control and Prevention.
Updated June 2012. This summary sheet only contains a subset of the recommendations from the US MEC. For complete guidance, see: http://www.cdc.gov/reproductivehealth/unintendedpregnancy/USMEC.htm.
Most contraceptive methods do not protect against sexually transmitted infections (STIs). Consistent and correct use of the male latex condom reduces the risk of STIs and HIV.
C, Continuation of contraceptive method; I, initiation of contraceptive method; NA, not applicable.
*Please see the complete guidance for a clarification to this classification: www.cdc.gov/reproductivehealth/unintendedpregnancy/USMEC.htm.
[‡]Condition that exposes a woman to increased risk as a result of unintended pregnancy.

TABLE 27-3

ROUTINE EXAMINATIONS AND TESTS NEEDED BEFORE INITIATION OF CONTRACEPTIVE METHODS BY HEALTHY WOMEN					
Examination Needed	IUD	Implant	Injectable	Combined Hormonal Contraceptive	Progestin-Only Pills
BP	C	C	C	A	C
BMI	C	C	C	C	C
Breast examination	C	C	C	C	C
Pelvic examination*	A	C	C	C	C

Adapted from Centers for Disease Control and Prevention: U.S. selected practice recommendations for contraceptive use, 2013. *MMWR Morb Mortal Wkly Rep* 62(5):1–46, 2013.
A, Essential and mandated; *BMI,* body mass index; *BP,* blood pressure; *C,* Does not contribute substantially to safe and effective method use; *IUD,* intrauterine device.
Laboratory tests: All methods were rated Category C for the following tests: glucose, lipids, liver enzymes, hemoglobin, presence of thrombogenic mutations, cervical cytology, and human immunodeficiency virus.
Note: Use of IUDs is the only contraceptive method for which sexually transmitted infection screening has any potential benefit; a woman may need risk- or age-related testing done at the time of placement if she has not previously had routine testing as recommended by the Centers for Disease Control and Prevention guidelines.
*Bimanual and speculum examinations.

LONG-ACTING REVERSIBLE CONTRACEPTION

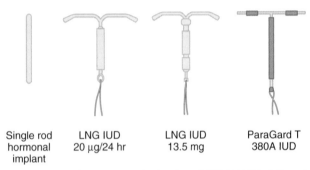

| Single rod hormonal implant | LNG IUD 20 µg/24 hr | LNG IUD 13.5 mg | ParaGard T 380A IUD |

FIGURE 27-1 The contraceptive implant (NEXPLANON; *left*) and the three intrauterine devices currently available in the United States: the levonorgestrel intrauterine system (LNG-IUD; *middle two*) and the ParaGard T 380A intrauterine copper contraceptive (*right*).

Immediate initiation of birth control and provision of adequate contraceptive supplies have both been shown to reduce unintended pregnancy rates and abortions.

TIER 1 REVERSIBLE CONTRACEPTIVE METHODS: IMPLANTS AND INTRAUTERINE DEVICES

The contraceptive implant (NEXPLANON) is a plastic rod mixed with the progestin etonogestrel. It measures 4 cm in length and 2 mm in diameter (Figure 27-1), and it releases the etonogestrel through a surrounding releasing membrane that is 0.06 mm thick. This contraceptive implant can be used by virtually any woman; only a history of recent breast cancer is an absolute contraindication. In addition, it has unsurpassed contraception effectiveness, is extremely convenient, and is rapidly reversible. It can be placed in a woman's arm in an office procedure that takes less than 5 minutes. This method provides 3 years of protection. In U.S. trials involving over 20,000 women-cycles, no pregnancies were seen when the implant was in place.

With counseling, the continuation rate for implants is considerably higher than for any of the Tier 2 methods.

The implant suppresses ovulation in all users for at least 30 months and in virtually all women (97%) for at least its full 36 months of approved life. The progestin also thickens cervical mucus to prevent sperm from ascending into the upper genital tract, which would prevent fertilization in any case where ovulation may occur. Decreased efficacy is demonstrated only in women taking medications that increase hepatic clearance of sex steroids, particularly anticonvulsants and St. John's wort. As with most progestin-only methods, the risk of endometrial cancer is reduced, but uterine bleeding may be more unpredictable.

IUDs are the most commonly used method of reversible contraception worldwide, but they have only recently started to regain popularity in the United States. A problem with infection that occurred years ago with one particular IUD that is no longer on the market resulted in decreased acceptance of the method. Like the implant, IUDs are also remarkably effective methods that provide convenient, uninterrupted contraception that is rapidly reversible.

Currently there are three different IUDs available in the United States. Their features are summarized in Table 27-4, and they are illustrated in Figure 27-1. Each of the IUDs can be used by most women; the only contraindications to all IUD use are pelvic infection, cancer of the uterus, or distortion or inappropriate size of the uterine cavity. In addition, copper IUDs should not be used by women with copper allergies or Wilson disease, and levonorgestrel IUDs should not be used by women with recent breast cancer. IUDs are placed into the endometrial cavity in a minor office-based procedure that takes less than 5 minutes.

The main differences among the three currently available IUDs are in their duration of action and their impact on uterine bleeding. **Levonorgestrel is used in each of the hormonal IUDs** because it is a potent and

TABLE 27-4

DISTINGUISHING FEATURES OF AVAILABLE INTRAUTERINE DEVICES

	ParaGard T 380A Intrauterine Copper Contraceptive IUD	Mirena LNG-IUS 20 µg/24 hr	Skyla LNG-IUS 13.5 mg
Duration of action	10 years	5 years	3 years
Mechanism of action	Functional spermicide	Thickens cervical mucus to block sperm entry	Thickens cervical mucus to block sperm entry
Impact on bleeding	Increased duration and flow*	Significant decrease in blood loss with increasing amenorrhea over time	Lighter flow over time
Noncontraceptive	Nonhormonal method	Treatment for heavy menstruation, dysmenorrhea, adenomyosis, and endometriosis	Smaller size for nulliparous women

IUD, Intrauterine device; LNG-IUS, levonorgestrel intrauterine system.
*Increases may be reversed by use of nonsteroidal antiinflammatory drugs.

long-acting progestin requiring the release of low doses into the uterus to thicken the cervical mucus. The levonorgestrel intrauterine system (LNG-IUS) 20 µg/24 hours is approved for up to 5 years of contraceptive use. It is associated with a 5-year cumulative pregnancy rate of less than 1%. It also is the most effective medical therapy for heavy menstrual bleeding because it induces high rates of amenorrhea by directly suppressing the endometrium, thus leaving estradiol levels in the normal range.

The lower-dose LNG-IUS 13.5 mg is a smaller IUD with a narrower diameter designed for up to 3 years of use. It can be more easily (and more comfortably) placed into a woman who has not delivered vaginally, and its lower progestin dose induces amenorrhea for fewer women (only about 12%).

The ParaGard T 380A intrauterine copper contraceptive IUD is the most effective nonhormonal contraceptive method. It is approved for 10 years of use, but may be effective for 12 to 20 years. The copper ions released from the IUD immobilize sperm and inactivate the sperm's acrosomal enzymes that are needed for the sperm to penetrate through the zona pellucida of the ovum. Union of the gametes is prevented. Because the copper IUD is known to increase menstrual blood loss by 35-50%, it is not recommended for women with heavy menstrual bleeding at baseline.

TIER 2 CONTRACEPTIVE METHODS: INJECTIONS, PILLS, PATCHES, AND RINGS

Although formal estimates of typical-use failure rates differ slightly between the injections and the other members of this group, in the Contraceptive CHOICE study in the United States, researchers found that the first-year failure rates for pills, patches, and rings were 20 times higher than those for IUDs or implants. The most common reason for the comparatively high failure rate was inconsistent use or nonuse. However, **Tier 2 methods remain the most popular in the United States,** partially for historical reasons and partially for the noncontraceptive benefits (e.g., acne improvement) that some of them offer.

In the United States, there are two types of progestin-only injections with depot medroxyprogesterone acetate (DMPA): one that is injected intramuscularly every 11 to 13 weeks and one that is administered subcutaneously every 12 to 14 weeks. Each offers very high efficacy if reinjected on time. Being progestin-only methods, the only contraindication (Category 4 condition) to their use in the US MEC is a history of recent breast cancer.

DMPA profoundly thickens cervical mucus and suppresses ovulation. Mean return to fertility is 9 months following injection, but it is delayed even longer in obese women. DMPA also thins the endometrium, which can initially cause irregular bleeding and **can increase rates of amenorrhea over time.** The label warns that use beyond 2 years is not recommended, because of potential bone loss. However, because the bone impacts have been shown to be reversible, professional organizations universally recommend that this warning should not affect long-term use. **Some women gain weight with DMPA use,** and experience with the first injection may help to predict future weight gain. **The noncontraceptive benefits of DMPA are impressive, including reduction of heavy bleeding, dysmenorrhea, sickle cell crises, pain from endometriosis, and future risk of endometrial hyperplasia and cancer.**

The combined hormonal contraceptives (CHCs) have both estrogen and a progestin to provide cycle control. There are over 90 different brands of combined oral contraceptives with different hormonal formulations, different regimens, and different doses. In addition, the transdermal patch and vaginal ring are more convenient delivery options.

The primary mechanisms of action of all CHCs are to thicken cervical mucus and suppress ovulation. Traditionally, combination birth control pills were given in packets with 21 active pills and 7 placebo pills to provide monthly scheduled bleeding. As the doses of hormones in the active pills dropped, it was noted that ovarian function returned after 4 days of placebo use, so the number of active pills in the low-dose formations was increased to at least 24, with 4 or fewer placebo pills. **Estrogen-containing pills significantly reduce menstrual blood loss and menstrual discomfort and offer noncontraceptive health benefits as well, including treatment of acne. These methods also significantly reduce the risk of endometrial and ovarian cancer.** Extended-cycle products provide distinct benefits to women with menstrual discomfort or medical problems that flare with bleeding (e.g., menstrual migraine and catamenial (monthly) seizures) by reducing the numbers of scheduled bleeding episodes.

The addition of estrogen to progestin adds rare but serious medical risks and more medical contraindications. **Risks that are clearly attributable to use of CHCs include increases in both venous and arterial thrombosis, resulting in pulmonary embolism, myocardial infarction, and stroke. Melasma** (facial pigmentation) and, uncommonly, **a reversible increase in blood pressure** are seen as a result of estrogen-containing contraceptive use.

Other side effects that have traditionally been attributed to oral contraceptive use, including headaches, breast tenderness, weight gain, mood changes, and gastrointestinal upsets, have been shown in prospective, double-blinded, placebo-controlled studies to occur at no higher frequency or with any greater intensity in pill users than in placebo users. It is not clear if the risk of gallbladder disease, hepatic adenoma, or breast cancer is increased with the use of oral contraceptives, because data derived from modern low-dose formulations are not consistent and at best show only minor impacts. Oral contraceptive use in *BRCA1* mutation carriers has not been shown to increase the incidence of breast cancer. Long-term studies have provided reassuring data that former use of oral contraceptives does not pose harm. In a large-scale study in which women who had ever used contraceptive pills were compared with never-users, those women who had ever used pills had lower overall mortality rates as well as lower mortality rates associated with cardiovascular disease and gynecologic and breast cancers.

The contraceptive patch and the vaginal ring were developed to relieve pill users of the requirement of daily administration. In the United States, consistent and correct use of oral contraception is infrequent. The once-a-week patch and the once-a-month vaginal rings demonstrated more consistent ongoing use in clinical trials than was seen with comparable pill users. **Both patches and the ring are designed to be used for 3 weeks and stopped for 1 week to induce scheduled bleeding.** When estrogen absorbed from the patch was found to be higher than doses absorbed from modern pills, the patch largely fell out of favor. The vaginal ring has increased in popularity as women have become more familiar with it. It is frequently used off-label without removal for 4 weeks at a time to induce amen-

orrhea. Newer formulations of both of these products may increase their use in the future.

Progestin-only pills (POPs) in the United States are generally reserved for breastfeeding women, but they have a much larger potential for use by women with medical problems. Because each pill in the packet is an active pill, instructions are easy to follow. For typical use, the failure rates of POPs are similar to those associated with any CHC. Because of their safety and rapid onset of action, POPs are clearly a "go to" choice for women whose evaluation for other methods is still pending.

TIER 3 CONTRACEPTIVE METHODS: BARRIERS AND BEHAVIORAL METHODS

There are several features of barrier and behavioral methods that set them apart from other methods. **They are generally available without a prescription** (except for diaphragms). That makes many of them available for episodic need when other methods are not available, as well as for ongoing use. However, their over-the-counter availability also shifts the burden of the cost onto the consumer (out-of-pocket expense) in the United States. **Tier 3 methods need to be used only at the time of intercourse, but that is the feature that most profoundly decreases their use and increases their failure rate.** Many offer varying levels of protection from sexually transmitted infections (STIs) as well as other noncontraceptive benefits, which can be very important to public health. They can generally be added to other methods or used together to enhance STI and/or pregnancy protection. The one notable exception is that male and female condoms should not be used together, because their effectiveness is decreased when they are combined.

Barrier Methods

When male condoms are used correctly and consistently, their first-year failure rate is 2%, but with typical use, their failure rate is 18%. Male condoms are the most commonly used method by adolescents at sexual debut. The use of condoms should continue to be supported as part of dual protection in that population for STI risk reduction.

Most male condoms used in the United States are made of latex. They are available in three sizes (snugger fit, large, and extra large), with variations in the diameter and lengths of the shaft as well as in the size and configuration of the portion of the condom that covers the glans. Some are smooth-tipped so that the man must leave room at the end to collect the ejaculate, whereas others are reservoir-tipped. Latex condoms are quite elastic, but they do not transmit heat and therefore can feel almost cold. **Latex allergies are found in 2-4% of the general population** and at greater rates in health care workers, people who work with latex, and those who need to self-catheterize. **Nonlatex**

condom options include a synthetic plastic isoprene (which has been used for years in surgical gloves) **and lamb cecum condoms.** The isoprene condoms are less elastic and are therefore available only in larger-sized condoms, but they do transmit heat. **The isoprene condoms also effectively block passage of the smallest viral particles and have high potential for reducing STI risk.** The so-called natural or cecum condoms block sperm and larger-size STI agents, but they do not block viruses as small as human immunodeficiency virus (HIV), human papillomavirus (HPV), or herpes simplex virus (HSV).

Female condoms have also been revised in recent years. To reduce costs, the FC2 female condom is now available in nitrite material. **Female condoms can also reduce STI risk.** They are best used by women whose partners will not use male condoms, because they have higher failure rates and are more expensive. **The FemCap is a silicone device shaped like a sailor's hat that applies spermicide to the cervix, which it covers with the bowl of the hat, while the brim of the hat is stabilized by the vaginal walls.** It is sized according to the patient's obstetrical history, "nulliparous," "parous" but no vaginal deliveries, and "parous" with "vaginal deliveries." The cap can be ordered online. Traditional diaphragms are rimmed silicone domes that need to be sized to fit across the vagina to cover the cervix with spermicide. A smaller, one-size diaphragm (SILCS) has been approved by the U.S. Food and Drug Administration (FDA). **The only available spermicide in the United States is nonoxynol-9 (N-9),** a detergent that disrupts the cellular membranes of sperm but also can disrupt vaginal epithelium and increase HIV transmission. **Spermicides are available as immediate-action foams and gels and delayed-action, but less messy, suppositories and films.** Newer, less destructive spermicides have been found to be as effective as N-9, and they may become available in the near future.

Behavioral Methods

Lactational amenorrhea is the most effective method in this category. Its low failure rate (2%) is limited to women who consistently (and exclusively) breastfeed during the first 6 months postpartum and who remain amenorrheic. After that time, pregnancy protection diminishes significantly, and ovulation often returns before the first menses. **Coitus interruptus (withdrawal) is one of the most commonly used behavioral methods historically.** Even for typical use, it works as well as many of the female barrier methods. Counseling about coital positioning is important to the success of coitus interruptus in that the man must learn to detect impending ejaculation and be able to withdraw his penis from the woman's vagina and direct the ejaculate away from her genital area before release.

Fertility awareness methods are designed to detect when a woman is at the greatest risk to conceive in her cycle. To be effective, these methods must take into account the life expectancy of sperm (5 to 7 days) and the duration of an ovum's ability to be fertilized (24 hours). Aids such as cycle beads for counting fertile days and smartphone apps can help a woman track her cycles and calculate her "at-risk days." **These methods work well only when cycles are reasonably regular (26 to 32 days).** The most easily implemented fertility awareness technique is called the *2-day method*. Each morning, the woman touches her vaginal introitus to determine if there is any moisture. Coitus is permitted only when her examination is dry of all secretions for 2 consecutive days.

Emergency Contraception

There are two FDA-approved hormonal methods for use following coitus. One is a series of products with high doses of the progestin levonorgestrel. Levonorgestrel suppresses ovulation up to the beginning of the luteinizing hormone (LH) surge. The efficacy of these products is inversely related to the time since exposure (4% failure rate at 72 hours) and to the woman's body mass index (BMI). These products are available by prescription or over the counter. The patient must pay full price for the over-the-counter packs. **The other hormonal product is the antiprogestin ulipristal acetate, which is given as a single dose within 5 days of exposure.** It is able to suppress ovulation until the peak of the LH surge. Its effectiveness does not diminish with time, although for obese women the pregnancy protection is less than for women with lower BMIs. It is available only by prescription.

The most effective method of postcoital pregnancy prevention (with a failure rate of 1 in 1000) is the placement of a copper IUD within 5 days of coitus. If placed late, after fertilization, it may work as an interceptive due to endometrial disruption caused during its placement. Another potential benefit with this placement is that the woman may enjoy up to 10 years of very effective contraception.

PERMANENT CONTRACEPTION

Also called *sterilization*, permanent contraceptive methods are available for both men and women. **Vasectomy is a safe, minor, office-based procedure that can be performed on men under local anesthesia in most situations.** There are various techniques available, but one of the most popular is the no-scalpel technique, in which the vas deferens is identified and grasped through the anesthetized skin. After it has been grasped, the vas deferens can be interrupted thermally, or it can be ligated. Complications include pain, hemorrhage, and infection, but long-term autoimmune problems have been disproven. Although no long-term efficacy trials have been done, **vasectomy is generally recognized to be a very effective method once azoospermia is achieved.** The man is asked to return 2 to 3 months after the procedure for a follow-up semen analysis. Couples must use other contraceptive methods until lack of sperm in the ejaculate is demonstrated.

Female permanent contraception is slightly more common in the Unites States, even though vasectomy is a safer procedure. Many tubal interruption procedures are performed at the time of delivery. With cesarean delivery, a partial salpingectomy can be done following closure of the uterine incision. Following a vaginal delivery, a small infraumbilical incision can be made just above the fundus. The fallopian tubes can be identified by tracing each tube out to the fimbria. A site along the fallopian tube without adjacent large vessels can be tented and the tube tied off and interrupted. Different techniques have been used to reduce the risk of fistula formation and future failure. **Figure 27-2 illustrates the Pomeroy method of tubal interruption (ligation) performed soon after delivery.**

Tubal interruption is also available as an interval procedure. Traditionally, women have had the procedure done while they are under general or regional anesthesia, with **laparoscopic techniques** used to thermally destroy, remove, or clamp a narrow portion of the tube on each side. The success rates for these permanent contraceptive methods vary with the woman's age (higher failure rates are seen in younger women) and with the technique used (interval procedures have higher failure rates). The chance of subsequent pregnancy associated with any of these techniques is low, but **if pregnancy should occur, the chance that it will be an ectopic pregnancy is increased to at least 20%.** The greatest mortality risk associated with interval sterilization is the anesthetic risk (3 deaths per 100,000 cases). Figure 27-3 illustrates interval tubal occlusion with the Hulka clip *(A)* and the Falope ring *(B)*.

Transcervical sterilization techniques have been introduced that can be done with local and intravenous anesthetic agents. Under hysteroscopic visualization, small coils are placed into the proximal ends of the fallopian tubes. These coils are filled with irritating fibers that induce local fibrosis of each tube. Complete tubal occlusion is documented 3 months later, usually with a hysterosalpingogram showing that none of the dye injected into the uterine cavity has entered into the tubes. Until tubal occlusion has been documented, couples must use other contraceptive methods.

Because it has been demonstrated that some serous ovarian and peritoneal carcinomas first develop in the fimbrial ends of the fallopian tubes, many have suggested that if a woman desires permanent contraception, it should be provided by fimbriectomy (removal of the distal end of the fallopian tube) or by salpingectomy (removal of the complete fallopian tube).

Abortion

Legal issues concerning the availability of abortion, the conditions under which consent for the procedure

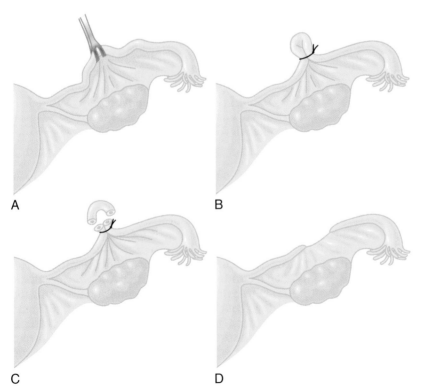

A

B

C

D

FIGURE 27-2 Pomeroy method of tubal ligation. **A,** Tube is grasped with Babcock forceps. **B,** A loop is ligated. **C,** The loop is excised. **D,** Several months later, the fibrosed ends of the tube separate.

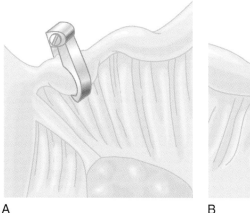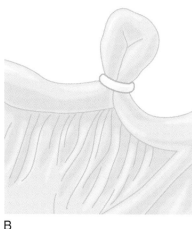

FIGURE 27-3 Tubal occlusion with **(A)** the Hulka clip and **(B)** the Falope ring. Cautery procedures use electric energy to destroy portions of each fallopian tube.

A   B

must be obtained, and governmental regulations of specifics of the procedure frequently change, and they vary from state to state. Some areas of the United States lack readily available abortion services.

From a medical standpoint, abortions are low-risk procedures with few serious adverse outcomes. Millions of abortions are performed each year in the United States, with mortality rates that are only a small fraction of the maternal mortality rate. Abortions also compare favorably in terms of complications with other routine procedures, such as tonsillectomy.

Before 49 days' gestational age, or with early failed pregnancies, both medical and surgical treatments are available. **Mifepristone 200 mg followed by misoprostol can induce complete abortion in 96-98% of pregnancies before 42 days' gestational age,** and success rates of 91-95% can be achieved in pregnancies from 42 to 49 days' gestation. Medical abortion is preferred in women at risk for surgical or anesthetic complications and in those presenting technical challenges, such as morbid obesity, cerebral palsy, or hip disorders.

Surgical management with vacuum aspiration (5 to 6 weeks' gestation) or dilation and curettage (6 to 13 weeks' gestation) is preferred over medical abortion in situations where anesthesia may help with anxiety and with pain or when mifepristone is contraindicated (e.g., adrenal insufficiency, hemorrhagic disorders, severe hepatic impairment, or renal failure). Women with medical problems should be referred to hospital-based providers. Antibiotic prophylaxis has been shown to significantly reduce the incidence of infectious complications associated with pregnancy termination. Softening the cervix mechanically (with laminaria, as illustrated in Figure 27-4) or pharmacologically (with misoprostol) reduces concerns about cervical damage and future cervical incompetence. **Cervical preparation is generally less of an issue in first-trimester pregnancy, but it may greatly facilitate**

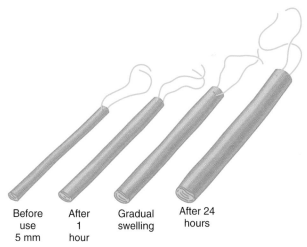

| Before use 5 mm | After 1 hour | Gradual swelling | After 24 hours |

FIGURE 27-4 Laminaria tents (osmotic dilators) used to gradually dilate the uterine cervix by absorbing body fluid. This technique reduces the risks of more rapid dilation during abortion procedures. Alternatively, prostaglandins placed vaginally can dilate the cervix medically.

surgical procedures done later in pregnancy. In the second trimester, both labor induction abortion with mifepristone and misoprostol (or with misoprostol alone if mifepristone is not available) and surgical dilation and evacuation procedures are available.

Women who present with septic abortion need emergency treatment with high-dose antibiotic therapy and surgical evacuation of the uterine contents by an experienced surgeon (see Chapter 22).

Abortion, with all of its controversial aspects, remains a safe and important method of family planning. The greater the availability of temporary and permanent methods of contraception, and the more informed women (and men) become about their safety and acceptability, the less demand there should be for abortion.

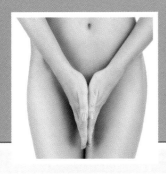

Sexuality and Female Sexual Dysfunction

JOSEPH C. GAMBONE

CLINICAL KEYS FOR THIS CHAPTER

- Sexuality and sexual expression are important aspects of human behavior. Recent liberalization of attitudes about sexuality and sexual expression has allowed the diversity of sexual behavior to be acknowledged. Although sexual expression is unlikely to begin before puberty, gender identity is expressed as early as 3 to 4 years of age. Gender identity disorder exists when children are unable to identify with their assigned gender.

- Studies document that physicians are mostly unaware of the sexual concerns of their patients. One survey showed that a high percentage of postmenopausal women with dyspareunia had never discussed this condition with their physician. The obstetrician gynecologist is in a unique position to inquire about, diagnose, initiate treatment of, or refer for sexual concerns and dysfunction, because women frequently report that sexual function is affected by reproductive events.

- Female and male physical sexual response cycles are similar, but they have some important differences. Most women need to experience a caring relationship and nongenital physical stimulation before satisfactory sexual arousal occurs. Men have a refractory phase during which no amount of stimulation will allow for an ejaculation and/or orgasm. Women may be capable of multiple orgasms, but an orgasm is not always necessary for sexual satisfaction.

- An assessment of sexual functioning is an important part of the complete medical evaluation. Including questions about sexual orientation and difficulties with sexual relations can lead to important information about female and male sexual dysfunction and may reveal episodes of intimate partner and childhood sexual abuse.

- Female sexual dysfunction may be primary (lifelong), secondary (acquired), or situational. The disorders include problems with desire, arousal, or orgasm, as well as pain during sexual activity. Referral to sex therapy specialists is appropriate for the first of those three disorders. The pain disorders frequently involve underlying gynecologic disease that the gynecologist can diagnose and treat. Lubricants and topical estrogen are often helpful. Investigations are underway to determine the safety and effectiveness of several androgenic preparations.

Sexuality **refers to how individuals express themselves as sexual beings.** Physically, sexuality encompasses sexual intercourse and other forms of sexual contact. Often patients may have medical concerns about their sexual feelings and behavior and how these activities may affect or be affected by disease. Obstetrician-gynecologists should be familiar with the physiology of the human sexual response and the types of sexual dysfunction that women may experience. Because female sexuality is most often expressed with another individual, and because that other individual is most often male, it is important for health care professionals who take care of women to know some basic aspects of the male sexual response and how it may differ from the female response. The sociology of human sexuality and sexual behavior, such as cultural, ethical, moral, religious, or legal aspects, are beyond the scope of this chapter.

Sexual Development

Although sexuality and sexual expression rarely begin before puberty, gender identity is experienced much earlier, starting at about 3 to 4 years of age. Children who are unable to identify with their assigned birth gender have **gender identity disorder (GID)** and may develop transgender issues later in life. **The diagnosis of GID can be made in an individual who has a strong** and persistent cross-gender identity and a discomfort about the assigned gender.

During puberty, many teens begin exploring their bodies and experiencing sexual activity with others. Many teens, especially males, have early intercourse and are not well educated about contraception or the risks of pregnancy or sexually transmitted infections (STIs). Young girls often engage in intercourse because of feelings of love, whereas boys are usually driven by curiosity. It is especially important for physicians to discuss sexuality with teens and to educate them about contraception and STI prevention. Teens are often apprehensive about discussing these issues and may fear parental discovery. They are usually more receptive to open-ended questions.

The early reproductive years are often the time when sexuality is explored and reproduction or its prevention becomes a priority. Infertility may be an issue in this age group, and many emotions may be evoked in infertile patients, often leading to sexual problems.

With increasing age, and especially after menopause, the frequency of and satisfaction with intercourse may decline. Decreased estrogen production causes progressive vaginal atrophy, which in turn leads to decreased vaginal lubrication, dyspareunia, and more difficulty in achieving orgasm. The decreased estrogen also decreases the acidity of the vaginal secretions, predisposing the woman to vaginal infections.

In many older couples, the frequency of intercourse declines because of the male partner's inability to have an erection. Illnesses or increased use of medications may also affect sexual functioning. A better understanding of the causes, as well as more effective treatment for male erectile dysfunction, is changing the sexual behavior of many older individuals.

Varied Sexual Expression

Human sexual expression is varied and often controversial. Health care professionals must be knowledgeable and nonjudgmental about healthy and legal sexual expression and lifestyles to facilitate open and comfortable communication.

Heterosexuals are individuals who engage in sexual activity with the opposite sex. Most individuals engage in heterosexual behavior, which is considered "normal." **Homosexuals are those who engage in sexual activities with members of the same sex.** Men who are homosexual are referred to as *gay,* whereas homosexual women are referred to as *gay* or *lesbian.* Whereas gay men tend to engage in more physical relationships and may have multiple partners, lesbians are generally inclined to be monogamous.

The reported incidence of homosexuality ranges from 6-20% in men and 3-18% in women. Several theories on homosexuality have been proposed, including a genetic predisposition, the maternal use of prenatal hormones, and other environmental factors. A multifactorial cause is likely.

Many homosexuals feel a need to conceal their sexuality for fear of loss of family, friends, or jobs. Familiarity with homosexuals has been shown to decrease the prejudice, and recently many homosexuals have "come out," revealing their sexual preference and expecting equal rights.

Bisexuals are those who engage in sexual activity with both men and women, either concomitantly or in different phases of their lives. The reported incidence of bisexuality is 1-7% of men and 1-2% of women. Many individuals briefly explore same-sex activity at some time in their lives but do not consider themselves bisexual.

Transgender or transsexual individuals are often confused with homosexuals. **They have a strong belief starting in childhood that they were born into a body with the wrong sex. Most are heterosexual in reference to their identified gender** (i.e., men who believe they are women are attracted to men), and few are homosexual. **Children with ambiguous genitalia who are assigned a particular gender may later show regret about their assignment.** Some experts recommend that these children be given a name that is appropriate to both genders to allow them to decide their gender for themselves later in life. Female-to-male transsexuals (FTM) are women who grow up as "tomboys" and often cross-dress. Male-to-female transsexuals (MTF) are men who grow up dressing as women. Transgender surgery is difficult to perform, especially for FTM transsexuals, and it is performed only in certain areas of the United States and the world.

Sexual Response

The process of sexual response was fully described by Masters and Johnson in 1966 based upon extensive research. They delineated the female and male physical sexual response cycles. Although modifications have been published, the original Masters and Johnson version remains the classic description of human sexual response. The female cycle is divided into four phases, whereas in men five phases are described. Generally, **clitoral tissue is the most sexually sensitive anatomic area for women.** Most women need to experience a caring relationship and nongenital physical stimulation before satisfactory sexual arousal can occur. A more recent conceptualization of the female (and male) sexual response recognizes the likelihood that a willingness to become aroused must come first and is followed by the sensation of desire (Figure 28-1). Box 28-1 lists the reproductive and life-cycle events that are known to affect a woman's sexual desire and response.

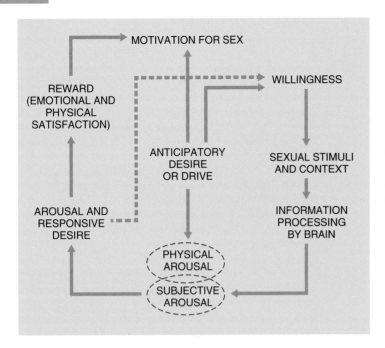

FIGURE 28-1 The circular sexual response cycle illustrating the probability that willingness is the essential first component. (From *Clin Updates Womens Health Care* 13[2], 2014, American College of Obstetricians and Gynecologists [ACOG], Washington, DC.)

BOX 28-1

POTENTIALLY DISRUPTIVE REPRODUCTIVE AND LIFE-CYCLE EVENTS ON SEXUAL FUNCTION

- Healthy pregnancy
- Complicated pregnancy precluding sexual intercourse and orgasm
- Postpartum period
- Miscarriage
- Therapeutic abortion
- Infertility
- Perimenopause
- Natural and premature menopause

Modified from *Clin Updates Womens Health Care* 13(2), 2014, American College of Obstetricians and Gynecologists (ACOG), Washington, DC.

FEMALE SEXUAL RESPONSE CYCLE

Excitement Phase

The excitement phase starts for females with physical or psychologic stimulation and may last minutes or hours. There is a sex flush, accompanied by erection of the nipples and engorgement of the breasts. A sex flush is an erythematous morbilliform skin change over the chest, neck, and face that occurs to a noticeable degree in 75% of women. In addition, the uterus elevates and vaginal lubrication begins. The clitoris and labia enlarge, and the heart rate and blood pressure increase. Most muscles become tense (Figure 28-2, *A*).

Plateau Phase

During the plateau phase, the breasts continue to enlarge and the clitoris may elevate and retract under its hood. The Bartholin glands may secrete fluid near the vaginal opening, and there is tenting of the uterus to allow easier passage of sperm. The vagina and labia become more engorged, and blood pressure, heart rate, respiratory rate, and muscle tension increase (see Figure 28-2, *B*).

Orgasmic Phase

During the orgasmic phase, there is release of sexual tension. This phase can occur without actual physical stimulation. It is concentrated in the clitoris, vagina, and uterus. There is contraction of vaginal, uterine, lower abdominal, and anal muscles, and usually there are 5 to 12 synchronized contractions 1 second apart. The first few contractions are the strongest and the closest together. Blood pressure, heart rate, and respiratory rate peak in this phase, and there is usually loss of voluntary muscle tone (e.g., most women curl their toes at orgasm). Women can have multiple orgasms before they enter the resolution phase (see Figure 28-2, *C*).

Resolution Phase

During the resolution phase, the nipples and breasts decrease in size and the vagina, clitoris, and uterus return to normal size and position. The sex flush disappears, and the blood pressure, heart rate, and respiratory rate also return to normal (see Figure 28-2, *D*).

MALE SEXUAL RESPONSE CYCLE

Excitement Phase

The excitement phase begins for males with physical or psychologic stimulation and may last minutes or hours. The nipples and penis become erect, and heart

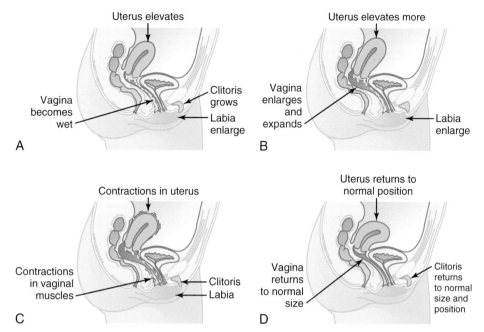

FIGURE 28-2 The four phases of the female sexual response cycle: **A,** The excitement phase. **B,** The plateau phase. **C,** The orgasmic phase. **D,** The resolution phase.

rate and blood pressure increase. The muscles become tense, and there is blood pooling in the extremities with vasocongestion in the penis and scrotum, as well as testicular swelling and elevation (Figure 28-3, *A*).

Plateau Phase

In the plateau phase, the testicles enlarge by 50%, and the prostate and penis also enlarge. There is increased blood flow, and the bulbourethral or Cowper gland secretes preejaculatory fluid, which may contain sperm. Blood pressure, heart rate, respiratory rate, and muscle tension increase. There is generally chest sex flushing (see Figure 28-3, *B*).

Orgasmic Phase

During the orgasmic phase, there is release of sexual tension; this phase is possible without actual physical stimulation. There are rhythmic contractions of the seminal vesicles, vas deferens, and prostate. The ejaculatory ducts push semen into the urethra, and ejaculation occurs with urethral contractions. The first few contractions are the strongest and the closest together. During this phase, the anal sphincter contracts. The **"point of imminence"** occurs a few seconds before ejaculation; this refers to the point when a man knows an orgasm is inevitable (see Figure 28-3, *C*).

Resolution Phase

In the resolution phase, the genitals and penis decrease in size and return to a flaccid state. The testes descend, and the sex flush disappears. The blood pressure, heart rate, and respiratory rate return to normal (see Figure 28-3, *D*).

Refractory Phase

The refractory phase occurs only in men. Because of this phase, men are not able to have multiple orgasms. During this phase, no amount of stimulation will cause another ejaculation. This phase lasts minutes in young men and hours to days in older men.

The similarity between the male and female cycles is apparent. Although the average time spent in each phase may differ (primarily as a result of learned behaviors), the elements of each cycle are the same. Because different neuronal circuits mediate each of these phases, sexual dysfunction may affect some phases without affecting the others.

Sexual Dysfunction

The overall prevalence of sexual dysfunction is not known, but female sexual dysfunction (FSD) is common. It has been estimated that **one-third of women experience decreased libido in situations where it is desired.** Comorbid conditions such as diabetes or obesity often play a causative role in sexual dysfunction, and not all women who lack interest in sexual activity are troubled by it.

EVALUATION OF SEXUAL FUNCTION

The assessment of sexual function should be an integral part of a complete medical evaluation, especially

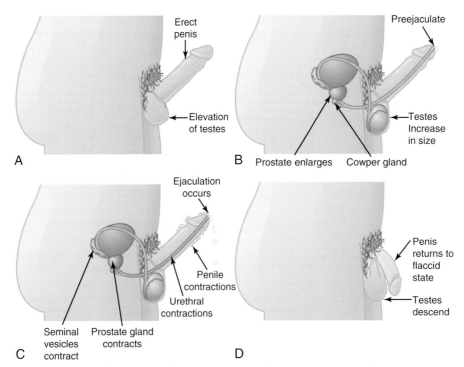

FIGURE 28-3 Four of the five phases of the male sexual response cycle. **A,** The excitement phase. **B,** The plateau phase. **C,** The orgasmic phase. **D,** The resolution phase. The refractory phase is not illustrated.

for the obstetrician-gynecologist. Skills needed for taking a sexual history are often overlooked in medical schools and sometimes are ignored by physicians. It is more difficult for a physician to inquire about a patient's sexuality if the physician is uncomfortable with the topic or is judgmental about sexual orientation. Clinicians may also be concerned about a patient's answers, not knowing what to say or do if a history of sexual trauma is revealed. They may also feel untrained to deal with problems related to and solutions for sexual inadequacies. Often they worry that the patient will misunderstand or be offended by the questions. **The acknowledgement and acceptance of diverse sexuality and sexual expression have changed in recent years, and it can be helpful to refer to** *sexual activity* **rather than intercourse and to a** *sexual partner* **rather than a husband.**

In taking a history, it is helpful to follow a routine pattern of questioning: (1) age of menarche, (2) menstrual patterns, (3) pregnancy history, (4) contraception use, (5) STI prevention, (6) sexual orientation, and (7) difficulties with sexual relations. Intimate partner violence and sexual abuse questions can then follow. Some sample questions include the following:

- Are you currently sexually active and, if so, with men, women, or both?
- Are you having any difficulties with sexual relations?

- Have you ever been in a situation where you have experienced unwanted or harmful sexual activity?

There are several factors that may affect taking a sexual history, including the physician's own sexuality. A gay physician may be either more thorough or afraid to inquire about a patient's sexual orientation. At times, clinicians of both sexes may find themselves attracted to patients. In these instances, acceptance of the feelings as normal is appropriate, as long as behavior is unaffected and a professional relationship is maintained.

FEMALE SEXUAL DYSFUNCTION

Sexual dysfunction is characterized by the Sexual Function Health Council of the American Foundation of Urologic Disease as failure of one or more of the phases of the sexual response cycle. Sexual dysfunction also includes pain disorders (Box 28-2).

FSD is a common condition and often increases with age. Sexual dysfunction can be subdivided into three categories, depending on whether it is **primary** (realistic sexual expectations have never been met under any circumstances), **secondary** (all phases have functioned in the past, but one or more no longer does), **or situational** (the response cycle functions under some circumstances, but not others). When a patient complains of hypoactive sexual desire, it is important to determine what her preferences are in

BOX 28-2

AMERICAN FOUNDATION FOR UROLOGIC DISEASE CONSENSUS CLASSIFICATION OF FEMALE SEXUAL DYSFUNCTION

I. Sexual desire disorders*
   A. Hypoactive sexual desire disorder
   B. Sexual aversion disorder
II. Sexual arousal disorder
III. Orgasmic disorder
IV. Sexual pain disorders
   A. Dyspareunia
   B. Vaginismus
   C. Other

*Each disorder can be subtyped as primary (lifelong) versus secondary (acquired), generalized versus situational, and by origin (organic, psychogenic, mixed, or unknown).

BOX 28-3

SOME DRUGS THAT CAN DIMINISH SEXUAL FUNCTION IN WOMEN

Antihypertensive agents: Reserpine, propranolol, methyldopa, atenolol, and spironolactone
Antidepressant medications: Tricyclics or selective serotonin reuptake inhibitors
Hypnotic agents: Alcohol, barbiturates, tranquilizers, and diazepam
Narcotics: Heroin and methadone
Antipsychotic agents: Fluphenazine and chlorpromazine
Stimulants: Cocaine and amphetamines
Hallucinogens: Lysergic acid (i.e., LSD) and mescaline
Diuretics: Acetazolamide

contrast to those of her partner. A woman who desires intercourse twice per week may be perfectly normal, but she may not function well in a relationship in which her partner desires coitus daily. Sexual dysfunction can occur in homosexual or heterosexual relationships, or even in masturbatory situations.

ETIOLOGY OF SEXUAL DYSFUNCTION

As a general rule, primary problems are predominantly psychogenic and tend to be of longer duration. Secondary problems are often associated with the onset of a disease process or the use of a pharmacologic agent. If such an association cannot be established, deterioration in the patient's relationship or some other chronologically related change in the patient's life experience should be inquired about. It is important to consider **psychologic causes,** such as depression or anxiety; **organic causes,** such as atherosclerosis, diabetes, or genital infections; and **pharmacologic causes** (Box 28-3). Factors initiating a problem may be different from those maintaining it. For example, drugs may

precipitate a problem, but if anxiety and fear of failure sustain the difficulty, discontinuation of the drug alone may not rectify the problem.

SEXUAL FUNCTION DISORDERS

Sexual Desire Disorders

Sexual desire appears to be an appetite similar to hunger, controlled by a dopamine-sensitive excitatory center in balance with a serotonin (5-hydroxytryptamine)-sensitive inhibitory center. **In both males and females, testosterone appears to be the hormone responsible for initially programming these centers during gestation and for maintaining their threshold of response.** Stimulation and ablation experiments in cats and other mammalian species have located these centers within the limbic system with significant nuclei in the hypothalamic and preoptic regions. For a woman, desire and interest in sexual activity result from a complex of both biologic and psychologic inputs, including her feelings about her partner.

    Disorders of sexual desire and/or interest include hypoactive sexual desire disorder and sexual aversion disorder. Lack of desire involves a decrease or absence of fantasy. **Sexual aversion disorder** may result from prior sexually associated trauma and personal aversion. In established relationships, decreased desire may result from sexual activity becoming too predictable and routine. Lack of privacy or external stresses, especially stress in the relationship, may initiate this disorder. Unrelated disease may also cause hypoactive desire. Women may fear sex with a partner who has had a heart attack or may have decreased desire themselves following a mastectomy or hysterectomy.

Arousal Phase Disorder

Sexual arousal disorder **is defined as the inability to attain or maintain sufficient sexual excitement, expressed as a lack of subjective excitement or somatic response such as genital lubrication. Estrogen is the hormone responsible for maintaining the vaginal epithelium and allowing transudation and lubrication to occur.** Its deficiency (with breastfeeding or after menopause) is by far the most common cause of excitement phase dysfunction in women. Extragenital changes during the excitement phase include an increase in heart rate and blood pressure, enhanced muscle tension throughout the body, an increase in breast size, nipple erection, engorgement of the surrounding areolae, and a sex flush. Some women do not recognize these symptoms as excitement and may experience arousal difficulty and even failure on that basis.

Orgasmic Phase Disorder

During the orgasmic phase, a series of reflex clonic contractions of the levator sling and related genital

musculature occur, mediated primarily via the sympathetic nervous system.

Orgasmic disorder is characterized by difficulty with or failure to attain orgasm following sufficient sexual stimulation and arousal. Anorgasmia may be situational. Many women experience orgasm only with manual or oral clitoral stimulation, and not with penile thrusting alone. If they are willing to increase direct clitoral stimulation before, during, or after penile penetration, they may achieve a wholly satisfactory sexual adaptation. Women who have been orgasmic in the past but have lost that capacity should be screened for organic or pharmacologic causes, and changes in their relationship or relationships should be carefully explored.

Most women with primary anorgasmia have had minimal or no effective stimulation from themselves or their partner. These patients should be encouraged to learn how to achieve orgasm through self-stimulation and then to share this new information with their partners. Increasing the intensity of stimulation should increase the intensity of response.

Sexual Pain Disorders

Dyspareunia is genital pain associated with sexual intercourse. It is helpful to categorize dyspareunia into three groups for easier diagnosis and treatment: (1) **pain with intromission** (often a result of vestibulitis, vaginismus, fissures, or other vulvar lesions), (2) **mid-vaginal pain** (often caused by lack of lubrication, surgical scars, or urethral diverticulosis), and (3) **deep-thrust dyspareunia** (often a result of endometriosis, interstitial cystitis, pelvic adhesions, or neoplasms).

Vaginismus is defined as severe pain and/or involuntary spasm of the distal vaginal and pelvic floor muscles during attempted penetration. A physical examination will reveal no organic condition, but the pubococcygeal muscles will be tight and vaginal penetration by speculum or examining finger will be painful and difficult, if not impossible. Often, affected women harbor fantasies about the inadequacy of their vaginas to accommodate a speculum or penis and fear that penetration will damage them. These women respond remarkably well to education and reassurance. Others may have been traumatized by early sexual or other abuse and require more intensive psychologic therapy. One important issue is whether they are motivated to participate with their partners in a stepwise **desensitization program.** This involves the slow, gentle vaginal insertion of dilators of gradually increasing size under the patient's own control. Once sufficient progress has been made, the partner's fingers and, ultimately, his penis may be substituted for the dilators. Alleviation of the problem is usually accomplished within 3 to 6 months.

Noncoital sexual pain disorder is pain that is induced by noncoital sexual stimulation.

MANAGEMENT OF SEXUAL DYSFUNCTION

Women with long-standing and complex sexual dysfunction disorders may need to be referred for treatment, but some sexual dysfunction problems can be managed effectively by the gynecologist. **Hormonal therapy is valuable in a limited number of situations.** Estrogen (orally or vaginally) may improve desire, arousal, and orgasm by decreasing dyspareunia that is caused by vaginal atrophy. **Testosterone may improve desire and arousal in some women, but it should be used with caution until newer formulations are tested for long-term effects.** Sildenafil (Viagra), which is used successfully in men with erectile dysfunction, inhibits cyclic guanosine monophosphate (cGMP) breakdown, thereby increasing clitoral and vaginal smooth muscle relaxation as well as improving lubrication. cGMP functions as a messenger in the nitric oxide–mediated relaxation of genital smooth muscle. **The use of sildenafil in women for sexual dysfunction has not been proven in controlled studies.** Dehydroepiandrosterone is currently being studied to determine its safety and effectiveness for desire and arousal disorders.

A clitoral vacuum device (the EROS-CTD) that has been approved by the U.S. Food and Drug Administration is said to improve clitoral blood flow and engorgement. **Fantasy therapy is helpful for hypoactive desire and sensate focusing therapy is helpful for excitement phase defects.**

Some of the most successful interventions for primary or lifelong FSD involve mindfulness-based and cognitive behavioral therapy supervised by sex therapists.

TREATMENT SUCCESS

As a group, orgasmic difficulties seem to respond to treatment most readily. For example, primary orgasmic difficulties may be resolved by means of guided masturbatory training and cognitive behavioral sex therapy. Secondary anorgasmia is more often associated with emotional or psychiatric disorders and relationship issues, so treatment is less effective. **Excitement phase dysfunctions do not have such positive outcomes, although problems with lubrication can nearly always be resolved satisfactorily. Lack of desire is the dysfunction most resistant to treatment.** Persons with little desire often have little internal motivation to seek more frequent sexual activity or to pursue help. Less than 50% of such patients show definite improvement. When the relationship is poor, behavioral approaches directed toward remedying the sexual problem are rarely successful. In contrast to erectile dysfunction and premature ejaculation in males, studies using medical and pharmacologic interventions for female arousal or orgasmic disorders are still ongoing, but they do show some promise.

Intimate Partner and Family Violence, Sexual Assault, and Rape

JOSEPH C. GAMBONE

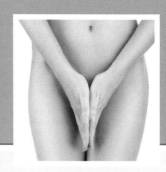

CLINICAL KEYS FOR THIS CHAPTER

- Intimate partner violence, formerly called *domestic violence*, is defined as intentionally abusive or controlling behavior by a person who is (or was) in an intimate or close relationship with the victim. The relationship may be heterosexual or between two people of the same sex. Most of the time a woman is the victim, but on occasion the abused person is a man.
- Although exact numbers for domestic violence events are not known, intimate partner violence, along with other types of family violence, are common. The enabling feature of these events is feelings of vulnerability that the victim cannot or will not attempt to overcome.
- Sexual assault includes sexual activity that ranges from sexual coercion to contact abuse, such as unwanted kissing or fondling, as well as rape.
- A medical consultation for sexual assault and rape should involve providing acute medical care, gathering evidence for possible prosecution, and transitioning the victim into longer-term care.
- The psychological consequences of intimate partner and family violence, as well as sexual assault, are significant, with lifelong problems reported. Providing social as well as psychological support and counseling are essential for adequate aftercare.

Domestic violence is now more commonly called *intimate partner violence.* The term *family violence* (covered only briefly in this chapter) also refers to abuse of other vulnerable persons such as the elderly, people with disabilities, or children. The American College of Obstetricians and Gynecologists (ACOG) Committee Opinion on Intimate Partner Violence (Number 518, February 2012) addresses these issues.

Sexual assault and rape are the most violent manifestations of sexual abuse. ACOG issued a recent committee opinion on the topic of sexual assault (Number 592, April 2014).

The obstetrician-gynecologist is in a unique position to identify the crimes of intimate partner violence and sexual abuse and help women deal with them.

Intimate Partner Violence and Family Violence

The obstetrician-gynecologist is the health care provider most likely to deal with the effects of abusive behavior directed against an intimate domestic partner. Intimate partner violence can include verbal abuse, intimidation, social isolation, and physical assault, such as a punch, a kick, a threat, a severe beating, an act of sexual assault, or even murder. It occurs in every age group, in all ethnic groups, in every occupation, and in every socioeconomic group. Although the obstetrician-gynecologist may be called to see a patient with acute injuries that result from partner violence or sexual assault, she or he is more likely to have to deal with the nonacute clinical manifestations of abuse (Box 29-1). Violence is most often perpetrated by a man against a woman; however, the gender relationship may occasionally be reversed. Intimate partner violence can also occur between same-sex partners.

EPIDEMIOLOGY

The prevalence and incidence of intimate partner violence are not known, but they are considerable. It has been estimated that as many as 2 million women are abused every year by someone they know. Any estimate of prevalence is likely to be understated, because of the likelihood that a significant number of

BOX 29-1

CLINICAL MANIFESTATIONS OF POSSIBLE INTIMATE PARTNER VIOLENCE*

Inadequately explained injuries, such as bruises and abrasions

Unusual difficulty during a gynecologic examination, such as excessive distress, discomfort, or avoidance behaviors

Chronic and unexplained pelvic pain, urinary symptoms, sexual dysfunction, or irritable bowel syndrome

Persistent or recurrent vaginitis or sexually transmitted infections in spite of appropriate treatment

Persistent vague complaints, such as headache, backache, palpitations, digestive, sleep, or eating disorders

Complaints or signs of depression, anxiety, phobias, panic attacks, or feelings of shame or worthlessness

Unintended pregnancy

Suicidal ideation

Modified from American College of Obstetricians and Gynecologists (ACOG): *Special issues in women's health—intimate partner and domestic violence,* Washington, DC, 2005, ACOG.
*No single presentation can confirm intimate partner and/or family violence.

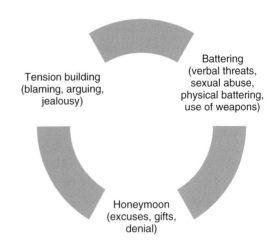

FIGURE 29-1 Cycle of violence. Elements of the cycle occur on a repetitive, unpredictable, and frequent basis. Verbal and emotional abuse are the most common forms of assault. An alternating kindness followed by abuse in an unpredictable manner contributes to the emotional distress and long-term psychological morbidity of victims. (From Gunter J: Intimate partner violence. *Obstet Gynecol Clin North Am* 34:367–388, 2007. Copyright 2007, with permission from Elsevier.)

victims are fearful of disclosing abuse. One study of the incidence of partner abuse found that of all women seeking care in an emergency room (ER), 54% said they had been threatened or injured at some time in their lives by a partner, and 24% said they had been injured by a current partner. One in three women presenting to an ER with injuries has symptoms related to partner violence. **More than 20% of violent crimes against women and 30% of female murders are committed by intimate partners.** Estimates of the number of pregnant woman who are victims of partner abuse range from less than 1% up to 20%.

Other forms of family violence are prevalent. The level of child abuse is epidemic, and it is estimated that nearly 500,000 elderly persons in domestic settings in the United States are abused or neglected. Seventy percent of cases of abuse of the elderly are perpetrated by a family member, including adult children.

In all cases of ongoing family and/or intimate partner abuse, the key enabling feature is some form of victim vulnerability that the victim cannot or will not attempt to overcome.

ADVERSE EFFECTS OF INTIMATE PARTNER VIOLENCE

The impact of intimate partner abuse and violence includes significant health, social, and economic effects. **Nearly one-third of female intimate partner violence victims have physical injuries** that require medical attention. **Many victims develop posttraumatic stress disorder** with all of its chronic symptoms and an increased risk of suicide. Women who are battered and abused have **lower overall health status and more depression and disability** than nonabused women.

Social services for women who are victims of intimate partner abuse **are inadequate.** Nearly one-third of battered women who request refuge are turned away because of a lack of space. Those turned away and their children often must return to a violent home. **Many become homeless and involved in substance abuse** as an escape mechanism or because they are forced into use and addiction by their partners.

The overall societal cost of intimate partner violence has been estimated to be in excess of $6 billion annually, and individual costs are increased because of higher insurance premiums paid by victims.

The abuser often provides for and is periodically in a caring and loving relationship with the victim, who may still love her partner despite the abuse. Other obstacles to leaving the abuser include (1) fear of more abuse, (2) loss of economic support, (3) fear of social isolation, (4) feelings of failure, (5) promises of change, (6) previously unanswered calls for help, and, in many cases, (7) fear of loss of child custody. Figure 29-1 illustrates the cycle of violence that exists in these abusive relationships.

ADDRESSING INTIMATE PARTNER/FAMILY VIOLENCE

Health care providers may have difficulty bringing up the topic of possible intimate partner violence. Because of the alarming frequency of this problem, **it is important to ask all women, when alone with them, if they feel safe in their own home. This should be a *routine practice* in taking a social history.** Even without a

BOX 29-2

MEDICAL PROFESSIONALS' RESPONSIBILITIES IN ADDRESSING INTIMATE PARTNER AND/OR FAMILY VIOLENCE

Implement a universal screening program
Acknowledge any trauma
Assess immediate safety of the patient and any children
Help to establish a safety plan
Review options
Offer educational materials and toll-free hotline information (Box 29-4)
Provide referrals
Document interactions
Provide ongoing support at subsequent visits
Inform authorities when appropriate (state medical societies can inform about legal requirements)

Modified from American College of Obstetricians and Gynecologists (ACOG): *Special issues in women's health—intimate partner and domestic violence,* Washington, DC, 2005, ACOG.

BOX 29-3

THE RADAR CHECKLIST APPROACH TO DOMESTIC VIOLENCE OR SEXUAL ABUSE

R: Remember to always ask about partner violence or sexual abuse in your practice.

A: Ask directly and clearly (in a private setting) about violence and abuse with questions such as, "At any time, has someone you live with hit, kicked, or otherwise physically abused or frightened you?"

D: Document all information about "suspected violence and abuse" in the patient's chart and file reports in accordance with local laws.

A: Assess the patient's safety, whether there are weapons in the house, and if any children are in danger.

R: Review possible options that your patient may have to increase safety, such as shelters and support groups.

Modified from Alpert EJ: *Intimate partner violence: the clinician's guide to identification, assessment, intervention, and prevention,* ed 4, Waltham, MA, 2004, Massachusetts Medical Society.

suspicion of physical abuse, the woman should be asked directly if a partner has ever hit, kicked, hurt, or threatened her. If a positive response is obtained, it is important to document any physical findings. Pictures and drawings should be used.

It is helpful and reassuring to tell the victim that she is not alone, that help is available to her, and that her partner's behavior is unacceptable. Nearly every victim believes that she is the only person to experience such abuse because of the isolating nature of abusive behavior. The perpetrator most likely will have convinced the victim that she is at fault and responsible for the abuse.

In addition to the need to comply with any reporting requirements (some states mandate reporting to appropriate authorities if there are acute injuries), social workers and other professionals should always be consulted when abuse is acknowledged or even if it is just suspected. Box 29-2 lists the responsibilities that health care providers have in addressing intimate partner and domestic violence. A useful checklist (**RADAR**) can be used to guide the practitioner during a patient encounter when domestic violence or other forms of abuse are suspected (Box 29-3).

Sexual Assault and Rape

Sexual assault and rape have different technical or legal definitions, depending on the state or country involved. However, **any sexual act performed on a person without his or her consent is classified as sexual assault.** Sexual assault includes any unwanted genital, anal, or oral penetration by a part of the attacker's body or by any object. **Rape,** on the other hand, **is generally a violent attack** that may or may not stem from the perpetrator's sexual desire. Very often, the perpetrator uses sex as a means of control over another person.

Whatever the rapist's intent, rape is definitely not a welcomed sexual experience for the victim. During any act of rape, the victim's predominant feeling is one of fear for her life or fear of mutilation.

Women of all ages, ethnicities, and socioeconomic groups can be victims of sexual assault, although the very young, people who have mental and/or physical disabilities, and the elderly are most vulnerable. **Nearly 75% of assaults are perpetrated by someone known to the victim,** such as husbands (marital or partner rape), boyfriends (date rape), fathers (incest), mothers' boyfriends, other relatives, or work associates. The American Medical Association reports that 20% of women under 21 years of age have been sexually assaulted. Other estimates are that 41% of women (of all ages) have been victims of actual or attempted sexual assault and that 50% of these women have been victims more than once. **Death occurs in about 1% of sexual assaults (including rapes), and serious injury occurs in 4%.**

MEDICAL CARE FOR SEXUAL ASSAULT

The medical consultation should proceed only after a supportive, caring relationship has been established. The adult or adolescent woman should be actively involved in the consultation so that she may regain a feeling of control over what has happened to her. **The purposes of the consultation are threefold: (1) to provide her acute medical care, (2) to gather evidence, and (3) to transition her into the long-term care she will need for psychological recovery from the extreme loss of control and great fear of death that nearly every rape victim experiences.** These objectives should be explained to her, and she should be allowed to dictate the pace of the questioning and the order of the examination.

During the interview and examination phases, a chaperone and/or patient advocate should be present.

Careful attention must be paid to the rules governing the chain of evidence to maintain the legal integrity and utility of all the specimens, photographs, and other materials collected. The woman should be asked about the detailed specifics of her assault to direct the collection of needed evidence and to address any risk of injury or infection. Information about her recent menstrual history, use of medications, recent immunizations, contraceptive use, and past medical and surgical history is important.

A thorough physical examination is needed to evaluate possible injuries, because **40% of all women who are sexually assaulted sustain injuries.** If possible, photographs or sketches of the injured areas should be obtained. The Centers for Disease Control and Prevention recommends routine testing for **gonorrhea** and **chlamydia** of specimens collected from any site of penetration or attempted penetration. Wet mounts and cultures for *Trichomonas* are routine, and a microscopic evaluation for **bacterial vaginosis** and **candidiasis** is prudent in a woman with a vaginal discharge. Serum tests for **human immunodeficiency virus (HIV), hepatitis B,** and **syphilis** are needed for baseline evaluation. Positive HIV status can be another clue to identifying victims of abuse.

Prophylaxis is suggested as preventive therapy. This includes hepatitis B vaccination (if previously unvaccinated) and appropriate antibiotics for sexually transmitted infections (see Chapter 22). **It is critical to provide any woman at risk for pregnancy with emergency contraception** (see Chapter 27). If prophylaxis for HIV is considered necessary, consultation with an HIV specialist is recommended. **Tetanus toxoid** should be administered to an unprotected, injured woman.

PSYCHOLOGIC SEQUELAE OF SEXUAL ASSAULT

Sexual assault is almost always associated with both immediate and long-term effects on victims. These effects have been termed the *rape trauma syndrome* and involve the following two phases:

1. **Acute/disorganization phase:** This phase lasts from days to weeks. **Immediately after the experience, victims frequently appear calm, although preoccupied and inattentive.** They are anxious, have difficulty sleeping, and commonly express shock, disbelief, fear, guilt, and shame. The **psychologic problems** that may result are varied and can mimic those seen in the aftermath of other kinds of traumatic experiences. Among the psychological problems expected in the acute phase of adjustment are **irritability, tension, anxiety, depression, fatigue, and persistent ruminations. Somatic symptoms** of a general nature may occur, such as **headaches or irritable bowel syndrome,** or symptoms may be more specific to the reproductive system, such as **vaginal irritation or discharge. Behavioral problems,** such as **overeating and alcohol or substance abuse,** may also surface, particularly when such problems have been evident in the past. **The long-term sequelae include changes in lifestyle, the occurrence of disturbing dreams and nightmares, and the persistence of phobic reactions. Fear persists as the predominant feeling.** These reactions often make it difficult for the victim to concentrate effectively on everyday activities and relationships.

2. **Integration and resolution phase:** During this phase, victims begin to accept the assault, but problems at work or with relationships may persist.

The management of the sexual assault victim in the acute phase influences long-term adjustment. Many rape victims may manifest **posttraumatic stress disorder.** The likelihood of this disorder developing is high, because of the abrupt nature of the crime, its violence, the passivity and helplessness imposed on the victim, and the high probability of sustaining physical and psychologic trauma. **The lifetime prevalence of posttraumatic stress disorder in rape victims is approximately 50%.**

In addition to attending to immediate physical and emotional needs in the initial evaluation, the obstetrician-gynecologist has an opportunity to prepare the victim for the long-term psychologic impact of the experience. This preparation is intended to diminish the long-term consequences and to enable the woman to recognize the common psychosocial sequelae when they occur, thus enabling her to seek professional help at an early stage. **Longer-term reactions involve nightmares, phobic reactions, and sexual fears.** Stimuli associated with the rape, such as a similar-looking man or similar surroundings, may be associated with flashbacks. **Flashbacks may also occur during pelvic examinations.**

Reactions to the sexual assault may result in problems with sexual behavior and functioning. Loss of libido is a common response to stressful or traumatic circumstances of any kind. Other complaints include vaginismus, impaired vaginal lubrication, and loss of orgasmic capability. These problems may be even more likely if the assault occurred at home while the woman was asleep. Preparing the woman for these eventualities can be extremely helpful in preventing sexual dysfunction from developing or persisting. Giving permission for a lower-than-usual sexual drive during the period following the assault may remove some performance anxiety. Explaining how anxiety and stress can inhibit sexual responsiveness and providing ways in which this can be overcome are also important.

Other Victims of Domestic Violence and Sexual Assault

The elderly, individuals with disabilities, and children may be particularly vulnerable to both domestic

violence and sexual abuse. In a recent study, researchers found that 14% of older adults who were not institutionalized had experienced physical, psychological, or sexual abuse during the previous year. This abuse included neglect and/or financial exploitation. In another study, investigators reported that women with disabilities were four times more likely to have been sexually assaulted than women without disabilities. Children are among the most vulnerable to domestic violence and sexual assault. All health care practitioners should be on the lookout for signs of these crimes in their patient populations.

Aftercare Planning

Careful follow-up must be arranged. If the woman uses the prophylactic therapies, a return visit is needed in 1 week to review the initial laboratory results and to monitor her progress. Repeat testing is needed only if the woman is symptomatic. If she did not receive prophylaxis, repeat testing for gonorrhea, chlamydia, and *Trichomonas* should be performed in 2 weeks and for syphilis in 6 weeks. Repeat serum tests for HIV should

---

BOX 29-4

KEY TELEPHONE NUMBERS FOR MEDICAL PROFESSIONALS AND VICTIMS OF FAMILY VIOLENCE AND SEXUAL ASSAULT

National Domestic Violence Hotline: 1-800-799-SAFE (7233 or 7234), TTY 1-800-787-3224 (hearing impaired)
RAINN (Rape, Abuse & Incest National Network) Hotline: 1-800-656-HOPE
National Child Abuse Hotline: 1-800-4-A-CHILD (1-800-422-4453)
Elderly Abuse Hotline: 1-800-922-2275
Disabled Person Abuse Hotline: 1-800-426-9009

---

be performed at 6, 12, and 24 weeks after the assault, regardless of whether prophylactic measures were taken.

Before discharging the patient, ensure that she has a safe place to go and a suitable means of transportation. She should also be given (in writing) the names, addresses, and telephone numbers of resources available in the community to meet her medical, legal, and psychosocial needs related to the assault (Box 29-4).

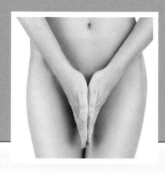

Breast Disease
A Gynecologic Perspective

NEVILLE F. HACKER • MICHAEL L. FRIEDLANDER

CLINICAL KEYS FOR THIS CHAPTER

- Mammographic screening of asymptomatic women after the age of 40 years decreases the mortality of breast cancer. About 40% of cancers detected by mammographic screening are not clinically apparent.
- Hyperplasia is the most common benign breast disorder. When associated with cellular atypia, there is an increased risk of subsequent malignant transformation.
- About 5-10% of breast cancers are hereditary and result from a germline mutation in the *BRCA1* or *BRCA2* gene. These genetic mutations also confer an increased risk of ovarian cancer.
- The modern approach to breast cancer management requires a multidisciplinary approach with breast-

conserving surgery and adjuvant radiation to the breast. Most patients are offered adjuvant chemotherapy and/or hormonal therapy, depending on the pathological features of the cancer and risk factors for recurrence.
- Although the single most important prognostic factor for breast cancer is the status of the axillary lymph nodes, this is an oversimplification, as it is now clear that breast cancer is a very heterogeneous disease. The patient's estrogen receptor status is an independent prognostic factor.

Breast cancer is not treated by gynecologists in most parts of the United States, but it is important that gynecologists be expert in breast examination, diligent about recommending screening asymptomatic women for breast cancer, familiar with common benign and malignant disorders of the breast, and conversant with the various therapeutic options available.

Screening of the Breast in Asymptomatic Women

SELF-EXAMINATION

Most breast cancers are detected by using medical screening techniques. Occasionally, a breast cancer is discovered by a woman during self-examination of her breasts. Because there is little scientific evidence that routine breast self-examination reduces mortality of breast cancer and may in fact lead to anxiety and unnecessary procedures, the United States Preventive Services Task Force (USPSTF) does not recommend routine breast self-examination. It seems reasonable,

however, to encourage women to be aware of any changes in their breasts and for them to seek professional evaluation of any noted changes.

BREAST EXAMINATION BY A PHYSICIAN

A complete breast examination should be performed by a physician at least every 3 years, especially for women older than 35 years of age. The breasts are first inspected with the patient in an upright position. The contour and symmetry are observed, and any skin changes or nipple retraction is noted. **Skin retraction, because of tethering to an underlying malignancy, may be highlighted by having the patient extend her arms over her head.**

Palpation of the breast, areola, and nipple is performed with the flat of the hand. If any mass is palpated, its fixation to deep tissues should be determined by asking the patient to place her hands over her hips and contract her pectoral muscles. Each axilla is then carefully examined while the patient's arm is supported. The supraclavicular fossae are also palpated for lymphadenopathy. **Following palpation with the** woman in the upright position, the examination is repeated with her in the supine position.

MAMMOGRAPHY

Several randomized controlled trials have demonstrated that mammographic screening of asymptomatic women older than 40 years of age can decrease the mortality of breast cancer. **Densities and fine calcifications constitute suspicious findings, and clinically inapparent malignancies of less than 1 cm in diameter may be detected.**

Mammograms of high quality can be made with about 0.3 cGy or less of radiation, so there is little, if any, risk of this technique causing breast cancer.

In 2009, the USPSTF estimated that screening was associated with 15%, 14%, and 32% reductions in breast cancer mortality for women 39 to 49, 50 to 59, and 60 to 69 years of age, respectively. The American Cancer Society recommends annual mammograms starting at age 40 years for women at normal risk.

ULTRASONOGRAPHY

Ultrasonography can differentiate cystic from solid masses and may demonstrate solid tissue that is potentially malignant within or adjacent to a cyst. It is also useful for imaging palpable focal masses in women younger than 30 years of age and in pregnant women, reducing the need for x-ray studies in this population.

MAGNETIC RESONANCE IMAGING

Magnetic resonance imaging is a useful adjunct in breast imaging. Reported advantages include improved staging and treatment planning, enhanced evaluation of the augmented breast, better detection of recurrences, and improved screening of high-risk women, including those with *BRCA* gene mutations.

Diagnosis of Breast Lesions

Physiologic nodularity and cyclic tenderness caused by the changing hormonal milieu must be distinguished from benign or malignant pathologic changes. **Definitive diagnosis of breast neoplasms may be made by open biopsy, by fine-needle (22-gauge) aspiration cytology, or by core biopsy.**

FINE-NEEDLE OR CORE BIOPSY

Fine-needle aspiration biopsy of a small, palpably suspicious lump in the breast can be performed in the outpatient clinic. Smears are prepared from the aspirate to allow cytologic evaluation. In experienced hands, the test is both sensitive and specific. **A negative result should never be accepted as definitive when there are clinical or mammographic and/or ultrasonic suspicions that the lesion may be malignant, and a core or open biopsy should be done.** In the presence of a large palpable lump, a core biopsy should make it possible to diagnose breast cancer without a formal excisional biopsy in at least 90% of cases, allowing the definitive management of the patient to be discussed preoperatively.

Relative indications for breast biopsy include those women with a clinically benign mass but a positive family or personal history of breast or ovarian cancer, a history of atypical hyperplasia, or an equivocal finding based on mammography or cytology.

Common Benign Breast Disorders

FIBROCYSTIC CHANGES

The earlier term *fibrocystic disease* has little clinical value, and the term was abandoned by the College of American Pathologists in 1985. Lesions formerly grouped together under the designation of fibrocystic disease represent a pathologically heterogeneous group of diseases that can be divided into three separate histologic categories: nonproliferative lesions, proliferative lesions (hyperplasia) without atypia, and atypical hyperplasias.

HYPERPLASIA

Hyperplasia is the most common benign breast disorder and is present in about 50% of women. Histologically, the hyperplastic changes may involve any or all of the breast tissues (lobular epithelium, ductal epithelium, and connective tissue). **When the hyperplastic changes are associated with cellular atypia, there is an increased risk for subsequent malignant transformation.**

It is postulated that the hyperplastic changes are caused by a relative or absolute decrease in production of progesterone or an increase in the amount of estrogen. Estrogen promotes the growth of mammary ducts and the periductal stroma, whereas progesterone is responsible for the development of lobular and alveolar structures. Patients with hyperplasia improve dramatically during pregnancy and lactation because of the large amount of progesterone produced by the corpus luteum and placenta and the increased production of estriol, which blocks the hyperplastic changes produced by estradiol and estrone.

The disorder usually occurs in the premenopausal years. Clinically, the lesions are usually multiple and bilateral and are characterized by pain and tenderness, particularly premenstrually.

Treatment depends on the age of the patient, the severity of the symptoms, and the relative risk of the development of breast cancer. Women older than 25 years of age should undergo baseline mammography to exclude carcinoma. **Cysts may be aspirated to relieve pain** (Figure 30-1). If the fluid is clear and the lump disappears, careful follow-up alone is indicated.

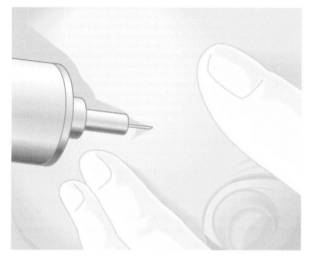

FIGURE 30-1 Aspiration of a breast cyst. Ultrasound may be used to differentiate a solid from a cystic breast mass.

TABLE 30-1	
ESTABLISHED RISK FACTORS FOR BREAST CANCER	
Risk Factor	**Relative Risk**
Age (≥50 yr vs. <50 yr)	6.5
Family history of breast cancer	
First-degree relative	1.4-13.6
Second-degree relative	1.5-1.8
Age at menarche (<12 yr vs. ≥14 yr)	1.2-1.5
Age at menopause (≥55 yr vs. <55 yr)	1.5-2.0
Age at first live birth (>30 yr vs. <20 yr)	1.3-2.2
Benign breast disease	
Breast biopsy (any histologic finding)	1.5-1.8
Atypical hyperplasia	4.0-4.4
Hormone replacement therapy	1.0-1.5

Data from Armstrong K, Eisen A, Weber B: Assessing the risk of breast cancer. *N Engl J Med* 342:564-571, 2000.

Open biopsy is required if the fluid is bloody or if there is any residual mass following aspiration.

FIBROADENOMA

Composed of both fibrous and glandular tissue, the fibroadenoma is the most common benign tumor found in the female breast. Clinically, these tumors are sharply circumscribed, freely mobile nodules that may occur at any age but are common before the age of 30 years. They usually are solitary and generally are removed when they reach 2 to 4 cm in diameter, although **giant forms up to 15 cm in diameter occasionally occur and have malignant potential.** Pregnancy may stimulate their growth, and regression and calcification usually eventuate postmenopausally. These larger tumors require surgical excision for definitive diagnosis and cure.

INTRADUCTAL PAPILLOMA

Papillary neoplastic growths may develop within the ducts of the breast, most commonly just before or during menopause. They are rarely palpable and are usually diagnosed because of a bloody, serous, or turbid discharge from the nipple. **Mammographic and cytologic examination of the fluid is helpful in investigating nipple discharge. Excisional biopsy of the lesion and involved duct is the treatment of choice.**

Histologically, there is a spectrum of lesions, ranging from those that are clearly benign to those that are anaplastic and give evidence of invasive tendencies.

GALACTOCELE

A galactocele is a cystic dilation of a duct that is filled with thick, inspissated, milky fluid. It presents during or shortly after lactation and implies some cause for ductal obstruction, such as inflammation, hyperplasia, or neoplasia. Often multiple cysts are present. **Secondary infection may produce areas of acute mastitis or abscess formation.** Needle aspiration is usually curative. If the fluid is bloody or the mass does not disappear completely, excisional biopsy is required.

Breast Cancer

Breast cancer is the most common female malignancy, accounting for 26% of malignancies in women. It is second only to lung cancer as the leading cause of cancer deaths in women. The estimate for 2013 was that 232,340 new cases of breast cancer would be diagnosed in the United States, which would be associated with approximately 39,620 deaths. **In the United States, there is a 1 in 8 chance that a woman will develop breast cancer during her lifetime if she lives to 90 years of age.**

ETIOLOGY

Established risk factors for breast cancer are shown in Table 30-1. However, 75% of women develop the disease despite having no apparently increased susceptibility.

The incidence and mortality rates for breast cancer are approximately five times higher in North America and northern Europe than they are in many Asian and African countries. Migrants to the United States from Asia (principally those of Chinese and Japanese ethnicity) do not experience a substantial increase in risk, but their first-generation and second-generation descendants have rates approaching those of the white population in the United States. The difference may be related to dietary customs.

Menopausal hormone replacement therapy produces a small increased risk of breast cancer, and the estrogen-progestin regimen increases the risk beyond that associated with estrogen alone.

About 5-10% of breast cancer cases are hereditary and result from mutations in the *BRCA1* or *BRCA2* gene. These genetic mutations also increase the risk of ovarian cancer. Hereditary breast cancer is particularly common in premenopausal women. Women with a mutated *BRCA1* or *BRCA2* gene have up to a 70% risk of developing breast cancer by age 65 years.

TUMOR TYPES

The mammary epithelium gives rise to a wide variety of histologic tumor types. **About 80% of all breast cancers are nonspecific infiltrating ductal carcinomas.** These tumors usually induce a significant fibrotic response and are often stony hard upon clinical palpation. **Less common types include infiltrating lobular, medullary, mucinous, tubular, and papillary tumors.** In many tumors, several patterns coexist.

Paget disease of the breast occurs in about 3% of patients with breast cancer. It represents a specific subtype of intraductal carcinoma that arises in the main excretory ducts of the breasts and extends to involve the skin of the nipple and areola, producing an eczematoid appearance. **The underlying carcinoma, although invariably present, can be palpated clinically in only about two-thirds of patients.**

Inflammatory breast cancer represents 1-4% of cases and typically occurs in younger women. It is characterized clinically by warmth and redness of the overlying skin and induration of the surrounding breast tissues. Biopsies of the erythematous areas reveal malignant cells in subdermal lymphatics, causing an obstructive lymphangitis. Inflammatory cells are rarely present. **Some patients with inflammatory breast cancer have palpable regional lymph nodes at initial presentation.**

TUMOR SPREAD

Breast cancer spreads by local infiltration as well as by lymphatic or hematogenous routes. Locally, the tumor infiltrates directly into the breast parenchyma, eventually involving the overlying skin or the deep pectoral fascia.

Lymphatic spread is mainly to the axillary nodes, involvement of which occurs in up to 50% of patients with symptomatic breast cancer and in 10-20% of patients with breast cancers detected by screening. The second major area for lymph node metastases is the internal mammary node chain. These nodes are most likely to be involved when the primary lesion is medially or centrally situated. **The supraclavicular nodes are usually involved only after axillary node involvement.**

Hematogenous spread occurs mainly to the lungs and liver, but other common sites of involvement include bone, pleura, liver, ovaries, and brain.

STAGING

Several systems of staging for cancer of the breast have been recommended. The one recommended by the American Joint Committee on Cancer is shown in Box 30-1.

CLINICAL FEATURES

Carcinoma of the breast is usually painless and may be freely mobile. A serous or bloody nipple discharge may be present. With progressive growth, the tumor may become fixed to the deep fascia. **Extension to the skin may cause retraction and dimpling, whereas ductal involvement may cause nipple retraction. Blockage of skin lymphatics may cause lymphedema and thickening of the skin, a change referred to as *peau d'orange*** (Figure 30-2).

TREATMENT

The modern management of breast cancer involves a multidisciplinary team approach. As much normal breast tissue as possible is left in women who have a wide local excision to conserve the cosmetic appearance of the breast while ensuring clear and uninvolved margins. Adjuvant radiation is given following the wide local excision, as well as chemotherapy or hormonal therapy, depending on the woman's pathological risk factors.

Surgery

The surgical management of breast cancer has been transformed over the last 50 years. This has occurred through an improved understanding of the biology of breast cancer, as well as earlier diagnosis through screening and increased awareness of the disease.

Radical mastectomy, as first described in 1894 by Halsted and Meyer, was for many years the standard operation for operable breast cancer, and it involved en bloc dissection of the entire breast, together with the pectoralis major and minor muscles and the contents of the axilla. It was based on a flawed understanding of the biology and mode of spread of breast cancer, and it was a mutilating procedure. It was superseded by less radical surgery 30 to 40 years ago. **Survival rates after conservative surgery with wide local excision in selected patients have been shown to be equal to those after modified radical mastectomy.** Although the size of the primary carcinoma alone is not a limiting factor for breast conservation, if the breast is small, breast conservation is unsatisfactory even for small tumors and is impractical for large tumors.

Routine axillary lymph node dissection has progressively been replaced by lymphatic mapping and sentinel lymph node biopsy as a less morbid means of determining the nodal status in the axilla. If the sentinel node is negative, the axillary nodes will be negative with an accuracy of about 95%, so axillary dissection

BOX 30-1

STAGING OF BREAST CANCER*

Primary Tumor (T)

- TX: Primary tumor cannot be assessed
- T0: No evidence of primary tumor
- Tis: Carcinoma in situ, intraductal carcinoma, lobular carcinoma in situ, or Paget disease of the nipple with no associated invasion of normal breast tissue
- T1: Tumor ≤2.0 cm in greatest dimension
  - T1mic: Microinvasion ≤0.1 cm in greatest dimension
  - T1a: Tumor >0.1 cm but not >0.5 cm in greatest dimension
  - T1b: Tumor >0.5 cm but not >1.0 cm in greatest dimension
  - T1c: Tumor >1.0 cm but not >2.0 cm in greatest dimension
- T2: Tumor >2.0 cm but not >5.0 cm in greatest dimension
- T3: Tumor >5.0 cm in greatest dimension
- T4: Tumor of any size with direct extension to (a) chest wall or (b) skin
  - T4a: Extension to chest wall
  - T4b: Edema (including *peau d'orange*) or ulceration of the skin of the breast or satellite skin nodules confined to the same breast
  - T4c: Both of the above (T4a and T4b)
  - T4d: Inflammatory carcinoma

Regional Lymph Nodes (N)

- NX: Regional lymph nodes cannot be assessed (e.g., previously removed)
- N0: No regional lymph node metastasis
- N1: Metastasis to movable ipsilateral axillary lymph node(s)
- N2: Metastasis to ipsilateral axillary lymph node(s) fixed or matted or in clinically apparent* ipsilateral internal mammary nodes in the *absence* of clinically evident lymph node metastasis
  - N2a: Metastasis in ipsilateral axillary lymph nodes fixed to one another (matted) or to other structures
  - N2b: Metastasis only in clinically apparent* ipsilateral internal mammary nodes and in the *absence* of clinically evident axillary lymph node metastasis
- N3: Metastasis in ipsilateral infraclavicular lymph node(s) with or without axillary lymph node involvement, or in clinically apparent* ipsilateral internal mammary lymph node(s) and in the *presence* of clinically evident axillary lymph node metastasis, or in ipsilateral supraclavicular lymph node(s) with or without axillary or internal mammary lymph node involvement
  - N3a: Metastasis in ipsilateral infraclavicular lymph node(s)
  - N3b: Metastasis in ipsilateral internal mammary lymph node(s) and axillary lymph node(s)
  - N3c: Metastasis in ipsilateral supraclavicular lymph node(s)

Pathologic Classification (pN)[†]

- pNX: Regional lymph nodes cannot be assessed (e.g., not removed for pathologic study or previously removed)
- pN0: No regional lymph node metastasis histologically and no additional examination for isolated tumor cells[‡]
- pN0(1–): No regional lymph node metastasis histologically, negative immunohistochemistry (IHC)
- pN0(1+): No regional lymph node metastasis histologically, positive IHC, and no IHC cluster >0.2 mm
- pN0(mol–): No regional lymph node metastasis histologically and negative molecular findings (reverse transcription polymerase chain reaction [RT-PCR])
- pN0(mol+): No regional lymph node metastasis histologically, and positive molecular findings (RT-PCR)
- pN1: Metastasis in one to three axillary lymph nodes, and/or in internal mammary nodes with microscopic disease, detected by sentinel lymph node (SLN) dissection but not clinically apparent[§]
  - pN1mi: Micrometastasis (>0.2 mm but not >2.0 mm)
  - pN1a: Metastasis in one to three axillary lymph nodes
  - pN1b: Metastasis in internal mammary nodes with microscopic disease detected by SLN dissection but not clinically apparent[§]
  - pN1c: Metastasis in one to three axillary lymph nodes and in internal mammary lymph nodes with microscopic disease detected by SLN dissection but not clinically apparent[§] (If associated with more than three positive axillary lymph nodes, the internal mammary nodes are classified as pN3b to reflect increased tumor burden.)
- pN2: Metastasis in four to nine axillary lymph nodes, or in clinically apparent* internal mammary lymph nodes in the *absence* of axillary lymph node metastasis to ipsilateral axillary lymph node(s) fixed to each other or to other structures
  - pN2a: Metastasis in four to nine axillary lymph nodes (at least one tumor deposit >2.0 mm)
  - pN2b: Metastasis in clinically apparent* internal mammary lymph nodes in the *absence* of axillary lymph node metastasis
- pN3: Metastasis in 10 or more axillary lymph nodes, or in infraclavicular lymph nodes, or in clinically apparent* ipsilateral internal mammary lymph node(s) in the *presence* of one or more positive axillary lymph node(s), or in more than three axillary lymph nodes with clinically negative microscopic metastasis in internal mammary lymph nodes, or in ipsilateral supraclavicular lymph nodes
  - pN3a: Metastasis in 10 or more axillary lymph nodes (at least one tumor deposit >2.0 mm) or metastasis to the infraclavicular lymph nodes
  - pN3b: Metastasis in clinically apparent* ipsilateral internal mammary lymph nodes in the *presence* of one or more positive axillary lymph node(s), or in more than three axillary lymph nodes and in internal mammary lymph nodes with microscopic disease detected by SLN dissection but not clinically apparent[§]
  - pN3c: Metastasis in ipsilateral supraclavicular lymph nodes

BOX 30-1

STAGING OF BREAST CANCER—cont'd

Distant Metastasis (M)

- MX: Presence of distant metastasis cannot be assessed
- M0: No distant metastasis
- M1: Distant metastasis

American Joint Commission on Cancer Stage Groupings

Stage 0

- Tis, N0, M0

Stage I

- T1[‖], N0, M0

Stage IIA

- T0, N1, M0
- T1[‖], N1, M0
- T2, N0, M0

Stage IIB

- T2, N1, M0
- T3, N0, M0

Stage IIIA

- T0, N2, M0
- T1[‖], N2, M0
- T2, N2, M0
- T3, N1, M0
- T3, N2, M0

Stage IIIB

- T4, N0, M0
- T4, N1, M0
- T4, N2, M0

Stage IIIC[¶]

- Any T, N3, M0

Stage IV

- Any T, Any N, M1

*Clinically apparent is defined as detected by imaging studies (excluding lymphoscintigraphy) or by clinical examination or grossly visible pathologically.
†Classification is based on axillary lymph node dissection with or without sentinel lymph node (SLN) dissection. Classification based solely on SLN dissection without subsequent axillary lymph node dissection is designated "(sn)" for sentinel node (e.g., pN0(1+) [sn]).
‡*Isolated tumor cells* (ITCs) are defined as single tumor cells or small cell clusters not larger than 0.2 mm, usually detected only by immunohistochemistry or molecular methods, but that may be verified by hematoxylin and eosin staining. ITCs do not usually show evidence of malignant activity (e.g., proliferation or stromal reaction).
§*Not clinically apparent* is defined as not detected by imaging studies (excluding lymphoscintigraphy) or by clinical examination.
‖T1 includes T1mic.
¶Stage IIIC breast cancer includes patients with any T stage who have pN3 disease. Patients with pN3a and pN3b disease are considered candidates for surgery and are managed as described in the section on Stages I, II, IIIA, and operable IIIC breast cancer. pN3c disease is considered inoperable, and patients with this stage of breast cancer are managed as described in the section on inoperable Stage IIIB or IIIC or inflammatory breast cancer.

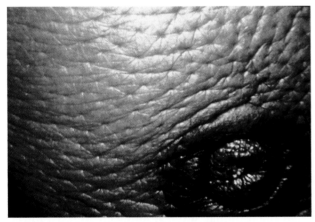

FIGURE 30-2 Carcinoma of the breast. Note the nipple retraction and the *peau d'orange* appearance. (From Swartz MH: *Textbook of physical diagnosis: history and examination,* ed 5, Philadelphia, 2006, Saunders.)

may be avoided. For a sentinel node that is positive, axillary dissection until recently was the standard of care, but this has been challenged by a number of trials in which researchers have found no evidence supporting a therapeutic benefit of routine axillary dissection in patients with positive sentinel nodes. This further illustrates just how much the surgical management of breast cancer has evolved over the last three decades.

Breast reconstruction after mastectomy is an integral part of the treatment of breast cancer. The procedure may be performed at the time of the mastectomy, or it may be delayed.

Radiation Therapy

Conservative surgery is always performed in conjunction with radiation therapy to the breast. This approach gives equivalent outcomes to a modified radical or simple mastectomy, and functional and cosmetic results are improved. External beam therapy is used, with 4500 to 5000 cGy delivered to the entire breast. **The ipsilateral supraclavicular and internal mammary nodes may be treated on the basis of their clinicopathologic characteristics, including size and nodal status.** A number of trials of postmastectomy radiation in women with involved lymph nodes have demonstrated not only a reduction in the risk of locoregional recurrence but also a survival benefit. The axilla is not routinely irradiated following an axillary node dissection, because of the high incidence of lymphedema.

Adjuvant Therapy

Adjuvant systemic therapy is used for most patients with early breast cancer, regardless of lymph node status. Overall, adjuvant therapy reducers the risk of relapse by at least one-third and reduces the risk of death by over 30%.

In the Early Breast Cancer Trialists' meta-analysis of adjuvant systemic therapy, authors reported mortality reductions of 38% (age <50 years) and 20% (age 50 to 69 years) associated with adjuvant chemotherapy, followed by a further reduction of 31% with tamoxifen therapy in patients with estrogen receptor (ER)–positive breast cancer. It was estimated that the final mortality reductions would be 57% and 45% for adjuvant chemotherapy and tamoxifen therapy, respectively. The absolute benefit of adjuvant systemic therapy depends on the risk of recurrence in an individual woman.

The recommendations regarding adjuvant systemic therapy are based on multiple clinicopathologic factors that cannot be summarized simply in a few lines. **These factors include age of the patient, tumor size, histological subtype, histologic grade, estrogen (ER) and progesterone receptor status, Ki67 and human epidermal growth factor receptor 2 (HER2) status, and nodal status.** It is essential that all these factors be taken into consideration and that the proportional reductions in recurrence and mortality, the absolute potential gains, and the potential adverse effects of treatment be discussed with patients.

The following is a simplified list of current recommendations for adjuvant chemotherapy and hormonal therapy:

- Premenopausal patients with ER-negative tumors should receive adjuvant systemic chemotherapy.
- Premenopausal patients with ER-positive tumors should receive hormonal therapy (tamoxifen) in addition to chemotherapy. There is a subset of patients in whom adjuvant hormonal therapy may be sufficient.
- Postmenopausal patients with ER-positive tumors who have negative nodes and low-risk features should be treated with adjuvant tamoxifen for 2 years, followed by an aromatase inhibitor (such as anastrazole) for 3 years or for 5 years. Those with positive nodes should receive hormonal therapy, and chemotherapy should also be considered.
- Postmenopausal patients with ER-negative tumors should receive adjuvant chemotherapy.
- Patients with HER2-positive breast cancers should be given anti-HER2-directed therapies such as trastuzumab, as well as chemotherapy and hormonal therapy if they are ER-positive.

An added benefit of adjuvant tamoxifen is a 50% reduction in the risk of cancer in the contralateral breast.

Adjuvant chemotherapy usually consists of so-called third-generation chemotherapy regimens with anthracycline and taxane combinations (e.g., 4 cycles of doxorubicin and cyclophosphamide followed by weekly paclitaxel for 12 weeks, or 5-fluorouracil, epirubicin, and cyclophosphamide every 3 weeks for 3 cycles followed by docetaxel every 3 weeks for 3 cycles, or docetaxel, doxorubicin, and cyclophosphamide every 3 weeks for 6 cycles). There are a subset of patients in whom four cycles of chemotherapy with docetaxel and cyclophosphamide is adequate therapy.

Approximately 30% of women with early breast cancer develop metastases. The 5-year survival of women with metastatic breast cancer is approximately 25%, and their median survival is 24 to 36 months, but there is a wide range. The most important prognostic factors include time to recurrence, ER status, HER2 status, site and number of metastases, and performance status. The median survival has increased over time related to more effective therapies and a wide range of available agents. Median survival rates are highest in women with luminal type A and HER2-positive breast cancers, and they are shortest in women with triple-negative metastatic breast cancers.

Trastuzumab (Herceptin), a humanized monoclonal antibody directed against *HER2/neu*, has been approved by the U.S. Food and Drug Administration for patients with early breast cancer in conjunction with chemotherapy, as well as for the treatment of patients with metastatic breast cancer. Its efficiency is predicted by *HER2/neu* gene amplification. It has transformed the prognosis of women with HER2-positive breast cancers, and there are now a number of new, very effective anti-HER2 therapies, including pertuzumab and ado-trastuzumab emtansine (T-DM1, Kadcyla).

PROGNOSIS

Although prognosis is related to the stage of the disease and the age of the patient (older patients have a better prognosis), **the status of the axillary lymph nodes has been considered to be the single most important prognosticator.** The ER status is also of independent prognostic significance; patients with ER-negative tumors have a poorer prognosis.

In the National Surgical Adjuvant Breast Project, patients with negative lymph nodes had an actuarial 5-year survival of 83%, compared with 73% for patients with 1 to 3 positive nodes, 45% for those with 4 or more positive nodes, and 28% for those with more than 13 positive nodes.

More recently, it has been appreciated that breast cancers are a very heterogeneous group of cancers. There are at least four different molecular subtypes that have a unique biologic behavior and prognosis, and nodal status alone is no longer considered to be the most important prognostic factor. The molecular subtypes include luminal A, which account for 40% of breast cancers. These cancers are typically of low grade, strongly ER-positive, and have a very good prognosis; luminal B, which are of higher grade, have lower expression of ER, and can be HER2-positive; HER2-enriched (10-15%); and basal-like, which are ER-negative, progesterone receptor–negative, and HER2-negative. This illustrates the complexity of breast cancers and how it is not possible to prognosticate on the basis of a diagnosis of breast cancer alone.

BREAST CANCER IN PREGNANCY

About 3% of breast cancers occur during pregnancy, complicating approximately 1 in every 3000 pregnancies. Diagnosis is usually delayed because small masses are more difficult to palpate in hypertrophied breasts. Needle aspiration or core biopsy, however, should be performed promptly upon discovery of any suspicious mass.

The surgical treatment is essentially the same as that for the nonpregnant patient. Postoperative irradiation is delayed until after delivery. **For patients with nodal metastases, termination should be considered if the patient is early in the first trimester of pregnancy because of the teratogenic risks of the adjuvant chemotherapy.** Adjuvant chemotherapy can be administered in the second and third trimesters of pregnancy. In the third trimester, chemotherapy can usually be delayed until after delivery, although surgery should occur promptly following diagnosis.

Stage for stage, the prognosis for pregnant patients is not much worse than that for nonpregnant patients. There is no indication to advise against subsequent pregnancy for patients with breast cancer who have no evidence of recurrence.

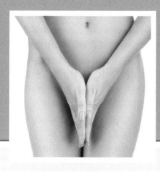

CHAPTER 31

Gynecologic Procedures
Imaging Studies and Surgery

JOSEPH C. GAMBONE

CLINICAL KEYS FOR THIS CHAPTER

- Imaging studies are used in gynecology to evaluate pelvic masses and also to assist in oocyte retrieval. Common modalities used include ultrasonography, sonohysterography, computed axial tomography, magnetic resonance imaging, mammography, and hysterosalpingography.
- Before any gynecologic procedure is performed, a process of informed consent should occur during which the patient collaborates and makes a choice with her surgeon. Most procedures are elective, allowing for several treatment options to be considered.
- Training for gynecologic procedures begins in residency and continues throughout a surgical career, with newer procedures being added as newer technologies are developed. *Privileging* refers to the process whereby surgeons are given the right to perform certain procedures in the hospital or clinic setting.
- Common gynecologic procedures range from minor biopsies of the vulva, cervix, and vagina to endoscopic procedures of the uterus and pelvic cavity and major surgeries such as adnexectomy and hysterectomy.
- New techniques in gynecology are less invasive and may involve the use of laser technology and surgical robots.

Imaging studies using sound wave energy (ultrasound), magnetic field energy (magnetic resonance imaging [MRI]), or radiation are often ordered, and sometimes the imaging is performed by the gynecologist to assist in the diagnosis and treatment of reproductive tract disorders. Gynecologic surgical procedures are becoming less invasive and safer, and advances in surgical techniques are resulting in more effective and more efficient reproductive health care for women. Table 31-1 lists the more common imaging modalities and procedures used in gynecologic practice.

Imaging Studies in Gynecologic Practice

Ultrasonography is widely used for diagnostic purposes and even to guide therapeutic applications such as oocyte retrieval for in vitro fertilization (IVF). The ultrasonic probe emits high-frequency sound waves that provide an image of tissues when reflected back to the sound source (a probe). Ultrasound is safe for both pregnant and nonpregnant women and should be used to assist but not replace adequate physical examina-

tion and history-taking. Ultrasound may be two-, three-, or even four-dimensional when movement is detected in real time. Two-dimensional technology is the most common, with three-dimensional imaging and movement detection and interpretation reserved for special studies, such as fetal cardiac evaluation. The sound-generating probe may be placed on the abdominal wall (transabdominally) or into the vaginal canal (transvaginally). Transvaginal insertion is more commonly used for gynecologic evaluation.

Figure 31-1 illustrates the transvaginal placement of the probe against the uterine cervix. This placement allows for excellent visualization of both normal anatomy and abnormal pelvic masses (uterine and adnexal). The size of ovarian follicular cysts can be measured and followed over time to assist fertility evaluation and treatment as well as oocyte retrieval (see Chapter 34). When saline is infused through a catheter into the uterine cavity during transvaginal ultrasonography, a **sonohysterogram** may be visualized and recorded.

Computed axial tomography (CAT or CT) uses computer algorithms to form cross-sectional x-ray images of pelvic tissues. Contrast media may be used

TABLE 31-1

COMMON IMAGING STUDIES AND PROCEDURES IN A GYNECOLOGIC PRACTICE

	Diagnostic Indications	Therapeutic Indications	Comments
Imaging Studies			
Ultrasonography (transvaginal)	Evaluation of pelvic cysts and tumors	Oocyte retrieval for in vitro fertilization	See Chapter 34 No radiation exposure
Sonohysterography	Evaluation of uterine cavity for polyps and/or tumors	None	Also called *saline infusion hysterography*
Computed axial tomography (CAT or CT)	Evaluation of pelvis and abdomen for cysts and tumors	None	Radiation exposure
Magnetic resonance imaging (MRI)	Evaluation of pelvis for cysts, tumors, and uterine abnormalities	None	No radiation exposure
Breast imaging (mammography)	Identification of breast pathology; screening criteria remain controversial	None	See Chapter 30 Ultrasound and MRI also used
Hysterosalpingography	Evaluation of uterine cavity and fallopian tubes for patency	Some studies show small increase in pregnancy rate with oil-based media	See Chapter 34
Procedures			
Endometrial sampling	Obtaining tissue for histopathologic examination	Intentional tissue damage is reported to increase implantation rate in some studies	Pipelle endometrial suction See Figure 31-2; see also Chapter 34
Biopsies Punch Cone (cold knife) Loop (electrosurgical excision)	Obtaining tissue for histopathology	Complete excision of pathologic tissue in some cases	Common sites for biopsy include the vulva, vagina, cervix, and endometrium
Colposcopy	Identification of cervical, vaginal, and vulvar pathology	None	See Chapter 38
Cryotherapy, electrotherapy, and laser therapy	Laser may be used for excisional cone biopsy of the cervix	Tissue destruction and ablation	See text, this chapter
Dilation and curettage (D&C)	Evaluation of endometrium	May temporarily control dysfunctional uterine bleeding	Polyps may be identified and removed
Sterilization and abortion procedures	NA	Prevent pregnancy or terminate existing pregnancy	See Chapter 27
Pelvic endoscopy (laparoscopy)	Multiple	Multiple	See text, this chapter
Pelvic floor procedures	NA	Surgical repair for stress urinary incontinence and organ prolapse	See Chapter 23
Hysteroscopy	Evaluate uterine cavity for the presence of polyps or tumors	Removal of polyps and/or tumors Ablation of tissue	See text, this chapter
Hysterectomy Abdominal Vaginal Laparoscopic and laparoscopically assisted	Primarily therapeutic but unexpected pathology may be found (e.g., undiagnosed endometrial or endocervical cancer or leiomyosarcoma)	See Table 30-2	See text, this chapter and Chapter 19 Morcellation of malignant uterine tissue can lead to spread of cancer
Adnexal surgery Cystectomy Oophorectomy Salpingectomy	Provision of tissue for histopathologic diagnosis of an adnexal mass	Treatment of adnexal masses, benign or malignant, with hysterectomy or with pathology (e.g., tubal pregnancy)	May be performed separately or at the same time as hysterectomy
Robotic procedures	Currently being studied	Multiple	No apparent advantage for benign indications See text, this chapter

NA, Not applicable.

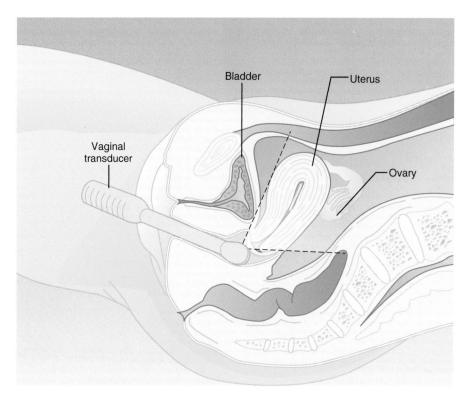

FIGURE 31-1 Placement of the transvaginal ultrasound probe against the uterine cervix to view the uterus and adnexal structures.

to enhance the images. CT scanning uses radiation and for this reason ultrasound or MRI may be preferred in pregnant patients.

MRI takes advantage of differing characteristics of body tissues when the tissues are exposed to magnetic field energy. By visually distinguishing between tissues such as fat and body fluids like blood and lymph, MRI is useful for the evaluation of uterine and ovarian structures. Uterine adenomyosis (see Chapter 25) and certain breast lesions may be detected using MRI.

Mammography uses radiation that penetrates compressed breast tissue to screen for breast cancer. There is both a false-positive and false-negative interpretation error associated with screening mammograms. Both MRI and ultrasound may be used to improve diagnostic accuracy (see Chapter 30).

Hysterosalpingography (HSG) employs fluoroscopy and radiopaque dyes injected transcervically to create an image of the uterine cavity and to verify fill and spill of dye out of the fallopian tubes (tubal patency). Uterine polyps and submucous uterine fibroids may be detected. Some studies show a statistically significant increase in the pregnancy rate after HSG, especially when oil-based media are used, suggesting therapeutic value. Figure 34-2 shows an HSG study.

Gynecologic Procedures

The gynecologic surgeon should have a high level of training during residency, followed by an ongoing commitment to retraining and retooling as effective procedures are added or substituted for outdated ones. Training methods now include computer-assisted simulations of procedures, providing for greater patient safety while the surgeon is learning and retraining. All facilities should have an active quality assessment program to continuously evaluate the safety and appropriateness of gynecologic care, including surgery.

Before any procedure or surgery begins, the most appropriate option (when more than one exists) for an individual patient must be selected, with optimal patient involvement in the decision-making process included as part of informed consent.

At least 80% of gynecologic surgical procedures are considered to be elective; that is, there are other alternative treatments to be considered. The appropriateness of performing these procedures should be evaluated by physician and patient on an individual basis (Box 31-1). **The trend toward minimal invasiveness in gynecologic surgery should not lead to minimal or questionable indications.**

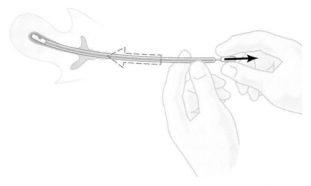

FIGURE 31-2 Endometrial sampling using the Pipelle endometrial suction instrument. A flexible, hollow plastic tube is inserted and held in the uterine cavity as the stylet is withdrawn, creating a vacuum and resulting in aspiration of tissue.

Credentialing, Privileging, and Ongoing Training

The rapid introduction of new technologies can present a challenge to the surgeon, who will need to keep up with the most advanced procedures, and to the institution, which is required to be certain that those who are granted surgical privileges have been properly trained and are currently qualified.

After a surgeon's credentials (diplomas, training certificates, and licenses) have been properly verified, a useful classification for the purpose of privileging stratifies procedures into the following levels:

- **Level 1:** procedures not requiring additional training after residency (e.g., dilation and curettage [D&C], cervical conization, adnexal excision, and abdominal or vaginal hysterectomy)
- **Level 2:** procedures requiring additional training (e.g., laparoscopic myomectomy)
- **Level 3:** procedures requiring advanced training and special skills generally acquired during subspecialty training (e.g., radical hysterectomy, tubal anastomosis, or oocyte harvesting)

As new procedures are incorporated into basic residency training, they can be reclassified.

Informed Consent and General Risks Associated with Procedures

The patient should be thoroughly counseled about surgical risks as part of the process of informed consent (see Chapter 1). In general, risks fall into three categories: risks of anesthesia, intraoperative risks, and postoperative complications. Risks of anesthesia depend on the type of anesthesia used (awake sedation, regional anesthesia, or inhalational agents). Regional anesthesia carries the risk of infection, postprocedural spinal headache, and failure, in which case an inhalational agent must be added to the regional anesthetic. Inhalational agents may be associated with the risks of aspiration pneumonia, allergic reaction to the agent, and damage to teeth or airways if intubation is necessary. Stroke, myocardial infarction, and death can result. The intraoperative risks include excessive bleeding and unintended damage to organs or tissues. Postoperative risks include infection, persistent bleeding, and thrombosis, all of which can lead to significant morbidity or even mortality. The specific risks of each procedure are described below.

Endometrial Sampling Procedures

One of the most common minor gynecologic surgical procedures is dilation of the cervix and curettage of the endometrium (D&C). Recent advances in office-based instrumentation for diagnosis (hysteroscopy, endometrial biopsy [Figure 31-2], and ultrasonic evaluation of endometrial thickness) have resulted in an appropriate decrease in the use of D&C. **However, if cancer of the cervix or endometrium is suspected, a thorough fractional curettage may be the best procedure to use to confirm its presence.**

INDICATIONS

D&C may be a diagnostic or a therapeutic procedure. A diagnostic D&C is performed for irregular menstrual bleeding, heavy menstrual bleeding, or postmenopausal bleeding, unless an endometrial biopsy has already revealed a diagnosis of malignancy. Irregularities in the contour of the endometrial cavity, either congenital (e.g., uterine septum) or acquired (e.g., submucous myomata), are sometimes determined during the operation. The finding of a thin endometrium on a transvaginal ultrasound (generally <5 mm) may eliminate the need for biopsy or D&C in some women. In

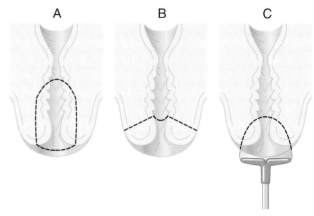

FIGURE 31-3 Cone biopsy of the cervix. **A,** Diagnostic conization performed when the squamocolumnar junction is not fully visualized colposcopically. **B,** Therapeutic conization performed for disease involving the exocervix (or ectocervix) and distal endocervical canal. **C,** Loop electrosurgical excision procedure. The goal of the procedure is to remove the cervical tissue to just above the squamocolumnar junction, including any visible lesions.

patients younger than 40 years of age who have irregular bleeding, hormonal manipulation preceded by office endometrial sampling frequently obviates the need for curettage.

The D&C may have a therapeutic effect in patients with heavy or irregular bleeding as a result of endometrial hyperplasia; endometrial polyps; or small, pedunculated submucous myomas. Unwanted first-trimester pregnancies are usually evacuated by dilation and suction curettage, although nonsurgical techniques are now available.

TECHNIQUE

The D&C operation is performed with the patient in the dorsal lithotomy position. Most D&Cs are now performed on an outpatient basis. Paracervical blocks and local anesthesia are frequently employed.

A pelvic examination is done under anesthesia, and after sterile preparation, a weighted speculum is placed in the posterior vagina. The cervix is grasped with a single-toothed or double-toothed tenaculum. A Kevorkian curette is used for curettage of the endocervical canal. The depth of the uterine cavity is determined with a uterine sound, and the cervix is then dilated with a set of graduated dilators. A small polyp or ovum forceps is introduced through the dilated cervix and gently rotated to remove any endometrial polyps. A thorough curettage is done with a sharp curette, proceeding with each stroke in either a clockwise or a counterclockwise manner to ensure that the entire uterine cavity has been covered. Potential complications of D&C are listed in Box 31-2.

Cervical Procedures

Conization of the cervix is a procedure in which a cone-shaped portion of the cervix is removed for diagnostic or, occasionally, for therapeutic purposes. The section of the tissue surrounding the external os represents the base of the removed specimen. The apex is either close to the internal os (Figure 31-3, *A*) or close to the external os (see Figure 31-3, *B*). Conization may also be performed in an office setting, using loop electrosurgical excision (see Figure 31-3, *C*) or large loop

excision of the transformation zone of the cervix. **Loop excision should not be performed before identification of a cervical intraepithelial lesion that requires treatment by colposcopically directed punch biopsy.** The technique and complications of cervical conization are also covered in Chapter 38.

Colposcopy is the use of magnification to view and evaluate the cervix and to determine optimal sites for biopsy. A more detailed description of this procedure is provided in Chapter 38.

The technique of **cryoablation** is commonly used to treat condylomas of the cervix, vagina, and vulva. These procedures almost always are office-based, and little if any anesthesia is required.

Laser instruments are sources of intense beams of light energy. The letters in the acronym *laser* stand for light amplification by the stimulated emission of radiation. When used in surgery, this radiant energy is converted inside the cell to thermal or acoustic energy, resulting in controlled vaporization or coagulation of tissue. Lasers come in longer wavelengths (carbon dioxide [CO_2]) or shorter wavelengths (neodymium:yttrium-aluminum-garnet [Nd:YAG], potassium-titanyl-phosphate [KTP], and argon) that can be propagated along flexible optical fibers. This allows delivery of energy for cutting, vaporization, and coagulation to tissues in locations unreachable by a CO_2 laser.

Because of the additional expense of laser equipment and the lack of evidence for improvements in outcome, **the use of this technology has been decreasing in recent years.** Nevertheless, laser technology has been applied to conization of the cervix, removal of leiomyomas (myomectomy), and destruction of the ectopic endometrial implants of endometriosis.

Pelvic Endoscopy

Gynecologic endoscopy **(laparoscopy and hysteroscopy)** is widely used for the diagnosis and treatment of reproductive organ disease and dysfunction. Laparoscopy and hysteroscopy have largely moved from the hospital operating room to the freestanding surgical outpatient unit and, with smaller instruments (needle scopes) and more refined fiberoptic technology, even into the office setting. **Because of the expense involved, the value of these techniques must be considered in terms of outcome, particularly with regard to the long-term health and functional status of the patient.**

Laparoscopy

The laparoscope is an instrument used for viewing the peritoneal cavity. Both pelvic and upper abdominal structures can be inspected. The attachment of a video camera to the lens of the laparoscope allows more than one surgeon to view the operative site on a video screen and thus to assist during procedures. Figure 31-4 is a typical laparoscopic image of the pelvic reproductive organs. Multiple puncture sites through the skin and into the abdominal cavity allow for the insertion of small rigid or flexible instruments directed toward the pelvis. Procedures that were once performed by laparotomy are now routinely carried out less invasively.

The indications for laparoscopy are both diagnostic and therapeutic. **Laser technology can be applied to operative laparoscopic procedures to excise and to vaporize areas of pathology.**

Absolute contraindications to laparoscopy include bowel obstruction and large hemoperitoneum with hypovolemic shock. In patients who have had multiple previous laparotomies, a history of peritonitis, previous bowel surgery, or a lower midline abdominal incision, open laparoscopy is preferable. In these conditions, the peritoneal cavity is opened through a small subumbilical incision under direct visualization before introduction of the trocar and sheath.

INDICATIONS

The following are indications for laparoscopy:

1. **Tubal sterilization:** The most common indication for the use of the laparoscope in gynecology is sterilization (see Chapter 27).

2. **Ectopic pregnancy:** The laparoscope is commonly used for the removal of tubal pregnancies that do not meet the criteria for medical therapy (see Chapter 24).

3. **Pelvic infection:** Although it is not routinely used for diagnosis of pelvic inflammatory disease (PID), the laparoscope can provide confirmation of a diagnosis when there is a diagnostic dilemma (see Chapter 22).

4. **Infertility:** Routine laparoscopic evaluation of an infertile woman is widely recommended, but it is controversial because of a lack of controlled evidence of improved outcome. Advanced assisted reproductive techniques, such as IVF and gamete intrafallopian transfer, may involve laparoscopic procedures, although the aspiration of oocytes for IVF is now almost always performed transvaginally using ultrasonic guidance (see Chapter 34).

5. **Pelvic pain:** Acute and chronic pelvic pain can be investigated by using the laparoscope (see Chapter 21).

6. **Endometriosis:** The laparoscope has become a widely used intervention for the diagnosis, staging, and treatment of ectopic endometrial tissue in both overtly symptomatic (pelvic pain) and silently symptomatic (infertility) patients. Laser coagulation, thermal vaporization, excision of endometriomas, and aspiration of endometriomas result in consistent, but sometimes temporary, improvement of pain and moderate improvement in fertility potential. Repeated procedures and the need for medical adjuvant treatment are common (see Chapter 25).

7. **Ovarian neoplasms:** Because of the need to rule out pelvic malignancies, the laparoscope can be used in a less invasive procedure to evaluate a persistent, small adnexal mass. Laparoscopic ovarian cystectomy or salpingo-oophorectomy allows a tissue diagnosis to be made. **Laparoscopic aspiration of cysts can be dangerous and may result in dissemination of an unsuspected ovarian cancer. Ovarian biopsy is seldom indicated, and in premenopausal patients with simple cystic enlargement, a trial of hormonal suppression or observation is indicated instead of immediate**

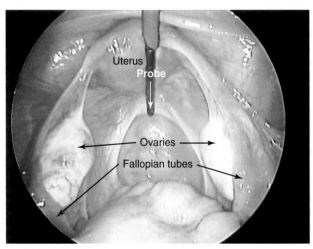

FIGURE 31-4 A typical image of normal reproductive organs seen through the laparoscope or on a video screen during diagnostic or operative laparoscopy. (Courtesy B. Beller, MD, Eugene, OR.)

surgical intervention. Most such lesions are functional cysts that spontaneously regress. The laparoscope in expert hands has been advocated for staging procedures in patients with ovarian cancer. These procedures have become feasible since the advent of laparoscopic lymphadenectomy, but port-site recurrences are a potential problem.

8. **Myomectomy:** Laparoscopic myomectomy remains controversial because of the possibility that smaller leiomyomas will be removed because they *can* be rather than because they *should* be. **Advocates of the procedure recommend that fibroids larger than 6 cm in diameter not be removed using the laparoscope and that morcellation of the fibroid not be used, due to the risk of dissemination of an occult sarcoma** (see Chapter 19).

9. **Urogynecologic procedures:** Urethropexy can be performed laparoscopically, with reported success rates comparable to those for procedures performed percutaneously (see Chapter 23).

10. **Hysterectomy:** The laparoscope is used by some surgeons to replace an abdominal procedure (laparoscopic hysterectomy), to assist in a vaginal hysterectomy, and to convert an abdominal hysterectomy to a vaginal hysterectomy. Adoption of laparoscopy-associated hysterectomy has been increasing in recent years.

TECHNIQUE

The procedure is performed with the patient in a modified dorsal lithotomy position (i.e., with knee crutches), usually with general anesthesia. An intrauterine manipulator is inserted to help in the visualization of the pelvic organs. A pneumoperitoneum is created by the insertion of a spring-loaded needle, such as a Veress needle, into the peritoneal cavity via the subumbilical fold, together with insufflation with either CO_2 or nitrous oxide. The trocar and surrounding sheath are then inserted through a small subumbilical incision.

The lighted telescope is inserted into the sheath and advanced slowly. With the patient in the Trendelenburg position (upper body lower than the pelvis), visualization of pelvic organs confirms that the peritoneal cavity has been entered. Gas may be added intermittently and automatically to maintain a sufficient pneumoperitoneum. To perform a second puncture, which is sometimes necessary, especially in laparoscopic surgical procedures, the abdominal wall is transilluminated to identify the position of the inferior epigastric vessels, and a 4- to 6-mm trocar and sheath are inserted under laparoscopic guidance through a small incision at the pubic hairline. A probe or other surgical instrument (e.g., surgical scissors) is passed through the second sheath.

Upon completion of the procedure, hemostasis is checked, the gas is released from the peritoneal cavity,

---

BOX 31-3

COMPLICATIONS OF LAPAROSCOPY

- Anesthetic complications caused by pneumoperitoneum
- Unintended insufflation of the abdominal wall instead of the peritoneal cavity
- Perforation of a viscus, such as bowel or bladder
- Bowel burns during fulguration of adjacent tissues
  - Less common with bipolar current

---

and the instruments are withdrawn. The small skin incisions are closed with a clip or single subcuticular suture. Common complications of laparoscopy are listed in Box 31-3.

Hysteroscopy

INDICATIONS AND USES

In recent years, the hysteroscope has seen progressive improvements in light sources, optical systems, distending media, and electronic equipment, and the instrument now has a wide variety of indications and benefits in clinical gynecology. Hysteroscopy has substantially improved accuracy compared with x-ray hysterography, and in some cases it may be more effective than diagnostic D&C in detecting intrauterine pathology such as endometrial polyps or submucous myomata.

INSTRUMENTATION

The hysteroscope (Figure 31-5, *A* and *B*) is a telescope consisting of light bundles and a sheath through which the telescope is inserted. For pure diagnostic use, the telescope is inserted alone, whereas for operative capabilities, it is inserted in conjunction with other instruments.

Two different types of telescopes are used today: rigid and flexible fiberoptic. Rigid telescopes are most commonly 1 to 5 mm in diameter for diagnostic procedures, and operative hysteroscopes typically range from 8 to 10 mm in diameter and contain a working element through which operative instruments are inserted.

Operating instruments such as rigid or flexible scissors, graspers, biopsy forceps, or even laser fibers are inserted through operating channels, which may be part of the outer sheath itself, or through separate devices interposed between the telescope and the outer sheath, which are called *bridges*. In addition to the standard operating instruments, some bridges have attachable electrodes and finger-controlled mechanisms to allow the performance of precise intrauterine surgery.

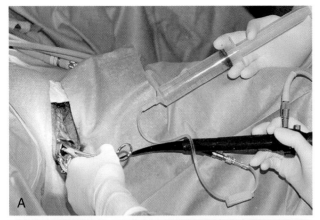

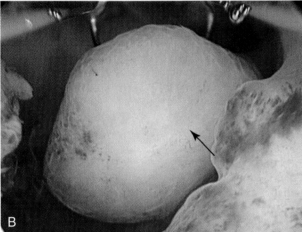

FIGURE 31-5 **A,** Hysteroscopy. **B,** View of an intrauterine polyp *(arrow).* (**A,** From Goldberg JM, Falcone T: *Atlas of endoscopic techniques in gynecology,* London, 2000, WB Saunders, p 185; **B,** from Goldberg JM, Falcone T: *Atlas of endoscopic techniques in gynecology,* London, 2000, WB Saunders.)

The uterine cavity needs distention for adequate visualization through the hysteroscope. Different distention media such as CO_2 gas and both low- and high-viscosity fluid may be used. It is critically important for the surgeon to know which media are compatible with electrosurgical or laser energy sources and which ones are prone to fluid overload or anaphylactic shock during the procedure.

As telescopes have become narrower, they can safely be inserted into the cervical canal with minimal pain. **Several manufacturers now have small, office-based telescopes that use physiologic low-viscosity distention fluids such as saline or Ringer lactate.** These allow the performance of hysteroscopy with little more than a paracervical block in patients who are bleeding, and they do not cause the shoulder pain and uterine spasm that often accompany use of CO_2 as a distention medium. **A significant number of hysteroscopies today are being performed as office procedures.**

COMPLICATIONS OF HYSTEROSCOPY

- Overall complication rate is about 2%
- Major complications occur <1% of cases
  - Uterine perforation, excessive bleeding, and distention media hazards
- Far less common; infection, cervical laceration, and cervical stenosis

INDICATIONS

Infertility

When abnormalities such as intrauterine synechiae or septa are found, hysteroscopic correction is associated with a high rate of success. Synechiae, which are almost always the result of trauma such as curettage or other uterine surgery, may vary from mild to severe, obliterating only a small part or almost all of the endometrial cavity. **One-third of patients with intrauterine synechiae have no apparent menstrual abnormalities.** Hysteroscopic scissors are most commonly used for incision of the adhesions, although lasers or electrical knife electrodes may also be used. **In infertile patients, conception rates up to 60% and a reduction of pregnancy wastage by 50% may be expected after incision of synechiae.**

Probably the most rewarding of all hysteroscopic procedures is the excision of an intrauterine septum, a congenital anomaly that occurs in up to 1% of women. Usually performed as an outpatient procedure, excision of the septum is a relatively short procedure, with minimal bleeding and minimal risks. It is best performed with mechanical scissors, as opposed to electrical or laser devices, to limit the spread of thermal injury to adjacent healthy myometrium.

In most cases, it is desirable to monitor the depth of incision by concomitant laparoscopy or ultrasonography to reduce the risk of uterine perforation (Box 31-4).

Abnormal Uterine Bleeding

The hysteroscopic evaluation of the patient with abnormal uterine bleeding frequently uncovers the presence of submucous myomas or endometrial polyps.

Small endometrial polyps can be removed very easily by using hysteroscopic scissors or grasping forceps inserted through an accessory channel of the operating hysteroscope, or they can be removed blindly with a polyp forceps followed by reinspection hysteroscopically to ensure complete removal. Because the endocervical canal is rarely dilated more than 10 mm to accommodate the operating instruments, polyps or myomas that are significantly larger than this may be difficult to remove without destruction or vaporization. Electrodes composed of thin wires, roller balls, roller cylinders, and grooved vaporization tips, coupled with continuous (cutting) electrical waveforms, may allow removal of such lesions.

Endometrial Ablation

Endometrial ablation is the destruction of the uterine lining for the treatment of chronic menorrhagia. It is performed when more conservative treatments, such as hormone therapy and curettage, are unsuccessful and when the more radical alternative of hysterectomy is undesirable or contraindicated.

Two general methods of endometrial ablation have emerged. The first type requires hysteroscopic visualization and employs electrical or laser energy to shave, vaporize, or coagulate the endometrial surface.

Following a preoperative drug regimen to suppress the endometrial thickness (danazol or leuprolide), hysteroscopic laser surgery can be performed in about 1 hour on an outpatient basis with the patient under general or regional anesthesia. A hysteroscope is introduced into the uterus, and a fiberoptic delivery system is passed through the operating channel. Resectoscopic endometrial ablation has become a more popular technique than laser ablation, and it appears to be at least as effective; its advantages are a significantly shorter operating time and much less expensive equipment.

Amenorrhea occurs in up to 70% of patients after resectoscopic ablation, whereas hypomenorrhea occurs in more than 90% of cases. Continued excessive bleeding is believed to be more likely when multiple myomas or severe adenomyosis exists.

A more recent method of endometrial ablation does not require hysteroscopic visualization. These techniques use either a reservoir for the delivery of heat to the endometrial surface or microwave energy directed at the endometrium to render it unresponsive to hormonal stimulation. Because they are narrower than operative hysteroscopes and their attachments, and because they can be inserted blindly into the uterine cavity, these methods are intended for office use and for use by surgeons who may not have the experience or skills needed for laser or resectoscopic surgery.

Hysterectomy

Hysterectomy is the most commonly performed major gynecologic operation, and it is among the top five most commonly performed major surgical procedures in the United States. It can be performed either abdominally or vaginally. Although some indications for hysterectomy remain controversial, high patient satisfaction levels and increasing safety of the procedure have been reported.

Table 31-2 provides a useful list of indications for abdominal or vaginal hysterectomy.

TABLE 31-2

HYSTERECTOMY: INDICATION LIST WITH CRITERIA

Acute Condition	
A-1*	Pregnancy catastrophe (e.g., severe hemorrhage)
A-2	Severe infection (e.g., ruptured tubo-ovarian abscess)
A-3*	Operative complication (e.g., uterine perforation)
Benign Disease	
B-1	Leiomyoma Symptomatic (e.g., bleeding, pressure) Asymptomatic ($\geq$12 wk size, confuses adnexal evaluation)
B-2	Endometriosis (distinct endometriosis, unresponsive to hormonal suppression or conservative surgery)
B-3	Adenomyosis (with symptomatic dysmenorrhea and bleeding unresponsive to treatment)
B-4	Chronic infection (e.g., recurrent pelvic inflammatory disease)
B-5	Adnexal mass (e.g., ovarian neoplasm)
B-6	Other (operator-defined, criteria-specified)
Cancer or Significant Premalignant Disease	
C-1	Invasive disease of reproductive organs
C-2	Significant preinvasive disease of the uterus (adenomatous hyperplasia of the endometrium with cellular atypia)
Discomfort (No Confirming Tissue Pathology Expected)	
D-1*	Chronic pelvic pain (negative laparoscopy and nonsurgical treatment attempted)
D-2*	Pelvic relaxation (symptomatic)
D-3*	Recurrent uterine bleeding (unresponsive to hormonal regulation, curettage, or endometrial ablation—normal-size uterus)
D-4*	Other (operator-defined, criteria specified)
Extenuating Circumstances (Not Specifically Indicated but Possibly Justified—Requires Preoperative Peer Review)	
E-1*	Sterilization (extenuating circumstances)
E-2*	Cancer prophylaxis (e.g., recurrent cervical intraepithelial neoplasia after cone biopsy or persistent adenomatous hyperplasia of the endometrium without atypia)
E-3*	Other: listing extenuating circumstances

Data from Gambone JC, Lench JB, Slesinski MJ, et al: Validation of hysterectomy indications and the quality assurance process. *Obstet Gynecol* 73:1045, 1989.
*Denotes indications for which tissue pathology is not expected to confirm the preoperative diagnosis.

ABDOMINAL HYSTERECTOMY

A total abdominal hysterectomy (Figure 31-6) is the most commonly performed procedure for benign uterine disease and involves the simple excision of the uterine corpus and cervix. It may be performed intrafascially, in which case the procedure is kept

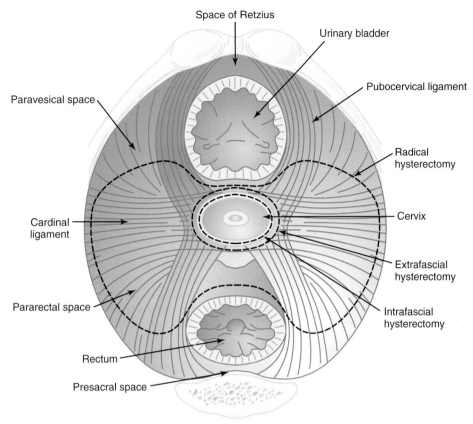

FIGURE 31-6 Types of hysterectomy: extrafascial, intrafascial, and radical. Note the extensive amount of parametrial tissue that is removed in a radical hysterectomy.

safely within the endopelvic fascia that surrounds the cervix and upper vagina, **or extrafascially,** in which case the investing fascia of the cervix and upper vagina is removed with the specimen. **A subtotal hysterectomy excises the uterine corpus,** usually at the level of the internal cervical os. **A radical hysterectomy involves the wide excision of the parametrial tissue laterally (see Figure 31-6), along with the uterosacral ligaments posteriorly,** after the rectum is dissected free and after each ureter is dissected out of its tunnel beneath the uterine artery.

Indications

The indications for **total abdominal hysterectomy** may include benign conditions such as uterine myomas, endometriosis, chronic PID, stage I endometrial cancer, and uterine bleeding that is unresponsive to more conservative measures. In some cases, a subtotal hysterectomy may be preferred if the bladder is densely adherent to the front of the cervix. Some women may request a subtotal hysterectomy because of possible involvement of the cervix in the sexual response.

A **radical hysterectomy** is indicated for stage IB and occasionally stage IIA cervical cancer. Endometrial cancer with gross cervical involvement may also be managed by radical hysterectomy.

In women who undergo hysterectomy at or after menopause, the uterine adnexa (fallopian tubes and ovaries) are usually removed. However, few studies weighing the risks and benefits of removing these normal organs have been done. Before menopause, the option of preserving the ovaries at the time of hysterectomy compared with the expense and possible dangers of hormone replacement therapy must be thoroughly discussed with the patient preoperatively. In general, the ovaries are preserved at hysterectomy for benign disease before menopause, unless there is a strong family history of breast or ovarian cancer. The choice of incidental oophorectomy with incidental appendectomy awaits a thorough, prospective quality-of-life analysis (economic and medical) to guide gynecologic surgeons and their patients.

Technique

Abdominal hysterectomy is carried out with the patient in the supine position, usually under general anesthesia. First, a thorough pelvic and abdominal examination is carried out and recorded with the patient under anesthesia. The choice of incision depends on the indication for the procedure. A vertical incision is advisable in patients who have had several prior abdominal operations, those who are extremely obese, or those in whom extensive adhesions or endometriosis is anticipated. In patients with restricted benign disease, incisions along the Langer lines (transverse in the lower abdomen) achieve a better cosmetic result. The various lower abdominal incisions and their anatomy are discussed in Chapter 3 and are depicted in Figure 3-12.

After the abdominal incision into the peritoneal cavity is made, the upper abdomen is manually explored with special reference to the liver, gallbladder, stomach, spleen, and paraaortic lymph nodes, and a reference to each must be recorded in the operative notes. The intestines are inspected in cases of cancer with careful attention to mesenteric lymph nodes and the vermiform appendix. The patient is then placed in the Trendelenburg position (tilted with upper body lower than the pelvis), and the abdominal viscera are packed out of the pelvis with laparotomy tapes.

Each round ligament is clamped, incised, and ligated. The peritoneum on both sides is incised lateral to the infundibulopelvic ligament. This allows entry to the retroperitoneum between the leaves of the broad ligament, exposing the ureter and pelvic vessels. The vesicouterine fold of the peritoneum is incised transversely between the incised round ligaments, and the bladder (adherent to the peritoneum) is reflected inferiorly off the fascia of the lower uterine segment, cervix, and upper vagina.

If the adnexa are to be removed, the ureters are identified and the infundibulopelvic ligaments with the ovarian vessels are clamped, cut, and tied. The medioposterior leaf of the broad ligament is incised toward the uterus, thus exposing the uterine artery and veins as they course superiorly toward the uteroovarian vascular anastomosis just below the ovarian ligament. If the uterine adnexa are to be preserved, the ovarian ligaments are clamped, incised, and ligated on each side.

The uterine vessels thus exposed are stripped of their adventitial tissue (skeletonized), clamped at the level of the internal cervical os, incised, and securely ligated bilaterally. The ligated uterine vessels are reflected laterally, allowing access to the cardinal ligament (Mackenrodt ligament). Operating medial to the ligated uterine vessels, the cardinal ligament on either side is clamped, incised, and ligated with a transfixion ligature. It may take several bites to free the cardinal ligaments from the lower cervix and upper vagina.

The peritoneum just below the posterior surface of the cervix is incised transversely between the uterosacral ligaments, and the rectum is reflected from the posterior aspect of the cervix and upper vagina. The uterosacral ligaments are clamped, incised, and ligated, which frees them from the cervix and upper vagina.

The total uterus (corpus and cervix) is removed by cutting across the vagina just below the cervix, with care taken to sufficiently reflect the urinary bladder and rectum inferiorly to avoid injury. **The vaginal cuff is normally closed with absorbable sutures,** incorporating the cardinal and uterosacral ligaments into each lateral angle of the vagina to preclude the later development of a vaginal vault prolapse. If the uterosacral ligaments are widely separated, they may be plicated to prevent the formation of an enterocele. **Progressive circular sutures (Moschcowitz sutures) may be placed to obliterate a particularly large pouch of Douglas, which also portends an increased risk of enterocele.**

Three points in the procedure present a particular risk for injury to the ureter: (1) as the infundibulopelvic ligaments are clamped and incised, (2) as the uterine vessels are ligated, and (3) as the cardinal ligaments are clamped if the urinary bladder is not sufficiently reflected inferiorly. **Use of the retroperitoneal approach, with identification of the ureters bilaterally and careful reflection of the bladder inferiorly, prevents ureteric injury.**

VAGINAL HYSTERECTOMY

Vaginal hysterectomy, if feasible, is preferable to the abdominal approach because it avoids a visible scar, is associated with less pain, affords an opportunity to correct pelvic relaxation, and generally requires less postoperative hospitalization and disability.

Indications

Ideally, vaginal hysterectomy is elected for benign disease when the uterus is mobile, is less than 12 gestational weeks in size, is characterized by some pelvic relaxation, and is expected to contain few or no adhesions caused by endometriosis, PID, or multiple prior lower abdominal operations. The procedure is most commonly performed in association with the correction of uterine prolapse, cystocele, rectocele, or enterocele in postmenopausal women.

The advent of laparoscopically assisted vaginal hysterectomy has greatly expanded the indications for the vaginal approach by freeing up adnexal adhesions, facilitating simultaneous removal of the tubes and ovaries, and identifying conditions that would not safely be managed at the time of vaginal hysterectomy.

Technique

The principles of the operation are similar to those of abdominal hysterectomy, except that ligation of the ligaments and vessels proceeds in the reverse order. The patient is placed in the dorsolithotomy position after induction of anesthesia. The bladder is emptied, and a thorough pelvic examination is performed. A weighted vaginal retractor is placed in the vagina, a tenaculum is placed on the cervix, and the uterus is drawn down toward the vaginal introitus and tested for descent and mobility. A transverse incision is made through the vaginal epithelium between the uterosacral ligaments at the posterior junction of the cervix and vagina. The peritoneum of the cul-de-sac is bluntly mobilized and sharply entered. Adhesions of the cul-de-sac and posterior uterine wall are excluded by finger exploration. The uterosacral ligaments are clamped, cut, and ligated, allowing additional descent of the uterus.

At this point, the vaginal epithelial incision is extended circumferentially around the cervix, and the bladder is advanced superiorly along the anterior uterine wall, exposing the anterior uterovesical fold of the peritoneum, which is sharply entered. The pubo-cervical ligaments (bladder pillars) containing the ureters are bluntly displaced laterally, and the cardinal ligaments are clamped, cut, and ligated, allowing further descent of the uterus.

An angle retractor (e.g., Heaney, Deaver) is placed into the opening of the anterior vesicouterine fold of the peritoneum, and the urinary bladder is retracted anteriorly. The uterine vessels are clamped, usually with a Heaney clamp, ensuring that the tips of the clamp include the peritoneal edge both anteriorly and posteriorly and that the tips are snug against the lateral uterine wall so as to include all of the uterine vessels. The clamped vessels are cut and securely ligated.

Downward traction on the uterus should allow full exposure of the round ligaments, fallopian tubes, ovarian ligaments, and utero-ovarian vascular anastomoses, and these structures are clamped as a group on each side, cut free of the uterus, and securely ligated. Because these pedicles are quite bulky, especially in premenopausal patients, it is wise to double clamp and ligate them, first with a loop hemostatic ligature and then with a transfixion ligature.

If the adnexa are to be removed, the suspensory ligament of the ovary is addressed instead of the ovarian ligament. With Allis clamps, the fimbriated end of the fallopian tube and ovary are drawn inferiorly into the operative field, which brings the suspensory ligament of the ovary into full view, allowing it to be clamped, cut, and ligated with special care taken to avoid the adjacent ureter. To visualize the ureter more clearly, the round ligament may be initially and separately clamped and ligated, which opens up the lateral extraperitoneal space. This phase of the procedure may be quite difficult in a premenopausal primigravida with good pelvic support, and it is most readily performed laparoscopically.

The peritoneum is then closed with a purse-string suture or one or more transverse U-sutures, leaving the pedicles in an extraperitoneal position. As with an abdominal hysterectomy, the uterosacral ligaments may be plicated with one or more sutures to avoid an enterocele. The ovarian and/or round ligaments may

be sutured together in the midline, but this is optional, as these ligaments add little or no pelvic support. The cardinal ligaments, however, should each be sutured to the lateral aspect of the vaginal cuff to provide vaginal support, to increase vaginal depth, and to prevent the later development of a vaginal vault prolapse. The cardinal ligaments should not be sutured together across the midline, as that might shorten the vagina. The vaginal epithelium is then closed with interrupted absorbable sutures. If the bladder pillars have been plicated to correct a cystocele or if a urethropexy has been employed to correct stress incontinence, catheter drainage of the bladder may be employed for 24 to 48 hours postoperatively.

COMPLICATIONS

Complications associated with any abdominal or pelvic surgery include anesthetic complications, hemorrhage, atelectasis, wound infection, urinary tract infection, thrombophlebitis, and pulmonary embolism. **Atelectasis occurs most commonly in the first 24 to 48 hours** and can be prevented and treated with aggressive pulmonary toilet. **Wound infection usually occurs about 5 days postoperatively** and is associated with redness, tenderness, swelling, and increased warmth around the wound.

Treatment may require systemic antibiotics, opening the incision, draining the discharge, local debridement, and wound care. **Urinary tract infection can occur at any time in the postoperative period,** and urine for microscopy and culture should be obtained from any patient with a postoperative fever. **Thrombophlebitis (with possible subsequent pulmonary embolism) is manifested by fever and leg swelling or pain; it usually occurs 7 to 12 days postoperatively.** A pulmonary embolism may occur even in the absence of signs of thrombophlebitis. **Wound disruption after abdominal hysterectomy with evisceration of intestines is generally heralded by a profuse serous discharge from the wound (peritoneal fluid) 4 to 8 days postoperatively.** When evisceration is suspected, the wound should be explored in the operating room.

The most common intraoperative complication of abdominal or vaginal hysterectomy is bleeding from the infundibulopelvic or utero-ovarian pedicles, the uterine vascular pedicle, or the vaginal cuff. When postoperative hemorrhage occurs, bleeding from the vaginal cuff can sometimes be identified and controlled vaginally. **If bleeding is sufficient to cause hypotension, a laparotomy may be required to tie off the bleeding vascular pedicle.**

Infection is common to both procedures and is manifested by fever and lower abdominal pain. Examination often reveals tenderness and induration of the vaginal cuff, which is indicative of pelvic cellulitis. This can usually be treated with antibiotic therapy. **Administration of prophylactic cephalosporin**

perioperatively has proven beneficial in controlling infection in vaginal hysterectomies performed in premenopausal patients.

Injury to the ureter is the most serious complication of hysterectomy. It usually occurs during the abdominal procedure, particularly during a difficult dissection for PID, endometriosis, or pelvic cancer. Ureteral injury can also occur during a vaginal hysterectomy. If not detected intraoperatively, fever and flank pain can develop postoperatively, and a ureterovaginal fistula or urinoma may become apparent 5 to 21 days after surgery. **If noted intraoperatively, a ureteral injury can be repaired by implanting the proximal cut end of the ureter into the bladder or by anastomosing the proximal and distal ends of the transected ureter over a ureteric stent.**

Intraoperative injury to the rectum or bladder, if recognized, should be repaired immediately. If a bladder repair is necessary, an indwelling catheter (suprapubic or transurethral) should be left on free drainage for 5 to 7 days. On rare occasions it may be necessary to protect the repair of an extensive rectal injury with a temporary loop colostomy.

Robotic Surgery in Gynecology

The role of computer-assisted or robotic surgery in gynecology is still evolving. Prospective studies are needed to compare the efficacy of this technology relative to conventional methods. In 2005, the da Vinci surgical system (Intuitive Surgical, Sunnyvale, CA) received U.S. Food and Drug Administration approval. As this new technology is introduced to improve surgical performance, its limitations (such as lack of tactile feedback and increased cost) will need to be addressed. Robot-assisted instrumentation is being used for hysterectomy, pelvic reconstructive surgery, gynecologic oncology, and urogynecology (see Chapter 23). Some studies have failed to show cost-effectiveness of this technology for benign gynecologic procedures.

Reproductive Endocrinology and Infertility

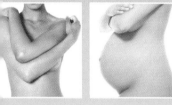
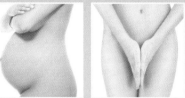
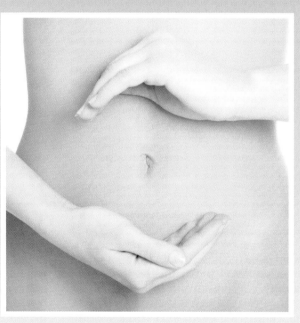
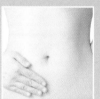

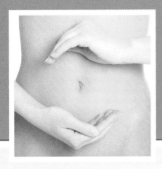

CHAPTER 32

Puberty and Disorders of Pubertal Development

SARA CHURCHILL • CAROLYN J. ALEXANDER

CLINICAL KEYS FOR THIS CHAPTER

- Both genetic and environmental factors determine the onset of pubertal change in young girls. Puberty may be delayed or may occur earlier, depending on nutrition-related factors and physical activity. Obesity causes earlier onset of puberty, and excessive exercise causes delay. Psychological disorders and chronic isolation may also affect the normal onset of puberty.

- The Frisch hypothesis states that an invariant mean weight (48 kg/106 lb) is essential for the initiation of the first menses (menarche). Leptin (a peptide hormone) secreted by adipose tissue may provide the "triggering link" for the initiation of menarche.

- The female fetus has the highest lifetime number of oocytes by mid-gestation. Brief follicular maturation and negative feedback on gonadotropin release due to follicular estradiol production also occurs in utero. Peak serum levels of gonadotropins are seen by 3 months after birth and then slowly decline, reaching their nadir at age 4 years. Between the ages of 4 and about 10 years, the "gonadostat" is said to regulate the hypothalamic–

pituitary–ovarian axis. A combination of high sensitivity to low levels of estradiol resulting in negative feedback on gonadotropin release, and an intrinsic central nervous system inhibition of gonadotropin-releasing hormone secretion, keep gonadotropins at low levels. By age 11 years (the usual onset of pubertal development), there is a gradual loss of the negative feedback to low levels of sex steroids, and pubertal development begins.

- The usual sequence of physical signs of puberty in girls is (1) thelarche (breast budding), (2) adrenarche and/or pubarche (axillary and pubic hair growth), (3) peak height velocity, (4) menarche (first menses), and (5) mature sexual hair and breast growth.

- Disorders of puberty include precocious development and delayed puberty. *Precocious puberty* refers to the development of any sign of secondary sexual maturation at an age earlier than 8 years in girls. Failure to undergo thelarche by the age of 14 years constitutes significant delay of pubertal development and requires evaluation.

Puberty encompasses the development of secondary sexual characteristics and the acquisition of reproductive capability. During this transition, usually between 10 and 16 years of age, a variety of physical, endocrinologic, and psychological changes accompany the increasing levels of circulating sex steroids.

The onset of pubertal changes is determined primarily by genetic factors, including race, **and is also influenced by geographic location** (girls in metropolitan areas, at altitudes near sea level, or at latitudes close to the equator tend to begin puberty at an earlier age) and **nutritional status** (obese children have an earlier onset of puberty, and those who are malnourished or have chronic illnesses associated with weight loss have a later onset of menses). **Excessive exercise** relative to the caloric intake can also delay the onset of

puberty. **It has been proposed that an invariant mean weight of 48 kg (106 lb) is essential for the initiation of menarche** in healthy girls. Leptin, a peptide secreted by adipose tissue, may be the link between weight and the initiation of menarche. **Psychological factors,** severe neurotic or psychotic disorders, and chronic isolation may interfere with the normal onset of puberty through a mechanism similar to adult hypothalamic amenorrhea.

In the United States and Western Europe, a decrease in the age of menarche (i.e., age at first menses) was noted between 1840 and 1970, from an estimated mean age of 17 years in 1840 down to a reported mean age of 13 years in 1970. This trend has plateaued since then, and currently **the mean age of menarche is approximately 12.4 years in the United States.**

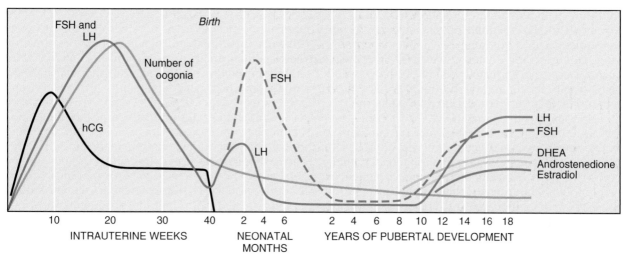

FIGURE 32-1 Changes in the concentration of gonadotropins (LH and FSH), sex steroids (DHEA, androstenedione, and estradiol), and the number of oogonia throughout fetal life and pubertal development. *DHEA,* Dehydroepiandrosterone; *FSH,* follicle-stimulating hormone; *hCG,* human chorionic gonadotropin; *LH,* luteinizing hormone. Adapted from Speroff L, Fritz MA: Neuroendocrinology. In Speroff L, Fritz MA, editors: *Clinical gynecologic endocrinology and infertility,* ed 7, Baltimore, MD, 2005, Lippincott Williams & Wilkins.

Endocrinologic Changes of Puberty

FETAL AND NEWBORN PERIOD

The fetal hypothalamic–pituitary–gonadal axis is capable of producing adult levels of gonadotropins and sex steroids. **By 20 weeks' gestation, levels of gonadotropins**—follicle-stimulating hormone (FSH) and luteinizing hormone (LH)—**rise dramatically in both male and female fetuses** (Figure 32-1). Late in gestation, a surge in levels of glucocorticoids in the fetal circulation occurs. This is essential for normal maturation of fetal lungs and critical for the development of the fetal thyroid, kidney, brain, and pituitary. Recently, it has been suggested that excessive exposure of the developing fetus to glucocorticoids or exposure at the wrong time may lead to lifelong alterations in the function of the hypothalamic–pituitary–adrenal axis.

The female fetus acquires the lifetime peak number of oocytes (in utero) by mid-gestation and also has a brief period of follicular maturation and sex steroid production in response to elevated gonadotropin levels in utero. This transient increase in serum estradiol (a sex steroid) acts on the fetal hypothalamic-pituitary unit, resulting in a reduction of gonadotropin secretion (a negative feedback effect), which in turn reduces estradiol production. This indicates that the inhibitory effect of sex steroids on gonadotropin release is operative before birth.

In both male and female fetuses, serum estradiol is primarily of maternal and placental origin. With birth and the acute loss of maternal and placental sex steroids, the negative feedback action on the hypothalamic-pituitary axis is lost, and gonadotropins are once again released from the pituitary gland, reaching adult or near-adult concentrations in the early neonatal period. **In the female infant, peak serum levels of gonadotropins are generally seen by 3 months of age, then they slowly decline until a nadir is reached by the age of 4 years.** In contrast to gonadotropin levels, sex steroid concentrations decrease rapidly to prepubertal values within 1 week of birth and remain low until the onset of puberty.

During fetal development, the adrenal glands are large in proportion to their size in adult life (similar to the fetal kidneys). Early in gestation, the fetal adrenal gland produces abundant dehydroepiandrosterone sulfate (DHEA-S), which serves as a precursor for estrogen production by the placenta and is also able to convert placental progesterone into cortisol. It is not until about 23 weeks' gestation that the fetal adrenal cortex expresses the enzyme to directly synthesize cortisol from cholesterol or pregnenolone. In the first few months of postnatal life, the innermost part of the adrenal cortex (the fetal zone) largely regresses, and there is a rapid decrease in the production of DHEA-S.

CHILDHOOD

The hypothalamic–pituitary–gonadal axis in the young child is suppressed between the ages of 4 and 10 years. The hypothalamic–pituitary system regulating gonadotropin release has been termed the *gonadostat.* Low levels of gonadotropins and sex steroids during this prepubertal period are a function of two mechanisms: **(1) maximal sensitivity of the gonadostat to the negative feedback effect of the low circulating levels of estradiol** present in prepubertal children, **and (2) intrinsic central nervous system**

inhibition of hypothalamic gonadotropin-releasing hormone (GnRH) secretion. These mechanisms occur independently of the presence of functional gonadal tissue. This is clearly demonstrated in children with gonadal dysgenesis. Agonadal children display elevated gonadotropin concentrations during the first 2 to 4 years of life, followed by a decline in circulating FSH and LH levels by 6 to 8 years of age. By 10 to 12 years of age, gonadotropin concentrations spontaneously rise once again, eventually achieving castration levels. This pattern of gonadotropin secretion in early childhood is similar to that of children with normal gonadal function. **These data suggest that an intrinsic central nervous system regulator of GnRH release is the principal inhibitor of gonadotropin secretion from 4 years of age until the peripubertal period.** Furthermore, after regression of the fetal zone of the adrenal gland (a few months after birth), very low concentrations of adrenal androgen precursors are available, resulting in decreased adrenal androgen production in early childhood.

LATE PREPUBERTAL PERIOD

In general, androgen production and differentiation by the zona reticularis of the adrenal cortex are the initial endocrine changes associated with puberty.

Serum concentrations of DHEA, DHEA-S, and androstenedione rise between the ages of 8 and 11 years. **This rise in adrenal androgens induces the growth of both axillary and pubic hair and is known as *adrenarche* or *pubarche*.** This increase in adrenal androgen production occurs independently of gonadotropin secretion or gonadal steroid levels, and the mechanism of its initiation is not understood at this time. Some studies have suggested that the morphologic and functional changes in the zona reticularis are induced by increasing cortisol levels. In cellular studies, human fetal adrenal cells exposed to cortisol in high concentrations produce DHEA, whereas in human studies, infants treated with high-dose adrenocorticotropic hormone for infantile spasms have been noted to have adrenal androgen production.

Recent studies indicate that **girls who undergo premature pubarche are more likely than other girls to develop polycystic ovarian syndrome (PCOS) as adults** (see Chapter 33).

PUBERTAL ONSET

By approximately the 11th year of life, there is a gradual loss of sensitivity by the gonadostat to the negative feedback of sex steroids (Figure 32-2). As a consequence, GnRH pulses (with their mirroring pulses

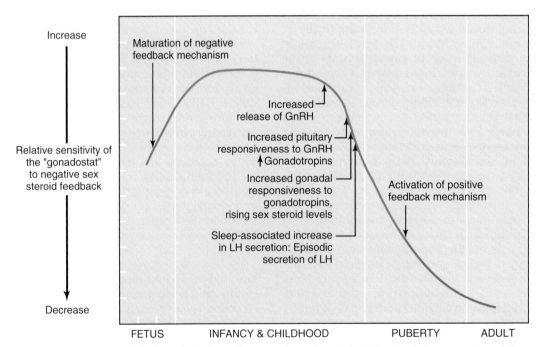

FIGURE 32-2 Changes in set point of the hypothalamic-pituitary unit (gonadostat) *(solid lines)* and the maturation of the negative and positive feedback mechanisms from fetal life to adulthood in relation to the normal changes of puberty. This figure does not illustrate the change in the sex steroid–independent intrinsic central nervous system inhibitory mechanism that is observed from late infancy to puberty. *GnRH,* Gonadotropin-releasing hormone; *LH,* luteinizing hormone. Adapted from Styne DM, Grumbach MM: Disorders of puberty in the male and female. In Yen SSC, Jaffe RB, editors: *Reproductive endocrinology: physiology, pathophysiology and clinical management,* ed 2, Philadelphia, Saunders, 1991.

of FSH and LH) increase in amplitude and frequency. The factors that reduce the sensitivity of the gonadostat are incompletely understood. **Some studies indicate that a rise in the concentration of leptin, a hormone produced by adipocytes (fat cells) that mediates appetite satiety, precedes and is necessary for this change.** This, in turn, supports the association between minimum weight or total body fat and the onset of puberty. The Frisch hypothesis suggests that a critical body weight is necessary for pubertal onset. Further investigations support the concept that fat stores might influence pubertal onset through several mechanisms. First, adipocytes secrete adipokines such as leptin. Leptin appears to serve as a signal to the hypothalamic GnRH pulse generator that there are sufficient energy stores for fertility to commence. Studies have shown that every 1-kg gain in body weight lowers the onset of menarche by 13 days and that every increase of 1 ng/ml in serum leptin lowers the age of menarche by 1 month. Second, aromatase activity in adipocytes is dependent on fat mass, and obesity results in greater peripheral conversion of androstenedione to estrone and of testosterone to estradiol. Last, increasing adipose tissue is related to increasing insulin resistance, which decreases serum levels of sex hormone binding globulin. This leads to an increased level of bioavailable sex hormones.

A further decrease in sensitivity of the gonadostat combined with the loss of intrinsic central nervous system inhibition of hypothalamic GnRH release is heralded by sleep-associated increases in GnRH secretion. This nocturnal dominant pattern gradually shifts into an adult-type secretory pattern, with GnRH pulses occurring every 90 to 120 minutes throughout the 24-hour day.

The increase in gonadotropin release promotes ovarian follicular maturation and sex steroid production, which induces the development of secondary sexual characteristics. By middle to late puberty, mat-

uration of the positive feedback mechanism of estradiol on LH release from the anterior pituitary gland is complete, and ovulatory cycles are established.

Somatic Changes of Puberty

Physical changes of puberty involve the development of secondary sexual characteristics and the acceleration of linear growth (gain in height). The Marshall and Tanner classification of breast and pubic hair development is employed for descriptive and diagnostic purposes (Figures 32-3 and 32-4). A useful acronym for remembering the usual chronologic order of the stages of female pubertal development is TAPuP ME (standing for thelarche, adrenarche, pubarche, peak growth velocity, and menarche).

STAGES OF PUBERTAL DEVELOPMENT

The first physical sign of puberty is usually breast budding (thelarche), followed by the appearance of axillary or pubic hair (adrenarche/pubarche). Unilateral breast development is not uncommon in early puberty and may last up to 6 months before the development of the contralateral breast. **Maximal growth or peak height velocity is usually the next stage, followed by menarche (the onset of menstrual periods).** The final somatic changes are the appearance of adult pubic hair distribution and adult-type breasts. In approximately 15% of normally developing girls, the development of pubic hair occurs before breast development. The sequence of pubertal changes generally occurs over a period of 4.5 years, with a normal range of 1.5 to 6 years (Figure 32-5).

Race plays a role in determining the age of the onset of puberty. African American girls begin puberty earlier than girls in other racial groups (on average between the ages of 8 and 9 years), followed by Mexican Americans and whites (Table 32-1). In African American girls, thelarche and adrenarche can occur as early as 6 years

TABLE 32-1

AGE AT ONSET OF PUBIC HAIR DEVELOPMENT, BREAST DEVELOPMENT, AND MENARCHE FOR THREE RACIAL/ETHNIC GROUPS OF U.S. GIRLS: NATIONAL HEALTH AND NUTRITION EXAMINATION SURVEY III, 1988-1994

Puberty Milestone	Non-Hispanic White (mean age*)	Black (mean age*)	Mexican American (mean age*)
Pubic hair[†]	10.5	9.5	10.3
Breast development[†]	10.3	9.5	9.8
Menarche[†]	12.7	12.1	12.2
Menarche[‡]	12.7	12.3	12.5

Modified with permission from Wu T, Mendola P, Buck GM: Ethnic differences in the presence of secondary sex characteristics and menarche among US girls: the Third National Health and Nutrition Examination Survey, 1988-1994. *Pediatrics* 110:752–757, 2002.
*Estimated with application of weights for the examination sample of the National Health and Nutrition Examination Survey III (NHANES III).
[†]Estimated using probit model for the status quo data of the puberty measurements.
[‡]Estimated using failure time model for the recalled age at menarche.

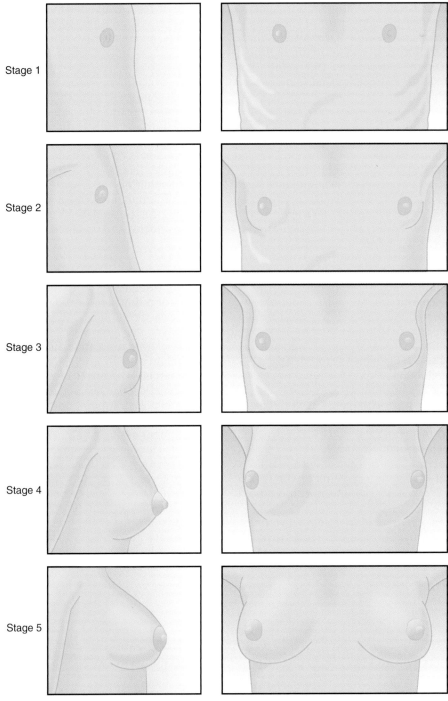

FIGURE 32-3 Stages of breast development as defined by Marshall and Tanner. *Stage 1,* Preadolescent; elevation of papilla only. *Stage 2,* Breast bud stage; elevation of breast and papilla as a small mound with enlargement of the areolar region. *Stage 3,* Further enlargement of breast and areola without separation of their contours. *Stage 4,* Projection of areola and papilla to form a secondary mound above the level of the breast. *Stage 5,* Mature stage; projection of papilla only, resulting from recession of the areola to the general contour of the breast. Adapted from Marshall WA, Tanner JM: Variations in pattern of pubertal changes in girls. *Arch Dis Child* 44:291, 1969.

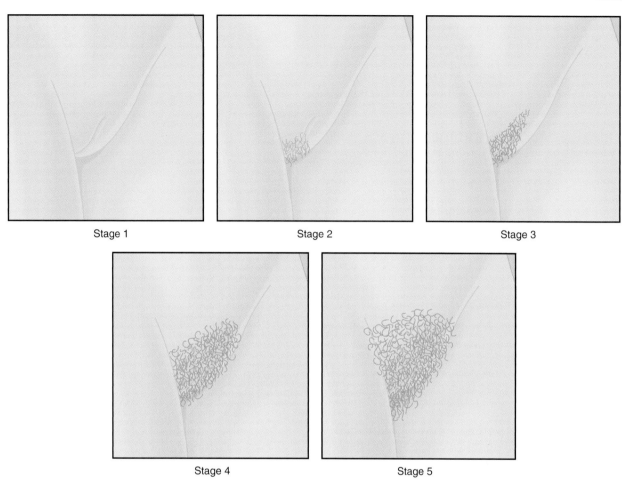

Stage 1   Stage 2   Stage 3

Stage 4   Stage 5

FIGURE 32-4 Stages of female pubic hair development according to Marshall and Tanner. *Stage 1,* Preadolescent; absence of pubic hair. *Stage 2,* Sparse hair along the labia; hair downy with slight pigmentation. *Stage 3,* Hair spreads sparsely over the junction of the pubes; hair is darker and coarser. *Stage 4,* Adult-type hair; no spread to the medial surface of the thighs. *Stage 5,* Adult-type hair with spread to the medial thighs assuming an inverted triangle pattern. Adapted from Marshall WA, Tanner JM: Variations in pattern of pubertal changes in girls. *Arch Dis Child* 44:291, 1969.

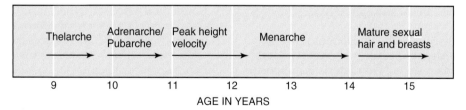

FIGURE 32-5 Sequence of physical changes during pubertal development. The acronym *TAPuP ME* has been used as a mnemonic device for **T**helarche, **A**drenarche/**Pu**barche, **P**eak height velocity, and **ME**narche, which precede mature sexual hair and breast development.

of age, whereas in whites, they can occur as early 7 years of age.

ADOLESCENT GROWTH SPURT

In general, the growth spurt is seen 2 years earlier in pubertal girls than in boys. Growth hormone, estradiol, and insulin-like growth factor 1 (formerly somatomedin C) are involved in the adolescent growth spurt. Peak height velocity occurs approximately 1 year before the onset of menarche. There is limited linear growth after menarche, as gonadal steroid production accelerates fusion of the long bone epiphyses.

BODY COMPOSITION AND BONE AGE

There are no significant differences in skeletal mass, lean body mass, or percentage of body fat between prepubertal boys and prepubertal girls. After attaining sexual maturity, girls generally have less skeletal and lean body mass and a greater percentage of body fat than boys do.

Bone age correlates well with the onset of secondary sexual characteristics and menarche. Bone age is determined by obtaining radiographs of the left (or nondominant) hand and wrist, elbow, or knee and comparing them with an index population. Osseous maturation is particularly useful in the evaluation of adolescents with delayed onset of puberty. Bone maturation, chronologic age, and height can also be used to predict the final adult stature based on standardized nomograms.

Precocious Puberty

Precocious puberty **refers to the development of any sign of secondary sexual maturation at an age 2.5 standard deviations earlier than the expected age of pubertal onset.** In North America, these ages are 8 years for girls and 9 years for boys. The incidence of precocious puberty is 1 in 10,000 children in North America, and it is approximately five times more common in girls. **In 75% of cases of precocious puberty in girls, the cause is idiopathic.** A thorough evaluation to eliminate a serious disease process, and to arrest potential premature osseous maturation that may affect the normal growth pattern, is mandatory.

The early development of secondary sexual characteristics may promote psychosocial problems for the child and should be addressed carefully. **Typically, these girls are taller than their peers as children but ultimately are shorter as adults, due to the premature fusion of the long bone epiphyses.** A classification system for female precocious puberty is shown in Box 32-1.

Precocious puberty may be divided into two major subgroups: **heterosexual precocious puberty (development of secondary sexual characteristics opposite those of the anticipated phenotypic sex) and isosexual precocious puberty (premature sexual maturation that is appropriate for the phenotype of the affected individual).**

Investigations for females with precocious puberty are shown in Box 32-2.

HETEROSEXUAL PRECOCITY

In females, heterosexual precocity results from virilizing neoplasms, congenital adrenal hyperplasia, or exposure to exogenous androgens.

Androgen-secreting neoplasms in females are either ovarian (most commonly an arrhenoblastoma)

BOX 32-1

CLASSIFICATION OF FEMALE PRECOCIOUS PUBERTY

Heterosexual Precocious Puberty

Virilizing neoplasm
   Ovarian
   Adrenal
Congenital   adrenal   hyperplasia   (adrenogenital syndrome)
Exogenous androgen exposure

Isosexual Precocious Puberty

Incomplete Isosexual Precocious Puberty

Premature thelarche
Premature adrenarche
Premature pubarche

Complete Isosexual Precocious Puberty

True isosexual precocious puberty
   Constitutional (idiopathic)
   Organic brain disease
      Central nervous system tumors
      Head trauma
      Hydrocephalus
      Central nervous system infection (abscess, encephalitis, meningitis)

Pseudoisosexual Precocious Puberty

Ovarian neoplasm
Adrenal neoplasm
Exogenous estrogen exposure
Advanced hypothyroidism
McCune-Albright syndrome
Peutz-Jeghers syndrome

Adapted from Brenner PF: Precocious puberty in the female. In Mishell DR Jr, Davajan V, Lobo RA, editors: *Infertility, contraception and reproductive endocrinology*, ed 3, Cambridge, MA, 1991, Blackwell Scientific, p 349.

---

or adrenal in origin and are exceedingly rare in childhood. They are diagnosed on the basis of physical and radiologic examinations of the abdomen and are treated by surgical removal.

Congenital adrenal hyperplasia most commonly results from a defect of the adrenal enzyme 21-hydroxylase that leads to excessive androgen production. More severe forms of this defect cause the birth of a female with ambiguous genitalia. If untreated, progressive virilization during childhood and short adult stature will result. The treatment of this disorder includes replacement of cortisol with a related glucocorticoid and surgical correction of any anatomic abnormalities in the first few years of life. A less severe form of this defect, referred to as *nonclassic (late onset) adrenal hyperplasia* can cause premature pubarche and an adult disorder resembling PCOS.

ISOSEXUAL PRECOCIOUS PUBERTY

Complete isosexual precocious puberty results in the development of the full complement of secondary sexual characteristics and increased levels of sex

BOX 32-2

LABORATORY TESTS USED SELECTIVELY TO EVALUATE FEMALE PRECOCIOUS PUBERTY

Radiologic

Serial bone age (isosexual precocity)

Magnetic resonance imaging (MRI) or computed tomography (CT) of the brain with optimal visualization of hypothalamic region and sella turcica (true isosexual precocity)

MRI, CT, or ultrasonography of abdomen, pelvis, or adrenal gland (heterosexual precocity, pseudoisosexual precocity)

Laboratory

Luteinizing hormone (LH) and follicle-stimulating hormone (FSH)

Dehydroepiandrosterone sulfate, testosterone (heterosexual precocity)

17-hydroxyprogesterone, 11-deoxycortisol (suspected congenital adrenal hyperplasia causing heterosexual precocity)

Thyroid function tests (thyroid-stimulating hormone, free thyroxine) (isosexual precocious puberty)

Gonadotropin-releasing hormone (GnRH) stimulation test: LH measurement after 100 μg of GnRH is given intravenously (to differentiate gonadotropin-dependent from gonadotropin-independent isosexual precocity)

steroids. It may arise from premature activation of the normal process of pubertal development involving the hypothalamic–pituitary–gonadal axis, which is called **true isosexual precocity.** Exposure to estrogen, independent of the hypothalamic–pituitary axis (such as from an estrogen-producing tumor), is called ***pseudoisosexual precocity.***

True Isosexual Precocity

In females, 75% of cases are constitutional. True isosexual precocity may be diagnosed by the administration of exogenous GnRH (a GnRH stimulation test) with a resultant rise in LH levels equivalent to those seen in older girls who are undergoing normal puberty. **In approximately 10% of girls with the true form of precocious puberty, a central nervous system disorder is the underlying cause.** This includes tumors, obstructive lesions (hydrocephalus), granulomatous diseases (sarcoidosis, tuberculosis), infective processes (meningitis, encephalitis, or brain abscess), neurofibromatosis, and head trauma. It is postulated that these conditions interfere with the normal inhibition of hypothalamic GnRH release. **Children with precocious puberty secondary to organic brain disease often exhibit neurologic symptoms before the appearance of premature sexual maturation.** Evaluation of true isosexual precocity should include MRI of the head for lesions.

Pseudoisosexual Precocity

Pseudoisosexual precocity occurs when estrogen levels are elevated and cause characteristic sexual maturation without activation of the hypothalamic–pituitary axis. In these girls, a GnRH stimulation test does not induce pubertal levels of gonadotropins. Causes include ovarian tumors and cysts, exogenous estrogenic compound use, McCune-Albright syndrome, severe prolonged hypothyroidism, and Peutz-Jeghers syndrome. Curiously, when the initial cause of pseudoisosexual precocity is eliminated, some girls go on to develop true isosexual precocity.

Some ovarian tumors can be felt on abdominal examination and are usually unilateral. Other lesions may require radiologic or ultrasonic imaging for diagnosis. Treatment of these lesions is surgical.

The McCune-Albright syndrome (polyostotic fibrous dysplasia) **represents 5% of cases of female precocious puberty.** This syndrome consists of sexual precocity, multiple cystic bone defects that fracture easily, café au lait spots with irregular borders (most frequently on the face, neck, shoulders, and back), and adrenal hypercortisolism. Hyperthyroidism and acromegaly may also occur in this syndrome. The pathophysiology involves a somatic mutation in affected postzygotic tissues that causes them to function independently of their normal stimulating hormones.

Prolonged, severe hypothyroidism has been hypothesized to cause pituitary gonadotropin release in response to the persistently elevated secretion of thyroid-releasing hormone. Concomitant elevation of prolactin may also occur with the development of galactorrhea. Ovarian cysts may occasionally develop, and bone age may be retarded. This is the only form of precocious puberty associated with delayed bone age. Treatment is with thyroid replacement therapy.

The Peutz-Jeghers syndrome has been associated with a rare sex cord tumor with annular tubules, which may secrete estrogen. Because this syndrome of gastrointestinal tract polyposis and mucocutaneous pigmentation has also been reported in association with granulosa-theca cell tumors, children with this disorder should be screened for the development of gonadal neoplasms.

Incomplete isosexual precocity is the early appearance of a single secondary sexual characteristic. These conditions include **premature thelarche,** the isolated appearance of breast development before the age of 4 years (unilateral or bilateral) that resolves spontaneously within months and that is probably secondary to transient estradiol secretion; **premature adrenarche,** the isolated appearance of axillary hair before the age of 7 years that is the result of premature androgen secretion by the adrenal gland; and **premature pubarche,** the isolated appearance of pubic hair in girls before the age of 8 years.

In general, premature thelarche and premature adrenarche are associated with appropriate sexual maturation, though they may be associated with the development of nonclassic adrenal hyperplasia and perhaps PCOS. Therapy for these conditions is not required. Both conditions are more common in girls than in boys. It is not possible to diagnose an incomplete form of sexual precocity on the basis of a single evaluation, and interval examinations of bone age are necessary to rule out true precocious puberty.

TREATMENT OF TRUE ISOSEXUAL PRECOCIOUS PUBERTY

Approximately 75% of cases of precocious puberty in girls prove to have a constitutional or idiopathic cause, and these patients are candidates for GnRH agonist therapy (e.g., leuprolide acetate). These girls require treatment to prevent further sex steroid release and accelerated epiphyseal fusion. Less than 50% of girls with idiopathic precocity will attain an adult height of 5 feet if the condition is left untreated.

GnRH agonists are the most effective therapy for idiopathic precocity. Long-term GnRH agonist treatment suppresses pituitary release of LH and FSH, resulting in decline of gonadotropin levels to prepubertal concentrations and arrest of gonadal sex steroid secretion. Clinically, normal gonadotropin release, sex steroid production, and pubertal maturation will resume 3 to 12 months after discontinuation of GnRH agonist therapy.

The final adult stature of girls with GnRH-dependent causes of precocious puberty is strongly influenced by their chronologic age at diagnosis and initiation of treatment. When GnRH agonist treatment is initiated before the chronologic age of 6 years, the final adult height is increased by 2-4%. In contrast, the final adult height is usually not affected when the chronologic age at diagnosis and treatment is greater than 6 years. Many studies have reported good long-term reproductive outcomes in GnRH-dependent precocious puberty after treatment with GnRH agonists and have shown no differences between regularity of menstrual cycles, pregnancy rates, and live births compared to a normal population. However, a few studies have suggested a higher prevalence (32% vs. 10%) of PCOS.

The majority of children with sexual precocity have few significant behavioral problems, but emotional support is important for these children. Behavioral expectations by family members and teachers should be based on the child's chronologic age, which determines psychosocial development, and not on the presence of secondary sexual characteristics.

Delayed Puberty

Although there is wide variation in normal pubertal development, the vast majority of girls in the United

---

BOX 32-3

RADIOLOGIC AND LABORATORY TESTS USED TO EVALUATE FEMALE DELAYED PUBERTY

Radiologic

Magnetic resonance imaging or computed tomography of the brain with optimal visualization of hypothalamic region and sella turcica (hypogonadotropic hypogonadism)

Laboratory

Follicle-stimulating hormone
Karyotype (delayed puberty, ambiguous genitalia)
Progesterone (delayed puberty secondary to 17-hydroxylase [P450c17] deficiency)
Prolactin (hypogonadotropic hypogonadism)

States begin pubertal maturation by the age of 13 years. If thelarche does not occur by age 14 years, an evaluation is required. A physiologic delay in the onset of puberty occurs in only 10% of girls with delayed puberty, and exclusion of other diagnoses is necessary. Physiologic delay in puberty tends to be familial. A careful history must be taken, with special attention to the patient's past general health, height, dietary habits, and exercise patterns. Details about the pubertal development of the patient's siblings and parents should be obtained. Box 32-3 lists tests that should be performed to evaluate girls with delayed puberty.

In general, the causes of delayed onset of puberty can be subdivided into two categories: hypogonadotropic hypogonadism and hypergonadotropic hypogonadism. Disorders resulting in hypogonadotropic hypogonadism that may cause primary or secondary amenorrhea are discussed in Chapter 33. Of note, anorexia nervosa, which can result in hypogonadotropic hypogonadism and delayed puberty, can affect 0.5-1.0% of young women. It is important to recognize this disorder in the evaluation of these patients. Chromosomal abnormalities or injury to the ovaries by surgery, chemotherapy, or radiation may cause hypergonadotropic hypogonadism. When the patient's abnormal karyotype includes the presence of a Y chromosome or the *SRY* gene in the sex-determining region, gonadectomy is recommended to prevent potential malignant neoplastic transformation.

A growing list of single-gene disorders resulting in delayed or absent female puberty is being documented in the literature.

Turner syndrome affects approximately 1 in 2500 live-born females and is characterized by loss or structural anomalies of an X chromosome. Its clinical features vary, and multiple organ systems may be affected. Often these patients present with hypergonadotropic hypogonadism and clinical features such as short stature and infertility.

roids, resulting in deficient or absent pubertal development. The accumulation of progesterone before the block leads to excessive synthesis of the mineralocorticoid 11-deoxycorticosterone, which generally causes hypertension and hypokalemia.

Mutations of leptin and leptin receptor gene are associated with retarded pubertal development and childhood morbid obesity.

Mutations in the steroidogenic acute regulatory (StAR) gene result in complete loss of adrenal steroidogenesis and delayed puberty, which is called ***congenital lipoid adrenal hyperplasia.*** The StAR protein is necessary for the transportation of cholesterol from the outer mitochondrial membrane to the inner mitochondrial membrane, which is the rate-limiting step in steroidogenesis.

Adolescents who present with permanent hypoestrogenism require estrogen therapy to complete the development of secondary sexual characteristics. Hormone therapy with estrogen plus a progestin or with a low-dose oral contraceptive after establishment of secondary sexual characteristics is required to avoid menopausal symptoms and to prevent osteoporosis. To further optimize gradual bone mineral deposition, 1500 mg of elemental calcium and 400 mg of vitamin D daily are recommended. This should be combined with regular weight-bearing exercises.

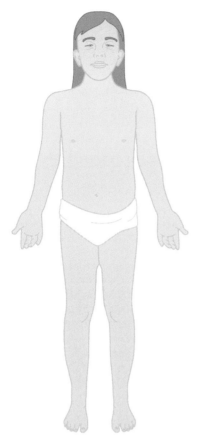

FIGURE 32-6 Kallmann syndrome is a genetic condition that results in hypogonadotropic hypogonadism caused by a defect in gonadotropin-releasing hormone (GnRH) production and release from the hypothalamus. Because the area in the hypothalamus where GnRH is produced is near the olfactory center, the sense of smell is usually affected, resulting in anosmia.

Kallmann syndrome (Figure 32-6) presents with hypogonadotropic hypogonadism and anosmia/hyposmia. It may result from a mutation of the *KAL* gene on the X chromosome or from autosomal mutations that prevent the embryologic migration of GnRH neurons into the hypothalamus. Individuals with this syndrome may have other anomalies of midline structures of the head. One in 50,000 females is affected.

Mutations of the GnRH receptor gene in females have resulted in low gonadotropin levels with primary amenorrhea or delayed puberty.

Mutations of the FSH β-subunit gene and the **FSH receptor gene** have been associated with primary amenorrhea and varying degrees of incomplete development of secondary sexual characteristics.

Females with **aromatase deficiency** present at puberty with progressive virilization, absence of thelarche, and primary amenorrhea.

17-Hydroxylase (P450c17) deficiency interferes with production of the androgenic and estrogenic ste-

Polycystic Ovarian Syndrome and Puberty

PCOS is the leading cause of female anovulatory infertility and is characterized by ovulatory dysfunction and hyperandrogenism. It is associated with obesity, insulin resistance, and metabolic dysfunction (see Chapter 33). During the transition from adrenarche/pubarche (adrenal androgen production dominance) to menarche, a relatively similar imbalance of hormones leads to irregular menses, polycystic ovaries, and a relative androgen excess. Because of these similar clinical findings, the diagnosis of PCOS in the adolescent population remains controversial.

Recently, it has been suggested that adolescents with congenital virilization, premature pubarche, or central precocious puberty are at higher risk of developing PCOS. **There is growing support for using a modified Rotterdam system to make a diagnosis of PCOS in adolescents.** This requires the presence of all three of the following criteria (rather than the standard two of three criteria): **oligo-ovulation or anovulation, hyperandrogenism, and polycystic ovaries visualized by pelvic ultrasonography.** Adolescent PCOS is associated with metabolic syndrome and sleep disorders, and treatment should include lifestyle modification. Other treatments commonly used to treat PCOS in an older population have not been studied thoroughly in adolescents.

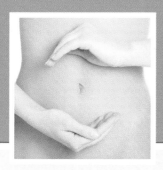

CHAPTER 33

Amenorrhea, Oligomenorrhea, and Hyperandrogenic Disorders

DANIEL A. DUMESIC • JOSEPH C. GAMBONE

CLINICAL KEYS FOR THIS CHAPTER

- *Amenorrhea* literally means the absence of menses. As a menstrual disorder, amenorrhea is *primary* when menstruation has never occurred by the age of 16 years (or 14 years with the absence of breast development) and is *secondary* when menses has occurred at least once and then has been absent for at least 6 months.
- A more clinically useful classification of these menstrual disorders is to characterize them based on the initial presentation (history and physical examination) as (1) primary amenorrhea without evidence of secondary sexual characteristics (sexual infantilism), (2) primary amenorrhea with breast development and müllerian anomalies, or (3) secondary amenorrhea or oligomenorrhea with breast development and normal müllerian structures.
- The most common cause of primary amenorrhea is gonadal dysgenesis and/or agenesis (50% of cases). Secondary amenorrhea occurs most commonly with pregnancy and menopause (physiologic), followed by pathologic conditions such as hypothalamic-pituitary dysfunction, premature ovarian failure, hyperprolactinemia, and hyperandrogenism, such as polycystic ovarian syndrome (PCOS).

- Amenorrhea or oligomenorrhea with elevated androgens (hyperandrogenism) may result from adrenal, pituitary, or ovarian disorders, including tumors and functional problems with these tissues. Congenital adrenal hyperplasia, Cushing syndrome, PCOS, and the hyperandrogenic insulin resistance and acanthosis nigricans syndrome have adrenal and/or ovarian causes. Tumors of the adrenal glands and ovaries may cause excess androgen levels that can disrupt the menstrual cycle. Some tumors may be malignant, and all such tumors are managed surgically.
- PCOS is the most common endocrinologic disorder in women of reproductive age in developed countries. It has been recognized recently as a complex endocrinologic and metabolic syndrome that is diagnosed when at least two of the following three findings are present: (1) hyperandrogenism (either clinical or biochemical), (2) oligomenorrhea, and/or (3) polycystic ovaries by morphology. Not all women with PCOS have polycystic ovaries, and some women with polycystic ovaries do not meet the criteria for PCOS.

Amenorrhea, or the absence of menses, is a common symptom of several pathophysiologic states. This condition traditionally has been divided into **primary amenorrhea,** in which menarche (the first menses) has not occurred, and **secondary amenorrhea,** in which menses has been absent for 6 months or more. A more functional or clinical division of menstrual disorders based on the initial history-taking and physical examination is **(1) primary amenorrhea with sexual infantilism** (absence of secondary sexual development), **(2) primary amenorrhea with breast development and müllerian anomalies,** and **(3) amenorrhea or oligomenorrhea with breast development and normal müllerian structures.** The last group of disorders causes secondary, rather than primary, amenorrhea,

including oligomenorrhea with and without hyperandrogenic states (Table 33-1).

Primary Amenorrhea

The diagnosis of primary amenorrhea is made when no spontaneous uterine bleeding has occurred by the age of 16 years. The workup should be initiated earlier if there is no evidence of breast development (thelarche) by age 14 years or if the patient has not menstruated (menarche) spontaneously within 2 years of thelarche. The presence of normal breast development confirms gonadal secretion of estrogen but not necessarily the presence of ovarian tissue. With androgen insensitivity, low levels of estrogen from the testicles

TABLE 33-1

CLINICAL CLASSIFICATION OF MENSTRUAL DISORDERS

Disorder	Notable Diagnostic Findings	Examples	Notable Clinical Features
Primary Amenorrhea with Sexual Infantilism			
Hypogonadotropic hypogonadism	Low FSH and LH, low estrogen; screening for other pituitary hormones is indicated; MRI of the hypothalamic and/or pituitary area is recommended	Central nervous system or pituitary tumor, constitutionally delayed puberty, Kallmann syndrome; rarely presents as secondary amenorrhea with late onset	Exclude serious causes before diagnosing constitutional delay (diagnosis of exclusion); anosmia/hyposmia with Kallmann syndrome
Hypergonadotropic hypogonadism	Elevated FSH and LH, low estrogen, karyotype indicated to rule out Y chromosome	Gonadal agenesis and/or dysgenesis (most common cause of primary amenorrhea), including Turner syndrome (45,XO) and pure gonadal dysgenesis (46,XX) or (46,XY)	May rarely present as secondary amenorrhea; streak gonads, short stature, and webbing of the neck with Turner syndrome
17-Hydroxylase (P450c17) deficiency	Low sex steroids (estrogens and androgens); a rare genetic disorder	Primary amenorrhea usually in 46,XX and female external genitalia in 46,XY	Hypertension and hypokalemia caused by mineralocorticoid excess (see Figure 33-1)
Primary Amenorrhea with Breast Development and Müllerian Anomalies			
Androgen insensitivity (46,XY)	Male levels of androgens in serum (which distinguishes androgen insensitivity from other müllerian anomalies)	Androgen insensitivity syndrome (formerly called *testicular feminization syndrome*)	Internal testicles, vaginal dimple, no uterus, and near-normal breast development with smaller areolae and/or nipples
Normal female karyotype (46,XX)	Female levels of androgens in serum	Anatomic defects resulting in outflow obstruction	Surgical correction possible in many, but not all, types
Imperforate hymen	Hematocolpos on abdominal ultrasound		Bulge at introitus, cyclic pain with absent vaginal bleeding
Transverse vaginal septum	Obstruction visible on MRI scan		Cyclic lower abdominal pain without menses, hematometra, decreased fertility potential
Cervical agenesis	Cervix absent on MRI scan		Hysterectomy likely
Müllerian agenesis and/or dysgenesis	Intravenous pyelogram or other renal imaging indicated	Mayer-Rokitansky-Küster-Hauser syndrome	Vaginal dimple only, absent uterus on rectal
Secondary (Rarely Primary) Amenorrhea and/or Oligomenorrhea with Breast Development and Normal Müllerian Structures			
Pregnancy	Positive pregnancy test		Always rule out first
Uterine defects	Intrauterine scarring visible on hysterosalpingogram	Asherman syndrome	Fertility problems
Hypoestrogenism	Low serum estrogen levels	Various types listed below	
Hypothalamopituitary dysfunction	Low FSH, LH, and prolactin; other hormone deficiencies should be ruled out	Excessive exercise (runner's amenorrhea); anorexia nervosa	Lean body mass; anorexia nervosa is primarily a psychiatric disorder with significant mortality (about 7%)
Premature ovarian failure	Elevated serum FSH, low serum estrogen, karyotype indicated if age <30 yr	Autoimmune premature ovarian failure	Age <40 yr
Hyperprolactinemia (serum estrogen level can vary)	Elevated serum prolactin	Pituitary adenoma, empty sella syndrome, primary hypothyroidism, drugs (for others, see Box 33-2)	Galactorrhea
Normal estrogen and amenorrhea and/or oligomenorrhea	Normal hormone levels	Mild hypothalamic amenorrhea: exercise, nutrition, stress, hypothyroidism	
Hyperandrogenism	Elevated androgens (variable)	Congenital adrenal hyperplasia, polycystic ovarian syndrome, HAIR-AN syndrome (for others, see Box 33-2)	Hirsutism, acne, insulin resistance, virilization in some severe cases

Modified from Gambone JC: *Student manual,* Los Angeles, 2003, David Geffen School of Medicine, University of California—Los Angeles.
FSH, Follicle-stimulating hormone; *HAIR-AN,* hyperandrogenic insulin resistance and acanthosis nigricans; *LH,* luteinizing hormone; *MRI,* magnetic resonance imaging.

may stimulate breast development in males (see Chapter 18). Normal amounts of pubic and axillary hair confirm gonadal or adrenal secretion of androgens as well as the presence of functional androgen receptors.

PRIMARY AMENORRHEA WITH SEXUAL INFANTILISM

Patients with primary amenorrhea and no secondary sexual characteristics (sexual infantilism) display an absence of gonadal hormone secretion. The differential diagnosis is based on whether the defect represents a lack of gonadotropin secretion (**hypogonadotropic hypogonadism**) or an inability of the ovaries to respond to gonadotropin secretion (**hypergonadotropic hypogonadism caused by gonadal agenesis/dysgenesis**). The distinction can be made by measuring a basal serum follicle-stimulating hormone (FSH) level.

Hypogonadotropic Primary Amenorrhea and Sexual Infantilism

Patients with hypogonadotropic hypogonadism have low serum FSH levels, whereas patients with hypergonadotropic hypogonadism (e.g., gonadal dysgenesis) have elevated serum FSH levels in the menopausal range (>20 to 40 mIU/L, depending on the assay used). The measurement of serum luteinizing hormone (LH) is of limited additional diagnostic value. The absence of breast development is indicative of inadequate secretion of estrogen.

Hypogonadotropic hypogonadism may be caused by lesions of the hypothalamus or pituitary gland or by functional disorders that suppress gonadotropin-releasing hormone (GnRH) synthesis and release. Kallmann syndrome is an example of lesions in the hypothalamus causing hypogonadotropic hypogonadism, usually with anosmia (see Chapter 32 and Figure 32-6). Because patients with sexual infantilism caused by hypogonadotropic hypogonadism may have a craniopharyngioma or other central nervous system (CNS) tumor, magnetic resonance imaging (MRI) or computed tomography (CT) of the hypothalamic-pituitary area is recommended.

Hypogonadotropic hypogonadism resulting in primary amenorrhea and sexual infantilism may also be caused by lesions of the pituitary, including prolactin-secreting adenomas, or a general process of pituitary failure. These patients should be screened for other pituitary hormone deficiencies by testing for thyroid-stimulating hormone (TSH), growth hormone, and adrenocorticotropic hormone (ACTH).

Finally, apparent hypogonadotropic hypogonadism may actually represent constitutionally delayed puberty. This delay in the normal onset of puberty is generally attributed to undefined hereditary factors because there is commonly a history of late puberty in family members. Constitutional delay of puberty is a diagnosis of exclusion.

Hypergonadotropic Primary Amenorrhea and Sexual Infantilism

Patients with hypergonadotropic hypogonadism have some form of failed gonadal development or premature gonadal failure and have elevated serum FSH levels. These patients may have gonadal agenesis (the absence or early disappearance of the normal gonad). An example in males, who may appear to be female in some cases, is **pure gonadal dysgenesis,** or the **testicular regression syndrome.** These patients have an apparently normal 46,XY karyotype but lack testicular development. If fetal testicular regression occurs between 8 and 10 weeks' gestation, these individuals may have female external genitalia with or without ambiguity in addition to a lack of gonads, a hypoplastic uterus (secondary to absent secretion of anti-müllerian hormone), and rudimentary genital ducts (Swyer syndrome). Regression of the testes after 12 to 14 weeks' gestation results in variable development of male external genitalia. Anorchia or streak gonads occur with testicular regression syndrome.

Other individuals with hypergonadotropic primary amenorrhea and sexual infantilism may have gonadal dysgenesis, or an abnormally developed gonad caused by chromosomal defects. The differential diagnosis includes 45,XO (Turner syndrome), a structurally abnormal X chromosome, mosaicism with or without a Y chromosome, and pure gonadal dysgenesis (46,XX and 46,XY). Although most affected patients show no signs of secondary sexual characteristics, occasionally an individual with mosaicism or Turner syndrome will have sufficient ovarian follicular activity and secrete enough estrogen to cause breast development, menstruation, ovulation, and rarely even pregnancy.

In individuals with the presence of a Y chromosome, there is a risk of developing a gonadoblastoma (a benign germ cell tumor of the gonad) and eventually a dysgerminoma (a malignant germ cell tumor). All patients with hypergonadotropic hypogonadism should have a karyotype performed. Because it is important to identify mosaicism, a greater number of white blood cells (>35) should be karyotyped.

Rarely, some patients with primary amenorrhea and sexual infantilism have a defect of estrogen and androgen production. One example of this is 17-hydroxylase (P450c17) deficiency, which prevents the synthesis of these sex steroids (Figure 33-1). These individuals have hypertension and hypokalemia caused by mineralocorticoid excess. Other patients, such as those with a 46,XY karyotype and Leydig cell agenesis, may lack the cells necessary for sex steroid production. Because Leydig cells in the testes are responsible for producing testosterone, these individuals are born with female external genitalia.

Patients with sexual infantilism may be treated to stimulate breast development by administering

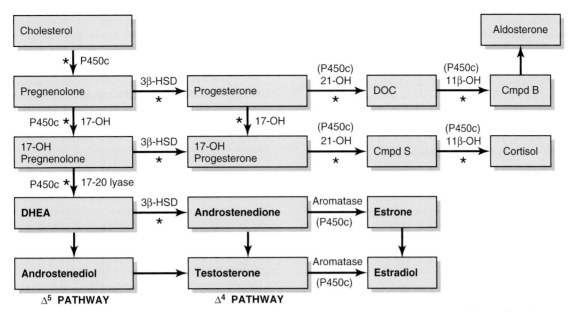

FIGURE 33-1 Diagrammatic representation of the steroid biosynthetic pathways. The *asterisks* denote specific enzyme defects that result in congenital adrenal hyperplasia. *Cmpd B,* Corticosterone; *Cmpd S,* 11-deoxycortisol; *DHEA,* dehydroepiandrosterone; *DOC,* deoxycorticosterone; *HSD,* hydroxysteroid dehydrogenase; *OH,* hydroxylase.

gradually increasing doses of estrogen. One commonly used regimen is to start with 0.3 mg of conjugated estrogen every other day and slowly increase the dose over 3- to 6-month intervals. This treatment should be guided by the presence or absence of mastalgia (breast tenderness) and the rate of breast development. The estrogen can safely be increased to 0.6 mg or more daily if necessary. Recently, skin patches that deliver 17β-estradiol (E2) in various comparable doses have been used.

Individuals with persistent hypogonadotropic hypogonadism who seek fertility require either human menopausal gonadotropin injections or pulsatile GnRH administered with an infusion pump. Patients with gonadal dysgenesis and 17-hydroxylase deficiency who have a normal uterus and cervix can achieve pregnancy only by in vitro fertilization (IVF) using donor oocytes.

PRIMARY AMENORRHEA WITH BREAST DEVELOPMENT AND MÜLLERIAN ANOMALIES

Patients with primary amenorrhea, breast development, and some defect of müllerian structures fall into two categories: (1) those with complete androgen insensitivity syndrome (AIS), formerly called *testicular feminization,* **and (2) those with müllerian dysgenesis or agenesis.** The distinction between these two diagnoses can be made by measuring serum testosterone and determining the karyotype.

Androgen Insensitivity Syndrome

Patients with complete AIS have a defect in the androgen receptor. Their karyotype is 46,XY, and they dem-

onstrate male levels of testosterone, although usually on the lower side of normal. They may also have mildly elevated FSH and LH levels, due to the location of their testes within the abdominal wall or cavity (cryptorchidism). This location, with greater body heat, typically does not allow for normal male hormone secretion. Breast development (with nipples and areolae smaller than a normal genotypical female's) is caused by the testicular secretion of estrogens and by the conversion of circulating androgen to estrogens in the liver and elsewhere. **The testes of individuals with AIS secrete normal male amounts of anti-müllerian hormone (AMH); therefore, patients have only a vaginal dimple and no uterus.** Treatment should consist of gonadal resection to avoid neoplasia (i.e., gonadoblastomas and dysgerminomas) once puberty is complete. The creation of a neovagina when the patient is prepared for sexual activity is possible by surgical and nonsurgical methods. Psychological counseling is an important component of care for these patients.

Müllerian Dysgenesis or Agenesis

Patients with primary amenorrhea, breast development, and a 46,XX karyotype have serum levels of testosterone appropriate for females. This clinical diagnosis may be caused by müllerian defects that cause obstruction of the vaginal canal (e.g., an imperforate hymen or a transverse vaginal septum) or by the absence of a normal cervix and/or uterus and normal fallopian tubes. An imperforate hymen should be suspected in adolescents who report monthly dysmenorrhea in the absence of vaginal bleeding. Clinically, these patients often present with a vaginal bulge and a midline cystic mass on rectal examination. Ultrasonography confirms the presence of a normal uterus and ovaries with a hematocolpos. These patients should be treated with hymenectomy.

Alternatively, females may present with similar symptoms, but without a vaginal bulge. When ultrasonography confirms a normal uterus and ovaries, **a transverse, obstructing vaginal septum or cervical agenesis should be suspected.** MRI is the diagnostic procedure of choice in these patients. If an MRI scan confirms a transverse septum, surgical correction is indicated. Surgical construction of a functional cervix is extremely difficult. In general, it is recommended that women with cervical agenesis undergo hysterectomy.

Finally, **rectal examination and ultrasonography may indicate the absence of a uterus, indicating müllerian agenesis or the Mayer-Rokitansky-Küster-Hauser syndrome.** This syndrome is characterized by a failure of the müllerian ducts to fuse distally and form the upper genital tract. These patients may have unilateral or bilateral rudimentary uterine tissues (anlagens), fallopian tubes, and ovaries. It is uncommon for an individual to have functional endometrial tissue within the anlagen. On occasion, the ovaries are not visible on ultrasonography because they have not descended into the pelvis. In these cases, CT or MRI may reveal them well above the pelvic brim. **Currently, the pathophysiology leading to müllerian dysgenetic defects is not known.**

Creation of a neovagina can be accomplished by using one of two general approaches. **The Frank method of vaginal dilation** uses dilation of the vaginal pouch with vaginal forms (usually thermoplastic acrylic resin [Lucite] dilators) over the course of weeks to months. Alternatively, a **McIndoe vaginoplasty,** which involves the surgical creation of a neovaginal space using a split-thickness skin graft, may be performed. Both of these methods should be initiated and/or performed close to the time when the patient anticipates having vaginal intercourse.

Congenital anatomic abnormalities of the uterus or vagina, or both, are often associated with renal abnormalities such as a unilateral solitary kidney or a double renal collecting system, among others. **Therefore, for these patients, an intravenous pyelogram or other diagnostic radiographic study should be obtained to confirm a normal urinary system.**

Amenorrhea or Oligomenorrhea with Breast Development and Normal Müllerian Structures

Disorders in which the patient has breast development and a demonstrable cervix and uterine fundus on physical examination may cause primary as well as secondary amenorrhea, or they may present as oligomenorrhea (less frequent menstruation). Typically, women with oligomenorrhea have fewer than nine menstrual cycles per year.

All patients with menstrual bleeding disorders should be tested for pregnancy. Once pregnancy has been excluded, these individuals can be characterized as shown in Table 33-1. The initial history-taking should include questions about the timing of thelarche, pubarche, and menarche. The timing and development of the menstrual disorder (present since puberty or new), significant weight change, strenuous exercise activities, dietary habits, sexual activity, concomitant illnesses or complaints, abnormal facial or body hair growth, scalp hair loss, acne, and the presence or absence of hot flashes and vaginal dryness should be noted. A comprehensive list of medications and dietary supplements taken should be obtained.

In addition to a pregnancy test, the initial investigation of the amenorrheic patient should include a serum FSH level and a progestin challenge test. If the patient does not have withdrawal bleeding after receiving a progestational agent, significant hypoestrogenism or hyperandrogenism, a uterine defect, or pregnancy are all possible. Progestogens that are used include medroxyprogesterone acetate 5 to 10 mg/day orally for 5 to 14 days, norethindrone acetate 2.5 to 10 mg/day orally for 5 to 14 days, oral micronized progesterone 100 to 300 mg/day for 5 to 14 days, or progesterone in oil 50 to 100 mg intramuscularly. To evaluate the estrogenic status, some clinicians prefer to order a serum estradiol (E2) instead of the progestin challenge test.

UTERINE DEFECTS

Women who do not have withdrawal bleeding after a hormonal challenge test and who have a history of uterine instrumentation, particularly a dilation and curettage following vaginal delivery or pregnancy termination, may have Asherman syndrome (AS). This interesting syndrome is characterized by intrauterine scarring (synechiae), and patients with AS may have normal ovulatory cycles with cyclic premenstrual symptoms. Patients with AS should be evaluated by hysterosalpingography or sonohysterography. Hysteroscopic treatment with excision of the synechiae and normalization of the uterine cavity is the treatment of choice.

AMENORRHEA OR OLIGOMENORRHEA ASSOCIATED WITH HYPOESTROGENISM

The differential diagnosis for patients with amenorrhea associated with low serum levels of estrogen includes hypothalamic and/or pituitary dysfunction (hypothalamic amenorrhea), premature ovarian failure, or hyperprolactinemia. Women in the first group have low serum FSH and prolactin levels; women in the second group have high serum FSH and normal serum prolactin levels; and women in the third group have high serum prolactin and low serum FSH levels.

Hypothalamic-Pituitary Dysfunction

Patients with hypothalamic amenorrhea include women with severe weight loss, women engaging in excessive exercise resulting in low body fat, and women experiencing severe psychological stress. Also included are those women with physical wasting caused by severe systemic diseases such as disseminated malignancies and patients with pituitary or CNS lesions. In the most severe and life-threatening form of hypothalamic amenorrhea, women may have pituitary failure or anorexia nervosa. All patients with hypogonadotropic hypogonadism and hypothalamic-pituitary dysfunction should be evaluated for the status of the other pituitary hormones. Evaluation should also include MRI of the hypothalamus and pituitary gland to exclude neoplastic and other lesions if it is uncertain whether the patient has one of the functional disorders described above.

When hypothalamic-pituitary dysfunction cannot be resolved by identifying a modifiable underlying cause (e.g., excessive exercise), combination estrogen and progestin therapy, usually in the form of a combined oral contraceptive pill or E2 skin patches with oral progestins, should be prescribed to reduce the risk of osteoporosis. This therapy is also recommended to maintain normal vaginal and breast development. In patients with anorexia nervosa (AN), ovarian hormone therapy without weight gain will not totally prevent osteoporosis.

Premature Ovarian Failure

Premature ovarian failure is defined as ovarian failure before the age of 40 years (see Chapter 35). When it occurs in patients younger than 30 years of age, ovarian failure may be caused by a chromosomal disorder. A karyotype should be performed to exclude mosaicism (i.e., some cells bearing a Y chromosome). If cells with a Y chromosome are present, a gonadectomy to prevent malignant transformation is indicated.

Other causes of premature ovarian failure include ovarian injury as a result of surgery, radiation, or chemotherapy; galactosemia; carrier status of the fragile X syndrome; and autoimmunity. When premature ovarian failure is secondary to autoimmunity, other endocrine organs may be affected as well. Because there are no specific laboratory tests available to diagnose autoimmune ovarian failure, all patients with unexplained ovarian failure should be screened for diabetes (fasting glucose), hypothyroidism (TSH and free thyroxine [T_4]), hypoparathyroidism (serum calcium and phosphorus), and hypocortisolism (fasting morning cortisol or cortisol response to ACTH stimulation). It is not unusual for patients with premature ovarian failure to have episodes of normal ovarian and menstrual function. **Patients with premature ovarian failure require hormone therapy (estrogen and a progestin) to reduce the risk of osteoporosis.**

AMENORRHEA OR OLIGOMENORRHEA WITH HYPERPROLACTINEMIA AND/OR GALACTORRHEA

The principal action of prolactin is to stimulate lactation. Hypersecretion of prolactin leads to gonadal dysfunction by interrupting the secretion of GnRH, which inhibits the release of LH and FSH and thereby impairs gonadal steroidogenesis. The primary influence on prolactin secretion is tonic inhibition of dopamine input from the hypothalamus. Any event disrupting this inhibition can result in a rise in prolactin levels.

The consequences of hyperprolactinemia that are clinically significant include menstrual disturbances and/or galactorrhea. About 10% of women with amenorrhea have elevated serum prolactin levels, and serum prolactin should be measured in all cases of amenorrhea of unknown cause. Potential causes of elevated serum prolactin are noted in Box 33-1. Normal serum prolactin levels are under 20 ng/dL, depending on the

---

BOX 33-1

CAUSES OF ELEVATED PROLACTIN

Pregnancy (10-fold increase from baseline)
Excessive exercise
Postprandial states
Stimulation of the chest wall or nipple
Medications
    Metoclopramide
    Phenothiazines
    Butyrophenones
    Risperidone
    Monoamine oxidase inhibitors
    Tricyclic antidepressants
    Serotonin reuptake inhibitors
    Verapamil
    Reserpine
    Methyldopa
    Estrogens
Craniopharyngiomas
Granulomatous infiltration of the pituitary or hypothalamus
Acromegaly
Severe head trauma
Prolactinomas
Pituitary stalk compression
Primary hypothyroidism
Chronic renal failure
Marijuana or narcotic use

laboratory used. In patients with prolactin-secreting tumors, levels are usually above 100 ng/dL. An elevated serum prolactin level should be confirmed by a second test, preferably with the patient in the fasting state, as food ingestion may cause transient hyperprolactinemia. At the same time that the repeat prolactin level is measured, a TSH level should be obtained to test for hypothyroidism because hyperprolactinemia may be seen in patients with primary hypothyroid conditions.

A biologically inactive complex of prolactin and immunoglobulin, called *big prolactin,* can produce a physiologically insignificant elevation. Hence, the presence of a clinical abnormality should initiate the decision to test for hyperprolactinemia. **If clinically significant hyperprolactinemia is not explained by primary hypothyroidism or drug use, CT or MRI of the sella turcica should be performed.**

Galactorrhea is the most frequently observed abnormality associated with hyperprolactinemia. The secretion of milk may occur spontaneously or only after breast manipulation. Both breasts should be examined gently by palpating the gland moving from the periphery to the nipple. To confirm galactorrhea, a smear may be prepared and examined microscopically for the presence of multiple fat droplets (indicating milk). **Besides galactorrhea, hyperprolactinemia frequently causes oligomenorrhea or amenorrhea.**

Prolactinomas

Pituitary adenomas may cause hyperprolactinemia, and they make up approximately 10% of all intracranial tumors. Their etiology is unknown. Prolactinomas can be divided into two categories: macroadenomas (≥10 mm in diameter) and microadenomas (<10 mm in diameter). This distinction is important because microadenomas are unlikely to cause new problems as a result of additional growth. About 50% of patients with hyperprolactinemia have radiographic changes in the sella turcica consistent with an adenoma. Most patients have normal or low baseline levels of FSH.

Other Central Nervous System Lesions Affecting Prolactin

About 60% of pituitary adenomas do not produce prolactin, but may cause hyperprolactinemia by compression of the pituitary stalk. Another interesting lesion, **the empty sella syndrome,** is caused by a herniation of the subarachnoid membrane into the pituitary sella turcica through a defective or incompetent sella diaphragm. An empty sella may coexist with a prolactin-secreting pituitary adenoma. **Hypothalamic tumors** may also cause hyperprolactinemia by damaging the hypothalamus or by compression of the pituitary stalk, thereby interfering with the production or transport of dopamine. **Craniopharyngiomas are the most common of these lesions.**

Pharmacologic Agents Affecting the Secretion of Prolactin

A number of drugs may cause hyperprolactinemia and nonphysiologic galactorrhea (see Box 33-1). The mechanism of drug-induced hyperprolactinemia is secondary to reduced hypothalamic secretion of dopamine, depriving the pituitary of a natural inhibitor of prolactin release. When clinically indicated, patients with hyperprolactinemia caused by medications should be encouraged to discontinue the medication for at least 1 month. If hyperprolactinemia persists, or if the patient cannot interrupt the medication, a complete evaluation is indicated.

Miscellaneous Causes of Hyperprolactinemia

Patients with **acute or chronic renal failure** may have hyperprolactinemia because of delayed clearance of the hormone. These patients rarely require treatment other than for their renal failure. Patients with scars from previous chest surgery, including breast implantation, may have galactorrhea caused by **peripheral nerve stimulation.** Herpes zoster of the area including the breasts, as well as other forms of breast stimulation, can cause galactorrhea and sometimes hyperprolactinemia by the same mechanism. In about 3-5% of patients with galactorrhea and hyperprolactinemia, **primary hypothyroidism** is the underlying cause. These patients have a low serum free T_4 level. Consequently, they lack negative feedback on the hypothalamic–pituitary axis, resulting in increased secretion of thyrotropin-releasing hormone (TRH). TRH in turn stimulates elevated levels of TSH and prolactin. **Patients with primary hypothyroidism should be given T_4 replacement therapy.** Rarely, cancers such as bronchogenic carcinoma or hypernephroma can result in elevated prolactin levels.

Treatment of Galactorrhea and Hyperprolactinemia

The objectives of therapy for galactorrhea and hyperprolactinemia include the elimination of lactation, the establishment of normal estrogen levels, and the induction of ovulation when fertility is desired. The recommended forms of management are periodic observation, medical therapy, and surgery.

OBSERVATION. Periodic observation is indicated in normally menstruating women with galactorrhea who have either normal serum prolactin levels or idiopathic elevations of prolactin. **As long as the galactorrhea is not socially embarrassing and the patient has regular menses (confirming normal estrogen levels), there is no need to institute treatment.** Patients with oligomenorrhea who do not desire fertility should be treated with periodic progestins, or if contraception is needed, with hormonal therapy, to induce regular uterine bleeding. Failure to induce withdrawal bleeding with progestins is suggestive of hypoestrogenism. When verified by low serum levels of estradiol (<30 pg/mL) and a negative pregnancy test, cyclic hormone therapy (estrogen and a progestin) should be initiated. **Long-term treatment with bromocriptine** (for hyperprolactinemia) **in women with normal estrogen levels is not indicated.**

Observation can be extended to some women with radiologic evidence of a pituitary microadenoma (<10 mm in diameter). **Because the growth rate of microadenomas is slow, an annual measurement of serum prolactin is appropriate in patients with normal estrogen levels.** Macroadenomas (≥10 mm in diameter) require further evaluation by periodic pituitary scanning and possible treatment.

MEDICAL THERAPY. Patients with hyperprolactinemia may have galactorrhea and anovulation with resulting infertility. In more severe cases, they may be hypoestrogenic, which places them at risk for developing osteoporosis. **Anovulatory patients without tumors demonstrable by MRI and for whom the only issues are prevention of osteoporosis and menstrual cycle regulation may be treated medically with combination hormonal contraceptives.**

The ergot compounds bromocriptine and cabergoline act as dopamine agonists to reduce prolactin secretion and allow for the restoration of cyclic, physiologic estrogen secretion. Bromocriptine has a high initial incidence of side effects such as headache, nausea, and orthostatic hypotension. As a consequence, it should be started at a dose of 1.25 to 2.5 mg at bedtime and slowly increased in divided doses to tolerance and restoration of normal prolactin levels. Some patients tolerate bromocriptine better when it is given vaginally. Cabergoline is taken in twice-weekly doses beginning at 0.25 mg and increasing to a maximum of 1 mg twice weekly. It is better tolerated and more convenient to take than bromocriptine, but it is also more expensive.

Ninety-five percent of women without radiographic evidence of an adenoma require 5 mg/day of bromocriptine, whereas about 50% of patients with adenomas require higher doses to resume regular menses. **Bromocriptine normalizes the secretion of prolactin in about 80% of women with microadenomas, and it restores menses and fertility in over 90%.** Usually, menses resume and galactorrhea resolves after about 6 weeks of bromocriptine therapy in women without adenomas. If an adenoma is present, it takes another 3 or 4 weeks for bromocriptine to become effective. Return of ovulation requires an average of 10 weeks without a tumor and 16 weeks with a microadenoma. Restoration of normal menstrual cycles and pregnancy may occur without complete normalization of the serum prolactin level. Discontinuation of therapy usually results in the return of hyperprolactinemia, leading to galactorrhea and amenorrhea.

Patients with macroadenomas (≥10 mm in diameter) should undergo visual field testing and screening for other pituitary hormonal deficiencies. A repeat MRI scan is obtained 6 months after the full therapeutic dose of bromocriptine is reached. As long as shrinkage of the adenoma is demonstrated, bromocriptine therapy is continued. **Surgery should be performed for patients with significant visual field defects or symptoms that cannot be relieved by medical therapy.**

Bromocriptine therapy is usually discontinued as soon as a pregnancy is confirmed. The risk of symptomatic enlargement of a microadenoma during pregnancy is only about 1%. When a macroadenoma is confined to the sella turcica, it is unlikely to enlarge significantly during pregnancy. **If there is extension of a macroadenoma beyond the sella turcica, there is a 15-30% risk of enlargement during pregnancy.** If possible, these larger lesions should be debulked before conception, then bromocriptine treatment should be initiated. Pregnant patients with macroadenomas should have their visual fields evaluated in each trimester. **When abnormalities in visual fields develop, bromocriptine treatment should be reinstituted or increased and maintained for the rest of the pregnancy.** There is no increase in fetal malformations as a result of bromocriptine treatment, and the drug can be discontinued after the pregnancy to allow for breastfeeding. Cabergoline has not been adequately evaluated for use in pregnancy.

SURGERY. When surgery is required, the transsphenoidal route for microsurgical exploration of the sella turcica gives the best results. **Recurrence rates for microadenomas after surgery approach 30%, and the rate increases to 90% for macroadenomas. For this reason, medical management is preferred,** with surgery reserved for cases with expansion outside the sella turcica or for compressive symptoms, such as visual field defects. Women who do not tolerate pharmacologic therapy may need surgery. Fifty percent of patients followed for 5 to 10 years after successful resection of an adenoma have recurrence of hyperprolactinemia without radiologic evidence of a tumor.

Amenorrhea or Oligomenorrhea with Normal Estrogen Levels

Patients with amenorrhea or oligomenorrhea who consistently have normal levels of estrogen have a mild form of hypothalamic anovulation that may be caused by low body weight and exercise issues, psychological stress, recent pregnancy, or lactation. They may also have been treated with Depo-Provera or combined hormonal contraceptives in the recent past. **These**

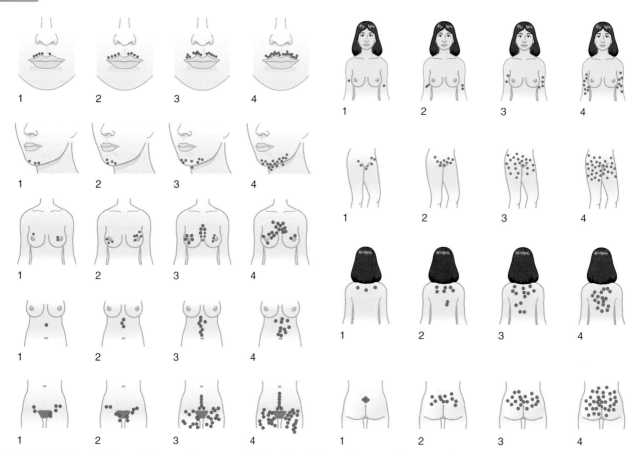

FIGURE 33-2 The Ferriman-Gallwey scoring system for hirsutism. (Adapted from Hatch R, Rosenfield RL, Kim MH, et al: Hirsutism: implications, etiology, and management. *Am J Obstet Gynecol* 140:815–830, copyright 1981, with permission from Elsevier.)

iatrogenic causes usually resolve spontaneously within 6 months. Some women with amenorrhea and/or oligomenorrhea and normal estrogen levels may have a subclinical androgen excess disorder, such as a mild form of polycystic ovarian syndrome (PCOS).

When contraception is not required in these anovulatory women and fertility is not desired, periodic progestin withdrawal to confirm normal estrogen levels and protect the endometrium is appropriate. When fertility is not desired, combination hormonal contraception is appropriate.

Amenorrhea or Oligomenorrhea with Hyperandrogenism

Hyperandrogenism is the clinical manifestation of elevated circulating levels of male hormones in women. **Features may range from mild, unwanted excessive hair growth and acne to alopecia (hair loss), hirsutism, and virilization.** *Hirsutism,* defined as excessive terminal hair appearing in a male-type pattern, represents exposure of hair follicles to androgen excess, either from a systemic origin and/or the local conversion of testosterone to the more potent dihydrotestosterone (DHT) by 5α-reductase in the hair follicle itself. Figure 33-2 illustrates a scoring system for hirsutism. ***Virilization (masculinization) refers to the acquisition of male characteristics (i.e., temporal balding, deepening of the voice, and enlargement of the clitoris).*** In females, it usually results from excessive male hormone production or exogenous hormone use. Signs of virilization also include defeminization or the loss of female body fat distribution (gluteofemoral fat deposits) and decreased breast size. Androgens in women are normally produced in the ovaries and the adrenal glands (see Figure 33-1). Therefore, hyperandrogenic disorders may be divided into nonneoplastic and neoplastic disorders of the adrenal glands or ovaries (Box 33-2).

NORMAL ANDROGEN METABOLISM

The formation of androgens results from the metabolism of cholesterol via the Δ^5 and Δ^4 pathways (see Figure 33-1). The stimulus for ovarian androgen production is LH.

BOX 33-2

HYPERANDROGENIC DISORDERS

Adrenal Disorders

Late-onset congenital adrenal hyperplasia
Cushing syndrome
Adrenal adenomas and carcinomas

Ovarian Disorders

Polycystic ovarian syndrome
HAIR-AN syndrome
Ovarian neoplasms
Sertoli-Leydig cell tumors
Hilar cell tumors
Lipoid cell tumors

Idiopathic Hirsutism

HAIR-AN, Hyperandrogenic insulin resistance and acanthosis nigricans.

Approximately one-half of serum androstenedione originates from the ovaries, whereas the other half arises from the adrenal glands. Approximately 50% of testosterone arises from peripheral conversion of androstenedione, whereas 25% is secreted by the ovaries and an additional 25% by the adrenal glands. Dehydroepiandrosterone (DHEA) and its sulfate DHEA-S are primarily products of the adrenal glands and serve as markers for the secretion of adrenal androgens. **Most circulating androgens are bound to proteins, such as albumin and sex hormone–binding globulin (SHBG). In the bound form, androgens are biologically inactive, although weak binding of testosterone to albumin allows some of this testosterone to become bioavailable for tissue activity.** The free fraction (that which is unbound to SHBG or albumin and is available for target tissue activity) represents only about 1-2% of total circulating testosterone.

When androgens reach a target tissue, they are further metabolized, which results in more potent intracellular hormones. **Testosterone is converted (via 5α-reductase) to DHT, which possesses greater biologic potency.** The skin, particularly its pilosebaceous unit (PSU), is capable of this conversion and is the reason why hirsutism can be accompanied by oily skin and acne. Alternatively, testosterone may be aromatized to estrogen, thereby modifying its action. Unlike testosterone, DHT is a potent, nonaromatizable androgen that cannot be converted to estrogen.

Hyperandrogenic Disorders

In general, hyperandrogenic disorders can be attributed to excessive secretion of androgens by the ovaries, the adrenal glands, or both. In addition, the inadvertent or accidental use or abuse of androgenic drugs should always be considered as a possible source of androgen exposure and generally can be excluded by history-taking and clinical evaluation.

ADRENAL DISORDERS

Congenital Adrenal Hyperplasia

Congenital adrenal hyperplasia (CAH) is a general term used to describe a group of disorders that arise from inborn glandular enzyme defects that cause overproduction of the immediate steroid precursor of the specific enzyme deficiency. **The most common cause of CAH is 21-hydroxylase deficiency,** an autosomal recessive disorder that exhibits a spectrum of severity, ranging from the severe salt-wasting form, to simple virilizing CAH, to nonclassic CAH. **Both salt-wasting and simple virilizing CAH are called *classic* because symptoms (e.g., salt loss or ambiguous genitalia in female newborns) are present at birth or shortly thereafter.** Alternatively, the nonclassic form (also called *late-onset CAH*) presents later in life, generally at the time of puberty or later. These patients do not present with genital abnormalities, but rather develop hirsutism, acne, and menstrual and/or ovulatory irregularities. Clinical manifestations of 21-hydroxylase deficiency depend upon the degree of enzyme deficiency, which is determined in part by the type of 21-hydroxylase genetic mutation that occurs on chromosome 6.

Because 21-hydroxylase is responsible for the conversion of 17-hydroxyprogesterone to 11-deoxycortisol (compound S), 21-hydroxylase deficiency causes excessive accumulation of 17-hydroxyprogesterone as the immediate steroid precursor for this enzyme. Consequently, 21-hydroxylase deficiency is characterized by an elevated serum 17-hydroxyprogesterone level as well as increases in its Δ^4 metabolites androstenedione and testosterone (see Figure 33-1).

The disease is inherited as an autosomal recessive trait. In patients with a positive family history and in ethnic groups with a high risk for nonclassic CAH (e.g., Ashkenazi Jews, with a prevalence of 1 in 27; Hispanics, with a prevalence of 1 in 40; and Slavs, with a prevalence of 1 in 50), this enzyme deficiency can be excluded by obtaining a follicular (preovulatory) phase serum 17-hydroxyprogesterone level, preferably in the morning. A level less than 2 ng/mL rules out late-onset CAH.

Cushing Syndrome

Another major adrenal disorder that leads to excessive androgen production is Cushing syndrome or persistent hypercortisolism. **Characteristic signs of Cushing syndrome include obesity; increased fat over the face (moon facies), trunk, and cervicodorsal as well as supraclavicular regions; hypertension; easy bruising resulting from thinning of the skin; impaired glucose tolerance; muscle wasting of the upper legs and arms; osteoporosis; and purple abdominal striae.** Other manifestations include hirsutism, acne, and irregular menses. Mental disturbances include excessive euphoria, irritability, insomnia, and depression. The depression may occur because of excess cortisol action on the CNS limbic system. Cushing syndrome may arise from a cortisol-producing tumor of the adrenal glands or from an ACTH-producing pituitary adenoma (called *Cushing disease*). These disorders are rare causes of androgen excess in women.

Adrenal Neoplasms

Adrenal tumors causing hyperandrogenism alone without evidence of glucocorticoid excess are very rare. More commonly, adrenal tumors produce large amounts of both glucocorticoids and androgens, with the predominant adrenal androgen being DHEA-S.

OVARIAN DISORDERS

Polycystic Ovarian Syndrome

According to recent guidelines (**Rotterdam criteria**), PCOS is defined by the inclusion of **at least two of the following three features: (1) clinical or biochemical hyperandrogenism, (2) oligomenorrhea or amenorrhea, and (3) polycystic ovaries,** excluding other endocrine disorders that mimic PCOS. The various PCOS phenotypes vary in severity, with the classic PCOS form (i.e., clinical or biochemical hyperandrogenism with oligo-ovulation) having the most severe reproductive and metabolic abnormalities. **PCOS affects about 6-10% of women worldwide on the basis of classic PCOS criteria, and even more individuals on the basis of the new Rotterdam criteria,** making it one of the most common human disorders and the single most common endocrinopathy among women of reproductive age. The clinical symptoms of PCOS usually develop at the time of puberty. PCOS is more prevalent among family members (20-40% of first-degree female relatives affected) than in the general population (prevalence: 6-10%), suggesting that **genetic factors influence development of the syndrome.** Because adolescent girls may have some of the features of PCOS without having the disorder, it is recommended that all three of the Rotterdam criteria be met in them (see Chapter 32).

The hyperandrogenism of PCOS results from an overproduction of male hormones by the ovary and often from the adrenal gland. A common clinical sign of hyperandrogenism in PCOS is hirsutism. Visual assessment of hirsutism is valuable because most women with PCOS of white or black race demonstrate excessive hair growth, although **hirsutism is less likely in women who have used hormonal contraceptives for prolonged intervals** and for many East Asian women. Obesity per se is not necessarily intrinsic to PCOS. Rather, the worldwide prevalence of obesity in most female populations has increased over the past two decades, and hyperinsulinemia caused by obesity-related insulin resistance worsens the symptoms of PCOS.

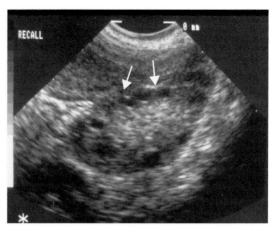

FIGURE 33-3 Transvaginal ultrasonogram of a woman with polycystic ovarian disease. The multiple subcapsular cysts, with their "string of pearls" appearance *(arrows),* are common in this syndrome.

In patients with PCOS, **ovarian hyperandrogenism, hyperinsulinemia caused by insulin resistance, and altered intraovarian signaling can disrupt follicular growth.** The consequent follicular arrest in PCOS is accompanied by menstrual irregularity, anovulatory subfertility, and the accumulation of small antral follicles within the periphery of the ovary, giving it a polycystic morphology (Figure 33-3). The ovarian stroma contains abundant theca cells that overproduce androgens. **Importantly, healthy women may also have polycystic-appearing ovaries, particularly in adolescence, when the ovaries normally contain a large number of follicles.**

LH hypersecretion increases serum LH levels in up to 70% of patients with PCOS, with elevated LH pulse amplitude and frequency inducing a two- to threefold elevation in circulating LH over FSH levels. Increased LH pulse frequency in PCOS, from enhanced hypothalamic GnRH pulsatile release, occurs as the result of reduced steroid hormone negative feedback on LH secretion from hyperandrogenism. As a result, **LH hypersecretion promotes ovarian hyperandrogenism in a feedforward mechanism, with androstenedione and testosterone undergoing peripheral aromatization to create tonic estrogen production without progesterone in the absence of ovulation.**

In women with PCOS, there is an association between hyperandrogenism and hyperinsulinemia because of insulin resistance. In approximately 60-70% of patients with PCOS, insulin sensitivity is impaired, leading to hyperinsulinemia. Consequently, the excessive amount of insulin perpetuates ovarian hyperandrogenism in several ways. The excess insulin stimulates the activity of CYP17A (cytochrome P450, 17A) in the theca cell. CYP17A is the enzyme responsible for androgen production in the theca cell. The excessive insulin also amplifies insulin-like growth factor 1 (IGF-1)–stimulated androgen production, elevating serum free testosterone levels through decreased hepatic SHBG production, which binds testosterone. Less binding results in more free testosterone. And finally, enhanced serum IGF-1 bioactivity results due to suppressed IGF-binding protein production. Thus, the physical manifestations of hyperandrogenism in PCOS may be dramatic in relation to the serum level of total testosterone.

Abdominal adiposity in women with PCOS preferentially worsens with weight gain, as does the prevalence of metabolic syndrome (elevated blood pressure and blood glucose with excess body fat around the waist). Metabolic syndrome, along with its underlying insulin resistance, occurs two to three times more frequently in women with PCOS than in age-matched controls, and it is 13.7 times more likely in PCOS women with the highest as opposed to the lowest BMI. **In the long term, the insulin resistance associated with PCOS may lead to an increased risk of cardiovascular disease,** most likely mediated through increased total and abdominal adiposity interacting with PCOS-related hyperandrogenism.

Women with PCOS also have a 2.7-fold increased risk of developing endometrial cancer. A major factor in this increased malignancy risk is the preceding development of endometrial hyperplasia caused by prolonged exposure to estrogen unopposed by progesterone in the absence of ovulation.

Hyperandrogenic Insulin Resistance and Acanthosis Nigricans Syndrome

The hyperandrogenic insulin resistance and acanthosis nigricans (HAIR-AN) syndrome is an inherited hyperandrogenic disorder of severe insulin resistance and is distinct from PCOS. HAIR-AN syndrome is characterized by extremely high circulating levels of insulin (>80 µU/mL basally and/or >500 µU/mL following an oral glucose challenge) caused by severe insulin resistance. Because insulin is also a mitogenic hormone, these extremely elevated insulin levels induce hyperplasia of the basal layers of the epidermal skin, leading to acanthosis nigricans, a velvety, hyperpigmented change in the creased areas of the skin (Figure 33-4). In addition, because of the effect of hyperinsulinemia on ovarian theca cells, the ovaries of many patients with the HAIR-AN syndrome develop hyperthecosis. Patients with HAIR-AN syndrome can be severely hyperandrogenic and present with virilization or severe, rapidly progressive hirsutism. In addition, these patients are at significant risk for dyslipidemia, type 2 diabetes mellitus, hypertension, and cardiovascular disease. These patients are particularly difficult to treat, although the use of long-acting GnRH analogs has been promising.

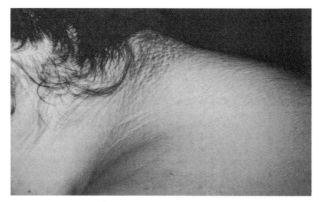

FIGURE 33-4 Acanthosis nigricans of the nape of the neck. These grayish brown velvety areas of the skin occur on the neck, groin, abdomen, or axillae and are markers of insulin resistance and hyperinsulinemia. (Courtesy Ricardo Azziz, MD, MPH, MBA, Cedars-Sinai Medical Center.)

Ovarian Neoplasms

Androgen-producing ovarian tumors are uncommon, occurring in only about 1 in 500 women with hirsutism. Ovarian tumors that produce androgens directly include **Sertoli-Leydig cell, hilus cell, and lipoid cell tumors.** Nevertheless, any large ovarian tumor (i.e., cystic teratomas, Brenner tumors, serous cystadenomas, and Krukenberg tumors) can produce androgens indirectly by causing hyperplasia of the surrounding normal stroma (see Chapter 20).

IDIOPATHIC HIRSUTISM

Some women exhibit mild to moderate hirsutism with normal ovulatory function and circulating androgen levels, a condition referred to as *idiopathic hirsutism.* This scenario may occur as a result of increased conversion of testosterone to the more biologically active DHT in the pilosebaceous units of the skin. Nevertheless, many conditions associated with hirsutism, including PCOS and CAH, have an inherited component, so hirsutism should be considered as a symptom of an underlying androgenic disorder in women until proven otherwise.

Evaluation of Patients with Signs of Hyperandrogenism

HISTORY

The evaluation of women with signs of androgen excess consists of diagnosing any serious underlying medical disease for which specific management may be necessary, assessing the emotional burden of hirsutism on the patient, and planning a personalized approach. **PCOS or late-onset CAH often initially appears during puberty and tends to progress slowly throughout**

adolescence into adulthood. Under these circumstances, the signs of androgen excess develop over the course of several years. In contrast, **neoplastic processes can occur at any time.** They most often arise years after puberty, and their manifestations appear abruptly. Progression is rapid, and these patients frequently present with recent onset of virilization. There is some overlap of symptoms between neoplastic and other androgen-related disorders in that 15% of patients with HAIR-AN syndrome can also exhibit signs of virilization, particularly severe hirsutism, temporal balding, and even clitoral enlargement.

PHYSICAL EXAMINATION

Patients should be asked about excessive facial hair, because they may conceal their hirsutism by waxing or electrolysis and may be too embarrassed to volunteer the information. The degree of hirsutism (see Figure 33-2), acne, or androgenic alopecia should be assessed. The thyroid should be palpated for any enlargement, and the breasts should be examined for galactorrhea. Any clinical evidence of Cushing syndrome should be noted. Acanthosis nigricans (see Figure 33-4) is a frequent marker of insulin resistance and hyperinsulinemia. A bimanual pelvic examination may reveal ovarian enlargement, with asymmetric ovarian enlargement accompanied by rapid onset of virilization suggestive of an androgen-producing tumor.

LABORATORY EVALUATION

It is important to test for elevated serum androgen levels in women with moderate or severe hirsutism or hirsutism of any degree when it is sudden in onset, rapidly progressive, or associated with menstrual dysfunction, obesity, or clitoromegaly.

On the basis of high-quality assay evidence, circulating total and free testosterone and DHEA-S are elevated in 50-75% of patients with PCOS. **Serum levels of DHEA-S above 7000 ng/mL or total testosterone in excess of 200 ng/dL raise suspicion of an adrenal or ovarian androgen-producing tumor, respectively. However, the best predictor of an androgen-secreting neoplasm is virilization,** which occurs with 98% of such tumors, regardless of circulating testosterone levels.

To exclude other disorders, measuring a **basal serum 17-hydroxyprogesterone level** is useful to exclude late-onset CAH due to 21-hydroxylase deficiency. A serum 17-hydroxyprogesterone level greater than 2 ng/mL requires an adrenal stimulation test to measure serum 17-hydroxyprogesterone before and 1 hour after intravenous infusion of the ACTH analog cosyntropin. If a 1-hour ACTH-stimulated serum 17-hydroxyprogesterone level exceeds 10 to 15 ng/mL, late-onset CAH is likely and can be confirmed by *CYP21* genotyping. Measurement of **serum prolactin and TSH levels** excludes hyperprolactinemia, with or without thyroid dysfunction. When Cushing syndrome is suspected, either a **24-hour measurement for free urinary cortisol** or an **overnight dexamethasone suppression test** should be performed. For the latter test, 1-mg dexamethasone is given orally at bedtime (11:00 pm), and serum cortisol is measured in an 8:00 am fasting specimen. Normal values are less than 5 µg/dL.

A pelvic ultrasound should be obtained to exclude any significant ovarian pathology. Androgen-secreting tumors of the adrenal gland can be detected by **CT or MRI.** If clinical or laboratory findings suggest an androgen-secreting tumor that cannot be located by these imaging techniques, **selective venous catheterization** may be performed to measure androgen levels in the venous blood from each adrenal gland and ovary, although this is not usually necessary.

A metabolic evaluation should be performed in patients with HAIR-AN syndrome or classic PCOS (particularly in those with a BMI >30 kg/m^2, lean with advanced age [>40 years], with a personal history of gestational diabetes, or with a family history of diabetes). Optimal screening for diabetes should include a **2-hour oral glucose tolerance test** because a 2-hour postprandial glucose level can be abnormal in the presence of a normal fasting glucose concentration. **Fasting serum lipid levels** also should be measured in these individuals.

TREATMENT OF HYPERANDROGENISM

Treatment should be guided by the nature of the underlying disease, the severity of clinical symptoms and signs, and the desires of the patient. **In the rare instance of an ovarian or adrenal neoplasm, surgical removal of the tumor is indicated.** In premenopausal women, unilateral salpingo-oophorectomy is sufficient for an ovarian tumor and preserves future childbearing potential. In postmenopausal women, the treatment is usually a total hysterectomy and bilateral salpingo-oophorectomy. **In patients with Cushing syndrome, treatment is surgical removal of the source of excessive cortisol or ACTH secretion** (adrenal or pituitary tumor).

PCOS is by far the most common ovarian abnormality causing hyperandrogenism, and its management depends on the patient's presentation and desires. **The initial therapy for hirsutism in patients with PCOS usually begins by suppressing ovarian androgen production with a combination oral contraceptive containing estrogen and a progestin.** Oral contraceptive therapy suppresses gonadotropins (both LH and FSH) and lowers circulating androgen levels, whereas its estrogen component stimulates SHBG production, which decreases free testosterone levels. There is no clinical advantage of one oral contraceptive over another.

A peripheral antiandrogen can be added to oral contraceptive therapy to treat hirsutism, regardless

of the source of the excessive androgen. This therapy also may improve idiopathic hirsutism. An antiandrogen is combined with an oral contraceptive for synergism and to prevent conception, because an antiandrogen would block normal sexual differentiation in a male fetus if used during pregnancy.

The antiandrogen most commonly used to treat hirsutism in the United States is spironolactone. This aldosterone antagonist competes for testosterone-binding sites, thereby exerting a direct antiandrogenic effect in target tissues. In addition, spironolactone interferes with steroid enzymes and decreases testosterone production. Because this medication opposes the action of aldosterone, serum potassium levels may rise and should be monitored. Other drugs that block the binding of androgens to their receptor include **flutamide** and **cyproterone acetate,** whereas **finasteride** blocks the conversion of testosterone to its more potent metabolite, DHT. It may take up to 6 months to begin to observe a cosmetic improvement in hirsutism, and the maximum effect may not be seen for up to 2 years.

Eflornithine hydrochloride cream, an irreversible inhibitor of epidermal androgenic activity, can be applied topically to treat facial hirsutism. It requires twice-daily application for up to 8 weeks for improvement to be seen and may be associated with rash, stinging, redness, and acne.

Suppression of excessive androgenic action generally diminishes further hair growth, but does not cause disappearance of existing hair. **To obtain good cosmetic results, some local hair removal is usually required in addition to medical therapy.** Mechanical methods of hair removal include shaving, depilatory creams, electrolysis, and laser therapy and/or intense pulsed light. Plucking of individual hairs should be discouraged because of discomfort and the risks of scarring and folliculitis. Regardless of the method of hair removal used, pharmacologic therapy should be continued in women with hyperandrogenemia to minimize hair regrowth.

All patients with PCOS who have chronic anovulation are at increased risk of developing menstrual irregularity. With tonic estrogen production without progesterone exposure, anovulatory women with PCOS also are at increased risk of developing endometrial hyperplasia as a precursor of endometrial cancer. **Medical management of abnormal vaginal bleeding or endometrial hyperplasia consists of estrogen-progestin oral contraceptives, cyclic or continuous oral progestins** (i.e., 5 to 10 mg of medroxyprogesterone

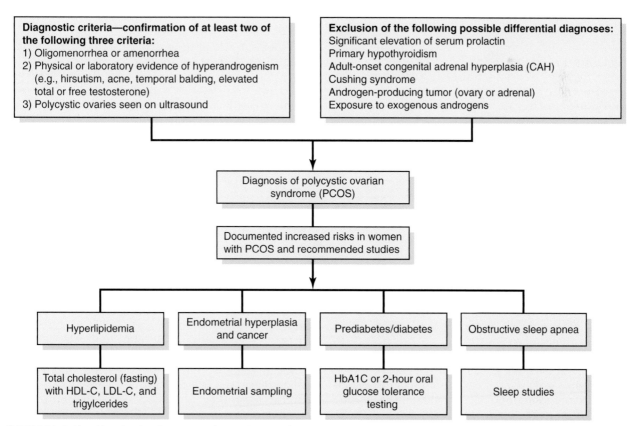

FIGURE 33-5 Algorithm for the diagnosis and investigation of patients with polycystic ovarian syndrome. *HbA1C,* Hemoglobin A1C; *HDL-C,* high-density lipoprotein cholesterol; *LDL-C,* low-density lipoprotein cholesterol.

acetate daily, 100 to 300 mg of micronized progesterone one to three times daily, **or 2.5 to 10 mg of norethindrone acetate daily), or a levonorgestrel-releasing intrauterine system (Mirena).**

INSULIN RESISTANCE AND POLYCYSTIC OVARIAN SYNDROME

Women with PCOS have a type of insulin resistance that is independent of, and additive with, that of obesity. Insulin resistance occurs in 50-70% of women with PCOS and in 95% of obese women with PCOS. Up to 40% of women with classic PCOS develop impaired glucose tolerance or type 2 diabetes mellitus by the fourth decade of life, with age and weight gain worsening glycemic control. **PCOS is associated with a fourfold increased prevalence of type 2 diabetes mellitus. Some patients with PCOS also may have several risk factors for cardiovascular disease, including increased abdominal adiposity, hypertension, hypertriglyceridemia, and low-density lipoprotein cholesterol levels and decreased high-density lipoprotein cholesterol levels.** Patients with PCOS with these findings should be counseled regarding weight loss, nutrition, exercise, and other lifestyle changes that will reduce their risk of developing diabetes mellitus and cardiovascular disease. In some cases, insulin-sensitizing agents such as **metformin** may be used to reduce insulin resistance and anovulation (see Chapter 34).

Controlling for body mass index, **women with PCOS are more likely to have sleep-disordered breathing and daytime sleepiness than healthy women,** which are additional risk factors for cardiovascular disease. Screening overweight and obese women with PCOS for symptoms of obstructive sleep apnea should be followed by polysomnography if necessary to make a definitive diagnosis. If obstructive sleep apnea is diagnosed, patients should be referred for appropriate therapy, including continuous positive airway pressure treatment. A flowchart for the diagnosis and investigation of patients with PCOS is shown in Figure 33-5.

Patients with adrenal hyperandrogenism, including late-onset CAH, can be treated with glucocorticoids (e.g., 0.25-mg dexamethasone every other day at bedtime). Many of these women, like those with PCOS, also require suppression of ovarian androgen secretion using combination oral contraceptives and antiandrogens.

Infertility and Assisted Reproductive Technologies

JOSEPH C. GAMBONE • INGRID A. RODI

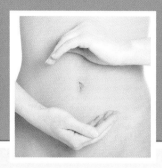

CLINICAL KEYS FOR THIS CHAPTER

- Eighty to eighty-five percent of fertile couples will conceive after 1 year of frequent attempts. *Infertility* is defined as an undesired absence of fertility for 1 year despite frequent intercourse. About 10-15% of couples in the United States are infertile. Most infertility is subfertility, and relatively few couples are sterile.
- A steady decrease in fertility begins at about age 24 years (female partner), when the fecundity (live-birth) rate is about 22% per monthly cycle, and declines to about 5% per cycle by 40 years of age. Evaluation for infertility should begin before 1 year when the female partner's age reaches 35 years or there is an obvious problem such as oligomenorrhea (fewer than nine menstrual cycles per year).
- The known causes of infertility include male coital problems, anatomic problems involving the uterus and/or the fallopian tubes, peritoneal problems such as endometriosis and/or pelvic adhesions, and problems with the quantity or quality of cervical mucus. About 10-15% of couples are found to have unexplained infertility.

- Evaluation of infertility in women younger than 35 years of age should begin at 1 year.
- Evaluation of sperm quantity and quality, ovulatory function, normal reproductive anatomy, and cervical mucus should occur after history-taking and physical examination are completed. Because about 40% of infertile couples have more than one factor present, the evaluation should be complete so that a second or third factor is not overlooked and thus left untreated. Conventional treatment includes ovarian stimulation with or without intrauterine insemination, destruction of endometriosis when found, and possible surgical intervention for uterine or tubal disease. About 50-60% of couples will conceive with adequate conventional treatments.
- Assisted reproductive technologies include in vitro fertilization, intracytoplasmic sperm injection, embryo transfer without or with embryo freezing, and oocyte donation for women with abnormal or absent ovarian function. Up to 85% of couples will conceive with the addition of adequate advanced treatment.

About 10-15% of couples in the United States are involuntarily infertile. **Couples are considered infertile after unsuccessfully attempting to achieve pregnancy for 1 year.** Most of these couples are more accurately described as have varying degrees of subfertility, with some of them conceiving spontaneously during and after episodes of fertility treatment. New assisted reproductive technologies (ARTs), such as controlled ovarian stimulation with or without intrauterine insemination (IUI), in vitro fertilization (IVF) and embryo transfer, and intracytoplasmic sperm injection (ICSI), are increasing the success of treatment for infertility and subfertility.

Infertility and the Physiology of Conception

Infertility is termed *primary* when it occurs without any prior pregnancy and *secondary* when it follows a previous conception. Some conditions, such as azoospermia (absence of sperm), endometriosis, and tubal occlusion are more common in couples with primary infertility, but virtually all conditions occur in both primary and secondary infertility.

For successful conception to occur, the male and female gametes must join at the optimal stage of maturation, followed by transportation of the newly

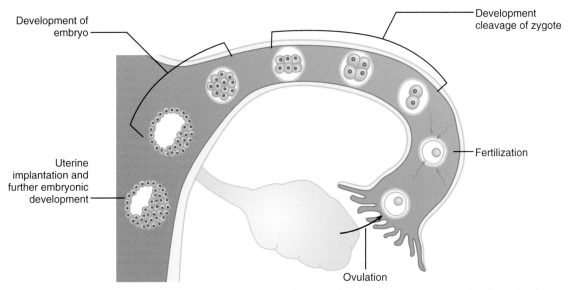

Development of
embryo

Development
cleavage of zygote

Fertilization

Uterine
implantation and
further embryonic
development

Ovulation

FIGURE 34-1 Sequence of events necessary for fertility: ovulation, fertilization, cleavage of zygote, continued embryo development, and implantation in the uterine cavity.

fertilized conceptus to the uterine cavity at a time when the endometrium is supportive of its continued development and implantation (Figure 34-1; see also Chapter 4). For these events to occur, the male and female reproductive systems must both be anatomically and physiologically intact, and coitus must occur with sufficient frequency for the semen to be deposited in close temporal relationship to the release of the oocyte from the follicle. **Even when fertilization occurs, it is estimated that more than 70% of resulting embryos are abnormal and fail to develop or become nonviable shortly after implantation.** According to the American Society for Reproductive Medicine (ASRM), early documented pregnancy loss (miscarriage) is considered a form of infertility when it is recurrent.

Considering the complexity of the reproductive process, it is remarkable that about **80-85% of couples achieve conception within 1 year.** More precisely, 25% conceive within the first month, 60% within 6 months, 75% by 9 months, and 90% by 18 months. The steadily decreasing rate of monthly conception demonstrated by these figures most likely reflects a spectrum of fertility extending from highly fertile couples to those with relative infertility (subfertility). After 18 months of unprotected sexual intercourse, the remaining couples have a low monthly conception rate without treatment, and many may have absolute defects that are preventing fertility (sterility). Table 34-1 lists the known causes of infertility as well as treatments for it, and Box 34-1 lists some important terms and definitions.

Evaluation of the Infertile Couple

Conception requires adequate function of multiple physiologic systems in both partners. **Infertility may result from either one major deficiency (e.g., tubal occlusion) or multiple minor deficiencies.** Failure to realize this important dictum may lead the inexperienced practitioner to overlook additional factors that might be more amenable to treatment than the one that has been identified. **Infertility in about 40% of infertile couples has multiple causes.** Therefore, for treatment to be most effective, a complete infertility evaluation should be performed for each couple. The psychological stress that is known to occur when conception is desired and is not occurring should not be overlooked or minimized. Participation in support groups such as **RESOLVE (www.resolve.org)** may help couples to cope with this stress and adjust to their situation. Couples should also be offered preconception counseling (see Chapter 7) and genetic screening for carrier status as part of their infertility care.

Age substantially decreases the rate of conception because of reduced embryo quality and likely reduced coital frequency. On the basis of a large study of donor insemination (ensuring proper timing of exposure), the strictly age-related reduction appears to be about one-third for women ages 35 to 45 years. It is reasonable to begin the basic evaluation at 6 months in older patients and to consider starting treatment for unexplained infertility earlier in women older than 35 years of age.

Evaluation and therapy may be started earlier (<1 year) when obvious defects are identified, or they may be delayed (e.g., when a correctable factor such as infrequent intercourse is identified).

In general, the first 6 to 8 months of evaluation involve relatively simple and noninvasive tests as well as the performance of a radiologic evaluation of tubal patency (hysterosalpingography [HSG]), which can sometimes have a therapeutic effect. **In some studies,**

TABLE 34-1

ETIOLOGIC FACTORS, DIAGNOSTIC TESTS, AND TREATMENT OPTIONS FOR INFERTILITY

Known Causes of Infertility	Diagnostic Tests and Procedures	Treatment Options	Comments
Male Factors (20-40%)	Semen analysis; testing for antisperm antibodies when suspected	IUI with washed sperm; IVF-ET with ICSI; donor insemination	Frequency of coitus without the use of toxic lubricants should be determined; paternal age could be a factor in miscarriage
Female Factors (50-65%)*			
Ovulation problems	Mid-luteal serum progesterone; LH predictor kits; serial ultrasounds	Clomiphene citrate or letrozole with or without hCG trigger for ovulation; lower-dose gonadotropins; IVF-ET; donor egg IVF-ET	Tests for ovulation are indirect and may be falsely positive; the only absolute proof of ovulation is pregnancy
Anatomic (uterine-tubal) problems	Hysterosalpingogram; saline infusion sonography; hysteroscopy; laparoscopy with chromotubation†	Tubal anastomosis to reverse sterilization procedures; tuboplasty for tubal damage; IVF-ET	When laparoscopy is performed, the tubes should be tested for patency; recent higher IVF-ET success rates make IVF-ET preferable to tubal surgery
Peritoneal problems (pelvic adhesions and endometriosis)	Laparoscopy with chromotubation† as part of infertility workup	Ablative procedures (electrocautery, laser) for endometriosis and lysis of adhesions; medical treatment for endometriosis (see Chapter 25); IVF-ET	Surgical removal of endometriomas may compromise ovarian reserve
Cervical mucus problems	Spinnbarkeit; postcoital test (Sims-Huhner); cultures for suspected infections	IUI with washed sperm; treatment for any detected infection	Postcoital test not performed by many practitioners, because of low predictive value
Unexplained Infertility (10-15%)	Laparoscopy to confirm diagnosis with negative findings	Ovarian stimulation; IVF-ET; donor insemination; donor IVF-ET; adoption	

hCG, Human chorionic gonadotropin; *ICSI*, intracytoplasmic sperm injection; *IUI*, intrauterine insemination; *IVF-ET*, in vitro fertilization and embryo transfer; *LH*, luteinizing hormone.
*Prevalence can vary in some populations due to differences in causes (e.g., infection or endometriosis).
†The use of a colored fluid such as indigo carmine to test for tubal patency.

BOX 34-1

IMPORTANT TERMS AND DEFINITIONS

- *Infertility:* Lack of fertility after 1 year of frequent attempts
- *Subfertility:* A decrease, but not an absence, of fertility potential
- *Sterility:* Complete inability to achieve fertility
- *Fecundity:* Probability of achieving a live birth in one menstrual cycle

---

use of an oil-based dye approximately doubled the success rate following HSG. Operative evaluation by laparoscopy is reserved for the small proportion of couples who have not conceived after 18 to 24 months or who have specific abnormalities or indications of a probable pelvic factor.

To keep the status of the evaluation in mind, it is helpful to arrange the workup under a series of five categories that can be mentally reviewed at each visit. Table 34-1 shows the approximate incidence and the tests involved in the evaluation of each factor. **In 10-15% of couples, no explanation can be found; their infertility is classified as unexplained.**

Etiologic Factors

MALE COITAL FACTORS

History

The evaluation of the male occurs early so that questions about coital frequency can be addressed and azoospermia or severe oligospermia or asthenospermia (low motility) can be identified. The history-taking from the male partner should cover any pregnancies previously sired; any history of genital tract infections, such as prostatitis or mumps orchitis; surgery or trauma to the male genitalia or inguinal region (e.g., hernia repair); and any exposure to lead, cadmium, radiation, or chemotherapeutic agents. Excessive consumption of alcohol or cigarettes or unusual exposure to environmental heat should be elicited. **Some medications, such as furantoins and calcium channel blockers, reduce sperm quality and/or function.**

Physical Examination

A physical examination is done upon referral to a urologist when semen analysis is abnormal. The normal location of the urethral meatus should be noted. An abnormal anatomic location could result in the deposition of semen in a less favorable location during intercourse. Testicular size should be estimated by comparison with a set of standard ovoids. The presence of a varicocele should be elicited by asking the patient to perform a Valsalva maneuver in the standing position.

Investigations

A semen analysis should be performed following a 2- to 4-day period of abstinence. The entire ejaculate should be collected in a clean, nontoxic container. Until relatively recently, the full range of normal variation was not appreciated. The characteristics of a normal semen analysis by percentile are shown in Table 34-2.

An excessive number of leukocytes (>10 per high-power field) may indicate infection, but special stains are required to differentiate polymorphonuclear leukocytes from immature germ cells. Semen quality varies greatly with repeated samples. **An accurate appraisal of abnormal semen requires at least three analyses.** Periodic reassessment is necessary.

Endocrinologic evaluation of the male with subnormal semen quality may uncover a specific cause. Hypothyroidism can cause infertility, but there is no place for the empirical use of thyroxine. **Low levels of gonadotropins and testosterone may indicate hypothalamic-pituitary failure. An elevated prolactin concentration may indicate the presence of a prolactin-producing pituitary tumor. An elevated level of follicle-stimulating hormone (FSH) generally indicates sub-**stantial parenchymal damage to the testes, as inhibin, produced by the Sertoli cells of the seminiferous tubules, provides the principal feedback control of FSH secretion. A response to any treatment is unlikely in the presence of an elevated level of FSH. However, the level of FSH is not helpful in predicting whether sperm will be recovered with testicular sperm extraction.

Treatment

The couple should be advised to have intercourse approximately every 1 to 2 days during the periovulatory period (e.g., days 12 through 16 of a 28-day cycle). **Because infrequent coitus is a common contributing factor, firm advice in this regard can be beneficial.** This "scheduled intercourse" can be disruptive and stressful, however, and insemination using the husband's or partner's sperm may relieve considerable pressure on a couple.

The woman should be advised to lie on her back for at least 15 minutes after coitus to prevent rapid loss of semen from the vagina. Lubricants may be toxic to sperm. **A nontoxic lubricant, Pre-Seed, has been developed for infertile couples.**

For optimal fertility, smoking and the use of alcohol or marijuana should be reduced or, preferably, stopped. The use of saunas, hot tubs, or tight underwear should be discouraged, as should exposure to other environments that raise scrotal temperature, because these factors may affect spermatogenesis.

Low semen volume may provide insufficient contact with the cervical mucus for adequate sperm migration to occur. When a high semen volume coexists with a low count, infertility may result because a lower density of sperm contacts the cervical mucus. **At present, these abnormalities of volume (as well as other factors mentioned below) are most commonly treated with sperm washing and IUI. Figure 34-2 illustrates the method of IUI.**

If low sperm density (oligospermia) or low motility (asthenospermia) is caused by hypothalamic-pituitary failure, injections of human menopausal gonadotropins (hMGs) may be effective. The suppressive effects of **hyperprolactinemia** on hypothalamic function **can be reversed by the administration of a dopamine agonist such as bromocriptine or cabergoline. When low semen quality coexists with a varicocele** (dilation and incompetence of the spermatic veins), **improved semen quality, particularly motility, may occur with ligation of this venous plexus.** Various medications (clomiphene, human chorionic gonadotropin [hCG], testosterone, letrozole, and hMG) have been tried when no cause is apparent (idiopathic oligoasthenospermia), but none has proved consistently effective. Because approximately 3 months is required for spermatogenesis and sperm transportation to occur, frequent semen checks during treatment are unnecessary and serve only to discourage the patient.

TABLE 34-2

WORLD HEALTH ORGANIZATION REFERENCE VALUES FOR SEMEN CHARACTERISTICS					
	Percentiles				
Characteristics	5th*	25th	50th	75th	95th
Semen volume (mL)	1.5	2.7	3.7	4.8	6.8
Sperm concentration (million/mL)	15	41	73	116	213
Total sperm (million/mL)	39	142	255	422	802
Total motility (%)†	40	53	61	69	78
Normal forms (%)	4	9	15	24.5	44

Data were generated from semen parameters of fertile men whose partners achieved a pregnancy within 12 months.
*Values in the 5th percentile are considered abnormal.
†Percentage of progressive plus nonprogressive.

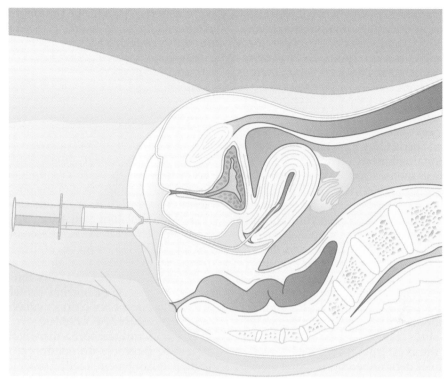

FIGURE 34-2 Illustration of the method of intrauterine insemination (IUI). Washed sperm are gently injected into the uterine cavity at the estimated time of ovulation. Untreated semen should not be used for IUI.

If semen quality cannot be improved, IUI with close timing of the insemination to the precise point of ovulation may be effective. By washing and concentrating the sperm into a small volume by centrifugation, large numbers of sperm can be placed into the uterus. When unwashed sperm is used it should be placed only on the cervix and not inside the uterus. Accurate timing may be accomplished either by measurement of daily luteinizing hormone (LH) concentrations or by controlled stimulation of the cycle with clomiphene or hMG, followed by administration of hCG when follicular diameter, as visualized by ultrasonography, indicates maturity. Insemination may then be carried out within a few hours of ovulation, which occurs 36 to 44 hours following the LH surge or hCG injection. When urinary LH testing is used, there is a delay of several hours between the onset of the surge and the positive urine test. It is advisable to test in the afternoon or evening, with insemination the following morning.

IVF is an effective treatment for the male factor because, with ICSI (intracytoplasmic sperm injection), only one motile sperm (with the tail removed) for each egg is required. Finally, insemination with donor sperm is effective when the male factor is refractory to treatment.

OVULATORY FACTORS

History

Most women with regular cycles (every 22 to 35 days) are ovulating, particularly if they have premenstrual molimina (e.g., breast changes, bloating, and mood change). Recent studies indicate reduced fecundity associated with very irregular cycles. A discussion of oligomenorrhea and its underlying causes is presented in Chapter 33.

Investigations

The simplest screening tests for confirming reasonably normal ovulation are serial measurement of urinary LH, which assesses the duration of luteal function, and the mid-luteal level of serum progesterone, which assesses the level of luteal function. The interval from the urinary LH surge to the onset of menses should be at least 12 days. An older test of ovulation, the basal body temperature, is now seldom used. A progesterone level of greater than 5 ng/mL indicates ovulatory activity, but mid-luteal concentrations usually exceed 10 ng/mL in cycles in which conception has occurred. Because of the marked pulsatile secretion of progesterone, a level between 5 and 40 ng/mL can be found in the normal luteal phase.

In spite of ovulation, an inadequate luteal phase may be responsible for infertility. **Endometrial biopsy, considered for many years to accurately reflect luteal function, has recently been shown to be a very imprecise test, causing most practitioners to abandon it as a tool for assessing ovulation.**

Treatment

Use of fertility drugs such as clomiphene citrate or gonadotropins will correct any luteal insufficiency in women with unexplained infertility.

In women whose menses are less frequent than every 35 days (oligomenorrhea), it is helpful to induce more frequent ovulation, thus increasing the opportunity for pregnancy and improving the ability to time coitus. Ovulation induction should always be preceded by a thorough workup for thyroid disease, hyperprolactinemia, and polycystic ovarian syndrome (PCOS) (see Chapter 33) because conditions causing anovulation (e.g., hypothyroidism) may be worsened by pregnancy or may complicate it. In addition, ovarian failure seldom responds to attempts to induce ovulation.

The choice of the most appropriate technique for ovulation induction is determined by the patient's specific diagnosis. With this approach, regular ovulation can be restored in more than 90% of anovulatory women. Provided that these patients persevere with treatment for an adequate period of time and no other infertility factors are present, their fertility should approximate that of normal women.

Pituitary insufficiency requires the injection of hMG (FSH and LH). Hypothalamic amenorrhea is caused by infrequent or absent pulsatile release of gonadotropin-releasing hormone (GnRH). GnRH is highly effective when administered in small pulses subcutaneously or intravenously in these patients every 90 to 120 minutes by using a small, portable infusion pump. Because this treatment is not currently available in the United States, hMG is used instead, but with a much higher risk of multiple pregnancy. **Hyperprolactinemia and its suppressive effect on the hypothalamus are specifically treated by use of dopamine agonists such as bromocriptine (Parlodel) or cabergoline (Dostinex).**

Most of the remaining patients with anovulation have some form of PCOS and generally respond to clomiphene, an orally active antiestrogen. Anovulation occurs in patients with polycystic ovaries because of chronic, mild suppression of FSH release. These women often have increased ovarian and adrenal androgen production. Clomiphene, by inhibiting the negative feedback effect of endogenous estrogen, causes a rise of FSH and stimulation of follicular maturation. One of the principal causes of excessive ovarian androgen production is higher circulating insulin concentrations because of insulin resistance. Metformin can also be used alone and may result in ovulation and pregnancy in some women. Recently, the aromatase inhibitor letrozole has been reported to be superior to clomiphene for ovulation induction, particularly in women with PCOS. Letrozole is currently not approved for this use by the U.S. Food and Drug Administration (FDA).

Other less frequently used treatments to induce ovulation in PCOS are laparoscopic "ovarian drilling," whereby multiple small craters are created by using a laser or cautery, and dexamethasone, which increases the ovarian response to clomiphene. Surgery is not often recommended, due to the possibility of causing scarring around the ovaries and tubes.

If ovulation does not occur with clomiphene or letrozole, follicular development may be occurring, but the normal LH surge may fail to occur. This results in lack of follicular rupture. **Assessment by serial pelvic ultrasonography and carefully timed hCG administration may lead to normal ovulation. If follicular maturation is not occurring, ovulation induction will require low-dose FSH or hMG.**

The main complications of ovulation induction are related to excessive stimulation of the ovaries. Substantial enlargement of the ovary with clomiphene citrate can generally be avoided by examining the ovaries before each treatment course and by using the lowest effective dose. Cystic ovarian enlargement is not an uncommon complication of hMG treatment, but it almost always regresses spontaneously. **The hyperstimulation syndrome is a serious illness associated with marked ovarian enlargement and exudation of fluid and protein into the peritoneal cavity.** The use of serum estradiol (E2) measurements, transvaginal ultrasonic scanning, and low-dose gonadotropin have greatly reduced the incidence of hyperstimulation syndrome. By starting at 50 to 75 U and increasing the dose by 25 to 50 U every 7 days if follicular maturation is not detected, a marked reduction in the incidence of multifollicular development, hyperstimulation, and multiple pregnancy can be achieved. **Multiple pregnancy occurs in 8-10% of clomiphene conceptions, with less than 1% of cases exceeding twins.** Multiple gestation occurs in 20-30% of hMG conceptions, and 5% of these conceptions are multiple births of more than two. Ultrasonic monitoring reduces this risk if the hCG is withheld in the presence of an excessive number of mature follicles. **Current use of a lower-dose regimen of hMG or pure FSH reduces the overall risk of multiple pregnancy to about 5%.**

CERVICAL FACTORS

During the few days before ovulation, the cervix produces profuse watery mucus (called *spinnbarkeit*) that exudes out of the cervix to contact the seminal ejaculate. To assess its quality, the patient must be seen during the immediate preovulatory phase (days 12 to

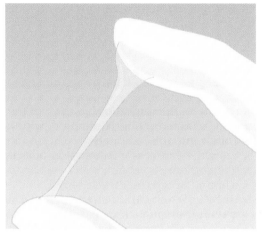

FIGURE 34-3 The cervix produces profuse watery mucus during the few days before ovulation. The *spinnbarkeit* refers to the ability of the mucus to "stretch" at least 6.5 cm.

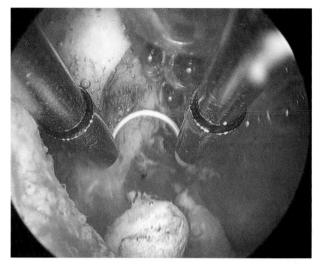

FIGURE 34-4 A significant submucosal polyp seen at the time of hysteroscopy.

14 of a 28-day cycle). Spuriously abnormal results can be reduced by timing the test to the morning after the urinary LH surge.

Investigations

The amount and clarity of the mucus is recorded. **The spinnbarkeit may be tested by touching the mucus with a piece of pH paper and lifting vertically. The mucus should extend in a thread to at least 6 cm (Figure 34-3).** The pH should be 6.5 or greater. **A post-coital (Sims-Huhner) test may be performed 2 to 12 hours after intercourse to assess the number and motility of spermatozoa that have entered the cervical canal.** The number of sperm, however, does not correlate well with semen quality, recovery of sperm from the cul-de-sac, or subsequent fertility. Consequently, the predictive value of this test for fertility is low, and many practitioners have abandoned this postcoital test. Empirical treatment with IUI for the cervical factor on a presumptive basis or when clomiphene is used (antiestrogenic effect) may avoid the morbidity and expense of injectable fertility drugs (gonadotropins).

Treatment

Any cervical infection should be treated by prescribing a 10-day course of doxycycline, 100 mg twice daily, for both partners. Persistent chronic cervicitis may be treated with cryotherapy if antibiotic treatment fails. Poor mucus quality can be treated with **washed sperm and IUI.**

UTERINE AND TUBAL FACTORS

Abnormalities of the uterine cavity are seldom the cause of infertility. Large submucosal myomas or endometrial polyps, as seen in Figure 34-4, may be associated with infertility and first-trimester spontaneous abortions (miscarriages). The role of intramural myomas is not clear, although myomectomy in some uncontrolled studies has been associated with conception in 40-50% of couples and some other studies with IVF have shown reduced conception with intramural myomas. Subserosal fibroids (see Figure 19-3) do not affect fecundity.

Tubal occlusion may occur at three locations: the fimbrial end, the mid-segment, or the isthmus-cornu. Fimbrial occlusion is by far the most common. Prior salpingitis is a common cause of tubal occlusion, although about one-half of cases are unassociated with any such history. Isthmic-cornual occlusion can be congenital or caused by mucus plugs, endometriosis, tubal adenomyosis, or prior infection. Mid-segment occlusion can be seen following surgery or infection with tuberculosis.

Investigations

Tubal abnormalities may be diagnosed by HSG (hysterosalpingography) or laparoscopy. To perform HSG, an occlusive cannula is placed in the cervix, and the instillation of a radiopaque dye is followed by image intensification under fluoroscopy. Selected radiographs are taken for permanent documentation (Figure 34-5). Anesthesia generally is not required. A water-soluble dye is used initially to confirm tubal patency because of the adverse effects of sequestration of an oil-based dye within the lumen of an occluded tube. If patency is confirmed, an oil-based dye (if available) may then be instilled because of its prominent therapeutic effect in women with unexplained infertility. If only one tube fills with dye, the HSG should be considered normal, as this finding is usually, although not

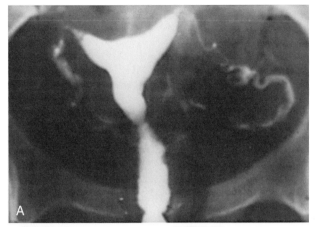

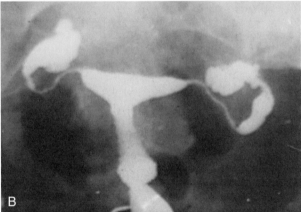

FIGURE 34-5 Normal hysterosalpingograms showing free spill of contrast material (**A**) and bilateral hydrosalpinges (**B**).

invariably, caused by the dye following the path of least resistance.

Serious infections can result from HSG. A normal pelvic examination and prophylactic doxycycline should reduce this risk to a minimum.

Treatment

In most circumstances, microsurgical tuboplasty is more effective than conventional surgical techniques for reversal of tubal occlusion. About 60-80% of patients achieve pregnancy after reversal of sterilization using microsurgical techniques. Tubal anastomosis may be carried out laparoscopically, with good results in experienced hands.

When performed for fimbrial occlusion, neosalpingostomy is associated with a success rate of 20-30%, although it has reached 40% with long-term follow-up. Most often this is done by laparoscopy. Because a hydrosalpinx reduces the success rate of IVF by about 50%, any hydrosalpinx not repaired should be removed, or its communication with the uterus can be interrupted by using cautery or clips.

For an isthmic-cornual occlusion caused by disease, clearing the obstruction with oral danazol has been reported when the occlusion coexists with peritoneal endometriosis. Selective catheterization has restored patency in the majority of proximal occlusions and should be the first line of therapy. Microsurgical resection and reanastomosis is associated with a 50-60% pregnancy rate. **If the intramural portion of the tube is occluded, reimplantation is required, with a new opening made into the endometrial cavity.** A substantially lower rate of success is achieved in this circumstance; a laparotomy is required; and similar success can be achieved with a single cycle of IVF.

At least 10% of conceptions after repair of diseased tubes are ectopic pregnancies. Anastomosis of healthy tubes carries a risk of ectopic pregnancy of about 3-5%. This possibility must always be considered in the management of an early pregnancy following tuboplasty. As IVF and embryo transfer success rates continue to increase and costs decrease, this procedure may be preferred to tubal surgery in most cases.

PERITONEAL FACTORS

Laparoscopy identifies previously unsuspected pathologic conditions in about 30% of women with unexplained infertility. Endometriosis is the most common finding. Periadnexal adhesions may be found and may hold the fimbriae away from the ovarian surface or entrap the released oocyte.

Endometriosis may interfere with tubal motility, cause tubal obstruction, or cause adhesions that directly disturb the pickup of the oocyte by the fimbriae. Other mechanisms of endometriosis-associated infertility must exist as well, because even minimal endometriosis has some negative effect. In a randomized study of laparoscopic cautery versus no treatment for minimal endometriosis, treatment resulted in one of eight affected women conceiving. These same women, however, may conceive with other treatments used for unexplained infertility. **There is a strong trend toward omitting laparoscopy in women who have no symptoms indicating peritoneal disease and who have a normal pelvic examination, a normal HSG result, and a normal pelvic ultrasound.** A serum titer for antichlamydial antibodies may be helpful if this approach is taken, to avoid overlooking occult pelvic adhesions.

Treatment of endometriosis depends on its extent; this is discussed fully in Chapter 25. **If substantial adhesions or endometriomas are present, laparoscopic surgery is preferable because these conditions generally do not respond to medical management. With advanced operative laparoscopic techniques, most endometriosis can be removed or ablated** without laparotomy by using advanced instrumentation, lasers, or fulguration.

Danazol, GnRH analogues (agonists and antagonists), or oral medroxyprogesterone acetate are effective treatments for symptomatic disease, with continuous oral contraceptive therapy being generally inferior. If minimal disease with scattered implants is found, simple cautery at the time of laparoscopy should suffice.

Periadnexal adhesions may be lysed by operative laparoscopy. Microsurgical techniques diminish adhesions. The most effective adjunct in preventing recurrent scarring is the placement of an artificial tissue barrier, separating the raw surfaces during the early period of healing.

Because of the current high success rate with IVF, that treatment is very often given as an alternative to the above surgeries. It is particularly important to conserve ovarian function as much as possible. IVF is preferable to removal of an endometrioma because of the compromised ovarian function that often results from ovarian surgery.

Unexplained Infertility

No cause is found for infertility in 10-15% of patients who have documented ovulation, normal semen analyses, and a normal HSG result. The problem may be primarily one of sperm transportation because IUI with washed sperm appears to increase the rate of conception. Some studies have shown subtle abnormalities of follicular growth and ovulation, partly explaining the increased fecundity associated with fertility drugs.

In other cases, a defect in the ability of the sperm to fertilize the egg may be present because a lower rate of fertilization is noted in couples with unexplained infertility who undergo IVF compared with couples in whom there is a tubal cause for infertility. Another male problem that may not be detected by routine evaluation is the presence of antisperm antibodies.

Other possible mechanisms of unexplained infertility include minimal endometriosis and mildly reduced ovarian reserve (reduced number of normal oocytes without hormonal abnormalities such as elevated FSH levels).

IUI, usually with controlled ovarian stimulation (stimulation of multiple follicles with clomiphene citrate or letrozole and/or gonadotropins and hCG timing of insemination), is employed next. The final therapeutic option is IVF.

Assisted Reproductive Technologies

The last resort for infertile couples with any of the aforementioned factors and failure of lesser treatments is the procedure of IVF and embryo transfer (Figure 34-6). In most cases of tubal occlusion in which the rate of success with tubal repair is low (<30%), IVF is preferable to surgery because of the more rapid conception rate and the lower ectopic pregnancy rate (<3% vs. >6% following tubal surgery). Even severe male factors can be effectively treated with IVF by using ICSI (intracytoplasmic sperm injection), with fertilization rates of 60-70% of injected oocytes and pregnancy rates similar to those of nonmale factor IVF (30-35%).

TECHNIQUE

A GnRH analogue, such as the GnRH agonist (GnRH-a), is given to prevent premature LH release. It is commonly started in the mid-luteal phase or overlapped with an oral contraceptive. After ovarian suppression (with GnRH-a), the ovaries are stimulated with FSH or hMG, or both, on the second or third day of the next cycle. Follicular size is assessed by transvaginal ultrasonic scanning.

An injection of hCG (usually 10,000 U) is given on the basis of follicular size and estradiol levels to induce the resumption of meiosis and completion of oocyte maturation. Thirty-five hours after the hCG injection, multiple oocytes are aspirated under transvaginal ultrasonic guidance. An antagonist (which is the FDA-approved analogue for use in IVF) may be used instead of the agonist and has the advantage of then allowing an agonist to be used to trigger ovulation rather than using hCG as the trigger. This has been shown to reduce the incidence of ovarian hyperstimulaton in some studies.

After a further period of in vitro maturation, washed sperm are added or a single sperm is injected (ICSI) into each oocyte. Fertilization may be identified 14 to 18 hours after insemination by the visualization of two pronuclei. The conceptus is then transferred to the uterine cavity 2 to 4 days after oocyte retrieval (early transfer) or at 5 to 6 days (blastocyst stage) by means of a tiny catheter (see Figure 34-6). In some cases, the hatching process is aided by making an artificial opening in the zona pellucida ("assisted hatching"). Surplus embryos not transferred at the time of the IVF treatment can be frozen, stored, and transferred in a later menstrual cycle in the event of failure or for additional pregnancies. As freezing-and-thawing methods have improved, many programs are not transferring fresh embryos in highly stimulated cycles when egg retrieval occurs. This "freeze-all" method can allow for the performance of preimplantation studies. Selected embryos are then thawed and transferred in more physiologic cycles. This technique may have other advantages in terms of pregnancy complications and does not decrease the overall success rate (see Figure 34-6, B).

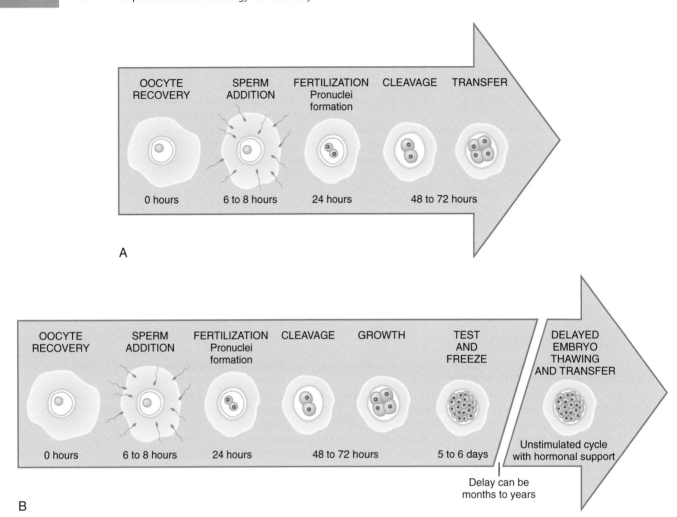

FIGURE 34-6 Approximate time-course for in vitro fertilization and embryo transfer in same cycle as stimulation (A) or delayed after embryo freezing and thawing (B).

OUTCOMES

The pregnancy rate with IVF is highly variable from center to center because of the complexity of the techniques required, whereas the pregnancy rate with gamete intrafallopian transfer, a technique whereby oocytes and washed sperm are mixed and placed into the fallopian tube or tubes, is more consistent. **The mean live delivery rate per retrieval with IVF currently approximates 30-40%, with about 2-3% of pregnancies being ectopic. This rate of ectopic pregnancy is at least double the rate with spontaneous conceptions (about 1%). The site of the ectopic pregnancy may also be affected by ARTs.** Most studies have not shown any significant increase of fetal abnormalities when treated couples are compared with subfertile couples (not fertile ones) who conceive without fertility treatment.

EGG DONATION

It is possible to achieve pregnancy with IVF and embryo transfer using donor eggs. This has a higher success rate than regular IVF (approximately 50%). The eggs generally come from young fertile women (known or anonymous volunteers). The recipient can be programmed for optimal uterine receptivity by replacement doses of estradiol and progesterone. Estradiol and progesterone must be continued until the placenta takes over late in the first trimester. **The excellent success of egg donation mandates the conservation of the uterus whenever future fertility is desired, even if the ovaries must be removed.**

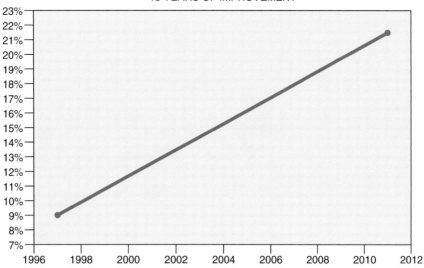

FIGURE 34-7 Average percentages of live-birth rates in women younger than 38 years of age resulting from nondonor, fresh embryo transfers from 1997 through 2011. (Data from Centers for Disease Control and Prevention (CDC), 1997-2012. Available from www.cdc.gov/art/reports/index.html.)

Overall Success of Infertility Therapy

Conventional therapies, when adequately performed, result in conception in about 50-60% of infertile couples, and the application of the advanced treat-ments described above should enable about 80-85% of couples who are infertile to conceive. The success rate of IVF as reported to the Centers for Disease Control and Prevention (CDC) has been improving each year, as shown in Figure 34-7.

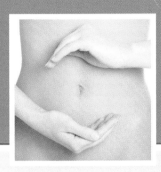

Menopause and Perimenopause

JOSEPH C. GAMBONE

CLINICAL KEYS FOR THIS CHAPTER

- The "climacteric" refers to the phase in a woman's reproductive life when a gradual decline in ovarian function results in decreased sex steroid production with its sequelae. Because this phase is a normal consequence of the aging process, it should not be considered an endocrinopathy. Menopause refers to the last menstrual period, and this occurs on average at age 51.5 years. The perimenopause refers to the several years of more gradually decreasing ovarian function that may be associated with the symptoms of reduced estrogen levels.

- Men produce gametes (sperm) frequently and well into their seventh and eighth decade of life. Women are born with all of the gametes (eggs) they will ever have. At birth, several million oocytes are present in both ovaries. Through a process of atresia (physiologic loss), about 400,000 oocytes remain in both ovaries at the time of menarche. Generally, only about 400 oocytes will ovulate during the reproductive life, which typically extends from age 15 to 50 years, when no more effective oocytes remain. Menopause represents the last uterine bleeding from hormones that have been produced by a responsive ovarian follicle. It also represents the end of a woman's reproductive life.

- The signs and symptoms of the perimenopause and menopause are related to progressively decreasing secretion of estrogen from the ovarian follicle. The symptoms and signs include hot flashes, insomnia, irritability, and memory loss early, with vaginal atrophy and dryness developing later. Calcium loss from bone is a frequent sign of the loss of estrogenic effect. Stress urinary incontinence and collagen loss from skin are widely reported.

- Widespread hormone replacement at or before the menopause has now evolved into more selective and shorter-term hormonal therapy for those women who have significant menopausal symptoms. Prospective studies in both the U.S. and the United Kingdom have confirmed some benefits (less hot flashes, mood changes, bone loss, and colorectal cancer) but have also documented increased risk of breast cancer and stroke when hormones (estrogen and progestin) are used to treat symptoms.

- First-line treatment for the menopause should begin with lifestyle changes such as diet and exercise to control mild to moderate symptoms, reserving hormonal therapy for those women who have significant problems. Women with a uterus need combined (estrogen and progestin) hormonal therapy to protect the uterine lining from unopposed estrogen that could lead to hyperplasia and cancer. Careful consideration of the risk to benefit ratio and adequate informed consent should precede menopausal hormonal therapy.

As average life expectancy increases, in the United States and elsewhere (Table 35-1), women and men are often living well into their ninth decade of life. The preservation of their quality of life in terms of both physical and mental activity is a high priority for them. Many women will live for 30 to 40 years after reproductive function ends.

The "climacteric" refers to a period of time when decreasing reproductive capacity occurs in both men and women. For women, this period in their lives is marked mostly by the last menstrual period or menopause and a variable time leading up to the last menses called the perimenopause.

Menopause and Perimenopause

Menopause literally refers to the last menstrual period. The exact time of menopause is usually determined in retrospect; that is, 1 year without menses. **In most women, menopause occurs between the ages of 50 and 55 years, with an average age of 51.5 years,** but some have their menopause before the age of 40

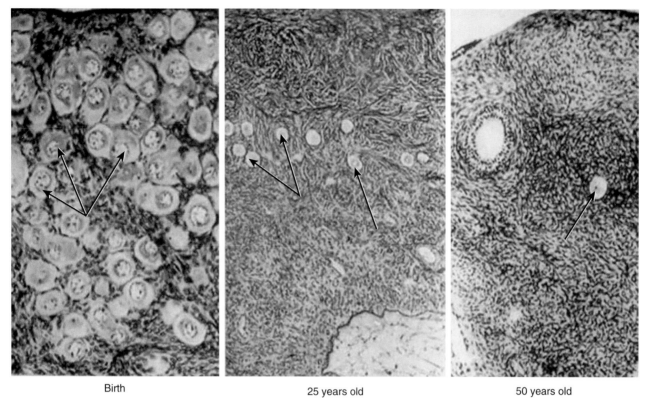

Birth   25 years old   50 years old

FIGURE 35-1 Histologic illustration of the density of oocytes *(arrows)* from birth to menopause. Note the abundance of eggs at birth and only an occasional one at or near menopause.

TABLE 35-1

INCREASING LIFE EXPECTANCY IN WOMEN, 1900-2015	
Year	Age
1900	48 yr
1950	72 yr
2000	79 yr
2015	>80 yr

(premature menopause), whereas a few may menstruate until they are in their 60s.

Women are born with between 1.5 and 2 million oocytes (primary ovarian follicles) and reach menarche (first menstruation) with about 400,000 potentially responsive eggs. Figure 35-1 illustrates the decreasing density of oocytes from birth until age 50 years. Most women ovulate about 400 times between menarche and menopause and during this time, nearly all other oocytes are lost through atresia. When the oocytes either have all ovulated or become atretic, the ovary becomes minimally responsive to pituitary gonadotropins, the ovarian production of estrogen and progesterone ends, and ovarian androgen production is reduced. These hormonal alterations often result in unpleasant and even harmful physical, psychological, and sexual changes in postmenopausal women, which can have a negative impact on their quality of life.

Menopause rarely occurs as a sudden loss of ovarian function. **For some years before menopause, the ovary begins to show signs of impending failure.** Anovulation becomes common, with resulting unopposed production of estrogen and irregular menstrual cycles. Occasionally, heavy menses, endometrial hyperplasia, and increasing mood and emotional changes may occur. In some women, hot flashes (or flushes) and night-sweats begin well before the last menses. **These perimenopausal symptoms may occur 3 to 5 years before there is complete loss of menses and postmenopausal levels of hormones are reached.**

Some women may suffer a more abrupt loss of estrogen. This usually occurs following a surgical intervention that removes or damages the ovaries or their blood supply or occasionally, following chemotherapy or radiotherapy for cancer. Women who are overweight may continue to produce estrogen indirectly in substantial amounts for many years after menopause. **Androstenedione from the ovary and the adrenal gland is converted in peripheral fat tissues to estrone, which is then capable of maintaining the vagina, skin,**

and bone in reasonable cellular tone and reducing the incidence of flashes. Although this unopposed estrogen may be beneficial to women in terms of symptom control, it is also responsible for the increased incidence of endometrial or breast cancer among obese women. It is important that all postmenopausal women have regular breast examinations and, if abnormal vaginal bleeding occurs, endometrial sampling.

PREMATURE MENOPAUSE

Women who reach menopause before the age of 40 years are said to have premature menopause or premature ovarian failure. Other causes of premature ovarian failure include abnormal karyotypes involving the X chromosome, the carrier state of the fragile X syndrome, galactosemia, and autoimmune disorders that may cause failure of a number of other endocrine organs.

Ovarian Senescence and Hormonal Changes

The ovary produces a sequence of hormones during a normal menstrual cycle. Under the influence of luteinizing hormone (LH), cholesterol from the liver is used to produce the androgens, androstenedione and testosterone, in the theca cells of the ovarian follicle. They, in turn, are converted in the granulosa cells immediately surrounding the oocytes into estrogen. Following ovulation, the luteal cells (luteinized granulosa cells) manufacture and secrete progesterone as well as estrogen. The synthesis of these sex hormones depends on the presence of viable follicles and ovarian stroma and the production of follicle-stimulating hormone (FSH) and LH in adequate amounts to induce their biosynthetic activity.

ESTROGEN

Following menopause, estradiol (E2) values decline (to only 10 to 50 pg/mL), **but estrone levels may increase.** Estrone (E1) can be produced by peripheral conversion of androstenedione from the ovary and the adrenal gland. In some women, the amount of postmenopausal estrogen may be considerable.

ANDROGENS

Women normally produce significant quantities of androgens by the metabolic conversion of cholesterol to both androstenedione and testosterone. Although the major portion of androgen is aromatized to estrogen, some androgen circulates. After menopause, there is a decrease in the level of circulating androgens, with androstenedione falling to less than half that found in normal menstruating young women, whereas testosterone gradually diminishes over about 3 to 4 years. **Even though postmenopausal women produce less**

androgens, they tend to be more sensitive to them because of the lost opposition of estrogen. This sometimes results in unwelcome changes such as excessive facial hair growth and decreased breast size.

PROGESTERONE

With anovulation during the climacteric and ovarian failure after the menopause, the production of progesterone declines to low levels. The minimal progesterone present is insufficient to induce those cytoplasmic enzymes (estradiol dehydrogenase and estrone sulfuryltransferase) that convert estradiol to the less potent estrone sulfate and to reduce the levels of cellular estrogen receptors. Altogether, this may result in increased estrogen-induced mitosis in the endometrium. The absence of progesterone also prevents the secretory histologic transformation in the endometrium and its subsequent sloughing. As a consequence, perimenopause is often associated with irregular vaginal bleeding, endometrial hyperplasia and cellular atypia, and an increased incidence of endometrial cancer.

GONADOTROPINS

The two gonadotropins, LH and FSH, are produced in the anterior pituitary gland. **When levels of estrogen are low, the arcuate nucleus and paraventricular nucleus in the hypothalamus are freed from negative feedback and are able to secrete increasing amounts of gonadotropin-releasing hormone (GnRH) into the pituitary portal circulation.** This, in turn, stimulates an increased release of LH and FSH into the circulation. The higher central nervous system neurotransmissions responsible for the increased pulsatile release of GnRH (and subsequent gonadotropin release) are also thought to have parallel effects elsewhere in the hypothalamus, especially in the body temperature control region. This leads to the sudden induction of increased skin blood flow and perspiration, the hot flash, which is so characteristic of the menopause. Typical levels of FSH in postmenopausal women are greater than 40 IU/L.

Clinical Manifestations

Loss of estrogen is associated with urogenital atrophy and osteoporosis (Table 35-2). Although postmenopausal women have a higher incidence of heart disease and of cancer, the relationship between these adverse events and reduced endogenous estrogen production, as well as the effects of hormonal therapy on these adverse events, remains controversial.

GENERAL SYMPTOMS

About 85% of women experience hot flashes as they pass through the climacteric, but about half of these women are not seriously disturbed by them. For about

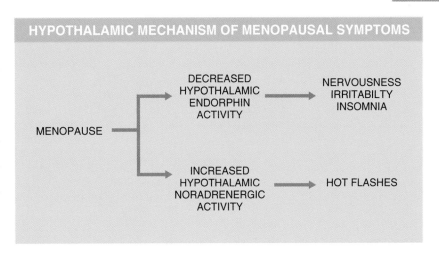

FIGURE 35-2 Combined effect of decreased endorphins and increased adrenergic activity at the time of decreasing estrogen (menopause and perimenopause). Although the exact mechanism of the menopausal (perimenopausal) hot flash is not known, evidence suggests that hypothalamic norepinephrine acts as a trigger for this temporary event that results in disordered thermoregulation. Core body temperature may actually decrease slightly at the time of the hot flash, with skin temperatures increasing from 2 to 10 degrees over a short period of time.

TABLE 35-2

CONSEQUENCES OF LOSS OF ESTROGEN

Symptoms (early)	Hot flushes (flashes) Insomnia Irritability Mood disturbances
Physical changes (intermediate)	Urogenital atrophy Stress (urinary) incontinence Skin collagen loss
Diseases (late)	Osteoporosis Dementia of the Alzheimer type (possible) Cardiovascular disease (unclear relationship) Cancers, for example, colon (unclear relationship)

40% of affected women, the hot flash is a most distressing experience. Flashes may occur as frequently as every 30 to 40 minutes, but more often they occur about 8 to 15 times daily. There may be associated sweating, dizziness, and palpitations. Often, the hot flash may awaken the woman at night and impair the quality of her sleep. Although the exact mechanism that triggers a hot flash is not known, they are probably caused by excessive noradrenergic activity. Studies show a significant rise in plasma norepinephrine before most hot flashes. There is also a related decrease in endorphin levels. **As a consequence of frequent flashes at night, the woman may experience increased fatigue, and irritability.** Figure 35-2 illustrates the combined effect of decreasing endorphins and increasing adrenergic activity on sleep-depriving hot flashes and mood.

Women are often given sedatives, hypnotics, or psychotropic drugs in an attempt to relieve the symptoms caused by deficiency of estrogen. **Some complain of confusion, loss of memory, lethargy, and inability to cope, as well as mild depression.** In addition, the hypoestrogenic state may be associated with a **loss of the sense of balance,** possibly resulting in an increased risk of falls. Many of these symptoms improve considerably when appropriate hormonal therapy (estrogen and a progestin or estrogen alone) is initiated. **Severe or even sustained moderate depression should never be attributed solely to climacteric hormonal changes.**

UROGENITAL SYMPTOMS

The vagina is very sensitive to estrogen, and it responds to this hormone by producing a thick moist epithelium with an acidic secretion (pH of about 4.0). The absence of estrogen results in a thin, dry epithelium with an alkaline secretion (pH > 7.0). **The postmenopausal vagina shrinks in diameter and splits and tears easily.** Atrophic vaginitis may result in unpleasant dryness, discharge, and severe dyspareunia.

Because the bladder and vagina are derived from the same embryologic tissue, it is not surprising that **some postmenopausal women also complain of urinary symptoms such as frequency, urgency, nocturia, and urinary incontinence.** Hormonal therapy markedly improves atrophic vaginitis but cannot prevent or treat urinary incontinence.

Osteoporosis

Remodeling of bone continues throughout life, but with estrogen deprivation, osteoclastic activity far exceeds the osteoblasts' ability to lay down bone. Under these conditions, osteopenia and finally osteoporosis occur. Figure 35-3 compares normal bone and bone with severe osteopenia. An early clinical sign of osteoporosis is a loss of height greater than 1.5 inches because of vertebral compression fracture, which may

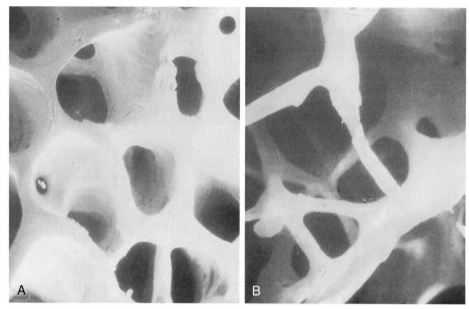

FIGURE 35-3 The appearance of normal bone **(A)** and bone with severe osteopenia **(B)** as seen on a dual-energy x-ray absorptiometry (DEXA) scan. Osteopenic bone is much more susceptible to fracture and deformity.

BOX 35-1

KNOWN RISK FACTORS FOR OSTEOPOROSIS IN WOMEN

- Family history of osteoporosis
- Reduced ovarian function (decreased estrogen production)
- Slender body composition
- Caucasian and Asian ethnicity
- Sedentary life style
- Cigarette smoking
- Thyroid excess
- Use of corticosteroid or anticonvulsant medications

BOX 35-2

BONE DENSITY SCREENING BEFORE THE AGE OF 65 YEARS

Recommended for women with any of the following risk factors:
- Body weight of <127 lb
- History of fragility fracture
- History of bone loss from medications or disease
- Family history of hip fracture
- Alcoholism
- Current smoker
- Rheumatoid arthritis

From American College of Obstetricians and Gynecologists (ACOG) Practice Bulletin 129 (Osteoporosis), September 2012.

be accompanied by acute and chronic back pain. Other important osteoporotic events include wrist and hip fractures. **Ten to 15 years after menopause, women begin to fracture their bones at a rate exceeding that of men by a factor of threefold to fivefold.** About 200,000 women break a hip each year in the United States, and the annual cost of osteoporotic fractures and their complications has been estimated to be in excess of $14 billion. The earlier women are deprived of estrogen in their lives, the earlier osteoporotic bone loss begins. **Most calcium is lost from trabecular bone, and as a consequence, the spinal column and femoral neck are the bones most commonly fractured. Box 35-1 lists the known risk factors for osteoporosis in women.**

The American College of Obstetricians and Gynecologists (ACOG) recommends bone mineral density screening for osteoporosis in women with risk factors (Box 35-2) who are under the age of 65 years, and in women without risk factors who are 65 years or older. The preferred screening modality is dual-energy x-ray absorptiometry measurements of the total hip and spine. The results of these studies are expressed in T scores, which are standard deviations (SDs) from the peak bone mineral density of normal young adults. Osteoporosis is defined as a T score of less than −2.5 SD. Drug therapy is recommended in postmenopausal women with a T score of less than −2.5 SD or a T score of −2.0 to −2.5 SD plus an additional risk factor for fracture. If bone mineral density measurements are used to monitor the effects of drug therapy, they should be repeated after at least 2 years of treatment.

Reducing the risk of osteoporotic fracture entails several changes of diet and lifestyle. **Postmenopausal** women should consume 1200 to 1500 mg of calcium and 400 to 600 U of vitamin D daily, which are contained in two to three portions of dairy products. Those who cannot or will not include dairy products in their meals should be encouraged to use calcium and vitamin D supplements. Excessive supplementation should be discouraged to avoid renal complications. **Walking and weight-bearing exercises both help to increase bone mineral mass and reduce the risk of fracture-causing falls.** The risk of falling can be reduced further by eliminating throw rugs in the home, placement of handrails in the bathroom, and minimizing the use of alcoholic beverages. **Smoking should be discouraged** for many other health reasons in addition to prevention of osteoporosis. Patients receiving replacement therapy for hypothyroidism should be tested to ensure that they are not receiving an excessive (and potentially bone density–depleting) dose.

Pharmacologic treatments for osteoporosis include estrogen (with or without a progestin), selective estrogen receptor modulators (SERMs), biphosphonates, calcitonin, and parathyroid hormone. Data from the Women's Health Initiative (WHI) study demonstrated that combined estrogen/progestin therapy reduced postmenopausal total fractures by 24% compared to controls, with a 34% reduction of hip fractures. This translates to a reduction of the hip fracture rate from 15 to 10 cases per 10,000 postmenopausal women per year. **SERMs, such as raloxifene, have been found to be beneficial for the prevention of vertebral fractures,** but data are lacking regarding the prevention of hip fracture. **Biphosphonates, such as alendronate, can effectively prevent and, at higher doses, treat osteoporosis** without requiring continued usage. In general, biphosphonates have few adverse side effects. However, they must be taken properly (empty stomach, upright position, and with a large glass of water) to minimize the risks of esophagitis and esophageal ulcers. **Both calcitonin and parathyroid hormone are second-line adjunctive treatments for osteoporosis.**

Ovarian Hormone Therapy

For over four decades, ovarian hormonal therapy (HT), called hormone replacement therapy (HRT) in the past, had been advocated for an expanding set of prophylactic indications. Initially, hormonal therapy was provided for the treatment of hot flashes and the symptoms of genitourinary atrophy. Later, increasing evidence revealed that prevention of osteoporosis was a specific benefit of ovarian hormonal therapy.

A number of large observational cohort and case–controlled studies had suggested ovarian hormonal therapy might prevent or delay the onset of arteriosclerotic heart disease and Alzheimer disease through a number of diverse mechanisms. On the other hand, observational studies had raised concerns about associated risks of venous thrombosis/pulmonary embolism and breast cancer.

Randomized controlled trials tend to minimize the biases of observational studies. However, they are difficult and time-consuming to do when the conditions being observed are relatively uncommon and all women who are studied are volunteers. In an attempt to control for most of the biases inherent in observational studies, the Women's Health Initiative (WHI) study was undertaken with a goal of sorting out the risks and benefits of ovarian hormonal therapy. Nearly 17,000 women were entered into one arm of the study comparing a combined preparation of conjugated estrogens and medroxyprogesterone acetate with placebo. There was also an estrogen only arm in the WHI study. After 5 years of follow-up, the combined ovarian hormonal arm was halted in July of 2002. **The previously reported protection from osteoporotic fracture was confirmed by the WHI study in all arms. In addition, a 37% reduction in the rate of colorectal cancer was found.** This would result in six fewer cases of colorectal cancer (10 vs. 16) per 10,000 women per year. **Combined ovarian hormone use, however, was found to increase the risks for coronary artery disease events (by 29%), stroke (by 41%), thromboses (by 100%), and breast cancer (by 26%).** Although most of the risks increased after 1 to 2 years of use, increased risk of breast cancer became apparent only after 4 years of use. **There was no significant increase in death rates between treatment and placebo groups.** Contrary to several previous studies, the WHI found an overall harmful rather than protective effect on cognitive decline and dementia.

In February 2004, the estrogen-only arm of the WHI was halted because of a significantly increased risk of stroke. It confirmed a protective effect against hip fracture, although none of the other significant findings in the combined arm were found to be present. **The risk of breast cancer was not increased in the estrogen-only arm of the WHI study.**

The WHI study has been widely criticized for examining women who, for the most part, were well past the age of menopause when they were entered into the study (average age 63). This was neither intentional nor desirable, but occurred because the study group was necessarily made up of those women who volunteered to participate in the study, and as a group they were older. Laboratory/animal studies have shown an atherosclerotic protective effect of estrogen after gonadectomy, when begun immediately. **Additional analyses of WHI data have failed to confirm increased coronary artery events in those subjects who began therapy less than ten years after the menopause.**

Although definite limitations of the WHI study have been identified, **the findings have had a significant effect on clinical practice, and the routine use of HT after the menopause is currently viewed with caution.**

The general consensus now is that combined ovarian hormonal therapy is indicated primarily for the relief of significant menopausal symptoms such as frequent hot flashes, genitourinary discomfort, and other quality-of-life issues. The length of treatment should be minimized, depending on the individual patient's clinical course and preference, and after informed consent. On the other hand, most experts recommend that younger hypoestrogenic women, such as those who undergo premature menopause or bilateral oophorectomy, should take HT.

A very large observational cohort study, the **Million Women Study (MWS)** also addressed the risks and benefits of hormonal therapy after menopause (age 50 years). Over one million women were enrolled in the United Kingdom, and long-term follow-up continues. After more than 4 years of follow-up, the MWS has also reported an increased breast cancer risk with hormonal therapy with and without progestin. Box 35-3 summarizes the goals and findings of the MWS.

The need for prevention and treatment of osteoporosis should be determined by bone densitometry studies rather than ovarian status, per se. Biphosphonates or raloxifene should be regarded as the first line of treatment in the absence of concomitant significant menopausal symptoms.

Management of Ovarian Hormonal Therapy

Women who still have a uterus should not be given unopposed estrogen for the treatment of menopausal symptoms because of the high risk of developing endometrial hyperplasia and endometrial adenocarcinoma. Concurrent progestin is protective for endometrial disease and may be given for 12 days per month or for 14 days per quarter with predictable uterine bleeding on withdrawal. **Patients who seek complete amenorrhea may use continuous combined estrogen/progestin** (e.g., conjugated estrogens, 0.625 mg, and medroxyprogesterone acetate, 2.5 mg daily). This latter regimen is characterized by unpredictable breakthrough bleeding, with a majority of patients achieving amenorrhea within a year. The estrogen-only arm of the WHI study (with lower breast cancer risk) suggested that progestins may be the more important element of risk for breast cancer in patients receiving hormonal therapy, so thought should be given to minimizing exposure to progestins.

There has been a recent trend toward the use of so-called bio-identical medications for hormonal treatment after menopause. This can be accomplished using U.S. Food and Drug Administration–approved estrogen patches (bio-identical to 17-beta estradiol) with progesterone suppositories (bio-identical to pro-

BOX 35-3

MILLION WOMEN STUDY

Study Goals

Recruit and study (with follow-up) at least one million women (aged 50 years and older) in the United Kingdom (UK) between 1993 and 2004, who are taking estrogens and progestogens with particular emphasis on breast cancer risk.

Study Design

Observational cohort study with 70% of those recruited participating in and completing the questionnaire and screening program.

Study Findings

Breast Cancer

Study included estrogen and progestogen in combination; estrogen only; and included oral, transdermal, and implanted hormones whether they were given continuously or sequentially.

Past users of hormones were not at increased breast cancer risk.

Current users of combination hormones (estrogen and progestogen) had a 2-fold increased risk of breast cancer.

Current users of estrogen only had a 1.3-fold increase in breast cancer risk.

Study authors estimated that 20,000 extra cases of breast cancer occurred between 1993 and 2004 in the UK because of hormone use.

Endometrial Cancer

Study confirmed that women with a uterus who used estrogen only had an increased risk of endometrial cancer and that the risk of endometrial cancer may be reduced in women taking estrogen and a progestogen in combination.

Ovarian Cancer

Study found no increased risk of ovarian cancer in former users of hormones. Current users have a 1.2-fold increase in ovarian cancer risk. Putting this risk into perspective, the study concluded that there would be one extra case of ovarian cancer for every 2500 women taking hormones and one extra death from ovarian cancer in 3300 hormone users over five years.

gesterone) added for women who still have a uterus. This method also avoids the oral route of delivery that has been shown to increase potentially harmful hepatic effects such as coagulation abnormalities. The use of a progestin-releasing intrauterine device (Mirena) has been suggested as a way to control irregular bleeding and protect the endometrium from the effect of unopposed estrogen.

Severe continuous bleeding or intermittent bleeding after more than 4 months of hormonal therapy should prompt a search for uterine pathology. Optimization of menopausal symptom control, although reducing adverse side effects of therapy, may be accomplished by using the lowest effective dose and by substituting continuous transdermal estrogen for oral preparations of estrogen when symptoms are not adequately controlled. When the patient's main concerns are with genitourinary symptoms, vaginal estrogen cream, tablets, or rings may be used on an "as needed" basis without necessarily adding a progestin.

Selective Estrogen Receptor Modulators

The biologic effect of estrogenic substances is mediated by the translocation of a ligand-estrogen receptor complex into the nucleus, where various estrogen-responsive genes are activated or repressed. **At least two estrogen receptors, α and β, are presently known to exist.** They exert different biologic effects and exist in different proportions in different tissues. In addition, different ligands bound in a complex with the same receptor manifest different biologic activity. The use of SERMs attempts to take advantage of these facts to produce some, but not all of the biologic effects of native estradiol. SERMs in use today include clomiphene, tamoxifen, and raloxifene. Unlike estradiol and other SERMs in current use, **raloxifene does not stimulate endometrial or breast duct epithelial proliferation.** However, **raloxifene does seem to reduce osteoclastic activity and prevent osteoporosis (at least in the spine).** Hence, raloxifene has some of the bone-sparing effect of estradiol without incurring the risk of endometrial hyperplasia/carcinoma. It may actually prove to be protective against breast cancer in the same way as tamoxifen. However, **raloxifene appears to worsen rather than ameliorate vasomotor symptoms.** Perhaps new SERMs will be discovered in the future that will provide symptom relief as well as skeletal protection.

Lifestyle Changes and Alternative Treatments for the Climacteric

Increasingly, an emphasis is being placed on the importance of lifestyle changes as a strategy for decreasing the inevitable effects of the aging process. **The most important change that anyone can make to increase longevity, reduce heart disease, and reduce calcium loss from bone is to stop smoking. Controlling weight, engaging in regular exercise, and eating a healthier, low-fat, and balanced diet should be strongly recommended,** especially in women with diabetes, hypertension, or significantly elevated blood lipids. All counseling about the effects of menopause should include a discussion of these issues, along with any possible medical therapies. In particular, **the statin drugs are important for postmenopausal women with an unfavorable lipid profile, as they significantly reduce the risk of cardiovascular disease and serendipitously protect against osteoporosis.**

Phytoestrogens (plant products that are functionally or structurally similar to estrogen) and herbal substances have been marketed to consumers as the "natural" alternative to traditional hormonal therapy for the symptoms of perimenopause and menopause. Women should be made aware that even placebos may decrease some of the symptoms, such as hot flashes, and that some herbal preparations have been shown to be ineffective or even harmful. Also, patients should be made aware of the less rigorous evaluation and regulation that these products undergo.

With proper counseling, appropriate screening, and professional care, the signs, symptoms, and sequelae of the climacteric can be managed successfully. Short-term use of hormonal therapy for symptom control, healthy lifestyle changes, appropriate monitoring, and medical or surgical interventions when necessary should provide a safe and effective level of care.

36

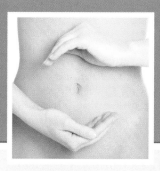

Menstrual Cycle–Influenced Disorders

JOSEPH C. GAMBONE

CLINICAL KEYS FOR THIS CHAPTER

- Premenstrual syndrome (PMS) and its more severe form, premenstrual dysphoric disorder (PMDD) are the quintessential menstrual cycle–influenced disorders. A common feature of these disorders is the inability to distinguish between affected women and normal controls by routine measurement of the traditional hypothalamic-pituitary-ovarian (HPO) hormones. Interestingly, in many cases, dramatic relief from the symptoms can be obtained by intentionally disrupting or abolishing regular menstrual function.

- Eight out of ten women with ovulatory cycles will have mild symptoms just before and during menses. This is referred to as molimina and should not be diagnosed as PMS. PMS causing moderate to severe symptoms that affect daily activities and relationships is reported by 5-10% of ovulatory women, and PMDD by less than 5%.

- The causative factors in these menstrual cycle–influenced disorders are not abnormal concentrations of the hormones of the HPO axis, but rather are atypical end organ responses to normal levels of gonadotropins and sex steroids. With the exception of recent evidence showing disruption of serotonin regulation in women with PMDD, alterations in hormone levels have been inconsistently documented.

- Because of the unclear and variable symptomatology associated with PMS/PMDD, an initial diagnostic tool is to have affected women keep a daily menstrual diary. This is done to establish the relationship between the symptoms and the luteal phase of the menstrual cycle. Once this relationship has been established, a number of effective treatments may be initiated.

- Other disorders that have been reported consistently to be influenced by the menstrual cycle include migraine headache, epilepsy, asthma, diabetes, rheumatoid arthritis, and irritable bowel syndrome. Less well studied problems include acne flare-ups, multiple sclerosis, glaucoma, and hereditary angioedema.

The human menstrual cycle is unique as a physiologic process in that it involves mechanisms that change on a daily basis rather than remaining stable. This process of change is carried out through the many intricate hormonal interactions between the hypothalamic region of the brain, the pituitary gland, the ovaries, and to some extent, the adrenal glands and the pancreatic islets of Langerhans (see Chapter 4).

The classic disorders that appear to be directly influenced by hormonal changes that occur during the menstrual cycle are **premenstrual syndrome (PMS)** and **premenstrual dysphoric disorder (PMDD).** Common symptoms reported by women with PMS and PMDD include significant bloating, mood changes, depression, and emotional lability that affect their daily activities. **There is a second group of menstrual** cycle–associated disorders, the hallmark of which is regular ovulatory cycles, that causes cyclical dysfunction of other organ systems.

Premenstrual Syndrome and Premenstrual Dysphoric Disorder

The acronyms PMS for premenstrual syndrome and PMDD for premenstrual dysphoric disorder refer to the same pathologic process at opposite ends of the symptom spectrum (Figure 36-1). **In both PMS and PMDD, patients experience adverse physical, psychological, and behavioral symptoms during the luteal phase of the menstrual cycle.** There is a crescendo of symptom intensity up to the time that menses begin,

Spectrum of Premenstrual Syndromes

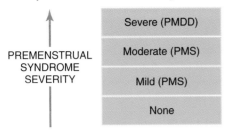

FIGURE 36-1 Spectrum of premenstrual syndromes. *PMDD,* Premenstrual dysphoric disorder; *PMS,* premenstrual syndrome.

BOX 36-1

CRITERIA FOR PREMENSTRUAL DYSPHORIC DISORDER

- Symptoms seriously interfere with usual functioning/relationships
- Premenstrual timing confirmed by menstrual calendar in two consecutive cycles
- Symptoms resolve after the onset of menses
- Symptoms are not an exacerbation of another disorder
- At least 5 premenstrual symptoms:
    1. At least one of the following:
       Depressed mood
       Marked anxiety
       Marked affective lability
       Marked irritability
    2. Other possible symptoms:
       Decreased interest in regular activities
       Difficulty concentrating
       Lethargy/fatigue
       Appetite change/food cravings
       Sleep disturbance
       Feelings of being overwhelmed
       Physical symptoms (breast swelling and tenderness, bloating, weight gain, edema, or headache)

From Diagnostic and Statistical Manual of Mental Disorders of the American Psychiatric Association for PMDD.

---

with quick resolution thereafter. Some patients have a brief surge of symptoms at the time of ovulation in midcycle.

As many as 80% of regularly ovulating women will experience some degree of physical and psychological premenstrual symptomatology. These mild "moliminal" symptoms are normal, and characteristic of ovulatory cycles. About 5-10% of these women have moderate symptoms that are disruptive to daily activities and are said to have PMS. In less than 5% of women, these symptoms are so severe that they seriously interfere with usual daily functioning and personal relationships. When these women meet the criteria outlined in Box 36-1, they may be diagnosed with PMDD.

Common symptoms reported by patients include depressed mood, anxiety, affective lability and irritability, decreased interest in regular activities, difficulty concentrating, fatigue, change of appetite, sleep disturbance, and feelings of being overwhelmed. Physical symptoms include breast swelling and tenderness, bloating (a sense of abdominal swelling), weight gain, edema, and headache. The diagnosis of these disorders is confirmed by the predominant occurrence of symptoms in the luteal phase, as documented on a menstrual calendar of two consecutive cycles.

A formal set of diagnostic criteria has been proposed in the fourth edition of **The Diagnostic and Statistical Manual (DSM-IV) of the American Psychiatric Association for PMDD** (see Box 36-1). Although the DSM-IV definition of PMDD specifies that this is not just an exacerbation of another disorder, the dividing line between PMDD and other neuropsychiatric disorders is not so clear cut. For example, **46% of PMDD patients have a history of a prior major depressive episode.** Moreover, patients with PMDD and clinical depression share similar alterations on a sleep electroencephalogram (EEG), and they are both responsive to the selective serotonin reuptake inhibitor (SSRI) antidepressants.

Although PMS/PMDD patients and controls do not differ in their average cyclic levels of sex steroids, gonadotropins, prolactin, or cortisol, **there exists a strong basis to believe that these disorders have a hormonal rather than a purely psychologic basis.** First, abolition of the menstrual cycle with gonadotropin-releasing hormone (GnRH) agonists, pregnancy, menopause, or spontaneous anovulation, provides symptomatic relief, whereas sequential ovarian hormonal therapy in hypogonadal patients can induce PMS/PMDD symptoms. Second, cycles with higher luteal phase levels of estradiol are associated with more severe symptoms.

The physiologic mechanism that results in the occurrence of PMS/PMDD is not well understood. Evidence exists that the phenomenon arises, in part, from atypical metabolism of progesterone that results in lower levels of the steroid allopregnanolone within the central nervous system. In turn, allopregnanolone interacts with the γ-aminobutyric acid (GABA) and serotonin neurons to influence the regions of the brain responsible for emotion and subjective perception. In addition, the GABA and serotoninergic neurons may be inherently dysfunctional in PMS/PMDD patients, especially in those with severe depressive symptoms, hence the overlap between PMDD and clinical depression. Major depressive disorder (MDD) persists, however, on a daily basis for weeks without a relationship to the menstrual cycle. **MDD may be exacerbated during the luteal phase of the menstrual cycle and can even coexist with PMDD in some women.** In such cases both PMDD and MDD need to be treated (Table 36-1).

Research performed to determine the best therapy for this disorder is problematic, because of the subjective nature of the condition, as well as the wide

TABLE 36-1

DISTINGUISHING PREMENSTRUAL DYSPHORIC DISORDER FROM PREMENSTRUAL SYNDROME AND MAJOR DEPRESSIVE DISORDER				
	Predominant Mood Symptoms	Premenstrual Physical Symptoms	Marked Social Impairment	Monthly Cyclicity
Premenstrual syndrome	–/+	+	–	Yes
Premenstrual dysphoric disorder	+	+	+	Yes
Major depressive disorder	+	–	+	No

variation in the severity of the symptoms from one cycle to the next. In addition, external influences at work and at home may affect the severity of the symptoms. Finally, placebo interventions produce significant initial benefits in most PMS/PMDD studies. All of these considerations necessitate prolonged studies, which are expensive and infrequently performed.

Because of the lack of clarity and consistency of symptomatology, the initial clinical approach to PMS/PMDD should be to obtain self-reported documentation that the symptoms only (or predominately) occur in the luteal phase of the menstrual cycle. **A detailed menstrual diary should be kept on a daily basis and reviewed for at least two cycles.** A number of paper-based and electronic tools (easy to use applications or apps) exist for keeping these diaries. When a major depressive disorder is suspected, the patient should be referred urgently for psychiatric care.

TREATMENT

The majority of women who could be characterized as having PMS should be treated individually and conservatively, with **reassurance and mild diuretics** for symptoms such as bloating. Aerobic exercise, reducing processed foods, refined sugars and trans-fats are reasonable lifestyle changes to recommend although studies do not show consistent improvement in PMS symptoms. The mild anxiety that frequently occurs with PMS may be treated with agents such as **buspirone.** At present, the most effective therapy studied for women with PMDD is the SSRI class of antidepressants. **Fluoxetine taken at dosages of 20 to 60 mg per day during the luteal phase of the cycle** provides significant symptomatic improvement in 50-60% of patients. **Sertraline at 50 to 150 mg per day** is equally effective. Side effects of the SSRIs are usually self-limited and include insomnia and sexual dysfunction.

Other preparations have been effective in at least one randomized controlled trial. They include **calcium carbonate, 1200 mg per day,** for control of mood and behavioral symptoms; **spironolactone, 100 mg per day,** for mood and bloating; and **buspirone, 25 to 60 mg per day,** for premenstrual anxiety. **Danocrine and bromocriptine** are effective for the treatment of cyclic mastalgia. Pyridoxine (vitamin B6), 50 to 100 mg a day, has demonstrated mixed results in clinical trials.

GnRH agonists, used with estrogen and progestin "add back" to minimize hot flashes, are effective in eliminating PMS/PMDD symptoms. However, this is an expensive therapeutic approach.

Treatments that have been demonstrated to be ineffective in randomized controlled trials include oral or vaginal progesterone and conventional use of combined oral contraceptives. With the latter, patients have PMS-like symptoms during the placebo week.

Recent studies have shown benefit from the continuous use, or 24 out of 28 day use, of an oral contraceptive containing the progestin drospirenone.

Other Menstrual Cycle–Influenced Disorders

MENSTRUAL MIGRANE HEADACHES

Migraine headaches, which are believed to result from sequential intracranial vasoconstriction and vasodilation, are known to be influenced by menstrual cycling. They are two to three times more common in women than in men. They improve in approximately 80% of patients during pregnancy but recur postpartum. Usually, migraines resolve following the onset of the menopause. **Sixty percent of women who suffer migraine link the occurrence of their attacks to the menstrual cycle,** and 7% exclusively have migraines on the 2 days before or after the onset of menstruation. Menstrual migraines usually occur without a preceding aura and are more long-lasting and resistant to treatment than migraines occurring at other times in the menstrual cycle.

The link between migraine headaches and the hormonal changes of the menstrual cycle is believed to be the phenomenon of estrogen withdrawal. Evidence for this derives from several observations: first, a small proportion of women with menstrual migraine have an upsurge in headache frequency following the pre-ovulatory estradiol surge; second, exogenous estrogen reduces the incidence of migraines; and third, exogenous progesterone may delay the onset of menstruation without preventing the migraine attacks.

Several mechanisms have been proposed to explain why estrogen withdrawal produces migraine headaches. They include abnormal platelet aggregation, central nervous system endogenous opioid dysregulation, and stimulation of increased synthesis of prostaglandin in the central nervous system.

Treatment

Standard treatment of migraine headaches includes triptans, nonsteroidal antiinflammatory drugs, and ergotamines. Drugs used for the short-term prophylaxis of menstrual migraines can be taken 3 to 5 days before and after the onset of menses. They include nonsteroidal antiinflammatory drugs and triptans. Monitoring of the menstrual cycle by basal body temperature charting or the use of a luteinizing hormone surge detector kit permits the initiation of these agents for more effective headache prevention.

Several hormonal protocols may also be effective in preventing menstrual migraines. For short-term prophylaxis, 100 mcg transdermal estrogen patches begun 48 hours before anticipated menses and continued for 3 to 6 days have been shown to be effective. Continuous oral contraceptive pills for intervals of 2 to 4 months (with symptomatic treatment during withdrawal between intervals) provide long-term prevention of migraines.

MONTHLY (CATAMENIAL) EPILEPSY

Seventy percent of female epileptics report an increased incidence of seizures premenstrually. Fourteen percent of female epileptics have catamenial epilepsy in which seizures only occur in the perimenstrual phase of the cycle. **This includes all varieties of epilepsy.** In these women, the onset of epilepsy is usually at the time of, or shortly after, menarche. Eight-four percent of catamenial epileptics have significant premenstrual syndrome symptoms, in contrast to a 22% incidence of PMS in epileptics whose seizures do not correlate with the menstrual cycle.

Two mechanisms are felt to underlie the phenomenon of catamenial epilepsy. The first is a direct effect on the neurons of the brain of the reduced progesterone/estradiol ratio. In vitro, estradiol lowers the seizure threshold of many varieties of neurons, whereas progesterone raises the threshold, making a seizure more likely. Thus, catamenial epilepsy reflects the effect of a reduced progesterone (and allopregnanolone) concentration or progesterone/estradiol ratio during the late luteal phase of the menstrual cycle. This correlates well with several clinical observations: first, some patients with catamenial epilepsy also suffer exacerbations during the preovulatory estradiol surge; second, seizure activity is prone to increase in anovulatory cycles, which may be managed with the use of clomiphene; and third, seizure activity may decrease in incidence after menopause.

A second mechanism explaining this disorder is a reduction in serum levels of anticonvulsants during the late luteal phase. This is believed to be mediated by increased hepatic mono-oxygenase activity, resulting directly from reduced sex steroid levels. This is the rationale for the treatment option of closely tracking the menstrual cycle and determining anticonvulsant concentrations in the late luteal phase, so that drug dosage may be altered when necessary.

Treatment

The anticonvulsant effect of progesterone is the basis for using Depo-Provera, progestin-only oral contraceptive pills, or premenstrual progesterone suppositories (50 to 400 mg BID) to reduce seizure activity. Ganaxolone, an allopregnanolone analog taken cycle days 21 through 3 of the next cycle, has also been found to be an effective seizure prophylactic. **GnRH agonist therapy** has been helpful for intractable cases. Combined oral contraceptives have inconsistent effects, with some patients suffering exacerbations during the placebo week. Moreover, pill efficacy is reduced by anticonvulsants, resulting in a 6% contraceptive failure rate with low-dose preparations.

PREMENSTRUAL ASTHMA

Eight to 40% of female asthmatics report increased symptoms or decreased peak expiratory flow rates in the premenstrual phase of their cycles. Progesterone has bronchodilatory and antiinflammatory effects, and the characteristic atypical metabolism of progesterone in PMS may be responsible for this phenomenon.

Treatment

Similar to other maneuvers with menstrual cycle–influenced disorders, monitoring of the cycle to modify glucocorticoid or leukotriene antagonist dosage may be helpful. There is little experience with hormonal-based therapies in asthma.

DIABETES MELLITUS

A high percentage of women with insulin dependent diabetes mellitus (IDDM) report changes in glycemic control premenstrually. Most women experience a worsening of glycemic control, although some report an improvement. Possible mechanisms for this effect include PMS-induced dietary binges and reduction of physical activity before and during menses. A direct hormonal effect on insulin sensitivity is also a possibility. The exact mechanism of menstrual cycle–related alterations in glycemic control has not been determined.

Treatment

The suggested management is intensified adherence to diet control, exercise, and glucose measurement. The SSRIs, which are commonly used to treat PMS and

PMDD, have been found to increase insulin resistance which may aggravate glycemic control. Metformin, which is used in conjunction with insulin for IDDM, acts as an insulin-sensitizing agent and may smooth out the glycemic control in some women.

RHEUMATOID ARTHRITIS

The connection between rheumatoid arthritis (RA) and menstruation is suggested by the facts that RA symptoms usually improve in the luteal phase of a menstrual cycle when sex steroids are highest, and RA is known to improve during pregnancy, with relapses common postpartum.

Treatment

Estrogen treatment alone, or with a progestin in the form of a lower-dose oral contraceptive, has provided effective relief for many women with RA. Interestingly, even lower dose hormonal treatment in postmenopausal women has not been shown to prevent or improve RA.

IRRITABLE BOWEL SYNDROME

Irritable bowel syndrome (IBS) affects women 3 to 20 times more frequently than men. It is well known that progesterone affects the gastrointestinal (GI) tract. In several studies, GI symptoms dramatically increased with menses when progesterone is lowest in the cycle.

Treatment

Symptomatic treatment for flare-ups is the usual treatment for IBS. There is some evidence for a prostaglandin link, based upon evidence that prostaglandin synthesis inhibitors are of benefit. GnRH agonists have been used to create a "medical oophorectomy" in women with severe IBS. After a trial of a GnRH agonist, surgical oophorectomy has been performed in rare cases.

Other Conditions

In some individuals, the following conditions may be influenced by the menstrual cycle on a cyclic basis: acne flare-ups, hereditary angioedema, aphthous ulcers, Behçet syndrome, acute intermittent porphyria, paroxysmal supraventricular tachycardia, multiple sclerosis, glaucoma, urticaria, erythema multiforme, and myasthenia gravis. Interestingly, in the case of myasthenia gravis, 25-50% of affected women improve premenstrually.

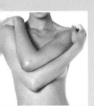
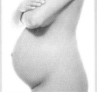
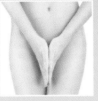
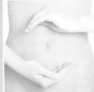

Gynecologic Oncology

5

PART

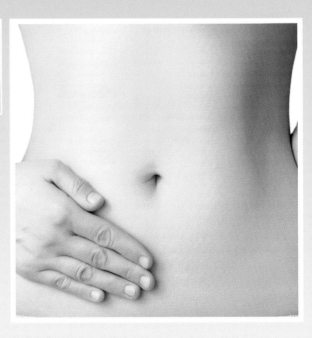

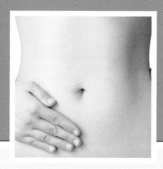

Principles of Cancer Therapy

NEVILLE F. HACKER

Modern gynecologic cancer management requires a multidisciplinary approach and includes surgery, chemotherapy, radiation therapy, hormonal therapy, and targeted therapy. In this chapter, the principles of the nonsurgical modalities are discussed, together with the principles of pain management and end-of-life issues.

Cellular Biology

The characteristic feature of malignant tumor growth is its uncontrolled cellular proliferation, which requires replication of deoxyribonucleic acid (DNA). There are two distinct phases in the life cycle of all cells: **mitosis** (M phase), during which cellular division occurs, and **interphase,** the interval between successive mitoses.

Interphase is subdivided into three separate phases (Figure 37-1). Immediately following mitosis is the G_1 **phase,** which is of variable duration and is characterized by a diploid content of DNA. DNA synthesis is absent, but ribonucleic acid (RNA) and protein synthe-

sis occur. During the shorter **S phase,** the entire DNA content is duplicated. This is followed by the G_2 **phase,** which is characterized by a tetraploid DNA content and by continuing RNA and protein synthesis in preparation for cell division. When mitosis occurs, a duplicate set of chromosomal DNA is inherited by each daughter cell, thus restoring the diploid DNA content. Following mitosis, some cells leave the cycle temporarily or permanently and enter the G_0 **or resting phase.**

The growth fraction of the tumor is the proportion of actively dividing cells. The higher the growth fraction, the fewer the number of cells in the G_0 phase and the faster the tumor-doubling time.

Chemotherapeutic agents and radiation kill cells by first-order kinetics, which means that a constant proportion of cells is killed for a given dosage, regardless of the number of cells present. Both therapeutic modalities are most effective against actively dividing cells because cells in the resting (G_0) phase are better able to repair sublethal damage. Unfortunately, both

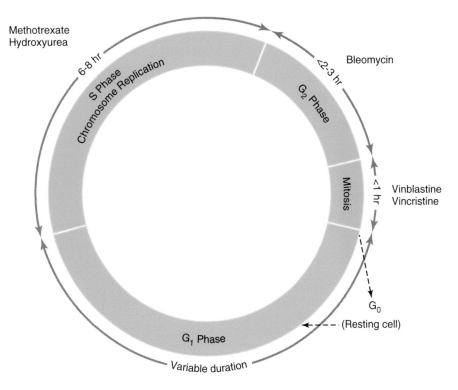

FIGURE 37-1 Phases of the cell cycle and sites of action of cell cycle–specific drugs.

therapeutic modalities also suppress rapidly dividing normal cells, such as those in the gastrointestinal mucosa, bone marrow, and hair follicles.

Chemotherapy

One of the major advances in medicine since the 1950s has been the successful treatment of certain disseminated malignancies, including choriocarcinoma and germ cell ovarian tumors, with chemotherapy.

CLASSIFICATION OF CHEMOTHERAPEUTIC AGENTS

Chemotherapeutic agents act primarily by disrupting nuclear DNA, and thus inhibiting cellular division. They may be subdivided into two categories according to their mode of action relative to the cell cycle:

1. **Cell cycle–nonspecific agents,** such as alkylating agents, cisplatin, and paclitaxel, which exert their damage at any phase of the cell cycle. They may damage resting as well as cycling cells, but the latter are much more sensitive.
2. **Cell cycle–specific agents,** which exert their lethal effects exclusively or primarily during one phase of the cell cycle. Examples include hydroxyurea and methotrexate, which act primarily during the S phase; bleomycin, which acts in the G_2 phase; and the vinca alkaloids, which act in the M phase.

PRINCIPLES OF CHEMOTHERAPY

Chemotherapeutic agents are selected on the basis of previous experience with particular agents for a given tumor, particularly after randomized controlled clinical trials. The drugs are usually given systemically so that the tumor can be treated regardless of its anatomic location. To increase the local concentration, certain drugs may occasionally be administered topically, by intraarterial infusion, or by intrathecal or intracavitary instillation (e.g., intraperitoneal therapy for ovarian cancer).

Chemotherapy is generally not administered if the neutrophil count is less than 1500/mm³ or if the platelet count is less than 100,000/mm³. Nadir blood counts are obtained 7 to 14 days after treatment, and subsequent doses may need to be reduced if there is significant myelosuppression or if the patient develops febrile neutropenia. Dosage reduction may also be necessary because of toxicity to other organs, such as the gastrointestinal tract, liver, or kidneys.

Resistance to chemotherapeutic agents may be temporary or permanent. Temporary resistance is mainly related to the poor vascularity of bulky tumors, which results in poor tissue concentrations of the drugs and an increasing proportion of cells in the relatively resistant G_0 phase of the cell cycle. Permanent resistance mainly results from spontaneous mutation to phenotypic resistance and occurs most commonly in bulky tumors. Permanent resistance may also be acquired by frequent exposure to chemotherapeutic agents.

CHEMOTHERAPEUTIC AGENTS

The common agents used in the management of gynecologic malignancies may be classified as shown in Table 37-1. This table also contains a summary of the main indications and side effects of these drugs.

Alkylating Agents

The cytotoxicity of alkylating agents results from their ability to cause alkylation to DNA, resulting in cross-linkage between DNA strands and prevention of DNA replication. There is cross resistance among the various alkylating agents.

Antimetabolites

Antimetabolites are compounds that closely resemble normal intermediaries, for which they may substitute in biochemical reactions, and thereby produce a metabolic block; for example, **methotrexate** competitively inhibits the enzyme dihydrofolate reductase, thus preventing the conversion of dihydrofolate to tetrahydrofolate. The latter is required for the methylation reaction necessary for the synthesis of purine and pyrimidine subunits of nucleic acid.

Antibiotics

Antibiotics are naturally occurring antitumor agents elaborated by certain species of *Streptomyces*. They have no single, clearly defined mechanism of action, but many agents in this group intercalate between strands of the DNA double helix, thereby inhibiting both DNA and RNA synthesis and causing oxygen-dependent strand breaks.

Plant Alkaloids

The most common plant alkaloids are the **vinca alkaloids,** which are derived from the periwinkle plant. These include vincristine and vinblastine. They are spindle toxins that interfere with cellular microtubules and cause metaphase arrest.

Other plant alkaloids include the **epipodophyllotoxins** such as etoposide (VP16), which are extracts from the mandrake plant, and **paclitaxel** (Taxol), an extract from the bark of the Pacific yew tree. **Docetaxel (Taxotere)** is the first semisynthetic analogue of paclitaxel. Etoposide appears to act by causing single-strand DNA breaks. Paclitaxel binds preferentially to microtubules, and results in their polymerization and stabilization.

Other Drugs

Cisplatin, one of the more important drugs in gynecologic oncology, causes inhibition of DNA synthesis by forming interstrand and intrastrand linkages. Carbo-platin is an analogue of cisplatin with a similar mechanism of action and efficacy, but with less gastrointestinal and renal toxicity.

Radiation Therapy

Radiation may be defined as the propagation of energy through space or matter.

TYPES OF RADIATION

There are two main types of radiation: electromagnetic and particulate.

Electromagnetic Radiation

Examples of electromagnetic radiation include the following:
- Visible light
- Infrared light
- Ultraviolet light
- X-rays (photons)
- Gamma rays (photons)

X-rays and gamma rays are identical electromagnetic radiations, differing only in their mode of production. X-rays are produced by bombardment of an anode by a high-speed electron beam; gamma rays result from the decay of radioactive isotopes, such as cobalt 60 (^{60}Co).

X-rays and gamma rays (photons) are differentiated from electromagnetic radiation of longer wavelength by their greater energy, which allows them to penetrate tissues and cause ionization.

Particulate Radiation

Particulate radiation consists of moving particles of matter. Their energy consists of the kinetic energy of the moving particles.

$$\text{Energy} = 0.5\, \text{mass} \times \text{velocity}^2$$

The particles vary greatly in size and include the following:
- Neutrons (no charge)
- Protons (positive charge)
- Electrons (negative charge)

The most commonly used particles are electrons. They may be derived from a linear accelerator, the beam of electrons being directed into the patient without first striking a metal target and producing x-rays. Alternatively, high-energy electrons (called beta particles) may be derived from the radiodecay of an unstable isotope, such as phosphorus 32 (^{32}P). Particulate radiation penetrates tissues less than photons but also produces ionization.

UNIT OF RADIATION MEASUREMENT

The Gray (Gy) is equivalent to an absorbed energy of 1 joule per kilogram of absorbing material.

TABLE 37-1

INDICATIONS, SIDE EFFECTS, AND PRECAUTIONS FOR COMMONLY USED CHEMOTHERAPEUTIC AGENTS

Drug	Main Indications	Side Effects	Precautions
Alkylating Agents			
Chlorambucil	Ovarian carcinoma	Bone marrow depression	
Melphalan	Ovarian and tubal carcinoma	Bone marrow depression, leukemia	Avoid prolonged courses (more than 12 cycles) to avoid leukemia
Cyclophosphamide	Ovarian carcinoma, germ cell tumors, squamous carcinomas, sarcomas	Bone marrow depression, nausea and vomiting, alopecia, hemorrhagic cystitis, sterility	Maintain adequate fluid intake to avoid cystitis
Antimetabolites			
Methotrexate	Gestational trophoblastic disease	Bone marrow depression, nausea and vomiting, stomatitis, alopecia, liver and renal failure, dermatitis	Ensure normal kidney and liver function
5-fluorouracil	Vaginal intraepithelial neoplasia (topical application)	Pain and ulceration	
Gemcitabine	Ovarian carcinoma	Bone marrow depression, flu-like illness, skin rash	IV infusion
Antibiotics			
Actinomycin-D	Gestational trophoblastic disease	Bone marrow depression, nausea and vomiting, diarrhea, stomatitis, alopecia, dermatitis, local tissue necrosis	Administer through running intravenous infusion to avoid extravasation
Doxorubicin	Ovarian carcinoma, recurrent endometrial carcinoma, sarcoma	Bone marrow depression, nausea and vomiting, cardiomyopathy, cardiac arrhythmias, alopecia, local tissue necrosis	Administer through running intravenous infusion; do not exceed total dose of 550 mg/m^2 to avoid cardiac toxicity; avoid if significant heart disease is present
Liposomal doxorubicin	Ovarian cancer	Hand-foot syndrome; less cardiotoxic than doxorubicin	IV infusion
Bleomycin	Germ cell tumors, squamous carcinomas	Pneumonitis and pulmonary fibrosis, alopecia, stomatitis, cutaneous reactions	Do not exceed total dose of 400 U; monitor pulmonary function with carbon monoxide diffusion capacity
Plant Alkaloids			
Vinblastine	Germ cell tumors, sarcomas	Bone marrow depression, nausea and vomiting, stomatitis, diarrhea, local tissue necrosis	Administer through running intravenous infusion
Vincristine	Germ cell tumors, sarcomas	Neurotoxicity, constipation, alopecia, local tissue necrosis; bone marrow depression less marked	Administer through running IV infusion; prophylactic cathartics may be helpful
Etoposide	Germ cell tumors	Bone marrow depression; nausea and vomiting	Administer slowly intravenously
Paclitaxel	Ovarian carcinoma, breast carcinoma	Myelosuppression, alopecia, allergic reactions, cardiac arrhythmias	Intravenously as a 3-24 hr infusion
Docetaxel	Ovarian and breast cancer	Myelosuppression, alopecia, dermatologic reactions	Intravenous infusion, IV dexamethasone to reduce fluid retention
Other Drugs			
Cisplatin	Ovarian carcinoma, germ cell tumors, squamous carcinomas	Renal toxicity, ototoxicity, neurotoxicity, severe nausea and vomiting, bone marrow depression less marked, hypokalemia, hypomagnesemia	Administer intravenous fluids to maintain urinary output of 100 mL/hr during infusion; discontinue if creatinine clearance <35 mL/hr
Carboplatin	Ovarian carcinoma, germ cell tumors	Bone marrow depression, less gastrointestinal toxicity, less renal toxicity, less neurotoxicity	Suitable for outpatient therapy because no need for high urinary output
Topotecan	Ovarian cancer	Bone marrow depression	IV for 5 days every 3 weeks

IV, Intravenous.

INVERSE SQUARE LAW

The intensity of electromagnetic radiation is inversely proportional to the square of the distance from the source. Thus, the dose of radiation 2 cm from a point source will be 25% of the dose at 1 cm.

BIOLOGIC CONSIDERATIONS

Ionization of Molecules

Radiation damage is caused by the ionization of molecules in the cell, with the production of free radicals. Because approximately 80% of a mammalian cell is water, most of the cellular radiation damage is mediated by ionization of water and the production of the free radicals H (hydrogen) and OH (hydroxide). **Free radicals may cause irreversible damage to DNA,** making it impossible for the cell to continue replication. Minor or sublethal damage to DNA, which the cell is capable of repairing, may also occur. RNA, protein, and other molecules in the cell are also damaged, but these molecules can be more readily repaired or replaced.

Oxygen Effect

In the absence of oxygen, cells show a two- or threefold increase in their capacity to survive radiation exposure. This means that **hypoxic cells are less radiosensitive than are fully oxygenated cells.** The enhancement of the lethal effects of radiation by oxygen is presumed to occur because the oxygen will combine with the free radicals split from cell targets by the radiation. This prevents the recombination of the free radicals with the targets, which would restore the integrity of the targets.

The effect of oxygen has important clinical implications. First, **anemic patients should undergo transfusion before radiation therapy.** Second, **bulky tumors are usually poorly vascularized and, therefore, are often hypoxic,** particularly in the center. Such areas are likely to be relatively resistant to radiation so that viable tumor cells may remain in spite of marked shrinkage of the tumor.

Pharmacologic Modification of the Effects of Radiation

A variety of chemical compounds are capable of enhancing the lethal effects of radiation. A series of randomized clinical trials has demonstrated a significant survival advantage, particularly in terms of local disease control, when cisplatin-containing chemotherapy is given concurrently with radiation for locoregionally advanced cervical cancer. Some of the regimens tested have included 5-fluorouracil in combination with cisplatin. This is called chemoradiation.

Time-Dose Fractionation of Radiation

Successful radiation therapy requires a delicate balance between dosage to the tumor and that to the surrounding normal tissues. A dose of radiation that is too high sterilizes the tumor but results in an unacceptably high complication rate because of the destruction of normal tissues.

Most normal tissues, such as gastrointestinal mucosa and bone marrow, have a remarkable capacity to recover from radiation damage by the division of stem cells as well as by repair of sublethal radiation damage. Tumors, in general, have less ability to repair and repopulate. This difference can be exploited by administering the radiation in multiple fractions, thereby allowing some recovery, particularly of normal cells, between fractions.

If the interval between each fraction increases, the total dose must increase to produce the same biologic effect because of the amount of recovery that will occur in the interval. **Cells that survive the acute effects of radiation usually repair sublethal damage within 24 hours;** therefore, conventionally fractionated radiation is usually given in daily increments.

When treating the pelvis with external radiation, each fraction is usually 180 to 200 centigray (cGy). In treating the whole abdomen, fractions are decreased to 100 to 120 cGy because the tolerance of normal tissues decreases as the volume irradiated increases. The major factors influencing the outcome of radiation therapy are summarized in Box 37-1.

MODALITIES OF RADIATION THERAPY

The modalities used to deliver radiation therapy are listed in Box 37-2. In general, there are two radiation techniques: teletherapy and brachytherapy. **In teletherapy, a device quite removed from the patient is used, as with external beam techniques. Figure 37-2 is a linear accelerator used to deliver external beam pelvic radiation. In brachytherapy, the radiation source is placed either within or close to the target tissue, as with intracavitary and interstitial techniques.** In contrast to external beam therapy, intracavitary and interstitial techniques allow a high dose of radiation to be delivered to the tumor, whereas dosages to surrounding normal tissues are considerably lower and are determined by the inverse square law.

BOX 37-1

MAJOR FACTORS INFLUENCING THE OUTCOME OF RADIATION THERAPY

Normal tissue tolerance
Malignant cell type
Total volume irradiated
Total dose delivered
Total duration of therapy
Number of fractions
Type of equipment used
Tissue oxygen concentration

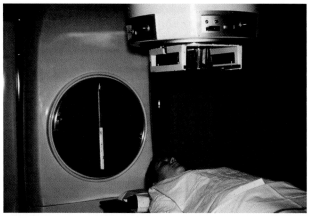

FIGURE 37-2 Linear accelerator used to deliver external beam pelvic radiation.

Teletherapy

EXTERNAL BEAM THERAPY. As the energy of the electromagnetic radiation increases, the penetration of the tissues increases, resulting in a relative sparing of the skin and an increased dosage to deeper tissues. At megavoltage energies (1 million electron volts or greater), there is no differential absorption of energy by bone.

Orthovoltage machines are no longer used except to treat skin cancers. Cobalt machines, developed in the early 1950s, have also been largely replaced by linear accelerators, which have a higher range of energies. The advantages of megavoltage therapy over the earlier orthovoltage machines are listed in Box 37-3.

External radiation allows a uniform dose to be delivered to a given field. The tolerance of the normal tissues (e.g., bowel, bladder, liver, kidneys) limits the total dosage that can be delivered. External radiation is usually used to shrink a large tumor mass before brachytherapy. When used alone, it is generally useful only when there is small residual macroscopic or microscopic disease following surgery. With highly radiosensitive tumors (e.g., dysgerminoma), external radiation alone may sterilize even bulky disease.

INTENSITY MODULATED RADIATION THERAPY. Computer technology and information systems have transformed delivery of external beam therapy in recent years. **Three-dimensional treatment planning based on computed tomographic (CT) imaging has allowed better definition of the specific target volume and the surrounding normal tissues.** Intensity modulated radiation therapy delivers radiation from multiple beam angles with nonuniform dose intensities, but the collective set of beams produces a more homogenous dose to the target volume. The multiple beams of variable intensity are achieved by the use of a multileaf collimator. **The end result is a high dose delivered to the target volume and acceptably low dose to the surrounding normal tissues.**

Brachytherapy

INTRACAVITARY RADIATION. Intracavitary therapy is used particularly in the treatment of cervical and vaginal cancer. **All applicators now in use should be "afterloaded,"** which means that they are placed in the patient and their position checked by radiography before the radioactive substance is loaded into the applicator. Traditionally, brachytherapy has been given at a low dose rate using radioactive substances such as cesium (^{137}Cs). Applicators for the management of cervical cancer are placed under general anesthesia. For low dose rate therapy, the applicators are left in situ for 48 to 72 hours. **Remote afterloading devices, such as the Selectron, allow the radioactive sources to be removed from the applicators when medical or nursing personnel enter the room,** thereby significantly limiting staff exposure to radiation. **More recently, high dose rate brachytherapy has been given, using radioactive sources such as iridium (^{192}Ir)** (Figures 37-3 and 37-4). Treatment is given as an outpatient, which is much more acceptable for patients.

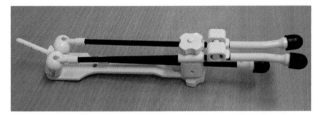

FIGURE 37-3 Intrauterine tandem and vaginal colpostats used for high dose rate intracavitary radiation in cervical cancer.

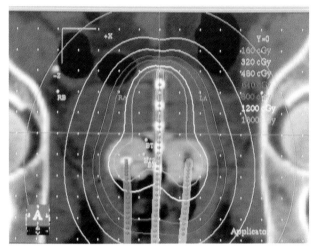

FIGURE 37-4 Posteroanterior view of brachytherapy applicator in situ, loaded with ^{192}Ir, **for the treatment of cervical cancer.** Note the isodose contours showing how the dose of radiation decreases with distance from the applicator.

Radioactive colloids, such as chromic phosphate (^{32}P), may be instilled directly into the peritoneal cavity to treat minimal residual disease, particularly in patients with ovarian cancer. To be effective, these agents must achieve a uniform distribution throughout the cavity, which is difficult to achieve, so such agents are rarely used at present. ^{32}**P is a pure beta (electron) emitter.**

INTERSTITIAL RADIATION. Interstitial therapy (in which the radioactive source is placed directly in the tumor) may be delivered by removable or permanent implants. **Permanent implants are used for inaccessible tumors. They use radioisotopes such as radon 222 (^{222}Rn) or iodine 125 (^{125}I) seeds** and are usually placed in an unresectable tumor nodule at the time of laparotomy.

Removable implants are placed in tumors that are accessible (e.g., cervical or vaginal tumors). Interstitial therapy has the theoretical advantage of better dose distribution within the tumor but the disadvantage that it is easier to overdose normal tissues, thereby increasing the complication rate. **The radioisotope of choice for afterloading interstitial implants is iridium**

192 (^{192}Ir), and afterloading devices are now available for interstitial therapy.

COMPLICATIONS ASSOCIATED WITH RADIATION

The success of radiation therapy depends on an exploitable gradient of susceptibility to injury in favor of normal tissue. Unfortunately, **most malignant tumors are only marginally more sensitive to radiation than are normal tissues,** so the total dose that can be delivered, and therefore the radiocurability, is limited by the associated complications.

Acute Complications

Acute reactions to radiation occur in the first 3 to 4 months, and include the following pathologic changes: rapid cessation of mitotic activity, cellular swelling, tissue edema, and tissue necrosis.

In the management of gynecologic tumors, these acute reactions may produce the following effects: **acute cystitis,** manifested by hematuria, urgency, and frequency; **proctosigmoiditis,** manifested by tenesmus, diarrhea, and passage of blood and mucus in the stool; **enteritis,** manifested by nausea, vomiting, diarrhea, and colicky abdominal pain; and **bone marrow suppression.** The latter is uncommon with pelvic radiation, but common with whole-abdominal radiation, particularly if the patient has had previous chemotherapy, or extended field (pelvic and paraaortic) radiation, particularly if the patient is given concurrent chemotherapy.

Chronic Complications

Chronic complications occur 6 months or more after completion of radiation and are characterized pathologically by the following changes: internal thickening and obliteration of small blood vessels **(endarteritis), fibrosis, and permanent reduction in the epithelial and parenchymal cell populations.**

Significant chronic complications occur in 5-10% of patients receiving 50c Gy or more of radiation, and they may be slowly progressive over several years.

Common chronic complications of radiation follow.

Radiation Enteropathy

Previous surgery, with resultant loops of small bowel adherent in the pelvis, predisposes the patient to **chronic radiation enteritis,** particularly when intracavitary or interstitial radiation is used in addition to teletherapy. **Small bowel injuries** usually present with cramping abdominal pain and vomiting, or with alternating diarrhea and constipation.

Large bowel injuries, which are best diagnosed by sigmoidoscopy or colonoscopy, may include: **proctosigmoiditis,** manifested by pelvic pain, tenesmus, diarrhea, and rectal bleeding; **ulceration,** manifested by rectal bleeding and tenesmus; **rectal or sigmoid stenosis,** manifested by progressive large bowel obstruction;

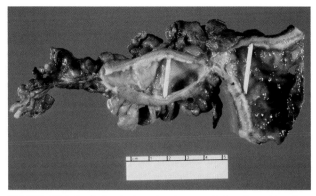

FIGURE 37-5 Radiation-induced stricture of the sigmoid colon. Note the tight fibrotic constriction, necessitating partial sigmoid colectomy for large bowel obstruction.

and **rectovaginal fistula,** manifested by passage of stool through the vagina. Figure 37-5 shows a radiation induced stricture of the sigmoid colon.

Vaginal Vault Necrosis

This is associated with severe pain and tenderness of the vaginal vault and a profuse vaginal discharge.

Urologic Injuries

The following are included in this category: **hemorrhagic cystitis,** which may necessitate frequent blood transfusions and, occasionally, urinary diversion; **ureteric stenosis,** which is manifested by progressive hydronephrosis; **vesicovaginal fistula,** manifested by the constant leakage of urine and demonstrable by cystoscopy; and **ureterovaginal fistula,** which is also manifested by constant leakage of urine and is demonstrable with an intravenous pyelogram.

Hormonal Therapy

The estrogen receptor (ER) status of primary and metastatic breast cancer has been shown to be of therapeutic and prognostic significance. The ER and progesterone receptor (PR) status of endometrial cancer also have prognostic and therapeutic significance.

MECHANISM OF ACTION OF HORMONAL RECEPTORS

Most steroid hormones influence their target tissues by the following series of steps: passive diffusion of the hormone through the cell membrane, specific binding in the cytoplasm with the hormone receptor, translocation of the receptor-hormone complex to the nucleus, binding of the receptor-hormone complex to an "acceptor" site on the chromatin, and transcription of DNA in a manner characteristic of the specific hormone–target cell interaction, eventually resulting in either an increase or a decrease in specific protein synthesis.

Tamoxifen binds with the ER and is translocated to the nucleus, where it binds to chromatin. It does not influence gene transcription, so functionally, tamoxifen acts as an antiestrogen.

Estrogen exposure increases the production of both ER and PR, whereas progesterone inhibits production of both ER and PR.

Aromatase inhibitors work by blocking aromatase, the enzyme that is responsible for the final step of estrogen synthesis. They prevent the production of estrogen, the substrate of the ER, in postmenopausal women.

Luteinizing hormone-releasing hormone agonists act by pituitary desensitization and receptor down-regulation, suppressing gonadotrophin release. They are as effective as surgical oophorectomy in premenopausal women with ER positive advanced breast cancer.

CLINICAL APPLICATIONS

Because tumor growth in patients whose tumors contain ER and PR is likely to be stimulated by estrogen exposure, tumor regression should occur if endogenous estrogen production is abolished or if the patient is exposed to a progestin or antiestrogen. **In breast cancer, patients whose tumors contain ER and PR have an 80% response rate to hormonal manipulation,** whereas fewer than 10% of receptor-poor tumors respond.

An objective response to progestin therapy occurs in about one-third of patients with recurrent or metastatic endometrial carcinoma. Progestin therapy is more likely to be effective in well differentiated endometrioid adenocarcinomas than in more poorly differentiated tumors because well differentiated tumors are the ones that are most likely to contain ER and PR.

ER and PR have been demonstrated in some ovarian adenocarcinomas, particularly endometrioid carcinomas. **Tamoxifen is effective in up to 30% of women with recurrent ovarian cancer,** and aromatase inhibitors are also active agents.

TARGETED THERAPIES

Targeted therapies are being increasingly used in patients with gynecologic cancers, and with the explosion in molecular biological research, their use will only increase further in the future. Unlike cytotoxic chemotherapy, which acts by preventing DNA replication and cellular division in general, so affects all rapidly dividing cells, **targeted therapies are directed against a particular signaling pathway within the cancer cell.**

A critical event for tumor growth is the formation of new blood vessels, or angiogenesis. The vascular endothelial growth factor (VEGF) and its receptors (VEGFR) are intimately involved in tumor angiogenesis. The major mediator is VEGF-A, which is upregulated in many tumors. **Bevacizumab (Avastin)** is a recombinant humanized monoclonal immunoglobulin G1 (IgG1) antibody that targets VEGF-A. It is being used for patients with ovarian cancer, either in conjunction with chemotherapy, or alone as maintenance therapy. Potential side effects include hypertension, thromboembolism, and an increased risk of bowel perforation.

Another very promising targeted approach in patients with ovarian cancer is use of **polyadenosine diphosphate-ribose polymerase (PARP) inhibitors.** These agents target DNA repair and are particularly effective in patients with BRCA 1 or 2 germline mutations.

Pain Management

More than 70% of patients with cancer will develop significant pain at some point in their disease. Proper pain management requires an understanding of pain physiology, pain mechanisms, and the pharmacology of analgesics.

Pain in gynecologic cancer may be the result of soft tissue infiltration, bone involvement, neural involvement, muscle spasm (e.g., psoas spasm), infection within or near tumor masses, or bowel colic.

Therapeutic approaches will vary according to the pain mechanism involved. Consideration must be given to the specific therapeutic measure that may be appropriate in the individual case, such as radiation therapy, chemotherapy, antibiotics, regional nerve block, or surgery.

Peripherally acting drugs such as acetaminophen (paracetamol) should rarely be omitted from analgesic regimens, and rectal suppositories are useful if oral intake is not appropriate. When pain is caused by bone metastases, nonsteroidal antiinflammatory drugs or bisphosphonates are helpful. Muscle spasm requires muscle relaxants such as diazepam, whereas bowel colic requires anticholinergics such as buscopan.

Opioid use will be necessary for severe pain, although nerve pain and muscle spasm are not well relieved by opioids. A variety of opioids is available, and in general, a low-potency opioid such as codeine or a high-potency opioid such as morphine is combined with a peripherally acting drug such as acetaminophen or aspirin.

Immediate release morphine, which is best given orally or subcutaneously, should be given at regular 4-hourly intervals. **Controlled-release morphine tablets are a significant advance in convenience of administration, as they need to be given only every 12 to 24 hours,** once the total 24-hour requirement has been determined from the use of an immediate release preparation. Constipation is a real problem with opioids, and prophylactic laxatives should be prescribed.

Alternative opioids (with equivalency to morphine 5 mg) include oxycodone (5 mg), hydromorphone (1 mg), pentazocine (45 mg), and meperidine (75 mg).

When pain is neurogenic in origin, an opioid and a peripherally acting drug should usually be supplemented by a tricyclic antidepressant, an anticonvulsant, or a corticosteroid.

End-of-Life Issues

When it becomes clear that the patient is dying, the goals are to control symptoms, maintain dignity, and allow time and privacy for communication with loved ones.

Medications should usually be given subcutaneously or rectally, any unnecessary tubes or equipment should be removed to facilitate contact with loved ones, and nursing care should particularly focus on pressure areas, mouth care, and "grooming." Sedation, for example, with sublingual lorazepam 0.5 to 2.5 mg every 4 to 6 hours, may be helpful if the patient is agitated.

Important issues from a patient's perspective are receiving adequate pain and symptom management, avoiding inappropriate prolongation of dying, achieving a sense of control, relieving the burden on caregivers, and strengthening relationships with loved ones.

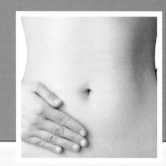

Cervical Dysplasia and Cancer

NEVILLE F. HACKER

Cervical cancer is the third most common cancer in women worldwide, after breast and colorectal cancer, but it is the major cause of death from cancer in women, killing around 275,000 women a year. About 80% of new cases occur in developing countries, where cervical screening programs are limited or nonexistent. **In developed countries, regular screening has markedly decreased the incidence of the disease,** and most cases now occur in women who have not had regular Papanicolaou smears. In the United States, cervical cancer now ranks only 13th among cancers in women, with 12,340 new cases expected in 2013, and 4030 deaths.

Studies have identified persistent infection with a high-risk human papillomavirus (HPV) as the cause of virtually all cervical cancers. Randomized clinical trials of prophylactic HPV vaccines have demonstrated dramatic efficiency in preventing HPV 16 and 18 infections, as well as precancerous cervical lesions. Although it will take several decades to demonstrate a decreased incidence of invasive cervical cancer, **with widespread use, HPV vaccination should markedly decrease the incidence of cervical cancer in future generations.**

Etiology and Epidemiology

There are 15 high-risk HPV types and types 16 and 18 are responsible for 70% of cervical cancers. Types 6 and 11 have been associated with cervical condylomas and low-grade cervical intraepithelial neoplasia (CIN).

The adolescent cervix is believed to be more susceptible to carcinogenic stimuli because of the active process of squamous metaplasia, which occurs within the transformation zone during periods of endocrine change. This squamous metaplasia is normally a physiologic process, but under the influence of the HPV, cellular alterations occur that result in an atypical transformation zone. These atypical changes initiate CIN, which is the preinvasive phase of cervical cancer.

Cervical cancer and its precursors have been associated with several epidemiologic variables (Box 38-1).

BOX 38-1

BOX 38-1

RISK FACTORS FOR CERVICAL CANCER

- Young age at first coitus (<17 yr)
- Multiple sexual partners
- Sexual partner with multiple sexual partners
- Young age at first pregnancy
- High parity
- Lower socioeconomic status
- Smoking

These risk factors basically increase the likelihood of exposure to a high-risk HPV type.

The disease is relatively rare before 25 years of age, and the mean age is about 47 years.

Primary Prevention

Two prophylactic vaccines are presently available. The **quadrivalent vaccine Gardasil,** which is manufactured by Merck and Co. and protects against HPV types 6, 11, 16, and 18, was approved by the U.S. Food and Drug Administration (FDA) in June 2006 for females aged 9 through 26 years. The **bivalent vaccine Cervarix,** which is manufactured by Glaxo Smith Kline and protects against HPV types 16 and 18, was approved by the FDA in October 2009, for use in females aged 10 through 25 years.

HPV vaccination is most effective if performed before the onset of sexual activity. Vaccination is still recommended after commencement of sexual activity, and even after prior abnormal cytology or CIN, but it is likely to be less effective after HPV exposure. In 2007, Australia was the first country in the world to introduce HPV vaccination into the National Immunization Program for all schoolgirls aged 12 years.

Screening of Asymptomatic Women

The American College of Obstetricians and Gynecologists (ACOG) has recommended that all women should undergo an annual physical examination, including a Papanicolaou (Pap) smear, within 3 years of sexual intercourse, or by age 21. The false-negative rate for conventional Pap smears for high-grade intraepithelial lesions is generally reported to be about 20%, but it is higher for glandular lesions and for invasive cancers.

New technologies have been developed to decrease the false negative rate. Thin Prep (Cytyc Corporation) and Surepath (TriPath Imaging) are automated liquid-based slide-preparation systems. With liquid-based cytology (LBC), the spatula or brush taking the smear is placed into a fixative solution, instead of smearing the cells directly onto a glass slide. Blood, mucus, and inflammatory cells are eliminated and a monolayer smear is then automatically prepared by a machine. Focal Point (Surepath) and ThinPrep Imager (Cytyc) are computerized image processors that select the most abnormal cells on a slide. They increase the sensitivity of slide reading, while decreasing the time needed by the cytotechnician to read each slide, thereby improving the cost effectiveness of screening.

The American Society for Colposcopy and Cervical Pathology (ASCCP) has recommended that screening with Liquid Based Cytology (LBC) should occur every 3 years from 21 to 30 years. Thereafter, they recommend continued screening every 3 to 5 years with LBC for HPV testing. Both the endocervical canal and the exocervix (or ectocervix) should be sampled when taking the Papanicolaou smear.

HPV deoxyribonucleic acid (DNA) testing is much more sensitive than cervical cytology, but less specific. It is presently being investigated as a primary screening test for women after the age of 25 to 30 in many developed countries. The negative predictive value of the HPV test is very high, so screening intervals could safely be extended to at least 5 years. If the HPV test is positive, reflex cervical cytology is performed to determine the need for referral for colposcopy.

Women should have regular cervical screening even if they have received the HPV vaccine, because the vaccine does not protect against all high-risk HPV viral types.

Cervical Topography

During early embryonic development, the cervix and upper vagina are covered with columnar epithelium. During intrauterine development, the columnar epithelium of the vagina is progressively replaced by squamous epithelium. At birth, the vagina is usually covered with squamous epithelium, and the columnar epithelium is limited to the endocervix and the central portion of the exocervix (or ectocervix). **In about 4% of normal female infants, the columnar epithelium extends onto the vaginal fornices.** Macroscopically, the columnar epithelium has a red appearance because it is only a single cell layer thick, allowing blood vessels in the underlying stroma to show through it.

The embryologic squamous and columnar epithelia are designated the original or native squamous and columnar epithelia, respectively. The junction between them on the exocervix (or ectocervix) is called the original squamocolumnar junction.

Throughout life, but particularly during adolescence and a woman's first pregnancy, metaplastic squamous epithelium covers the columnar epithelium so that a new squamocolumnar junction is formed more proximally. This junction moves progressively closer to the external os and then up the endocervical canal. **The**

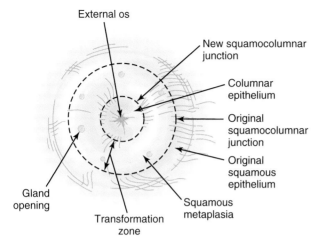

External os
New squamocolumnar junction
Columnar epithelium
Original squamocolumnar junction
Original squamous epithelium
Squamous metaplasia
Gland opening
Transformation zone

FIGURE 38-1 Schematic representation of the transformation zone.

transformation zone is the area of metaplastic squamous epithelium located between the original squamocolumnar junction and the new squamocolumnar junction (Figure 38-1).

Classification of an Abnormal Papanicolaou Smear

In 1988, a consensus meeting was convened by the Division of Cancer Control of the National Cancer Institute to review existing terminology and to recommend effective methods of cytologic reporting. As a result of this meeting, **the Bethesda system** was devised and requires **(1) a statement regarding the adequacy of the specimen** for diagnosis, **(2) a diagnostic categorization** (normal or other), and **(3) a descriptive diagnosis.** A revised Bethesda system was developed in 2001 and is shown in Box 38-2.

CERVICAL INTRAEPITHELIAL NEOPLASIA

CIN represents a spectrum of disease, ranging from LSIL, low-grade squamous intraepithelial lesion (formerly called CIN I or mild dysplasia) to HSIL, high-grade squamous intraepithelial lesion (formerly called CIN II and III, or moderate and severe dysplasia). At least 35% of patients with HSIL will develop invasive cancer within 10 years, whereas LSIL often spontaneously regresses. With CIN, there is abnormal epithelial proliferation and maturation above the basement membrane. Involvement of the inner one-third of the epithelium represents LSIL, while involvement of the outer two-thirds represents HSIL (Figure 38-2). The disease is asymptomatic.

COLPOSCOPY

The colposcope is a stereoscopic binocular microscope of low magnification, usually 10× to 40×. Illumination

---

BOX 38-2

THE 2001 BETHESDA CLASSIFICATION OF CYTOLOGIC ABNORMALITIES (ABRIDGED)

Specimen Adequacy

Satisfactory for evaluation (note presence/absence of endocervical/transformation zone component)
Unsatisfactory for evaluation (specify reason)
Specimen rejected/not processed (specify reason)
Specimen processed and examined, but unsatisfactory for evaluation of epithelial abnormality because of (specify reason)

General Categorization (Optional)

Negative for intraepithelial lesion or malignancy
Epithelial cell abnormality
Other

Interpretation/Result

Negative for Intraepithelial Lesion or Malignancy

Organisms (e.g., *Trichomonas vaginalis*)
Reactive cellular changes associated with inflammation (includes typical repair), radiation, intrauterine contraceptive device
Atrophy

Epithelial Cell Abnormalities

Squamous Cell

Atypical squamous cells of undetermined significance (ASCUS) cannot exclude high-grade squamous intraepithelial lesions (ASC-H)
Low-grade squamous intraepithelial lesion (LSIL) encompassing: human papillomavirus/mild dysplasia/cervical intraepithelial neoplasia (CIN I)
HSIL encompassing: moderate and severe dysplasia, carcinoma in situ; CIN 2 and CIN 3
Squamous cell carcinoma

Glandular Cell

Atypical glandular cells (AGC) (specify endocervical, endometrial, or not otherwise specified)
Atypical glandular cells, favor neoplastic (specify endocervical or not otherwise specified)
Endocervical adenocarcinoma in situ (AIS)
Adenocarcinoma

Other

For example, endometrial cells in a woman ≥40 years of age

---

is centered, and the focal length is between 12 and 15 cm.

To perform a colposcopic examination, an appropriately sized speculum is inserted to expose the cervix, which is cleansed with a cotton pledget soaked in 3% acetic acid to remove adherent mucus and cellular debris. A green filter can be employed to accentuate the vascular changes that frequently accompany pathologic alterations of the cervix.

At colposcopy, the original or native squamous epithelium appears gray and homogeneous. The

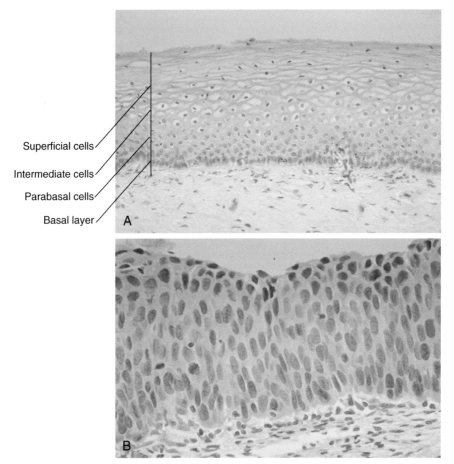

FIGURE 38-2 Histologic appearance of normal cervical squamous epithelium **(A)** and high-grade squamous intraepithelial lesion (HSIL) **(B)** of the cervix. In the normal epithelium, note the orderly maturation from the basal layer to the parabasal cells, glycogenated intermediate cells, and flattened superficial cells. In the HSIL, the entire thickness of the epithelium is replaced by immature cells that are variable in size and shape and have irregular nuclei. Mitotic figures are seen in the lower two-thirds of the epithelium.

columnar epithelium appears red and grapelike. **The transformation zone can be identified by the presence of gland openings that are not covered by the squamous metaplasia and by the paler color of the metaplastic epithelium compared with the original squamous epithelium. Nabothian follicles may also be seen in the transformation zone. Normal blood vessels branch like a tree.**

Evaluation of a Patient with an Abnormal Papanicolaou Smear

An algorithm for the evaluation of patients with abnormal Papanicolaou smears is presented in Figure 38-3.

Any patient with a grossly abnormal cervix should have a punch biopsy performed, regardless of the results of the Papanicolaou smear.

Patients with atypical squamous cells of undetermined significance (ASCUS) found on their smear may have a repeat smear in 6 months. Alternatively,

HPV testing, such as with the Hybrid Capture assay (Digene Diagnostics, Silver Spring, MD) may be used to triage such patients. About 6-10% of patients with an ASCUS smear will have high-grade CIN on colposcopy, and 90% of these can be detected by HPV testing for high-risk viral types.

The colposcopic hallmark of cervical intraepithelial neoplasia is an area of sharply delineated acetowhite epithelium—that is, epithelium that appears white after the application of acetic acid. It is thought that the acetic acid dehydrates the cells and that there is increased light reflex from areas of increased nuclear density. **Within the acetowhite areas, there may or may not be abnormal vascular patterns.**

There are two basic changes in the vascular architecture in patients with CIN: punctation and mosaicism (Figure 38-4). Punctation is caused by single-looped capillaries lying within the subepithelial papillae, seen end-on as a "dot" as they course toward the surface of the epithelium. Mosaicism is caused by a fine network of capillaries disposed parallel to the

Evaluation of an abnormal Papanicolaou smear
in a patient with a grossly normal cervix

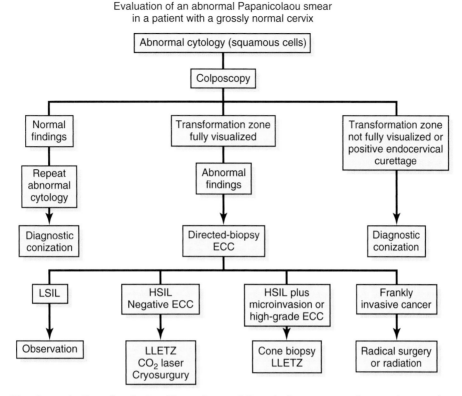

FIGURE 38-3 Algorithm for evaluation of patients with an abnormal Papanicolaou smear and a grossly normal-appearing cervix. *ECC,* Endocervical curettage; *HSIL,* high-grade squamous intraepithelial lesion; *LLETZ,* large loop excision of the transformation zone; *LSIL,* low-grade squamous intraepithelial lesion.

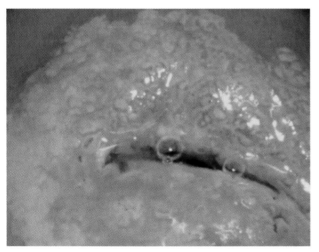

FIGURE 38-4 Colposcopic appearance of a patient with high-grade squamous intraepithelial lesion. Note the densely acetowhite epithelium with sharply demarcated borders, and the coarse mosaic vascular pattern.

surface in a mosaic pattern. Punctate and mosaic patterns may be seen together within the same area of the cervix. The more dilated and irregular the punctate and mosaic capillaries and the greater the intercapillary distance, the more atypical is the tissue on histologic examination. Similarly, the whiter the lesion, the more severe the dysplasia.

With microinvasive carcinoma, extremely irregular punctate and mosaic patterns are found, as are small atypical vessels. **The irregularity in size, shape, and arrangement of the terminal vessels becomes even more striking in frankly invasive carcinoma, with exaggerated distortions of the vascular architecture producing comma-shaped, corkscrew-shaped, and dilated, blind-ended vessels.**

BIOPSY AND ENDOCERVICAL CURETTAGE

If the colposcopic examination is satisfactory, which implies that the entire transformation zone has been visualized, a punch biopsy is taken from the worst area or areas, together with an endocervical curettage. The endocervical curettage is not performed in patients who are pregnant.

A diagnostic cone biopsy of the cervix is indicated in the following circumstances:
1. **Pap smear shows a high-grade lesion and the colposcopic examination is unsatisfactory.**
2. **Endocervical curettings show a high-grade lesion.**
3. **Pap smear shows a high-grade lesion that is not confirmed on punch biopsy.**

4. **Pap smear shows adenocarcinoma in situ.**
5. **Microinvasion is present on the punch biopsy.**

Treatment of Intraepithelial Neoplasia

It is reasonable to observe biopsy-proven LSIL without active treatment, as many cases will spontaneously regress. Active treatment is indicated for HSIL.

Superficial ablative techniques, such as large loop excision of the transformation zone (LLETZ), cryosurgery, or carbon dioxide laser are appropriate if the entire transformation zone is visible.

LARGE LOOP EXCISION OF THE TRANSFORMATION ZONE

LLETZ has gained popularity because **the equipment is relatively cheap, it can be performed on an outpatient basis under local anesthesia, and tissue is obtained for histologic evaluation.** Hence, occult invasive lesions should be more readily diagnosed. In unskilled hands, diathermy artifact may make histologic interpretation impossible.

LASER

Destruction of the transformation zone by carbon dioxide laser (light amplification by stimulated emission of radiation) ablation can be performed as an outpatient procedure, under local anesthesia. Bleeding may sometimes occur, but scarring is minimal and large lesions may be destroyed with low failure rates (in the order of 5-10%). **The equipment is expensive, so laser has lost favor in most centers.**

CRYOSURGERY

The cryosurgery technique is a relatively painless outpatient procedure that can be performed without anesthesia. There is no bleeding, and the equipment is cheap. However, **there is a high failure rate for large lesions and for lesions extending down glandular crypts.** It is mainly useful for lesions involving 1 or 2 quadrants. The major side effect is a rather copious vaginal discharge that persists for several weeks.

CERVICAL CONIZATION

Cervical conization is mainly a diagnostic technique, but it may also be therapeutic if the surgical margins are clear. **Bleeding, infection, cervical stenosis, and cervical incompetence are the major complications. Laser conization decreases the risk of cervical stenosis compared with cold knife conization.**

HYSTERECTOMY

Hysterectomy is rarely necessary for the treatment of HSIL. It may be applicable when there is concomitant uterine or adnexal disease.

Persistence and recurrence rates combined are approximately 2-3% after hysterectomy. This number should be significantly reduced by using colposcopy and Schiller staining (Lugol iodine) preoperatively to exclude intraepithelial neoplasia in the upper vagina.

Invasive Cancer

SYMPTOMS

Invasive cancer usually presents with postcoital, intermenstrual, or postmenopausal vaginal bleeding. In patients who are not sexually active, bleeding from cervical cancer usually does not occur until the disease is quite advanced (unlike patients with endometrial cancer, who almost always bleed early). **Persistent vaginal discharge, pelvic pain, leg swelling, and urinary frequency are usually seen with advanced disease.** In developing countries, it is not uncommon for patients to present with loss of urine or stool from the vagina, because of fistula formation.

PHYSICAL FINDINGS

Patients with cervical cancer usually have a normal general physical examination. Weight loss occurs late in the disease. With advanced disease, there may be enlarged inguinal or supraclavicular lymph nodes, edema of the legs, or hepatomegaly, but these are not commonly seen.

On pelvic examination the cervix may be ulcerative or exophytic (Figure 38-5). It usually bleeds on palpation and there is often an associated serous, purulent, or bloody discharge. The lesion may involve the adjacent vagina and extend toward the introitus.

A rectovaginal examination is essential to determine the extent of disease. **The diameter of the primary cancer and spread to the parametria are much more easily detected with a finger in the rectum, as is extension into the uterosacral ligaments.**

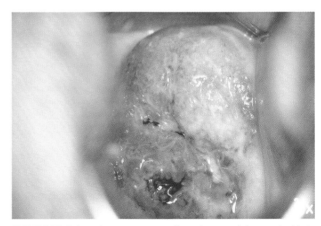

FIGURE 38-5 Invasive squamous cell carcinoma of the cervix. Note the irregular, ulcerated surface of the exocervix (or ectocervix). A biopsy of such a lesion is mandatory.

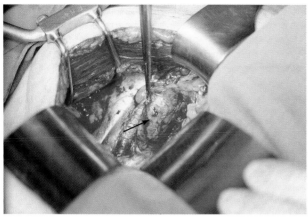

FIGURE 38-6 Grossly enlarged lymph node *(arrow)* at the bifurcation of the common iliac artery in a patient with stage IB2 carcinoma of the cervix. Large nodes such as this can cause ureteric obstruction.

PATHOLOGIC FEATURES

Most uterine cervical cancers are squamous in origin. Adenocarcinomas and adenosquamous carcinomas are increasing in incidence and account for about 20-25% of cases. Melanomas and sarcomas occur rarely.

PATTERNS OF SPREAD

Invasive cervical cancer spreads by direct invasion to involve the cervical stroma, corpus, vagina, and parametrium; lymphatic spread to pelvic and then paraaortic lymph nodes (Figure 38-6); and hematogenous spread, particularly to the lungs, liver, and bone.

PREOPERATIVE INVESTIGATIONS

The official International Federation of Gynecology and Obstetrics (FIGO) staging for cervical cancer was changed in 2009. It remains a clinical staging method based on physical examination and noninvasive testing, because most patients with cervical cancer worldwide are treated with radiation therapy (Table 38-1). **Studies allowed include biopsies, cystoscopy, sigmoidoscopy, chest and skeletal radiographs, intravenous pyelography, and liver function tests.**

An abdominal and pelvic computed tomographic (CT) scan or a magnetic resonance imaging scan (MRI) may be helpful in planning management, but the results do not influence the FIGO stage. The MRI is particularly helpful in defining the extent of the primary lesion, including any extension into the parametrium, bladder, or rectum. Neither is particularly sensitive for detecting lymph node metastases, and **positron-emission tomographic (PET) scanning is being increasingly used** for this purpose. **The incidence of paraaortic lymph node metastases is approx-**imately 20% in patients with stage II disease and 30% in those with stage III. The status of the paraaortic nodes is the single most important prognostic factor.

Laboratory studies may reveal abnormalities with advanced disease, the most common being anemia from blood loss, elevated blood urea nitrogen and creatinine levels from ureteric obstruction, and abnormal liver function tests if there are liver metastases. **Ureteric obstruction occurs in about 30% of patients with stage III disease and in 50% of patients with stage IV disease.** Hypercalcemia may denote bone metastases.

TREATMENT OF INVASIVE CANCER

Stage IA (Microinvasive Carcinoma)

A preoperative diagnosis of microinvasive carcinoma can be made only on the basis of a cone biopsy of the cervix with clear surgical margins, which allows multiple-step sections to be taken at 2-mm intervals. With a punch biopsy, the sampling of the cervix is too limited, and a more frankly invasive focus may be missed. The concept of microinvasive carcinoma also applies to glandular lesions, although an occasional adenocarcinoma will have a skip lesion higher in the endocervical canal.

When the depth of invasion on cone biopsy is 3 mm or less, horizontal dimension is 7 mm or less (stage IA1), and there is no lymphatic or vascular space involvement, an extra-fascial abdominal or vaginal hysterectomy is appropriate treatment. Cervical conization alone may suffice if the patient desires to maintain her fertility, as long as the cone margins are free of disease and the endocervical curettings (taken after the conization) are negative. **For stage IA2 disease, or if there is lymphatic or vascular space involvement, most gynecologic oncologists recommend modified radical hysterectomy and pelvic lymph node dissection.** If childbearing is desired, large-cone biopsy or radical trachelectomy combined with pelvic lymphadenectomy may be offered.

Stages IB1 and IB2

Stage IB disease may be treated by either primary surgery (radical hysterectomy and bilateral pelvic lymphadenectomy) or primary chemoradiation therapy. The advantages of surgery are that the ovaries may be spared in younger women, surgical staging may be carried out, and chronic radiation complications may be avoided, particularly vaginal stenosis, radiation proctitis, and radiation cystitis. Primary surgery is regarded as the treatment of choice for Stage IB1 cervical cancer.

The results of treatment by either method are similar when both the surgeon and the radiotherapist are knowledgeable and skilled. Chemoradiation is often chosen for Stage IB2 lesions, but primary surgery followed by tailored external beam therapy is a valid

TABLE 38-1

INTERNATIONAL FEDERATION OF GYNECOLOGY AND OBSTETRICS STAGING OF CARCINOMA OF THE CERVIX UTERI (2009)

Stage	
I	The carcinoma is strictly confined to the cervix (extension to the corpus would be disregarded)
IA	Invasive carcinoma which can be diagnosed only by microscopy, with deepest invasion ≤5.0 mm and largest extension ≤7.0 mm
IA1	Measured stromal invasion of ≤3.0 mm in depth and extension of ≤7.0 mm
IA2	Measured stromal invasion of >3.0 mm and not >5.0 mm with an extension of not >7.0 mm
IB	Clinically visible lesions limited to the cervix uteri or preclinical cancers greater than stage IA*
IB1	Clinically visible lesion ≤4.0 cm in greatest dimension
IB2	Clinically visible lesion >4.0 cm in greatest dimension
II	Cervical carcinoma invades beyond the uterus, but not to the pelvic wall or to the lower third of the vagina
IIA	Without parametrial invasion
IIA1	Clinically visible lesion ≤4.0 cm in greatest dimension
IIA2	Clinically visible lesion >4.0 cm in greatest dimension
IIB	With obvious parametrial invasion
III	The tumor extends to the pelvic wall and/or involves lower third of the vagina and/or causes hydronephrosis or nonfunctioning kidney[†]
IIIA	Tumor involves lower third of the vagina, with no extension to the pelvic wall
IIIB	Extension to the pelvic wall and/or hydronephrosis or nonfunctioning kidney
IV	The carcinoma has extended beyond the true pelvis or has involved (biopsy proven) the mucosa of the bladder or rectum; a bullous edema, as such, does not permit a case to be allotted to stage IV
IVA	Spread of the growth to adjacent organs
IVB	Spread to distant organs

From FIGO Committee on Gynecologic Oncology: Revised FIGO staging for carcinoma of the vulva, cervix, and endometrium. *Int J Gynecol Obst* 105:103–104, 2009.
*All macroscopically visible lesions—even with superficial invasion—are allotted to stage IB carcinomas. Invasion is limited to a measured stromal invasion with a maximal depth of 5.00 mm and a horizontal extension of not >7.00 mm. Depth of invasion should not be >5.00 mm taken from the base of the epithelium of the original tissue—squamous or glandular. The depth of invasion should always be reported in mm, even in those cases with "early (minimal) stromal invasion" (≈1 mm). The involvement of vascular/lymphatic spaces should not change the stage allotment.
[†]On rectal examination, there is no cancer-free space between the tumor and the pelvic wall. All cases with hydronephrosis or nonfunctioning kidney are included, unless they are known to be due to another cause.

alternative approach. Patients with deep stromal penetration and extensive vascular space invasion but negative lymph nodes may receive a "small field" of pelvic radiation, whereas patients with positive common iliac or paraaortic nodes may receive extended field radiation, usually combined with cisplatin.

RADICAL HYSTERECTOMY. In this procedure, the uterus is removed along with adjacent portions of the vagina, cardinal ligaments, uterosacral ligaments, and bladder pillars.

The most common complication of radical hysterectomy is bladder dysfunction, which occurs because of interruption to the autonomic nerves traversing the cardinal and uterosacral ligaments. Normal bladder function is usually restored within 1 to 3 weeks, but 1-2% of patients have permanent dysfunction necessitating lifelong self-catheterization. A nerve-sparing radical hysterectomy has been described and is increasingly used.

The most serious complication of radical hysterectomy is ureteric fistula or stricture, which occurs in 1-2% of cases. A less common but life-threatening complication is **deep venous thrombosis,** with or without **pulmonary embolism.** The incidence of venous thromboembolism can be reduced with the use of external pneumatic calf compressors at the time of surgery, early ambulation, and prophylactic anticoagulants. Some degree of **lymphedema** occurs in 15-20% of patients having a pelvic lymphadenectomy.

RADICAL TRACHELECTOMY. For young women with early cancer (up to 2 cm diameter), radical vaginal or abdominal trachelectomy and pelvic lymphadenectomy may allow fertility preservation, without significantly compromising survival.

RADIATION THERAPY. For patients with stage IB2 disease, most centers use primary chemoradiation, using weekly cisplatin as the radiation sensitizer. **Therapy usually begins with external radiation in an attempt to shrink the central tumor and improve the dosimetry of the subsequent intracavitary therapy (brachytherapy).**

If primary radical hysterectomy is performed, external radiation may be used postoperatively for patients with lymph node metastases or inadequate surgical margins, but brachytherapy may be avoided, thereby decreasing the incidence of vaginal stenosis. The addition of weekly cisplatin (40 mg/m^2 intravenously) during external beam therapy has been shown to improve survival.

Stage IIA1 or IIA2

In patients with minimal involvement of the posterior vaginal fornix (up to 1 cm), radical hysterectomy, upper vaginectomy and pelvic lymphadenectomy is appropriate, particularly for patients with stage IIA1 disease. With more extensive posterior forniceal involvement, chemoradiation therapy is the treatment of choice, because surgery would leave the patient with a much shortened vagina. If there is involvement of the anterior fornix, surgical margins on the bladder would be close, and treatment should be with chemoradiation therapy. Most patients with stage IIA2 disease will be treated with chemoradiation.

Stage IIB

Most patients with stage IIB lesions are treated with a combination of external beam chemoradiation and intracavitary brachytherapy. **If positive paraaortic or high common iliac lymph nodes are detected preoperatively on imaging, extended-field radiation may be employed** to treat all of the paraaortic lymph nodes up to the diaphragm.

Stages IIIA and IIIB

Patients with stage IIIA and stage IIIB disease are treated with chemoradiation therapy, usually external beam followed by intracavitary brachytherapy. In patients with locally advanced disease, distortion of the cervix and vagina may make brachytherapy difficult to apply. Therefore, a higher dose of external therapy, up to 7000 centigray (cGy), may be necessary. Alternatively, interstitial radiation may be given to get a better dose distribution than would be possible with intracavitary therapy.

Stage IVA

Pelvic chemoradiation therapy is used in most patients with stage IVA lesions. If radiation therapy results in only partial tumor regression, a "salvage" pelvic exenteration may be performed. **Primary pelvic exenteration is performed only rarely,** usually when the patient presents with a rectovaginal or vesicovaginal fistula.

Stage IVB

These patients basically require palliative care and control of symptoms, because they are not curable. Control of symptoms will usually necessitate some pelvic radiation therapy to palliate bleeding from the vagina, bladder, or rectum. Bone metastases may require radiation, and chemotherapy may be offered for systemic metastases to prolong survival.

Recurrent or Metastatic Disease

CHEMOTHERAPY. The effectiveness of chemotherapy is limited for metastatic cervical cancer.

Several drugs have been tested and found to be active in up to 35% of cases. Most responses are partial, and the patients usually progress within 12 months. **The most active agents are cisplatin, bleomycin, mitomycin C, methotrexate, and cyclophosphamide.**

PELVIC EXENTERATION. Pelvic exenteration is generally reserved for patients who have a central recurrence following pelvic irradiation. **Total exenteration involves removal of the pelvic viscera, including the uterus, tubes, ovaries, vagina, bladder, and rectum** (Figure 38-7). Depending on the site and extent of the disease, the operation may be limited to an anterior exenteration, which spares the rectum, or a posterior exenteration, which spares the bladder.

Following the extirpative surgery, pelvic reconstruction is necessary. If the bladder is removed, the ureters must be implanted into a portion of the small or large bowel that has been isolated from the remainder of the gastrointestinal tract to form a conduit. **A continent conduit may be created,** particularly in younger patients. When the disease is confined to the upper vagina and rectovaginal septum, the lower rectum and anal canal may be preserved and reanastomosed to the sigmoid colon. A temporary colostomy is often required to protect the reanastomosis because of the prior irradiation. **Vaginal reconstruction can be performed using a split-thickness skin graft, bilateral gracilis myocutaneous grafts, a rectus abdominus myocutaneous flap, or a segment of large intestine.**

Relatively few patients with recurrent cancer of the cervix are suitable to undergo pelvic exenteration because most have metastases outside the pelvis or fixation of the tumor to structures that cannot be removed, such as the pelvic side wall. All patients should have a preoperative PET/CT scan to exclude nodal or other systemic metastases.

In selecting patients who may be suitable for pelvic exenteration, the triad of unilateral leg edema, sciatic pain, and ureteral obstruction is ominous and usually indicates unresectable disease in the pelvis.

Cervical Carcinoma in Pregnancy

Carcinoma of the cervix associated with pregnancy usually implies diagnosis during pregnancy or within 6 months postpartum. It is relatively uncommon, invasive carcinoma occurring in approximately 1 in 2200 pregnancies.

SYMPTOMS

The symptoms are similar to those in nonpregnant patients, with painless vaginal bleeding being the most common. During pregnancy, this symptom can readily

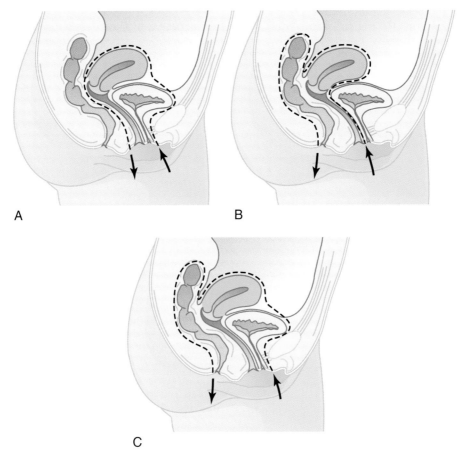

A   B

C

FIGURE 38-7 Organs removed in anterior exenteration (**A**), posterior exenteration (**B**), and total pelvic exenteration (**C**).

be attributed to conditions such as threatened abortion or placenta previa, so there is often an unnecessary delay in diagnosis.

Diagnosis

A prenatal Pap smear leads to the diagnosis in most cases. **Pregnancy tends to exaggerate the colposcopic features of SIL so that overdiagnosis is more likely than the reverse.** Endocervical curettage should not be performed during pregnancy because of the risk of rupturing the membranes. **Cone biopsy, if required, is best performed during the second trimester to avoid the possibility of induced abortion in the first trimester and severe hemorrhage and premature labor in the third trimester.** Unfortunately, about half of the patients are not diagnosed until the postpartum period. The later the diagnosis is made, the more likely the cancer is to be in an advanced stage.

MANAGEMENT

HSIL diagnosed during pregnancy should be managed conservatively, with the pregnancy allowed to proceed to term, vaginal delivery anticipated, and appropriate therapy carried out 6 to 8 weeks postpartum.

Microinvasive carcinoma of the cervix diagnosed by conization of the cervix during pregnancy may also be managed conservatively, the pregnancy being allowed to continue to term. At term, vaginal delivery or cesarean delivery may be appropriate based on obstetrical considerations, followed by appropriate surgical management 6 to 8 weeks later. If further childbearing is not desired, appropriate surgical management may occur at the time of cesarean delivery.

Frankly invasive cancer requires relatively urgent treatment. The risks and benefits of all treatment options must be carefully discussed with the parents, particularly the mother. Some mothers are unwilling to sacrifice their fetus, even if continuing the pregnancy would significantly impair their own prognosis. Such patients are best treated with neoadjuvant chemotherapy.

For early lesions, radical hysterectomy and pelvic lymphadenectomy may be performed. Before 20 weeks' gestation, this is performed with the fetus in situ.

TABLE 38-2

SURVIVAL BY THE INTERNATIONAL FEDERATION OF GYNECOLOGY AND OBSTETRICS STAGE (N = 11,639)

Stage	Patients	Overall Survival Rates (%)				
		1-Year	2-Year	3-Year	4-Year	5-Year
IA1	829	99.8	99.5	98.3	97.5	97.5
IA2	275	98.5	96.9	95.2	94.8	94.8
IB1	3020	98.2	95.0	92.6	90.7	89.1
IB2	1090	95.8	88.3	81.7	78.8	75.7
IIA	1007	96.1	88.3	81.5	77.0	73.4
IIB	2510	91.7	79.8	73.0	69.3	65.8
IIIA	211	76.7	59.8	54.0	45.1	39.7
IIIB	2028	77.9	59.5	51.0	46.0	41.5
IVA	326	51.9	35.1	28.3	22.7	22.0
IVB	343	42.2	22.7	16.4	12.6	9.3

Data from the 26th Annual Report on the Results of Treatment in Gynecological Cancer: Patients treated 1999-2001. *Int J Gynecol Obstet* 95:543–S103, 2006, with permission. These data are based on the 1994 FIGO Staging in which stage IIA is not divided into IIA1 and IIA2.

Between 20 and 25 weeks, hysterotomy through a high incision in the uterine fundus is performed to remove the fetus before the radical surgery. After about 25 weeks, it is usual to await fetal viability at about 34 weeks. Classical cesarean delivery followed immediately by radical hysterectomy and bilateral pelvic lymphadenectomy is then undertaken.

For some patients with early disease and for all patients with advanced disease, the alternative to radical surgery is radiation therapy. Treatment begins with external beam therapy to shrink the tumor. Abortion usually occurs spontaneously during the course of external therapy; if it does not, uterine curettage should be performed in the first trimester or hysterotomy through a high incision in the corpus in the second trimester before brachytherapy is given.

If a decision is made to await fetal viability, it is important to be certain by ultrasonography that the fetus is apparently healthy and to obtain a mature lecithin-to-sphingomyelin ratio to ensure fetal lung maturity before delivery. Neoadjuvant chemotherapy is increasingly used to try to "contain" the disease, and about 10% of patients will have a complete response to the chemotherapy.

Because of the increased risk of hemorrhage and infection likely to be associated with delivery through a cervix containing gross cancer, classic cesarean delivery is the preferred method of delivery. **For patients in whom inadvertent vaginal delivery has occurred, there is no evidence to indicate that the prognosis is altered.**

Prognosis for Cervical Cancer

Prognosis is related directly to clinical stage (Table 38-2). With higher stage disease, the frequency of nodal metastasis escalates, and the 5-year survival rate diminishes. Adenocarcinomas and adenosquamous carcinomas have a somewhat lower 5-year survival rate than do squamous carcinomas, stage for stage.

Matched, controlled studies have demonstrated identical survivals for pregnant and nonpregnant patients.

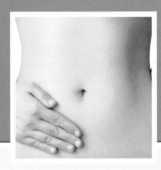

CHAPTER 39

Ovarian, Fallopian Tube, and Peritoneal Cancer

JONATHAN S. BEREK

CLINICAL KEYS FOR THIS CHAPTER

- Ovarian cancer is the fifth most common cancer among women in the United States, accounting for one-fourth of all gynecologic cancers. It is the leading cause of death resulting from gynecologic cancer because it is difficult to detect before it disseminates.
- Most ovarian neoplasms (80-85%) are derived from coelomic epithelium and are called *epithelial carcinomas.* The most common type of ovarian and fallopian tube cancer is serous adenocarcinoma. On the basis of relatively recent molecular, genetic, and pathologic data, many high-grade serous carcinomas formally designated as "ovarian cancers" have been shown to arise in the fimbrial end of the fallopian tubes.
- Approximately 10% of epithelial ovarian cancers occur in women with a known hereditary predisposition.
- The diagnosis of ovarian cancer requires a laparotomy or laparoscopy. In patients with no gross evidence of disease

beyond the ovary and fallopian tube, the standard operation is total abdominal hysterectomy, bilateral salpingo-oophorectomy, infracolic omentectomy, and thorough surgical staging. In patients with advanced disease, cytoreductive surgery ("debulking") is required. The objectives are to remove the primary tumor and all of the metastases, if possible.
- Germ cell tumors of the ovary account for only about 2-3% of all ovarian malignancies, and they occur predominantly in young patients. They frequently produce either human chorionic gonadotropin or α-fetoprotein, which serve as tumor markers. The most common germ cell tumors are the dysgerminoma and immature teratoma.

Ovarian cancer is the fifth most common cancer among women in the United States, accounting for one-fourth of all gynecologic cancers. It is the leading cause of death from gynecologic cancer because it is difficult to detect before it disseminates. In 2013, 22,240 new cases and more than 14,030 deaths were expected from this disease. Most women with ovarian cancer are in their fifth or sixth decade of life.

Epithelial ovarian cancers have been thought to arise from a single layer of cells that covers the ovary or lines cysts immediately beneath the ovarian surface. **There is now molecular, genetic, and pathologic evidence that as many as 60-80% of high-grade serous cancers actually arise in the fimbrial ends of the fallopian tubes.** Peritoneal cancers arise in the tissues lining the peritoneal cavity, and most are histologically identical to serous carcinomas arising in the ovaries or fallopian tubes. Because the treatment of these malignancies is identical, they are now grouped together in

the same International Federation of Gynecology and Obstetrics (FIGO) staging classification.

Epithelial Ovarian Cancer

ETIOLOGY AND EPIDEMIOLOGY

The cause of ovarian cancer is unknown. The patient characteristics found to be associated with an increased risk for epithelial ovarian cancer include white race; late age at menopause; family history of cancer of the ovary, breast, or bowel; and prolonged intervals of ovulation uninterrupted by pregnancy. There is an increased prevalence of ovarian cancer in nulliparous women and those who have been infertile.

The incidence of ovarian cancer varies in different geographic locations. Western countries, including the United States, have rates that are three to seven times higher than those in Japan. Second-generation Japanese immigrants to the United States have an incidence of ovarian cancer similar to that of American women. White Americans experience ovarian cancer about 1.5 times more frequently than do black Americans.

Approximately 10% of epithelial ovarian cancers occur in women with a hereditary predisposition. Although women with hereditary cancers may have two or more first-degree relatives on either the paternal or maternal side who have had breast or ovarian cancer, recent studies have shown that 30-40% of patients with a *BRCA* germline mutation have no family history of disease. It is recommended that all patients with a high-grade serous or endometrioid ovarian cancer be referred for genetic counseling and possible genetic testing. **The pattern of inheritance is autosomal dominant. Breast cancers generally occur in young premenopausal women, whereas ovarian cancers occur at a median age of approximately 50 years.**

The breast-ovarian cancer syndrome is caused by germline mutations in *BRCA1,* **which is located on chromosome 17, or** *BRCA2,* **which is located on chromosome 13. Lynch II syndrome, a nonpolyposis colorectal cancer syndrome, is associated with mutations in the mismatch repair genes.** Adenocarcinomas of the ovary, breast, colon, stomach, pancreas, and endometrium are seen in the families of these individuals.

The use of oral contraceptives has been found to protect against ovarian cancer, possibly because of suppression of ovulation. It has been postulated that **incessant ovulation may predispose to malignant transformation in the ovary.**

Patients with a known germline mutation (e.g., *BRCA1* or *BRCA2* mutation) may be offered prophylactic salpingo-oophorectomy once childbearing has been completed, and this operation is highly protective for ovarian and fallopian tube carcinomas. The risk of subsequent breast cancer is also significantly reduced in these women. There is still a small risk of peritoneal carcinoma after prophylactic salpingo-oophorectomy.

The results of some case-control studies suggest that the use of postmenopausal estrogen replacement therapy may increase the risk of ovarian cancer, but these data are controversial.

It has also been postulated that a causative agent could enter the peritoneal cavity through the lower genital tract. For example, the perineal use of asbestos-contaminated talc has been linked to the development of epithelial ovarian cancer. This possibility remains controversial, although **tubal ligation and hysterectomy are both associated with a decreased risk of the disease.**

SCREENING FOR OVARIAN CANCER

Population screening for ovarian cancer is not feasible, because ultrasonography and available tumor markers, such as cancer antigen (CA)-125, lack specificity and sensitivity for early-stage disease. CA-125 is more useful in postmenopausal women because false-positive measurements occur commonly in premenopausal women in association with endometriosis, pelvic inflammatory disease, or uterine fibroids. Patients with a strong family history of epithelial ovarian cancer may benefit from surveillance with serial transvaginal ultrasonography and serum CA-125 level measurements.

Clinical Features of Epithelial Ovarian, Fallopian Tube, and Peritoneal Cancer

SYMPTOMS

Unfortunately, many patients in whom ovarian cancer develops have only nonspecific symptoms before dissemination takes place. In early-stage disease, vague abdominal pain or bloating is common, although symptoms of a mass compressing the bladder or rectum, such as urinary frequency or constipation, may bring the patient to a physician. Sometimes the patient complains of dyspareunia. Premenopausal women may experience menstrual irregularity. Only rarely does a patient present with acute symptoms, such as pain secondary to torsion, rupture, or intracystic hemorrhage.

In advanced-stage disease, patients most often present with abdominal pain or swelling. The latter is usually caused by ascites. Careful questioning usually reveals that there has been a history of vague abdominal symptoms, such as bloating, constipation, nausea, dyspepsia, anorexia, lethargy, or early satiety. Premenopausal patients may complain of irregular menses or heavy vaginal bleeding.

Clinically, **patients with fallopian tube cancer can present with a vaginal discharge that is typically watery in nature,** as well as with vaginal bleeding, pelvic pain, or some combination of symptoms. In postmenopausal patients, the vaginal discharge may be yellow, watery, and similar to that seen with a urinary fistula. **A fallopian tube cancer should be suspected in a postmenopausal patient whose bleeding or abnormal cytologic findings are not explained by endometrial or endocervical curettage.** In most patients, the diagnosis is not made preoperatively.

Peritoneal carcinomas usually present with abdominal swelling caused by ascites.

SIGNS

These malignancies are frequently misdiagnosed for several months because of the nonspecific nature of the symptoms. **With ovarian cancer, a vaginal or rectal examination will usually reveal a solid, irregular,** fixed pelvic mass; if combined with an upper abdominal mass, ascites, or both, the diagnosis is almost certain.

Preoperative Evaluation

The diagnosis of ovarian, fallopian tube, and peritoneal cancer requires a laparotomy or laparoscopy. Routine preoperative hematologic and biochemical studies should be obtained, as should a chest radiograph. A pelvic and abdominal computed tomographic (CT) scan will exclude liver metastases and may demonstrate retroperitoneal lymphadenopathy.

Endometrial biopsy and endocervical curettage are necessary in patients with abnormal vaginal bleeding, because concurrent primary tumors occasionally occur in the ovary and endometrium. In the presence of ascites, abdominal paracentesis for cytologic evaluation should be performed to confirm the diagnosis of malignancy if neoadjuvant chemotherapy is planned. **In patients with occult blood in the stool or significant intestinal symptoms, a barium enema or lower gastrointestinal endoscopy should be obtained** to rule out a primary colonic cancer with ovarian metastasis. Similarly, **an upper gastrointestinal endoscopy is important if significant gastric symptoms are present.** Breast cancer may also metastasize to the ovaries, so **bilateral mammograms should be obtained if there are any suspicious breast masses.**

Pelvic ultrasonography, particularly transvaginal ultrasonography with or without color Doppler studies, **may be useful** for small (<8 cm) masses in premenopausal women. Masses that are predominantly solid or multilocular have a high probability of being neoplastic, whereas unilocular cystic masses are generally functional cysts. In postmenopausal women, ultrasonography may also be useful because small, unilocular cysts (<5 cm) that are stable are generally benign.

Several tumor markers have been investigated, but none has been consistently reliable. **The tumor-associated antigen CA-125 is elevated in only about 50% of women with stage I ovarian cancer.** When this assay is elevated, it is useful for monitoring the clinical course of the disease.

Differential Diagnosis

Ovarian and fallopian tube malignancies must be differentiated from benign neoplasms and functional cysts of the ovaries and fallopian tubes. In addition, a variety of gynecologic conditions can simulate a neoplastic process, including tubo-ovarian abscess, endometriosis, and a pedunculated uterine leiomyoma. Nongynecologic causes of pelvic tumor must also be excluded, such as an inflammatory or neoplastic disease of the colon, or a pelvic kidney.

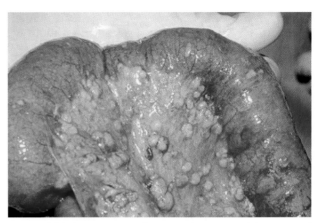

FIGURE 39-1 Numerous small metastatic tumor nodules scattered around the mesentery of the small bowel.

Mode of Spread

Ovarian and fallopian tube cancers typically spread by exfoliating cells that disseminate and implant throughout the peritoneal cavity. The distribution of intraperitoneal metastases tends to follow the circulatory path of peritoneal fluid, so **metastases are commonly seen on the posterior cul-de-sac, paracolic gutters, right hemidiaphragm, liver capsule, and omentum.** Implants are also common on the bowel serosa and its mesenteries (Figure 39-1). In general, they grow around the intestines, encasing them with tumor without invading the bowel lumen. Widespread bowel metastases can lead to a functional obstruction known as *carcinomatous ileus.*

Lymphatic dissemination to the pelvic and para-aortic nodes is common, particularly in patients with advanced disease. Extensive blockage of the diaphragmatic lymphatics is at least partially responsible for the development of ascites. Hematogenous metastases are not common, and parenchymal metastases to the liver and lungs are seen in only about 2% of patients at initial presentation.

Death caused by ovarian cancer usually results from progressive encasement of abdominal organs, leading to anorexia, vomiting, and inanition. The bowel obstruction caused by tumor growth is often incomplete and intermittent and may last for several months before the patient's death.

Staging

The 2013 FIGO staging system for ovarian, fallopian tube, and peritoneal cancer is presented in Table 39-1. Even though all macroscopic (visible) disease may appear to be confined to the ovaries and/or fallopian tubes at the time of laparotomy, microscopic spread may have already occurred; thus, patients must

TABLE 39-1

INTERNATIONAL FEDERATION OF GYNECOLOGY AND OBSTETRICS STAGING FOR CANCER OF THE OVARY, FALLOPIAN TUBE, AND PERITONEUM (2014)

International Federation of Gynecology and Obstetrics (FIGO)		Tumor, Node, Metastasis (TNM)
Ov	**Primary tumor, ovary**	**Tov**
FT	**Primary tumor, fallopian tube**	**Tft**
P	**Primary tumor, peritoneum**	**Tp**
X	**Primary tumor cannot be assessed**	**Tx**

Designate histologic type:
High-Grade Serous (HGS), Endometrioid (E), Clear Cell (CC), Mucinous (M), Low-Grade Serous (LG), Other or cannot be classified (O), Germ Cell (GC), Sex-Cord Stromal Cell Tumor (SC)

Stage I	**Tumor confined to ovaries or fallopian tube(s)**	**T1**
IA	Tumor limited to one ovary (capsule intact) or fallopian tube No tumor on ovarian or fallopian tube surface No malignant cells in the ascites or peritoneal washings	**T1a**
IB	Tumor limited to both ovaries (capsules intact) or fallopian tubes No tumor on ovarian or fallopian tube surface No malignant cells in the ascites or peritoneal washings	**T1b**
IC	Tumor limited to one or both ovaries or fallopian tubes, with any of the following:	**T1c**
IC1	Surgical spill intraoperatively	
IC2	Capsule ruptured before surgery or tumor on ovarian or fallopian tube surface	
IC3	Malignant cells in the ascites or peritoneal washings	
Stage II	**Tumor involves one or both ovaries or fallopian tubes with pelvic extension (below pelvic brim) or peritoneal cancer (Tp)**	**T2**
IIA	Extension and/or implants on the uterus and/or fallopian tubes/and/or ovaries	**T2a**
IIB	Extension to other pelvic intraperitoneal tissues	**T2b**
Stage III	**Tumor involves one or both ovaries, fallopian tubes, or peritoneal cancer, with cytologically or histologically confirmed spread to the peritoneum outside the pelvis and/or metastasis to the retroperitoneal lymph nodes**	**T3**
IIIA	Metastasis to the retroperitoneal lymph nodes with or without microscopic peritoneal involvement beyond the pelvis	**T1, T2, T3aN1**
IIIA1	Positive retroperitoneal lymph nodes only (cytologically or histologically proven)	
IIIA1(i)	Metastasis ≤10 mm in greatest dimension	
IIIA1(ii)	Metastasis >10 mm in greatest dimension	
IIIA2	Microscopic extrapelvic (above the pelvic brim) peritoneal involvement with or without positive retroperitoneal lymph nodes	**T3a/T3aN1**
IIIB	Macroscopic peritoneal metastases beyond the pelvic brim ≤2 cm in greatest dimension, with or without metastasis to the retroperitoneal lymph nodes	**T3b/T3bN1**
IIIC	Macroscopic peritoneal metastases beyond the pelvic brim >2 cm in greatest dimension, with or without metastases to the retroperitoneal nodes (Note 1)	**T3c/T3cN1**
Stage IV	**Distant metastasis excluding peritoneal metastases**	**Any T, Any N, M1**
IVA	Pleural effusion with positive cytology	
IVB	Metastases to extraabdominal organs (including inguinal lymph nodes and lymph nodes outside of abdominal cavity)	

Note 1: Includes extension of tumor to capsule of liver and spleen without parenchymal involvement of either organ

Note 2: Parenchymal metastases are stage IVB

Additional notes:
1. The primary site—that is, ovary, fallopian tube, or peritoneum—should be designated where possible. In some cases, it may not be possible to clearly delineate the primary site, and these should be listed as "undesignated."
2. The histologic type should be recorded.
3. The staging includes a revision of the stage III patients, and allotment to stage IIIA1 is based on spread to the retroperitoneal lymph nodes without intraperitoneal dissemination, because an analysis of these patients indicates that their survival is significantly better than the survival of those who have intraperitoneal dissemination.
4. Involvement of retroperitoneal lymph nodes must be proven cytologically or histologically.
5. Extension of tumor from omentum to spleen or liver (stage IIIC) should be differentiated from isolated parenchymal splenic or liver metastases (stage IVB).

From FIGO Committee on Gynecologic Oncology. Pratt J on behalf of FIGO committee: Staging classification for cancer of the ovary, fallopian tube, and peritoneum. *Internal J Gynaecol Obstet* 124(1):1–5, 2014.

BOX 39-1

REQUIREMENTS FOR STAGING OPERATIONS*

Peritoneal Washings for Cytology

Multiple Intraperitoneal Biopsies

Pelvis

Cul-de-sac peritoneum
Bladder peritoneum
Pedicles of infundibulopelvic ligaments
Any adhesions

Abdomen

Both paracolic gutters
Bowel serosa and mesenteries
Omentum
Any adhesions

Extraperitoneal Biopsies

Pelvic and paraaortic lymph nodes

*Procedures performed in patients with no visible evidence of metastatic disease.

TABLE 39-2

HISTOGENETIC CLASSIFICATION OF PRIMARY OVARIAN NEOPLASMS

Derivation	Type of Tumor

Epithelial origin (80-85%)	"Common" epithelial tumors: benign, borderline, malignant
	  Serous tumor
	  Mucinous tumor
	  Endometrioid tumor
	  Clear cell (mesonephroid) tumor
	  Brenner tumor
	Undifferentiated carcinoma
	Carcinosarcoma or malignant mixed mesodermal tumors

Germ cell origin (10-15%)	Teratoma
	  Mature teratoma
	  Solid adult teratoma
	  Dermoid cyst
	  Struma ovarii
	  Malignant neoplasms secondarily arising from teratomatous tissues (squamous carcinoma, carcinoid tumor, sarcoma)
	  Immature teratoma
	Dysgerminoma
	Endodermal sinus tumor
	Embryonal carcinoma
	Choriocarcinoma
	Gonadoblastoma*
	Mixed germ cell tumors

Specialized gonadal-stromal origin (3-5%)	Granulosa-theca cell tumors
	  Granulosa cell tumor
	  Thecoma
	Sertoli-Leydig tumors
	  Arrhenoblastoma
	  Sertoli cell tumor
	Gynandroblastoma
	Lipid cell tumors

Nonspecific mesenchymal origin (<1%)	Fibroma, hemangioma, leiomyoma, lipoma Lymphoma Sarcoma

Data from Hart WR, Morrow CP: The ovaries. In Romney SL, Gray MJ, Little AB, et al, editors: *Gynecology and obstetrics: the health care of women,* ed 2, New York, 1981, McGraw-Hill.
*Combined germ cell and specialized gonadal-stromal elements.

undergo a thorough "surgical staging." Procedures necessary to stage these cancers are shown in Box 39-1.

Classification of Ovarian Neoplasms

The histologic classification system for ovarian neoplasms is listed in Table 39-2. These lesions fall into four categories according to their tissue of origin. **The most common type of epithelial ovarian cancer is serous adenocarcinoma. Most fallopian tube cancers are serous adenocarcinomas.** Less common ovarian tumors are derived from primitive germ cells, specialized gonadal stroma, or nonspecific mesenchyme. In addition, the ovary can be the site of metastatic carcinomas, most often from the gastrointestinal tract or the breast.

PATHOLOGIC FEATURES

The main histologic subtypes of epithelial carcinomas are serous (about 55%), mucinous (about 20%), endometrioid (about 15%), and clear cell (about 5%) tumors. Malignant Brenner tumors and undifferentiated carcinomas are uncommon.

Serous tumors resemble fallopian tube epithelium histologically, and many lesions that used to be classified as ovarian cancer arise in the fallopian tubes. About 30% of patients with stage I and stage IIA disease have bilateral involvement. On gross examination, serous carcinomas have an irregular and multilocular appearance (Figures 39-2 and 39-3).

Mucinous tumors histologically resemble endocervical epithelium and are often large, measuring 20 cm or more in diameter. They are bilateral in 10-20% of patients.

Endometrioid tumors closely resemble carcinomas of the endometrium and arise in association with primary endometrial cancer in about 20% of patients. In early-stage disease, they are bilateral in about 10% of cases. Approximately 10% of endometrioid ovarian carcinomas are associated with endometriosis, although malignant transformation of endometriosis occurs in less than 1% of patients.

Clear cell carcinomas of the ovary are uncommon. **In about 25% of cases, they occur in association with endometriosis.**

Psammoma bodies

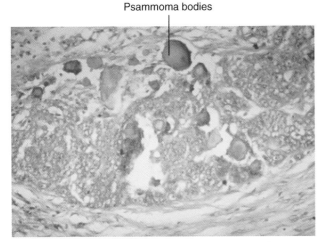

FIGURE 39-2 Papillary serous cystadenocarcinoma. This tumor frequently contains numerous psammoma bodies, which are shown here. Their origin is uncertain, but it has been suggested that they may reflect an immune reaction against the tumor or, more simply, represent alteration of the secretions from the malignant cells. There is no relationship between the presence of psammoma bodies and the malignancy of the tumor.

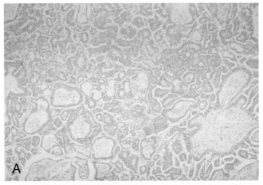

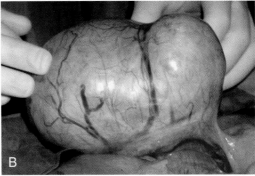

FIGURE 39-4 **A,** Serous tumor—borderline. (Papillary serous cystadenocarcinoma of low malignant potential.) The papillary pattern filling the cyst lumen is very complex, and the epithelium is, in places, more than one cell thick. Mitotic figures are present, although not abundant. **B,** Large borderline tumor mobilized out of the pelvis. Note the smooth surface and large blood vessels coursing over the surface.

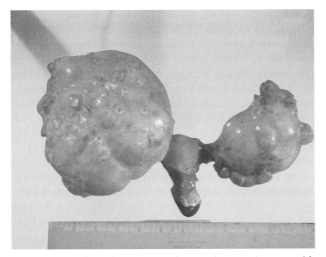

FIGURE 39-3 Bilateral serous cystadenocarcinomas. A uterus with both ovaries grossly enlarged by multilocular tumors with papillary excrescences on their serosal surfaces.

trioid, clear cell, and Brenner tumors are only rarely borderline.

Management of Epithelial Ovarian, Fallopian Tube, and Peritoneal Cancer

The initial approach to all patients with ovarian, fallopian tube, and peritoneal cancer is surgical exploration of the abdomen and pelvis.

EARLY-STAGE DISEASE

Definitive diagnosis requires an intraoperative frozen section. In patients with no gross evidence of disease beyond the ovary and fallopian tube, the standard operation is total abdominal hysterectomy, bilateral salpingo-oophorectomy, infracolic omentectomy, and thorough surgical staging, as shown in Box 39-1. Patients who wish to preserve their fertility may have a unilateral salpingo-oophorectomy. **In patients with grade 1 or grade 2 tumors confined to one or both ovaries after surgical staging, no further treatment is**

The Brenner tumor represents only 2-3% of all ovarian neoplasms, and less than 2% of these tumors are malignant. **About 10% of Brenner tumors occur in conjunction with a mucinous cystadenoma or dermoid cyst in the same or opposite ovary.**

Tumors of low malignant potential or borderline histologic appearance exist for each histologic type. **Approximately 5-10% of malignant serous tumors are borderline (Figure 39-4), whereas 20% of malignant mucinous tumors fall into this category.** The endome-

necessary. Patients with poorly differentiated (grade 3) tumors are subsequently treated with systemic chemotherapy.

ADVANCED-STAGE DISEASE

In patients with advanced disease, cytoreductive surgery ("debulking") is required. The objectives are to remove the primary tumor and all of the metastases, if possible. **If all macroscopic disease cannot be removed, an attempt should be made to reduce individual tumor nodules to 1 cm or less in diameter.** Patients in whom this goal is achieved are said to have had "optimal" cytoreduction, which can be achieved in about 70% of patients. In addition to a total or subtotal abdominal hysterectomy, bilateral salpingo-oophorectomy, omentectomy, and resection of peritoneal metastases, optimal cytoreduction may necessitate bowel resection.

In retrospective studies, patients whose individual residual tumor nodules are 1 cm or less in diameter before the commencement of chemotherapy have been shown to have longer median survival and a more complete response to therapy. The longest survival is seen in patients in whom all visible tumor has been removed before treatment.

In patients who are medically unfit or have a poor performance status, usually because of a large pleural effusion and massive ascites, it may be prudent to give two or three cycles of neoadjuvant chemotherapy before undertaking radical surgery. If the disease does not respond to chemotherapy, as evidenced by the failure to resolve the malignant effusions, the patient should be offered palliative care only. **Usually, the effusions resolve completely, and an "interval" cytoreductive operation can safely be undertaken.**

Following primary cytoreductive surgery, combination chemotherapy is given, most commonly intravenous carboplatin and paclitaxel, or intraperitoneal cisplatin and paclitaxel. Intraperitoneal treatment is useful only for patients with minimal residual disease. Single-agent therapy with paclitaxel or carboplatin is occasionally used for frail or elderly patients.

During chemotherapy, **the patient's response is monitored with serum CA-125 titers.** If the values rise or plateau within 6 months, it is advisable to change to second-line drugs, such as liposomal doxorubicin, topotecan, etoposide, gemcitabine, bevacizumab, or experimental chemotherapeutic agents. If the progression-free interval has been longer than 6 to 12 months, the patient may respond to further paclitaxel or carboplatin chemotherapy. The response rate for second-line chemotherapy is in the range of 20-50%, but patients are not considered to be curable after their initial relapse. **Secondary cytoreduction may be appropriate if the disease-free interval is 24 months or longer or if the recurrent disease is amenable to complete surgical resection.**

Prognosis

Patients with stage I disease have 5-year survival rates of 75-95%, depending on the histologic grade.

Almost all patients with carefully staged IA, grade 1 ovarian and fallopian tube cancer are cured surgically, whereas the 5-year survival rate for patients with poorly differentiated bilateral lesions is as low as 75%. The 5-year survival rate for patients with stage II disease is about 65%. Despite aggressive primary surgery and combination chemotherapy, **the 5-year survival rate for patients with advanced-stage disease is only about 20%, although the median survival is between 2 and 3 years.** Patients whose tumors are associated with *BRCA1* and *BRCA2* mutations have a somewhat better prognosis.

Patients who have borderline ovarian tumors can be expected to have a prolonged survival. If the disease is confined to the ovary, the vast majority of tumors never recur. Five- and 10-year survival rates are 95-100%, but late recurrences may occur, and 20-year survival rates are approximately 85-90%. Patients who initially present with metastatic disease are more likely to exhibit subsequent clinical evidence of disease, although the rate of progression is slow; most live at least 5 years.

Germ Cell Tumors

Germ cell tumors of the ovary account for only about 2-3% of all ovarian malignancies. They occur predominantly in young patients and frequently produce either human chorionic gonadotropin (hCG) or α-fetoprotein (AFP), which serve as tumor markers. The most common germ cell tumors are the dysgerminoma and immature teratoma. Endodermal sinus tumors, embryonal tumors, and nongestational choriocarcinomas are less common. Mixed germ cell tumors are not uncommon.

DYSGERMINOMAS

Dysgerminomas occur predominantly in children and young women. About 10% are bilateral. **These tumors, of varying malignant virulence, are occasionally seen in patients with gonadal dysgenesis or the testicular feminization syndrome.** In such patients, the dysgerminoma may arise in a gonadoblastoma. In about two-thirds of patients, the disease is confined to the ovaries at the time of diagnosis. About 10% of dysgerminomas are associated with other germ cell malignancies. **Pure dysgerminomas do not produce the tumor markers hCG and AFP, but they do commonly produce lactate dehydrogenase.**

Treatment

In most patients, the contralateral ovary and the uterus can be preserved. **Surgical staging,** as outlined earlier in this chapter, **is less important because these tumors** are very sensitive to chemotherapy, even when meta-static. **Any spread is commonly to the paraaortic lymph nodes.** This region should be carefully palpated, and any enlarged nodes should be removed.

If disease extends beyond one ovary, metastatic disease that can be removed with minimal morbidity should be resected and chemotherapy promptly initiated. **The regimen employed for these patients is usually bleomycin, etoposide, and cisplatin.** Carboplatin and paclitaxel are also being tested in these patients. Dysgerminomas are uniquely radiosensitive, and radiotherapy was previously the treatment of choice. However, it is now best reserved for the management of recurrent, chemoresistant disease.

Prognosis

The 5-year survival rate for patients with stage IA pure dysgerminoma treated with unilateral oophorectomy is about 95%, whereas it is 80% for stage II and 60-70% for stage III disease. Recurrences following conservative surgery have at least an 80% 5-year survival rate.

IMMATURE TERATOMAS

Immature teratomas are the second most common malignant ovarian germ cell tumor. About 75% of malignant teratomas are encountered during the first two decades of life. Bilateral lesions are rare, although the other ovary may contain a benign dermoid cyst in about 5% of cases. Like other germ cell tumors, immature teratomas grow fairly rapidly, cause pain early, and are found to be confined to the ovary in about two-thirds of cases at the time of diagnosis. **Pure immature teratomas do not produce hCG or AFP.** Histologically, the tumors can be graded from 1 to 3 according to the degree of differentiation, with grade 3 tumors being the least differentiated. Neural elements are most frequently seen, but cartilage and epithelial tissues are also common.

Treatment

The primary tumor should be removed. **In young patients, the uterus and contralateral ovary should be preserved to maintain fertility.** All patients with other than stage IA, grade 1 immature teratomas should receive postoperative chemotherapy using bleomycin, etoposide, and cisplatin. Three cycles of chemotherapy are usually given for stage I disease.

Prognosis

Survival correlates with grade and stage of disease. The 5-year survival rate for patients with grade 1 immature teratomas is about 95%, compared with 80% for grade 2 and 60-70% for grade 3 disease.

OTHER GERM CELL TUMORS

The endodermal sinus tumor is a rare malignancy. It is also referred to as a *yolk sac tumor.* **Endodermal sinus tumors produce AFP,** which can serve as a useful serum marker for this neoplasm. **Embryonal carcinomas produce both hCG and AFP, whereas nongestational choriocarcinomas produce hCG only.** All occur in children and young women, and all grow rapidly. **Bilateral tumors are rare.**

Therapy for these lesions includes surgical resection of the primary tumor, followed by systemic combination chemotherapy with bleomycin, etoposide, and cisplatin. Before the advent of effective chemotherapy, these tumors were usually fatal. The overall 5-year survival rate is now about 70-80%.

Specialized Gonadal-Stromal Tumors

A group of relatively uncommon tumors is derived from the specialized ovarian stroma. As such, they are often endocrinologically functional, many of them being capable of synthesizing gonadal or adrenal steroid hormones. Because the ovarian stroma has sexual bipotentiality, hormones that are secreted can be either female or male. **Estrogen and progesterone are typically associated with granulosa-theca cell tumors, whereas testosterone and other androgens may be secreted by many Sertoli-Leydig cell tumors. Rarely, lipid cell tumors,** which are usually virilizing, **produce adrenal corticoids** and a clinical cushingoid syndrome.

PATHOLOGIC FEATURES

Granulosa cell tumors are the most common stromal carcinomas. They have a distinct histologic pattern: **small groups of cells called *Call-Exner bodies* are the hallmark.** They may secrete large amounts of estrogen and can be associated with endometrial cancer in adults or with sexual pseudoprecocity in children.

Thecomas, which are only one-third as common as granulosa cell tumors, are rarely malignant. Mixtures of the two types of tumor may exist.

Sertoli-Leydig cell tumors (arrhenoblastomas) contain both Sertoli-type and Leydig-type stromal cells and are classically associated with masculinization. **Only 3-5% of these tumors are malignant.**

Lipid cell tumors are often referred to as *hilar cell tumors* because they are located in the ovarian hilus. **Only a rare lipid tumor, usually larger than 8 cm in diameter, behaves in a malignant fashion.**

TREATMENT

Most stromal tumors occur in postmenopausal women, and they are best treated by performing a total abdominal hysterectomy and bilateral salpingo-oophorectomy. Conservation of the uterus and contralateral ovary is appropriate for carefully staged young patients with stage I disease, provided that the possibility of an associated adenocarcinoma of the endometrium has been excluded by dilation and curettage. The tumors are not very chemosensitive.

PROGNOSIS

Granulosa cell tumors, which tend to grow slowly, are usually confined to one ovary at the time of diagnosis. **The 5-year survival rate is approximately 90% for stage I disease. Recurrences are usually detected late** and may result in death 15 to 20 years after removal of the primary lesion.

Metastatic Cancers

About 4-8% of ovarian malignancies are metastatic, most commonly from either the gastrointestinal tract or the breast. **The Krukenberg tumor is a specific type of metastatic tumor in which "signet-ring" cells are seen in the ovarian stroma histologically.** Most Krukenberg tumors are bilateral and metastatic from the stomach. Rarely, it has not been possible to locate a primary focus, and removal of the ovarian disease has produced apparent cures.

Vulvar and Vaginal Cancer

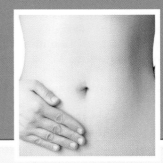

NEVILLE F. HACKER

CLINICAL KEYS FOR THIS CHAPTER

- Most vulvar cancers are squamous cell carcinomas, and, etiologically, there are two different types. The more common type occurs in older women and is frequently related to long-standing lichen sclerosus. The less common type occurs in younger women and is related to infection with the human papillomavirus and smoking.
- Invasive vulvar cancer spreads initially to adjacent organs, such as the urethra, vagina, or anus, and also by lymphatic embolization to the inguinofemoral lymph nodes. About 30% of patients with vulvar cancer have lymph node metastases.
- Modern management of vulvar cancer should be individualized and requires a multidisciplinary team

approach. Radical local excision is usually appropriate for the primary lesion, with the emphasis on vulvar conservation.
- Carcinoma in situ of the vagina, or vaginal intraepithelial neoplasia (VAIN), is much less common than its counterparts on the cervix or vulva. Most lesions occur in the upper third of the vagina, and women are usually asymptomatic. VAIN appears to be related to infection with the human papillomavirus.
- The diagnosis of VAIN is usually considered because of an abnormal Papanicolaou smear in a woman who either has had a hysterectomy or has no demonstrable cervical abnormality.

Vulvar and vaginal cancers are considered to be lower genital tract carcinomas along with carcinoma of the cervix. At all three sites, the predominant cancer is squamous cell histologically, and the human papillomavirus (HPV) plays a role in carcinogenesis. A patient who develops cancer at one site is at risk of developing cancer at another lower genital tract site, so colposcopy of the cervix, vagina, and vulva should be part of the diagnostic workup for vulvar and vaginal cancers.

Vulvar Neoplasms

Vulvar cancer is uncommon, representing 4% of malignancies of the female genital tract. Because the vulva is an external genital organ, the treatment of vulvar cancer usually causes significant psychosexual distress.

Most tumors are squamous cell carcinomas, and they occur mainly in postmenopausal women. A history of chronic vulvar itching is common.

EPIDEMIOLOGY

The mean age at diagnosis of squamous cell carcinoma of the vulva is 65 years. Recent studies suggest two different etiologic types of vulvar cancer. **One type is seen mainly in younger patients, is related to HPV infection and smoking, and is commonly associated with vulvar intraepithelial neoplasia (VIN) of the basaloid, warty, or usual type. The more common type is seen mainly in elderly women and is unrelated to smoking or HPV infection. It is frequently related to long-standing lichen sclerosus.** Concurrent VIN is uncommon, but when present, it is of the differentiated type.

Although rarely seen in the United States, **vulvar cancer may also occur in association with the venereal diseases syphilis, lymphogranuloma venereum, and granuloma inguinale.** In such cases, the cancer occurs at an earlier age and carries a graver prognosis.

Intraepithelial Neoplasia

The International Society for the Study of Vulvovaginal Disease recognizes two varieties of intraepithelial neoplasia: **squamous cell carcinoma in situ (Bowen disease), or VIN;** nonsquamous intraepithelial neoplasia, including **Paget disease;** and **noninvasive tumors of melanocytes.** With the introduction of the HPV vaccines, there should be a significant reduction in the incidence of VIN and invasive vulvar cancer, particularly in young patients, in the future.

VULVAR INTRAEPITHELIAL NEOPLASIA

During the last 30 years, the incidence of VIN has increased markedly. Younger patients are being affected, and the mean age at diagnosis is approximately 45 years.

Clinical Features

Itching is the most common symptom, although some patients present with palpable or visible abnormalities of the vulva. Approximately half of the patients are asymptomatic. There is no absolutely diagnostic appearance. Most lesions are elevated, but the color may be white, red, pink, gray, or brown (Figure 40-1). **Approximately 20% of the lesions have a "warty" appearance, and the lesions are multicentric in about two-thirds of cases.**

Diagnosis

Diagnosis requires biopsy of suspicious lesions, which can be done in the office with the patient under local anesthesia. Careful inspection of the vulva under a bright light, with the aid of a magnifying glass if necessary, is the most useful technique for detecting abnormal areas. Colposcopic examination of the entire vulva after the application of 5% acetic acid will sometimes highlight additional acetowhite areas.

Management

Most cases of VIN can be treated adequately by local superficial surgical excision with primary closure. The microscopic disease seldom extends significantly beyond the colposcopic lesion, so **margins of about 5 mm are usually adequate. For extensive lesions involving most of the vulva, a "skinning" vulvectomy,** in which the vulvar skin is removed and replaced by a split-thickness skin graft, **may be used.**

Laser therapy is effective for multiple small lesions or for lesions involving the clitoris or perianal area. No specimen is available for histologic study after laser ablation, so a liberal number of biopsies must be taken before treatment to exclude invasive cancer.

PAGET DISEASE

Paget disease of the vulva predominantly affects postmenopausal white women. Paget disease also occurs in the nipple areas of the breast.

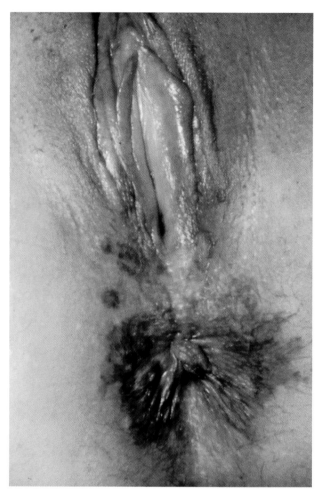

FIGURE 40-1 Vulvar intraepithelial neoplasia (grade III) or carcinoma in situ of the vulva. Note the pigmented and multicentric nature of the lesions and the extensive perianal involvement in this patient.

Clinical Features

Itching and tenderness are common and may be longstanding. **The affected area is usually well demarcated and eczematoid in appearance,** with the presence of white, plaquelike lesions (Figure 40-2). As growth progresses, extension beyond the vulva to the mons pubis, thighs, and buttocks may occur; rarely, it may extend to involve the mucosa of the rectum, vagina, or urinary tract. **In 10-20% of cases, Paget disease is associated with an underlying adenocarcinoma.**

Histologic Features

The disease is an adenocarcinoma in situ and is characterized by large, pale, pathognomonic Paget cells that are seen within the epidermis and skin adnexa. They are rich in mucopolysaccharide, a diastase-resistant substance that stains positive with periodic acid-Schiff stain. The intracytoplasmic mucin may also be demonstrated by Mayer mucicarmine staining. **The**

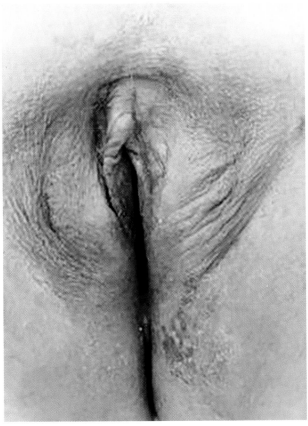

FIGURE 40-2 Paget disease of the vulva. Note the eczematoid appearance, particularly on the left.

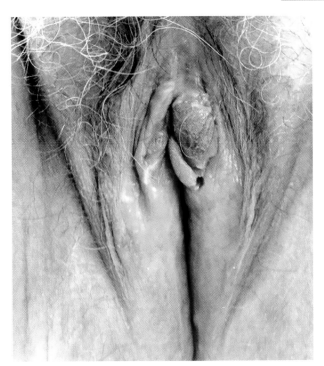

FIGURE 40-3 A large squamous cell carcinoma of the clitoris. Note the ulcerated surface.

Paget cells are typically located adjacent to the basal layer, both in the epidermis and in the adnexal structures.

Management

If the disease involves the anus, colonoscopy should be undertaken to exclude an underlying rectal cancer, whereas if the urethra is involved, cystoscopy should be performed to exclude an underlying urothelial cancer.

The histologic extent of Paget disease usually extends well beyond the visible lesion. **Local superficial excision with 5- to 10-mm margins is required to clear the gross lesion, exclude underlying invasive cancer, and relieve symptoms.** Recurrences are common and may be treated by further excision or laser therapy.

If an underlying invasive carcinoma is present, the treatment should be the same as for other invasive vulvar cancers.

Invasive Vulvar Cancer

SQUAMOUS CELL CARCINOMA

Squamous cell carcinoma accounts for about 90% of vulvar cancers.

Clinical Features

Patients generally present with a vulvar lump, although long-standing pruritus is common. The lesions may be raised, ulcerated, pigmented, or warty in appearance, and **definitive diagnosis requires biopsy of the lesion with the patient under local anesthesia.** Most lesions occur on the labia majora; the labia minora are the next most common sites. Less commonly, the clitoris or the perineum is involved (Figure 40-3). Approximately 5% of cases are multifocal.

Methods of Spread

Vulvar cancer spreads by direct extension to adjacent structures, such as the vagina, urethra, and anus; **by lymphatic embolization to regional lymph nodes;** and **by hematogenous spread to distant sites,** including the lungs, liver, and bone. In most cases, the initial lymphatic metastases are to the inguinal lymph nodes, located between the Camper fascia and the fascia lata. From these superficial nodes, spread occurs to the femoral nodes located medial to the femoral vein. The Cloquet node, which is situated beneath the inguinal ligament, is the most cephalad of the femoral node group. **From the inguinofemoral nodes, spread occurs to the pelvic nodes, particularly the external iliac group** (Figure 40-4).

The incidence of lymph node metastases in vulvar cancer is approximately 30%. Metastasis is related to the size of the lesion (Table 40-1). **Approximately 5% of patients have metastases to pelvic lymph nodes.**

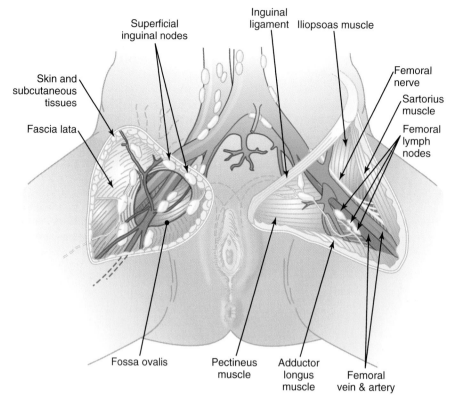

FIGURE 40-4 Lymphatic drainage of the vulva. Inguinal nodes are displayed on the right side of the groin, and femoral nodes are seen on the left side of the groin.

TABLE 40-1

INCIDENCE OF LYMPH NODE METASTASES IN RELATION TO LESION SIZE IN VULVAR CANCER

Lesion Size (cm)	Number	Positive Nodes	Percent
0-1	43	3	7.0
1-2	63	14	22.2
2-4	52	14	26.9
>4	41	14	34.1

Data from Gonzalez Bosquet J, Kinney WK, Russell AH, et al: Risk of occult inguinofemoral lymph node metastasis from squamous carcinoma of the vulva. *Int J Radiat Oncol Biol Phys* 57:419-424, 2003.

Such patients usually have three or more positive unilateral inguinofemoral lymph nodes. Hematogenous spread usually occurs late in the disease and rarely occurs in the absence of lymphatic metastases.

Staging

A clinical staging system was introduced by the International Federation of Gynecology and Obstetrics (FIGO) in 1969, and this was changed to a surgical staging system in 1988. The present FIGO staging system is shown in Table 40-2.

Management

Since the 1980s, a vulva-conserving approach has been used for most primary lesions, and the groin dissection has usually been performed through a separate groin incision. Unilateral tumors are now treated with unilateral groin dissection.

Groin seromas, wound breakdown, and cellulitis are common acute complications, whereas chronic complications include lower-limb lymphedema, genital prolapse, and urinary stress incontinence.

The major long-term morbidity associated with groin dissection is lower-limb lymphedema, which occurs in 50-60% of patients and is a lifelong affliction. The incidence of lymphedema may be markedly reduced with the use of sentinel node biopsy. After the injection of a blue dye and a radiocolloid around the primary tumor, the sentinel node or nodes are identified and resected. They are subjected to thorough histopathologic analysis to detect any small micrometastasis. Patients with negative sentinel nodes are at very low risk for disease in other nodes, so full groin dissection may be avoided. There is a small but definite false-negative rate, and most patients who experience recurrence in an undissected groin die as a result of their disease. Properly informed, most but not all

TABLE 40-2

INTERNATIONAL FEDERATION OF GYNECOLOGY AND OBSTETRICS STAGING OF CARCINOMA OF THE VULVA (2009)

Stage	Description
I	Tumor confined to the vulva
IA	Lesions ≤2 cm in size, confined to the vulva or perineum and with stromal invasion ≤1.0 mm,* no nodal metastasis
IB	Lesions >2 cm in size or with stromal invasion >1.0 mm,* confined to the vulva or perineum, with negative nodes
II	Tumor of any size with extension to adjacent perineal structures (one-third lower urethra, one-third lower vagina, anus) with negative nodes
III	Tumor of any size with or without extension to adjacent perineal structures (one-third lower urethra, one-third lower vagina, anus) with positive inguinofemoral lymph nodes
IIIA	(i) With 1 lymph node macrometastasis (≥5 mm), or (ii) 1-2 lymph node micrometastases (<5 mm)
IIIB	(i) With 2 or more lymph node macrometastases (≥5 mm), or (ii) 3 or more lymph node micrometastases (<5 mm)
IIIC	With positive nodes with extracapsular spread
IV	Tumor invades other regional (two-thirds upper urethra, two-thirds upper vagina) or distant structures
IVA	Tumor invades any of the following: (i) Upper urethral and/or vaginal mucosa, bladder mucosa, rectal mucosa, or fixed to pelvic bone, or (ii) Fixed or ulcerated inguinofemoral lymph nodes
IVB	Any distant metastasis including pelvic lymph nodes

From Pecorelli S: Revised FIGO staging for carcinoma of the vulva, cervix, and endometrium. *Int J Gynaecol Obstet* 105:103-104, 2009.
*The depth of invasion is defined as the measurement of the tumor from the epithelial-stromal junction of the adjacent most superficial dermal papilla to the deepest point of invasion.

patients prefer to develop lymphedema than take a small risk of dying because of a groin recurrence.

EARLY VULVAR CANCER

Modern management of vulvar cancer should be individualized. The most appropriate management for the primary lesion and for the groin nodes should be determined independently. In determining the management of the primary cancer, the following two factors are taken into account:
1. The presence of any multifocality
2. The condition of the remainder of the vulva

For patients whose tumor is unifocal and the remainder of the vulva is normal, radical local excision with surgical margins of at least 1 cm is the treatment of choice. If there is associated VIN or multifocality, a radical or modified radical vulvectomy may be necessary.

With respect to the lymphadenectomy, **patients with a 2-cm tumor in whom the depth of penetration is less than 1 mm from the overlying basement membrane do not need groin dissection.** All other patients require at least an ipsilateral inguinal–femoral lymphadenectomy. For patients with midline lesions invading more than 1 mm, bilateral groin dissection is necessary.

Sentinel node biopsy may be considered in selected patients with a primary lesion up to 4 cm, as long as the patient gives properly informed consent.

ADVANCED VULVAR CANCER

If the cancer involves the proximal urethra, anus, or rectovaginal septum, radical surgery will necessitate a bowel or urinary stoma. For such patients, preoperative radiation or chemoradiation should be used to shrink the primary tumor, followed usually by a more conservative surgical resection of the tumor bed. Bilateral groin node dissection is usually performed before the radiation therapy, or alternately the nodes may be included in the radiation fields. If there are palpably enlarged nodes, these should be removed before any radiation therapy. Most patients can be spared a stoma with this approach.

MANAGEMENT OF PATIENTS WITH POSITIVE NODES

Patients with more than one nodal micrometastasis (≤5 mm diameter), one or more macrometastases, or evidence of extranodal spread should receive postoperative radiation to both groins and to the pelvis.

Prognosis

The overall survival rate for vulvar carcinoma is about 70%. The most important prognostic factor is the status of the groin lymph nodes. **Patients with positive nodes have a 5-year survival rate of about 50%, whereas those with negative nodes have a 5-year survival rate of about 90%.** Patients with only one involved node without extracapsular spread have a good prognosis.

MALIGNANT MELANOMA

Malignant melanoma is the second most common type of vulvar cancer. Melanomas may arise de novo or from a preexisting junctional or compound nevus. They occur predominantly in postmenopausal white women and most commonly involve the labia minora or clitoris (Figure 40-5).

Diagnosis and Staging

Any pigmented lesion on the vulva, unless it has been known to be present for a long time, should be excised for histologic diagnosis. The prognosis correlates more closely with the depth of penetration into the dermis. **Those lesions that penetrate to a depth of 1 mm or less from the granular layer of the epidermis rarely metastasize.** Clark levels are not readily applicable to vulvar melanomas.

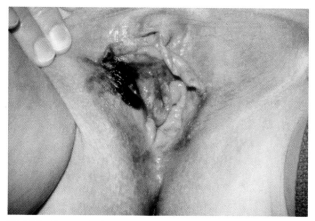

FIGURE 40-5 Malignant melanoma arising from the right labium minus.

Management

For lesions invading less than 1 mm, radical local excision alone, with margins of at least 1 cm, is adequate therapy. For lesions with 1 mm or greater invasion, **radical local excision of the primary tumor is usually combined with at least ipsilateral inguinofemoral lymphadenectomy.**

Prognosis

The overall 5-year survival rate for vulvar melanomas is approximately 30%.

VERRUCOUS CARCINOMA

Verrucous carcinoma is a variant of squamous cell carcinoma and was originally described as occurring in the oral cavity. The lesions, which are cauliflower-like in nature, may occur in the cervix, vulva, or vagina. Invasion occurs with a broad "pushing" front, and unless the base of the lesion is submitted for histologic examination, these tumors may be difficult to differentiate from a condyloma acuminatum or squamous papilloma. **Metastasis to regional lymph nodes is rare,** but the tumors are locally aggressive and prone to local recurrence unless wide surgical margins are obtained. **Radiation therapy may induce anaplastic transformation and is contraindicated.**

BARTHOLIN GLAND CARCINOMA

Adenocarcinomas, squamous cell carcinomas, and, rarely, transitional cell carcinomas may arise from the Bartholin gland and its duct. A history of preceding inflammation of the Bartholin gland is present in about 10% of patients, and malignancies may be mistaken for benign cysts or abscesses. Current management consists of hemivulvectomy and ipsilateral inguinofemoral lymphadenectomy. **Postoperative vulvar irradiation appears to decrease the local recurrence rate for patients with large lesions.**

BASAL CELL CARCINOMA

Basal cell carcinomas of the vulva are rare. They commonly present as a rolled-edged "rodent" ulcer, although nodules and macules may occur. They are locally aggressive but do not metastasize, so wide local excision is adequate treatment.

VULVAR SARCOMA

Vulvar sarcomas represent 1-2% of vulvar malignancies. Many histologic types have been reported, including leiomyosarcomas, fibrosarcomas, neurofibrosarcomas, liposarcomas, rhabdomyosarcomas, angiosarcomas, and epithelioid sarcomas. Leiomyosarcomas are the most common, and recurrences are most likely with lesions that are larger than 5 cm, have infiltrating margins, and have 5 or more mitotic figures per 10 high-power fields.

Vaginal Neoplasms

INTRAEPITHELIAL NEOPLASIA

Carcinoma in situ of the vagina (vaginal intraepithelial neoplasia [VAIN]) is much less common than its counterparts on the cervix or vulva. Most lesions occur in the upper third of the vagina, and the patients are usually asymptomatic.

Etiology

VAIN appears to be related to infection with the wart virus in many cases, and vaccination against HPV should decrease the incidence of VAIN and vaginal cancer in the future. Patients with a past history of in situ or invasive carcinoma of the cervix or vulva are at increased risk. Some lesions may occur after irradiation for cervical cancer.

Diagnosis

The diagnosis is usually considered because of an abnormal Papanicolaou smear in a woman who either has had a hysterectomy or has no demonstrable cervical abnormality. Definitive diagnosis requires vaginal biopsy, which should be directed by colposcopy or Lugol iodine staining. Colposcopic findings are similar to those seen with cervical lesions, although thorough colposcopy of all vaginal walls is technically more difficult. **In postmenopausal patients, a 4-week course of topical estrogen before colposcopy is indicated to enhance the colposcopic features and eliminate those patients with Papanicolaou smear abnormalities caused by inflammatory atypia.**

Management

When the lesion involves the vaginal vault, surgical excision is indicated to treat the VAIN and to exclude invasive cancer. For multifocal disease, laser therapy or topical 5-fluorouracil cream may be used. Extensive disease may require total vaginectomy and creation of a neovagina using a split-thickness skin graft.

SQUAMOUS CELL CARCINOMA OF THE VAGINA

Squamous cell carcinoma of the vagina is uncommon. The mean age of patients at presentation is about 60 years. **Up to 30% of patients with primary vaginal cancer have a history of in situ or invasive cervical cancer that was treated at least 5 years earlier.** Symptoms consist of abnormal vaginal bleeding, vaginal discharge, and urinary symptoms. During a physical examination, ulcerative, exophytic, and infiltrative growth patterns may be seen. About half of the lesions are in the upper third of the vagina, particularly on the posterior wall. Punch biopsy is required to confirm the diagnosis.

Patterns of Spread

Vaginal cancer spreads by direct invasion as well as by lymphatic and hematogenous dissemination. **Direct tumor spread may result in involvement of the bladder, urethra, or rectum or in progressive lateral extension to the pelvic side wall.** The lymphatic drainage from the upper vagina is to the obturator, hypogastric, and external iliac nodes, whereas the lower third of the vagina drains primarily to the inguinofemoral nodes. Hematogenous spread is uncommon until the disease is advanced.

Staging

The FIGO staging for vaginal cancer is clinical, as shown in Table 40-3. In practice, all patients should have at least a chest, pelvic, and abdominal computed tomographic scan or magnetic resonance imaging scan to detect evidence of metastatic spread, including bulky pelvic or paraaortic lymph nodes. Positron emission tomography is increasingly being used to look for metastatic disease.

Management

Chemoradiation is the main method of treatment for primary vaginal cancer. Initial treatment usually consists of 4500- to 5000-centigray (cGy) external irradiation to the pelvis to shrink the primary tumor and treat the pelvic lymph nodes and paravaginal tissues. Brachytherapy is then given, either with intracavitary vaginal applicators or by using interstitial techniques. **When the lower third of the vagina is involved, the groin nodes should either be included in the treatment field or surgically removed.**

Radical surgery has a limited role in the management of vaginal cancer. **Radical hysterectomy, partial vaginectomy, and pelvic lymphadenectomy may be performed for early lesions in the posterior fornix.** Pelvic exenteration with creation of a neovagina may be required for medically fit patients in whom a central recurrence develops following irradiation.

Prognosis

The overall 5-year survival for vaginal cancer is about 50%. When corrected for deaths resulting from intercurrent disease, 5-year survival rates should be approximately 85-90% for stage I, 55-65% for stage II, 30-35% for stage III, and 5-10% for stage IV.

RARE VAGINAL CANCERS

Adenocarcinoma

Most adenocarcinomas of the vagina are metastatic, usually from the cervix, endometrium, or ovary, but occasionally from more distant sites such as the kidney, breast, or colon. **About 10% of primary vaginal carcinomas are adenocarcinomas.** They are more common in younger women, regardless of whether or not they are related to diethylstilbestrol (DES) exposure in utero (see later in this chapter). Primary adenocarcinomas of the vagina may arise in residual glands of müllerian (paramesonephric) origin, originate in the Gartner duct (a remnant of the embryonic wolffian or mesonephric duct), or develop from foci of endometriosis.

Malignant Melanoma

Vaginal melanomas account for less than 2% of vaginal malignancies. The mean age at diagnosis is 55 years. The carcinoma usually occurs on the distal anterior wall. **Radical surgery has been the traditional treatment, but comparable local control and overall survival may be obtained with conservative tumor resection and postoperative radiation therapy.** The use of high-dose fractions (>400 cGy) may be beneficial. The prognosis is poor, with an overall 5-year survival rate of 5-10%.

Sarcoma

Vaginal sarcomas are rare. In adults, leiomyosarcomas are most common, whereas **in infants and children, sarcoma botryoides predominates.** The latter term comes from the Greek *botrys* (bunch of grapes), which these lesions usually grossly resemble. The mean age at

TABLE 40-3		
INTERNATIONAL FEDERATION OF GYNECOLOGY AND OBSTETRICS STAGING OF VAGINAL CANCER		
Stage	**Description**	
I	Carcinoma limited to the vaginal wall	
II	Carcinoma has involved the subvaginal tissue but has not extended onto the pelvic side wall	
III	Carcinoma has extended to the pelvic side wall	
IV	Carcinoma has extended beyond the true pelvis or has involved the mucosa of the bladder or rectum	
IVA	Spread to bladder or rectum	
IVB	Spread to distant organs	

diagnosis of sarcoma botryoides is 2 to 3 years, and the age range at diagnosis is 6 months to 16 years. **Histologically, the tumor is an embryonal rhabdomyosarcoma. Treatment consists of conservative surgical resection followed by adjuvant chemotherapy, with or without radiation therapy.**

DIETHYLSTILBESTROL EXPOSURE IN UTERO

In 1971, an association between in utero exposure to DES and the later development of clear cell adenocarcinoma of the vagina was reported. Since that time, numerous nonneoplastic uterine and vaginal anomalies have been reported in young women exposed in utero to DES. **Vaginal adenosis (vaginal columnar epithelium) is the most common anomaly and is present in about 30% of exposed females.** This tissue behaves similarly to the columnar epithelium of the cervix and is replaced initially by immature metaplastic squamous epithelium. With progressive squamous maturation, complete resolution of this anomaly usually occurs.

Structural changes of the cervix and vagina occur in about 25% of exposed females. Possible changes include a transverse vaginal septum, cervical collar, cockscomb (a raised ridge, usually on the anterior cervix), or cervical hypoplasia. Most of these changes tend to disappear as the individual matures. The risk is insignificant if the drug was given after the 22nd week of gestation.

In addition to these changes in the lower genital tract, upper genital tract anomalies occur in at least half of the patients and may be associated with exposure later in pregnancy. **The most common abnormalities are a T-shaped uterus and a small uterine cavity** (<2.5 cm in length). Exposed individuals have an increased risk of miscarriage, premature delivery, or ectopic pregnancy, but most are able to deliver a viable infant successfully.

Prescribing DES in pregnancy was discontinued in the 1970s, so DES-related clear cell adenocarcinomas are now rarely seen in clinical practice. The mean age at diagnosis of these tumors was 19 years.

Uterine Corpus Cancer

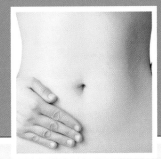

NEVILLE F. HACKER

CLINICAL KEYS FOR THIS CHAPTER

- There are two different clinicopathologic types of endometrial cancer. Type I endometrial cancers are caused by unopposed estrogenic stimulation, are endometrioid in histologic type, and generally have a good prognosis. Type II endometrial cancers are unrelated to estrogenic stimulation, are often nonendometrioid histologically (serous or clear cell), and have a poor prognosis.
- About 5% of endometrial cancers occur in women with Lynch syndrome, which is also called *hereditary nonpolyposis colon cancer* (HNPCC) *syndrome*. This syndrome is caused by germline mutations in the DNA mismatch repair genes. Women with HNPCC syndrome have about a 40% risk of developing endometrial cancer, which is similar to their risk of developing bowel cancer.
- The commonest presenting symptom of patients with endometrial cancer is postmenopausal bleeding. A transvaginal ultrasound will reveal an endometrial stripe that is wider than 4 mm, and an endometrial biopsy done in the office will usually allow histologic diagnosis. If the office biopsy is negative or shows endometrial

hyperplasia, hysteroscopy and uterine curettage will be necessary to definitively exclude endometrial cancer.
- Total hysterectomy and bilateral salpingo-oophorectomy is the basic treatment for stage I endometrial cancer, and this is usually performed by laparoscopic or robotic surgery. Any enlarged pelvic or paraaortic lymph nodes should be resected in all patients. Formal surgical staging, including at least pelvic lymphadenectomy, should be performed in high-risk patients, including those with serous, clear cell, or grade 3 histology, outer-half myometrial invasion, or cervical extension.
- For patients with advanced disease, treatment must be individualized. The uterus, tubes, and ovaries should be removed, if possible, for palliation of bleeding and other pelvic symptoms. Some cases of advanced disease are a result of delayed diagnosis. If the patient has an advanced grade 1 or 2 tumor with positive estrogen or progesterone receptors, good responses and prolonged survival may be seen with the use of high-dose progestins or tamoxifen.

Cancer of the endometrium is the most common gynecologic malignancy in the United States. For 2013, it was estimated that there would be 45,560 new cases and 8190 deaths. It is the fourth most common malignancy found in American women after breast, colorectal, and lung cancers, and it is predominantly a disease of affluent, obese, postmenopausal women of low parity.

Epidemiology and Etiology

There are two different clinicopathologic types of endometrial carcinoma (Table 41-1): an estrogen-dependent and a non–estrogen-dependent type.

Any factor that increases exposure to unopposed estrogen increases the risk for type I endometrial cancer. If the proliferative effects of estrogen are not counteracted by a progestin, endometrial hyperplasia and possibly adenocarcinoma can result.

Obesity results in an increased extraovarian aromatization of androstenedione to estrone. Androstenedione is secreted by the adrenal glands, whereas the increased peripheral conversion occurs predominantly in fat depots, as well as in the liver, kidneys, and skeletal muscles. **Granulosa-theca cell tumors of the ovary produce estrogen,** and up to 15% of patients with these tumors have an associated endometrial cancer.

Unopposed estrogenic stimulation from anovulatory cycles occurs in patients who have polycystic ovarian syndrome (Stein-Leventhal syndrome) **and in patients with a late menopause.** In postmenopausal women taking estrogen replacement without a progestin for menopausal symptoms, the risk of cancer

TABLE 41-1

CLINICOPATHOLOGIC TYPES OF ENDOMETRIAL CARCINOMA	
Type I	Type II
Endometrioid	Non endometrioid (serous, clear cell)
Mean age 63 yr	Mean age 67 yr
Estrogen-related	Non–estrogen-related
Microsatellite instability	Chromosomal instability
Mutations in *PTEN, PIK3CA, KRAS*	*TP53* mutations
Good prognosis	Poor prognosis

TABLE 41-2

ETIOLOGY OF POSTMENOPAUSAL BLEEDING	
Factor	Approximate Percentage
Exogenous estrogens	30
Atrophic endometritis, vaginitis	30
Endometrial cancer	15
Endometrial or cervical polyps	10
Endometrial hyperplasia	5
Miscellaneous (e.g., cervical cancer, uterine sarcoma, urethral caruncle, trauma)	10

developing appears to be both dose-dependent and duration-dependent. This increased risk varies from 2- to 14-fold compared with nonusers. The addition of progestin in a cyclic fashion for 10 to 14 days of the month or in a continuous fashion daily throughout the month eliminates this increased risk. **Women taking tamoxifen for breast cancer have a two- to threefold increased risk of endometrial cancer.** Young women who use oral contraceptives have been shown to have a lower incidence of subsequent endometrial cancer.

About 5% of endometrial cancers occur in women with Lynch syndrome, which is also called the *hereditary nonpolyposis colon cancer* (HNPCC) *syndrome.* This syndrome is caused by germline mutations in the DNA mismatch repair genes. Women with the HNPCC syndrome have about a 40% risk of developing endometrial cancer, usually before the menopause. Their risk of developing bowel cancer is also about 40%.

Screening of Asymptomatic Women

Population screening for endometrial cancer is not feasible, because there is no simple method of cancer detection available. However, screening may be justified for high-risk women, including those with a family history of HNPCC syndrome, those with polycystic ovarian disease, and any woman with an intact uterus taking unopposed estrogen. **Only about 50% of women with endometrial cancer will have malignant cells on a Papanicolaou smear.**

Since the 1990s, transvaginal ultrasonography has increasingly been used for endometrial evaluation. Almost all women with endometrial hyperplasia or carcinoma will have an endometrial thickness of 5 mm or more. **Tamoxifen produces a confusing ultrasonic image, which leads to frequent false-positive reports.**

Symptoms

The most common symptom of endometrial cancer is abnormal vaginal bleeding, which is present in 90% of patients. **Postmenopausal bleeding is always abnormal and must be investigated.** The most common conditions associated with postmenopausal bleeding are listed in Table 41-2. In the premenopausal or perimenopausal patient, diagnosis is often delayed because frequent or heavy bleeding is usually thought to be dysfunctional in nature.

As menopause approaches, menstruation often becomes lighter and less frequent. If the bleeding becomes heavier or more frequent, it should be investigated.

Signs

A general physical examination may reveal obesity, hypertension, and the stigmata of diabetes mellitus. Evidence of metastatic disease is unusual at initial presentation, but the chest should be examined for any effusion and the abdomen carefully palpated and percussed to exclude ascites, hepatomegaly, or evidence of upper abdominal masses.

On pelvic examination, the external genitalia are usually normal. The vagina and cervix are also usually normal, but they should be inspected and palpated carefully for evidence of involvement. **A patulous cervical os or a firm, expanded cervix may indicate extension of disease from the corpus to the cervix.** The uterus may be of normal size or enlarged, depending on the extent of the disease and the presence or absence of other uterine conditions, such as adenomyosis or fibroids. The adnexa should be palpated carefully for evidence of extrauterine metastases or an ovarian neoplasm. **A granulosa cell tumor or an endometrioid ovarian carcinoma may occasionally coexist with endometrial cancer.**

Diagnosis

Any woman who presents with postmenopausal bleeding should undergo transvaginal ultrasonography. If the endometrial thickness is greater than 4 mm, endometrial evaluation is necessary. An outpatient endometrial biopsy is usually feasible with a sampling device such as a Pipelle, GynoSampler, or Vabra aspirator. Outpatient endometrial biopsy has a diagnostic accuracy of about 95%. If the endometrial biopsy reveals endometrial cancer, definitive treatment can be arranged. **If the endometrial biopsy is negative for cancer or reveals endometrial hyperplasia, a hysteroscopy and fractional dilation and curettage should be performed with the patient under general anesthesia.** Specimens from the endometrium and endocervix should be submitted separately for histologic evaluation to determine whether the tumor has extended to the endocervix.

In a premenopausal patient with high-risk factors and abnormal uterine bleeding, the endometrium must be sampled. If there are no high-risk factors present, failure to respond to medical management or a suspicious transvaginal ultrasound is also an indication for hysteroscopy and uterine curettage.

STAGING

In 1988, the International Federation of Gynecology and Obstetrics (FIGO) changed from a clinical to a surgical staging system for endometrial cancer. This surgical staging system was further revised in 2009. The latest FIGO staging system is shown in Table 41-3.

Preoperative Investigations

In addition to a thorough physical examination, blood studies should include a complete blood count; determinations of hepatic enzymes, serum electrolytes, blood urea nitrogen, and serum creatinine; and a coagulation profile. A routine urinalysis should be performed. **It is usual to perform computed tomography (CT) of the chest, pelvis, and abdomen, particularly in high-risk cases,** to detect any enlarged lymph nodes, liver or lung metastases, hydronephrosis, or adrenal masses. **Magnetic resonance imaging is useful for differentiating superficial from deep myometrial invasion or detection of cervical involvement.** It may be useful for triaging patients to a gynecologic oncologist.

Pathologic Features

About 75% of endometrial cancers are pure adenocarcinomas. When squamous elements are present, the tumor is called an *adenocarcinoma with squamous differentiation*. Such tumors are graded on the glandular component of the lesion. Less often, **clear cell,**

TABLE 41-3

INTERNATIONAL FEDERATION OF GYNECOLOGY AND OBSTETRICS SURGICAL STAGING FOR CARCINOMA OF THE ENDOMETRIUM (2009)

Stage	Description
I*	Tumor confined to the corpus uteri
IA*	No or less than half myometrial invasion
IB*	Invasion equal to or more than half of the myometrium
II*	Tumor invades cervical stroma, but does not extend beyond the uterus†
III*	Local and/or regional spread of the tumor
IIIA*	Tumor invades the serosa of the corpus uteri and/or adnexa‡
IIIB*	Vaginal and/or parametrial involvement‡
IIIC*	Metastases to pelvic and/or paraaortic lymph nodes‡
IIIC1*	Positive pelvic nodes
IIIC2*	Positive paraaortic lymph nodes with or without positive pelvic lymph nodes
IV*	Tumor invades bladder and/or bowel mucosa, and/or distant metastases
IVA*	Tumor invasion of bladder and/or bowel mucosa
IVB*	Distant metastases, including intraabdominal metastases and/or inguinal lymph nodes

From Pecorelli S: Revised FIGO staging for carcinoma of the vulva, cervix, and endometrium. *Int J Gynaecol Obstet* 105:103-104, 2009.
*Either Grade 1, Grade 2, or Grade 3.
†Endocervical glandular involvement should be considered only as stage I and no longer as stage II.
‡Positive cytology has to be reported separately without changing the stage.

squamous, or serous carcinomas occur, and all carry a worse prognosis.

Invasive adenocarcinoma of the endometrium demonstrates proliferative glandular formation with minimal or no intervening stroma. Tumor grade is determined by both the degree of abnormality of the glandular architecture and the degree of nuclear atypia. A lesion that is well differentiated (grade 1) forms a glandular pattern similar to normal endometrial glands (Figure 41-1). A moderately well-differentiated lesion (grade 2) has glandular structures admixed with papillary, and occasionally solid, areas of tumor. In a poorly differentiated lesion (grade 3), the glandular structures have become predominantly solid with a relative paucity of identifiable endometrial glands (Figure 41-2).

Pattern of Spread

Endometrial cancer spreads by (1) direct extension, (2) exfoliation of cells that are shed through the fallopian tubes, (3) lymphatic dissemination, and (4) hematogenous dissemination.

The most common route of spread is direct extension of the tumor to adjacent structures. The tumor may invade through the myometrium and eventually

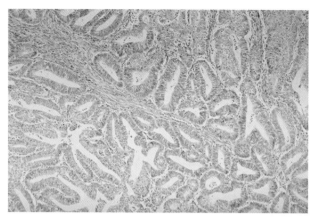

FIGURE 41-1 Well-differentiated endometrial adenocarcinoma. Note the back-to-back glands with minimal intervening stroma and the gland-within-gland pattern.

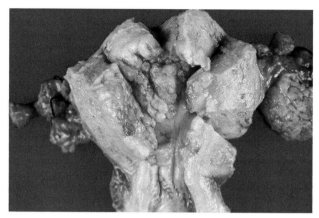

FIGURE 41-3 Specimen from a total abdominal hysterectomy and bilateral salpingo-oophorectomy. The uterus has been opened to reveal an exophytic carcinoma on the posterior wall of the corpus.

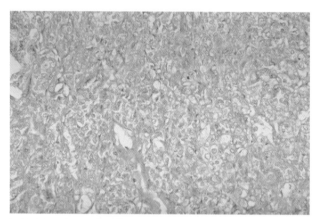

FIGURE 41-2 Poorly differentiated endometrial adenocarcinoma. Note the predominantly solid nature of the tumor with minimal gland formation.

penetrate the serosa. It may also grow downward and involve the cervix. Although uncommon, progressive growth may eventually involve the vagina, parametrium, rectum, or bladder.

Exfoliated cells may pass through the fallopian tubes and implant on the ovaries, the visceral or parietal peritoneum, or the omentum.

Lymphatic spread occurs most commonly in patients with deep myometrial penetration. **Spread occurs mainly to the pelvic nodes and subsequently to the paraaortic nodes, although simultaneous spread to both nodal groups may occur.** About 50% of patients with positive pelvic nodes will have positive paraaortic nodes, but isolated paraaortic nodal metastases occur in only about 2-3% of cases.

In stage I endometrial cancer, the overall incidence of pelvic lymph node metastases is about 12%, and paraaortic metastases occur in about 8% of cases. **In patients with deeply invasive, poorly differentiated**

stage I adenocarcinomas, pelvic lymph node metastases occur in up to 40% of cases. Lymphatic spread is also responsible for vaginal vault recurrences.

Hematogenous dissemination is less common, but it results in parenchymal metastases, particularly in the lungs or liver, or both.

Treatment

STAGE I

Surgery

Total hysterectomy and bilateral salpingo-oophorectomy are performed on all patients, unless there are absolute medical contraindications (Figure 41-3). This is usually performed by laparoscopic or robotic surgery, although some cases will still require open laparotomy. Upon entering the abdomen, peritoneal washings are taken with normal saline for cytologic evaluation, although the status of the washings is no longer part of the FIGO staging. Retroperitoneal spaces should be opened and evaluated, and any enlarged pelvic or paraaortic lymph nodes should be resected. **Formal surgical staging, including at least pelvic lymphadenectomy, should be performed on high-risk patients, including those with serous, clear cell, or grade 3 histology; outer-half myometrial invasion; or cervical extension.**

Radiation Therapy

With the advent of surgical staging, less reliance has been placed on adjuvant radiation therapy in the management of patients with endometrial cancer.

Recommendations are as follows (Figure 41-4):
1. Patients with grade 1 or 2 endometrioid carcinomas confined to the inner half of the myometrium may be followed **without adjuvant therapy** (i.e., **stage IA, grade 1 or 2**).

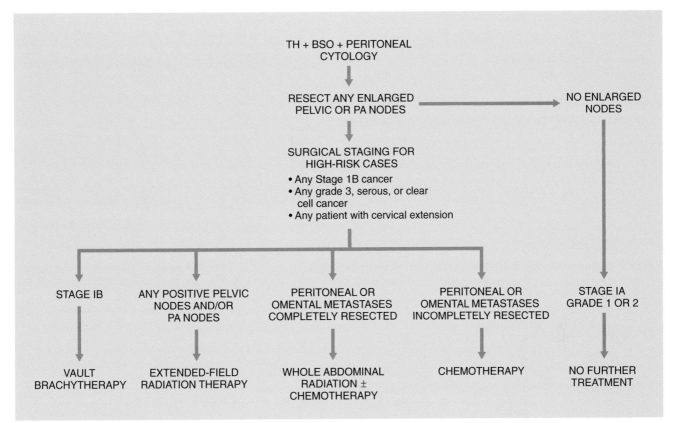

TH + BSO + PERITONEAL
CYTOLOGY

↓

RESECT ANY ENLARGED
PELVIC OR PA NODES → NO ENLARGED NODES

↓

SURGICAL STAGING FOR
HIGH-RISK CASES
• Any Stage 1B cancer
• Any grade 3, serous, or clear
  cell cancer
• Any patient with cervical extension

STAGE IB	ANY POSITIVE PELVIC NODES AND/OR PA NODES	PERITONEAL OR OMENTAL METASTASES COMPLETELY RESECTED	PERITONEAL OR OMENTAL METASTASES INCOMPLETELY RESECTED	STAGE IA GRADE 1 OR 2
VAULT BRACHYTHERAPY	EXTENDED-FIELD RADIATION THERAPY	WHOLE ABDOMINAL RADIATION ± CHEMOTHERAPY	CHEMOTHERAPY	NO FURTHER TREATMENT

FIGURE 41-4 Algorithm for the treatment of stage I and occult stage II endometrial cancer. *BSO,* Bilateral salpingo-oophorectomy; *PA,* paraaortic; *TH,* total hysterectomy.

2. Patients with **high-risk carcinomas with negative pelvic nodes** (i.e., any stage IB cancer; any grade 3, clear cell, or serous cancer; or any stage II cancer) may have **vault brachytherapy** (without external beam pelvic radiation).
3. Patients with any positive pelvic nodes or proven positive paraaortic nodes should receive **extended-field radiation** (i.e., pelvic and paraaortic).
4. For patients with pelvic peritoneal or upper abdominal metastases completely resected, whole abdominal radiation may be given.

In patients medically unfit for surgery, radiation therapy alone may be employed. A combination of intracavitary plus external beam radiation is used. The overall 5-year survival rate is about 20% lower than that for patients treated with hysterectomy.

Hormone Therapy

Endometrial cancer occasionally occurs **in women younger than 40 years of age.** These tumors are usually at an early stage and of low grade, and there is frequently a desire to preserve fertility. **High-dose medroxyprogesterone acetate** (200 mg twice daily) **for 3 to 6 months will reverse the changes in about 75% of patients,** but recurrences are common, so careful monitoring is essential. A levonorgestrel-releasing intrauterine device (Mirena) may also be useful in these patients.

STAGE II

If the cervix is grossly normal and involvement is detected only on the histologic evaluation of the endocervical curettage material (occult stage II disease), treatment may be the same as that for stage I disease (i.e., total hysterectomy, bilateral salpingo-oophorectomy, surgical staging, and tailored postoperative radiotherapy).

Alternatively, regardless of the size of the cervix, primary radical hysterectomy, bilateral salpingo-oophorectomy, together with pelvic and paraaortic lymphadenectomy, may be performed. If the lymph nodes are negative, no brachytherapy is required. If they are positive, postoperative external beam extended-field radiation is required.

ADVANCED STAGES

For advanced disease, treatment must be individualized. The uterus, tubes, and ovaries should be removed, if possible, for palliation of bleeding and other pelvic symptoms. If gross disease is present in the upper abdomen, tumor metastases that are readily removable, such as an omental "cake," should be extirpated in an attempt to improve the patient's quality of life by temporarily decreasing abdominal discomfort and ascites. In addition, patients with advanced disease will also require chemotherapy and/or radiation therapy.

Some cases of advanced disease are a result of delayed diagnosis. **If the patient has an advanced grade 1 or 2 tumor with positive estrogen receptors (ERs) or progesterone receptors (PRs), good responses and prolonged survival may be seen with high-dose progestin or tamoxifen therapy.**

Chemotherapy

The role of chemotherapy in patients with advanced endometrial cancer remains controversial. **Platinum-based regimens are the most effective,** but increased pelvic recurrence rates have been reported when adjuvant chemotherapy is used alone in patients with high-risk or advanced disease.

RECURRENT DISEASE

Seventy-five percent of recurrences develop within 2 years of treatment. If recurrent disease is detected, the patient should undergo a complete physical examination and metastatic workup. Careful follow-up is particularly important for patients treated without adjuvant therapy. The majority of recurrences in these patients are at the vaginal vault, and 70-80% of isolated vault recurrences can be salvaged by radiation therapy.

Metastases in other sites, such as the upper abdomen, lungs, or liver, are treated initially with high-dose progestins or antiestrogens. About one-third of recurrent endometrial carcinomas contain ERs and PRs, with the more well-differentiated tumors more likely to contain such receptors. As with breast cancer, the likelihood of response to progestin treatment is increased in patients whose tumor contains ERs and PRs. Approximately 80% of such patients respond to progestin therapy, compared with fewer than 10% of patients whose tumor is receptor-negative.

Medroxyprogesterone acetate (Provera 50 mg three times daily; Depo-Provera 400 mg intramuscularly weekly) or megestrol acetate (Megace 80 mg twice daily) may be given. **If disease progresses while the patient is receiving progestins, chemotherapy may be offered.** The combination of carboplatin and paclitaxel (Taxol) gives a response rate of about 50%.

Prognosis

The patient's prognosis is dependent on several variables, including histologic type, grade of tumor, depth of myometrial penetration, status of lymph nodes, and presence or absence of occult adnexal or upper abdominal metastases. **Serous and clear cell endometrial carcinomas have a particularly poor prognosis, and**

TABLE 41-4

CARCINOMA OF THE CORPUS UTERI: PATIENTS TREATED FROM 1999 TO 2001 WITH SURVIVAL RATES BY FIGO SURGICAL STAGE (N = 7990)

Strata	Patients	Overall Survival (%)		
		1-Year	3-Year	5-Year
IA	1054	98.2	95.3	90.8
IB	2833	98.7	94.6	91.1
IC	1426	97.5	89.7	85.4
IIA	430	95.2	89.0	83.3
IIB	543	93.5	80.3	74.2
IIIA	612	89.0	73.3	66.2
IIIB	80	73.5	56.7	49.9
IIIC	356	89.9	66.3	57.3
IVA	49	63.4	34.4	25.5
IVB	206	59.5	29.0	20.1

Modified from Creasman WT, Odicino F, Maisonneuve P, et al: Carcinoma of the corpus uteri. FIGO 26th Annual Report on the Results of Treatment in Gynecological Cancer. *Int J Gynaecol Obstet* 95(Suppl 1):S105-S143, 2006.
These results are based on the 1988 FIGO staging system. Stages IA and IB are now officially combined as stage IA, and there is no stage IIA.

both of these histologic types are prone to early dissemination. Five-year survival rates for these tumor types are less than 50%.

Five-year survival rates for each FIGO stage of endometrioid endometrial cancer are presented in Table 41-4.

Follow-up

Follow-up examinations should be performed every 3 months for 2 years, then every 6 months for a further 3 years. It is important to take a vault Papanicolaou smear from patients who have not had radiation therapy.

Uterine Sarcomas

Uterine sarcomas account for about 3% of uterine cancers. They are mesodermal tumors, which have a tendency for hematogenous dissemination and a poor prognosis.

CLASSIFICATION

A classification system for uterine mesodermal tumors is presented in Table 41-5.

Uterine sarcomas may also be classified as homologous, implying that the tissue that is malignant is normally present in the uterus (e.g., endometrial stroma, smooth muscle), **or heterologous,** implying that the tissue that is malignant is not normally present in the uterus (e.g., bone or cartilage). The majority of pure uterine sarcomas are leiomyosarcomas and endometrial stromal sarcomas.

TABLE 41-5

UTERINE MESODERMAL TUMORS WITH MALIGNANT POTENTIAL

Tumor Type	Percentage of Tumors
Smooth Muscle Tumors	30-40%
Leiomyosarcomas	
Smooth muscle tumors of uncertain malignant potential	
Endometrial Stromal Tumors	15-25%
Endometrial stromal sarcomas	
Undifferentiated uterine sarcomas	
Carcinosarcomas	40-50%
Homologous	
Heterologous (malignant mixed müllerian tumors)	
Adenosarcomas	5%

TABLE 41-6

INTERNATIONAL FEDERATION OF GYNECOLOGY AND OBSTETRICS STAGING FOR LEIOMYOSARCOMAS (2009)

Stage	Definition
I	Tumor limited to uterus
IA	<5 cm
IB	>5 cm
II	Tumor extends to the pelvis
IIA	Adnexal involvement
IIB	Tumor extends to extrauterine pelvic tissue
III	Tumor invades abdominal tissues (not just protruding into the abdomen)
IIIA	One site
IIIB	More than one site
IIIC	Metastasis to pelvic and/or paraaortic lymph nodes
IV	
IVA	Tumor invades bladder and/or rectum
IVB	Distant metastasis

From FIGO Committee on Gynecologic Oncology: FIGO staging for uterine sarcomas. *Int J Gynaecol Obstet* 104:179, 2009.

TABLE 41-7

INTERNATIONAL FEDERATION OF GYNECOLOGY AND OBSTETRICS STAGING OF ENDOMETRIAL STROMAL SARCOMAS AND ADENOSARCOMAS (2009)

Stage	Definition
I	Tumor limited to uterus
IA	Tumor limited to endometrium/endocervix with no myometrial invasion
IB	Less than or equal to half myometrial invasion
IC	More than half myometrial invasion
II	Tumor extends to the pelvis
IIA	Adnexal involvement
IIB	Tumor extends to extrauterine pelvic tissue
III	Tumor invades abdominal tissues (not just protruding into the abdomen)
IIIA	One site
IIIB	More than one site
IIIC	Metastasis to pelvic and/or paraaortic lymph nodes
IV	
IVA	Tumor invades bladder and/or rectum
IVB	Distant metastasis

From FIGO Committee on Gynecologic Oncology: FIGO staging for uterine sarcomas. *Int J Gynaecol Obstet* 104:179, 2009.
Note: Simultaneous tumors of the uterine corpus and ovary/pelvis in association with ovarian/pelvic endometriosis should be classified as independent primary tumors.

present with pelvic pain, abnormal uterine bleeding, or a pelvic or lower abdominal mass. A sensation of pressure on the bladder or rectum may also be noted.

Most cases are not diagnosed preoperatively; they are often discovered at the time of exploratory surgery for a probable fibroid. Curettings are usually normal. **If a known fibroid uterus appears to be rapidly enlarging, especially postmenopausally, malignancy should be suspected.**

The treatment of a uterine leiomyosarcoma consists of total abdominal hysterectomy and bilateral salpingo-oophorectomy. Adjuvant pelvic radiation appears to decrease local pelvic recurrence; it does not prolong survival, however, because most patients die with distant metastases.

Response rates to chemotherapy are very low.

LEIOMYOSARCOMA

Leiomyosarcomas usually arise de novo from the uterine muscle, although rarely they may arise from a preexisting leiomyoma. The risk of malignant transformation in a benign fibroid is less than 1%. **The histologic criteria for distinguishing leiomyosarcomas from leiomyomas are the mitotic count (usually >10 per 10 high-power fields), the presence or absence of coagulative necrosis, and the presence or absence of cellular atypia.** Leiomyosarcomas were officially staged by FIGO in 2009 (Table 41-6).

Clinically, the mean age of patients with leiomyosarcoma is about 55 years. Patients with this disease may

ENDOMETRIAL STROMAL TUMORS

The three types of stromal tumors are (1) endometrial stromal nodule; (2) endometrial stromal sarcoma, previously known as endolymphatic stromal myosis; and (3) high-grade endometrial sarcoma. The first of these, **the stromal nodule, is a rare, benign condition.** There are typically 3 or fewer mitoses per 10 high-power fields. A hysterectomy is curative. These tumors were officially staged by FIGO in 2009 (Table 41-7).

Endometrial stromal sarcoma is a low-grade lesion. Histologically, there is minimal to no cellular atypia, with usually fewer than 5 mitoses per 10 high-power fields. There is always evidence of vascular channel invasion. These patients usually present with abnormal vaginal bleeding and often with pelvic pain.

Most patients are cured with total abdominal hysterectomy and bilateral salpingo-oophorectomy. Local and distant recurrences may occur, even 10 to 20 years later, and require reexploration and resection of disease. Prolonged survival is possible after resection of recurrent disease, and response to progestins is good. Pelvic disease may respond to radiation therapy.

Undifferentiated endometrial sarcoma generally causes abnormal uterine bleeding, and more than half the patients are premenopausal. **The diagnosis can often be made by endometrial biopsy or uterine curettage.** Histologically, there are 10 or more mitoses per 10 high-power fields, and the lesion is composed of very poorly differentiated cells. Aggressive myometrial invasion occurs, and hematogenous spread is common at the time of diagnosis.

The treatment of high-grade endometrial sarcoma is total abdominal hysterectomy and bilateral salpingo-oophorectomy. A thorough exploration of the peritoneal cavity and retroperitoneum should be done for evidence of metastases. **Postoperative pelvic irradiation improves local control but does not improve survival.** In patients with metastatic disease, progestogens or chemotherapy may be offered. The best chemotherapeutic agents are cisplatin, doxorubicin, and ifosfamide, but the prognosis is poor.

ADENOSARCOMAS

Adenosarcomas are typically low-grade tumors characterized by a benign epithelial component and a malignant mesenchymal component. The latter is commonly a low-grade endometrial stromal sarcoma. These tumors are usually seen in postmenopausal women, and the treatment and prognosis are consistent with that of the mesenchymal component.

MALIGNANT MIXED MESODERMAL TUMORS

Malignant mixed mesodermal tumors or carcinosarcomas are believed to be metaplastic carcinomas, and they behave, and should be managed, as a grade 3 endometrioid carcinoma. They usually occur in postmenopausal patients and present with vaginal bleeding or discharge. About one-third of patients have tumors growing through the cervix into the vagina as a polypoid mass. The tumors aggressively invade the myometrium and disseminate via the lymphatics and the bloodstream. **Up to 50% of patients have evidence of metastatic disease at the time of diagnosis if surgically staged.**

Prognosis

The prognosis for uterine leiomyosarcomas and endometrial sarcomas is poor because of the propensity for hematogenous dissemination. The overall 5-year survival rate is about 35%. Patients with endometrial stromal sarcomas have a good prognosis, whereas patients with stage I or II carcinosarcomas have a 5-year survival of about 70% if treated with surgical staging and adjuvant radiation and chemotherapy.

Gestational Trophoblastic Diseases

JONATHAN S. BEREK

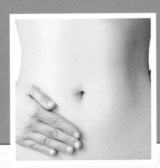

Gestational trophoblastic diseases (GTDs) represent a broad spectrum of disorders that includes **molar pregnancy** (complete and partial), which usually goes into spontaneous remission, as well as persistent tumors designated **gestational trophoblastic neoplasms (GTNs).** The latter include **invasive moles,** which can metastasize, and the frankly malignant **choriocarcinoma.** GTNs are some of the rare human malignancies that are curable with chemotherapy, even in the presence of extensive metastatic disease.

Most molar pregnancies are sporadic, but a familial syndrome of recurrent hydatidiform mole has been described and is reported to be strongly associated with a mutation in the *NLRP7* gene. **The majority of patients (80-90%) with GTD have a benign course.** This diverse group of diseases has a **sensitive tumor marker, human chorionic gonadotropin (hCG),** that allows accurate follow-up and assessment of the diseases.

Epidemiology and Etiology

The incidence of molar pregnancy is about 1 in every 1500 to 2000 pregnancies among white women in the United States. There is a much higher incidence among Asian women in the United States (1 in 800) and an even higher incidence among women in Asia. For example, in Taiwan, 1 in every 125 to 200 pregnancies is a molar pregnancy. **The risk of the development of a second molar pregnancy is 1-3%,** or as much as 40 times greater than the risk of developing the first molar pregnancy. Although the cause of GTN is unknown, it is **known to occur more frequently in women younger than age 20 years and in those older than 40 years of age.** It appears that GTN may result from defective fertilization, a process that is more common in both younger and older individuals. Diet may play a causative role. **The incidence of molar pregnancy has been noted to be higher in geographic** areas where people consume less β-carotene (a retinoid) and folic acid.

Genetics of Gestational Trophoblastic Disease

The cytogenetic analysis of tissue obtained from molar pregnancies offers some clues to the genesis of these lesions. Figure 42-1 illustrates the genetic composition of molar pregnancies.

COMPLETE MOLE

The majority of hydatidiform moles are "complete" moles and have a 46,XX karyotype. Specialized studies indicate that both of the X chromosomes are paternally derived. This androgenic origin probably results from fertilization of an "empty egg" (i.e., an egg without chromosomes) by a haploid sperm (23 X), which then duplicates to restore the diploid chromosomal complement (46,XX). Only a small percentage of lesions are 46,XY. **Complete molar pregnancy is only rarely associated with a fetus, and this may represent a form of twinning.**

PARTIAL MOLE

In the "incomplete" or partial mole, the karyotype is usually a triploid, often 69,XXY (80%). The majority of the remaining lesions are 69,XXX or 69,XYY. Occasionally, mosaic patterns occur. **These lesions, unlike complete moles, often present with a coexistent fetus.** The fetus usually has a triploid karyotype and is defective.

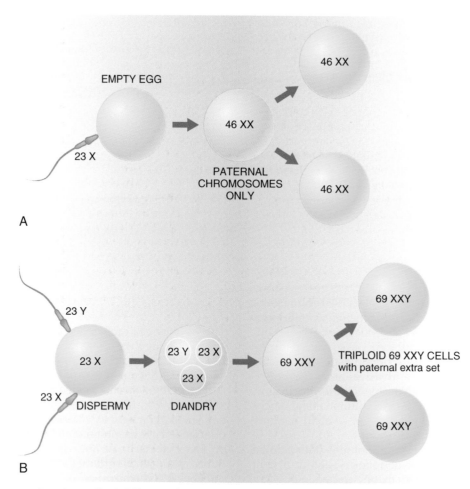

FIGURE 42-1 Cytogenetic makeup of hydatidiform mole. **A,** Chromosomal origin of a complete mole. A single sperm fertilizes an "empty egg." Reduplication of its 23 X set gives a completely homozygous diploid genome of 46,XX. A similar result follows fertilization of an empty egg by two sperms with two independently drawn sets of 23 X or 23 Y; note that both karyotypes, 46,XX and 46,XY, can ensue. **B,** Chromosomal origin of the triploid, partial mole. A normal egg with a 23 X haploid set is fertilized by two sperms that can carry either sex chromosome to give a total of 69 chromosomes with a sex chromosome configuration of XXY, XXX, or XYY. A similar result can be obtained by fertilization with a sperm carrying the unreduced paternal genome 46,XY (resulting sex complement, XXY only). (Adapted from Szulman AE: Syndromes of hydatidiform moles: partial vs. complete. *J Reprod Med* 29:789–790, 1984.)

CLASSIFICATION OF GESTATIONAL TROPHOBLASTIC DISEASES

Benign

Hydatidiform mole
- Complete mole
- Incomplete ("partial") mole

Malignant

Invasive mole ("chorioadenoma destruens")
Choriocarcinoma
Malignant GTN, which may be
- Nonmetastatic
- Metastatic
  - Good prognosis
  - Poor prognosis

GTN, Gestational trophoblastic neoplasia.

CLINICAL FEATURES OF METASTATIC GESTATIONAL NEOPLASIA WITH A POOR PROGNOSIS

- Urinary hCG level >100,000 IU/24 hr or serum hCG level >40,000 IU
- Disease presents >4 mo from the antecedent pregnancy
- Metastasis to the brain or liver (regardless of hCG titer or duration of disease)
- Prior failure to respond to single-agent chemotherapy
- Choriocarcinoma after a full-term delivery

hCG, Human chorionic gonadotropin.

CHORIOCARCINOMA

Genetic analysis of choriocarcinomas usually reveals aneuploidy or polyploidy, typical for anaplastic carcinomas.

Classification

The term *gestational trophoblastic neoplasia* is of clinical value because often the diagnosis is made and therapy instituted without definitive knowledge of the precise histologic pattern. GTD may be benign or malignant and nonmetastatic or metastatic (Box 42-1).

The benign form of GTD is called *hydatidiform mole.* Although this entity is usually confined to the uterine cavity, trophoblastic tissue can occasionally embolize to the lungs. **The malignant forms, called *GTNs,* are invasive mole and choriocarcinoma. Invasive mole is usually a locally invasive lesion,** although it can be associated with metastases. This lesion accounts for the majority of patients who have persistent hCG titers following molar evacuation. **Choriocarcinoma is the frankly malignant form of GTN.**

Metastatic GTN can be subdivided into "good prognosis" and "poor prognosis" groups, depending on the sites of metastases and other clinical variables (Box 42-2).

Pathologic Features

Grossly, a hydatidiform mole appears as multiple vesicles that have been classically described as a "bunch of grapes" (Figure 42-2). **The characteristic histopathologic findings associated with a complete molar pregnancy are (1) hydropic villi, (2) absence of fetal blood vessels, and (3) hyperplasia of trophoblastic tissue** (Figure 42-3). Invasive mole differs from hydatidiform mole only in its propensity to invade locally and to metastasize.

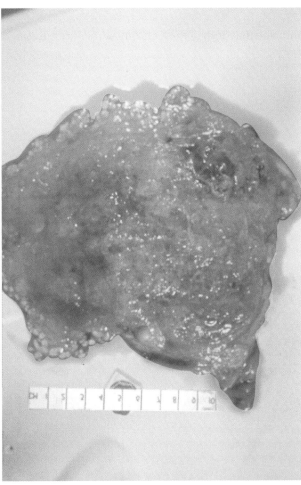

FIGURE 42-2 Complete hydatidiform mole. Multiple hydropic villi (vesicles), resembling a "bunch of grapes," are admixed with areas of necrosis *(white areas)* and hemorrhage. Note the absence of a fetus.

A partial mole has some hydropic villi, whereas other villi are essentially normal. Fetal vessels are seen in a partial mole, and the trophoblastic tissue exhibits less striking hyperplasia.

Choriocarcinoma in the uterus appears grossly as a vascular-appearing, irregular, and "beefy" tumor, often

Edge of chorionic villus

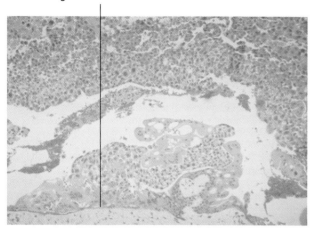

FIGURE 42-3 Histologic appearance of a complete hydatidiform mole. Note the marked trophoblastic proliferation.

Hydatidiform Mole

SYMPTOMS

Most patients with hydatidiform moles present with irregular or heavy vaginal bleeding during the first or early second trimester of pregnancy (Box 42-3). The bleeding is usually painless, although it can be associated with uterine contractions. In addition, **the patient may expel molar "vesicles" from the vagina and occasionally may have excessive nausea, even "hyperemesis gravidarum."** Irritability, dizziness, and photophobia may occur, because **some patients experience preeclampsia. Patients may occasionally exhibit symptoms related to hyperthyroidism,** such as nervousness, anorexia, and tremors.

SIGNS

The patient's vital signs may reveal tachycardia, tachypnea, and hypertension, reflecting the presence of preeclampsia or clinical hyperthyroidism. Funduscopic examination may show arteriolar spasm. In the rare case of trophoblastic emboli to the pulmonary system, wheezing and rhonchi may be noted on chest examination. Abdominal examination may reveal an enlarged uterus. **Auscultation of the uterus is typically remarkable for the absence of fetal heart sounds.**

On pelvic examination, the grapelike vesicles of the mole may be detected in the vagina. Blood clots may be present. **About half of patients with molar pregnancy present with a uterus that is bigger than expected based on their last menstrual period,** whereas about one-fourth have a uterine size compatible with or smaller than gestational age. **Theca lutein cysts occur in about one-third of women with molar pregnancies,** but they may be difficult to detect until the uterus has been evacuated.

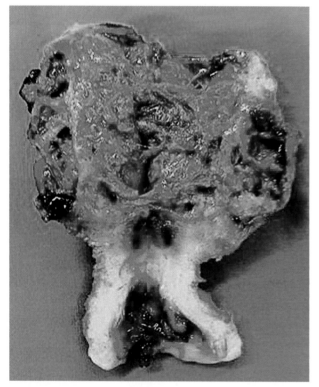

FIGURE 42-4 Uterine choriocarcinoma that has penetrated the serosa. The patient presented with a hemoperitoneum.

growing through the uterine wall (Figure 42-4). Metastatic lesions appear hemorrhagic and have the consistency of currant jelly. **Histologically, choriocarcinoma consists of sheets of malignant cytotrophoblast and syncytiotrophoblast with no identifiable villi.**

DIAGNOSIS

The β-hCG levels can be high for early pregnancy. This should alert the physician that the patient might have GTD or a multiple gestation. The condition must also be distinguished from a threatened spontaneous abortion or an ectopic pregnancy.

Definitive diagnosis of hydatidiform mole can usually be made ultrasonographically. Ultrasonography is noninvasive and reveals a "snowstorm" pattern that is diagnostic.

CLINICAL INVESTIGATIONS

Patients who have the presumptive or definitive diagnosis of hydatidiform mole should have a complete blood count done to exclude anemia, which might require a transfusion. They require an assessment of platelet count, prothrombin time, partial thromboplastin time, and fibrinogen level, because an occasional patient may experience disseminated intravascular coagulation. Liver and renal function tests should be performed. Blood should be typed and cross-matched in the event that excessive bleeding is encountered at the time of evacuation of the mole. A chest film should be obtained, as should an electrocardiogram if tachycardia is present or if the patient is older than 40 years of age.

STAGING

The International Federation of Gynecology and Obstetrics (FIGO) staging system for gestational trophoblastic tumors is shown in Table 42-1.

Stage I: Patients with persistently elevated hCG levels and tumor confined to the uterine corpus.
Stage II: Patients with metastases to the vagina or pelvis or to both.
Stage III: Patients with pulmonary metastases with or without uterine, vaginal, or pelvic involvement. The diagnosis is based on a rising hCG level in the presence of pulmonary lesions on chest films.
Stage IV: Patients with advanced disease and involvement of the brain (Figure 42-5), liver, kidneys, or gastrointestinal tract. These patients are in the highest risk category because their disease is most likely to be resistant to chemotherapy. The histologic pattern of choriocarcinoma is usually present, and disease commonly follows a nonmolar pregnancy.

TREATMENT

Evacuation

The standard therapy for hydatidiform mole is suction evacuation followed by sharp curettage of the uterine cavity, regardless of the duration of pregnancy. This should be performed in the operating

TABLE 42-1

Stage	Definition
I	Disease confined to uterus
IA	Disease confined to uterus with no risk factors
IB	Disease confined to uterus with one risk factor
IC	Disease confined to uterus with two risk factors
II	Gestational trophoblastic tumor extending outside uterus but limited to genital structures (adnexa, vagina, broad ligament)
IIA	Gestational trophoblastic tumor involving genital structures without risk factors
IIB	Gestational trophoblastic tumor extending outside uterus but limited to genital structures with one risk factor
IIC	Gestational trophoblastic tumor extending outside uterus but limited to genital structures with two risk factors
III	Gestational trophoblastic disease extending to lungs with or without known genital tract involvement
IIIA	Gestational trophoblastic tumor extending to lungs with or without genital tract involvement and with no risk factors
IIIB	Gestational trophoblastic tumor extending to lungs with or without genital tract involvement and with one risk factor
IIIC	Gestational trophoblastic tumor extending to lungs with or without genital tract involvement and with two risk factors
IV	All other metastatic sites
IVA	All other metastatic sites without risk factors
IVB	All other metastatic sites with one risk factor
IVC	All other metastatic sites with two risk factors

Risk factors affecting staging include the following: (1) human chorionic gonadotropin greater than 100,000 IU/mL and (2) duration of disease longer than 6 months from termination of antecedent pregnancy. The following factors should be considered and noted in reporting: (1) prior chemotherapy has been given for known gestational trophoblastic tumor, (2) placental-site tumors should be reported separately, (3) histologic verification of disease is not required.

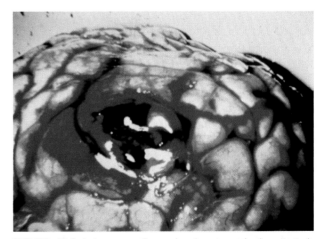

FIGURE 42-5 Autopsy specimen showing a cerebral metastasis from choriocarcinoma. Brain metastases carry a high mortality.

room with general or regional anesthesia. **Intravenous oxytocin is given simultaneously to help stimulate uterine contractions and reduce blood loss.** This technique is associated with a low incidence of uterine perforation and trophoblastic embolization.

Most patients have an uncomplicated course in the immediate postoperative period. Some require transfusion, however, because of excessive blood loss. Abnormal clotting parameters should be treated with fresh frozen plasma and platelet transfusions, as indicated. Rarely, a patient can experience acute respiratory distress from trophoblastic embolization or fluid overload. Such patients may require respiratory support via a ventilator and careful cardiopulmonary monitoring.

Monitoring Levels of the β-Subunit of Human Chorionic Gonadotropin

Following the evacuation of a hydatidiform mole, the patient must be monitored with weekly serum assays of β-hCG until three consecutive levels have been normal. Monthly β-hCG levels should then be followed until three consecutive levels have been normal. Because β-hCG drops to a low level, a nonspecific pregnancy test cannot be used, because of the possibility of cross-reactivity with luteinizing hormone. The radioimmunoassay, sensitive to levels of 1 to 5 mIU/mL, should be used. Following the evacuation, the β-hCG levels should steadily decline to undetectable levels, usually within 12 to 16 weeks. A normal regression curve for β-hCG levels following evacuation of a molar pregnancy is shown in Figure 42-6.

Chemotherapy

Prophylactic chemotherapy is not indicated in patients with molar pregnancy, because 90% of these individuals have spontaneous remissions. If the β-hCG levels plateau or rise at any time, chemotherapy should be initiated. This is discussed later in this chapter.

Partial Mole

The incomplete or partial mole is usually associated with a developing fetus. **Patients with a partial mole display most of the pathologic and clinical features of patients with a complete mole, although usually in a less severe form.** Partial moles are usually diagnosed later than are complete moles, and they generally present as a spontaneous or missed abortion.

It is unusual for a partial mole to be detected before the spontaneous termination of a pregnancy. **Ultrasonography performed for other indications may indicate possible "molar degeneration" of the placenta associated with the developing fetus. Under these circumstances, amniocentesis should be performed to determine whether the karyotype of the coexisting fetus is normal.**

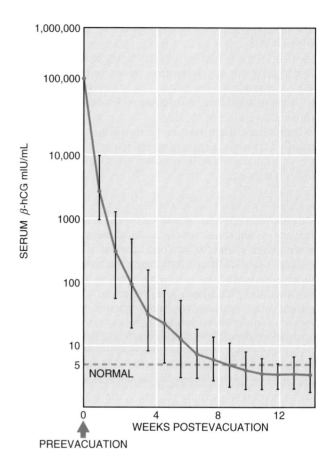

FIGURE 42-6 Normal regression curve of β-human chorionic gonadotropin (β-hCG) following molar evacuation. (Adapted from Morrow CP, Kletzky OA, Disaia PJ, et al: Clinical and laboratory correlates of molar pregnancy and trophoblastic disease. *Am J Obstet Gynecol* 128:428, 1977.)

Uterine enlargement is much less common; **most patients with partial moles are actually "small for dates."** When preeclampsia occurs with a partial mole, it may be severe, but the condition usually occurs between 17 and 22 weeks' gestation, about 1 month later than with a complete mole. The most striking difference between partial and complete moles is related to the malignant potential of the two lesions. **Partial moles rarely metastasize, and only rarely is there the need for chemotherapy because of β-hCG levels that have plateaued or risen.**

Invasive Mole

An invasive mole is usually a locally invasive tumor. It constitutes about 5-10% of all molar pregnancies, representing the majority of those with persistent β-hCG levels after molar evacuation. The lesion may penetrate the entire myometrium, rupture through the uterus, and result in hemorrhage into the broad ligament or peritoneal cavity. **Rarely is an invasive mole associated** with metastases, particularly to the vagina or lungs, although brain metastases have been documented.

Histologic confirmation of an invasive mole is almost always made at the time of hysterectomy. The latter is usually performed in patients with persistent β-hCG levels following evacuation of a molar pregnancy or in patients with persistent titers despite chemotherapy who have no evidence of metastatic disease. The hysterectomy is usually curative.

Placental Site Trophoblastic Tumor

Placental site trophoblastic tumor is an uncommon but important variant of GTD that consists predominantly of an intermediate trophoblast and a few syncytial elements. These tumors produce small amounts of hCG and human placental lactogen relative to their mass, tend to remain confined to the uterus, and metastasize late in their course. In contrast to other trophoblastic tumors, placental site tumors are relatively insensitive to chemotherapy, so surgical resection of disease is important.

Choriocarcinoma

The frankly malignant form of GTN is choriocarcinoma. **About one-half of patients with gestational choriocarcinoma have had a preceding molar pregnancy. In the remaining patients, the disease is preceded by a spontaneous or induced abortion, ectopic pregnancy, or normal pregnancy.** Trophoblastic disease following a normal pregnancy is always choriocarcinoma. The tumor has a tendency to disseminate hematogenously, particularly to the lungs, vagina, brain, liver, kidneys, and gastrointestinal tract.

SYMPTOMS

Most patients with choriocarcinoma present with symptoms of metastatic disease. Vaginal bleeding is a common symptom of uterine choriocarcinoma or vaginal metastasis. Because of the gonadotropin excretion, amenorrhea may develop, simulating early pregnancy. **Hemoptysis, cough, or dyspnea** may occur as a result of lung metastasis. In the presence of central nervous system metastases, the patient may complain of **headaches, dizzy spells, "blacking out,"** or other symptoms referable to a space-occupying lesion in the brain. **Rectal bleeding** or "dark stools" could represent disease that has metastasized to the gastrointestinal tract.

SIGNS

The signs, like the symptoms, are common to many pathologic entities.

Uterine enlargement may be present, with blood coming through the os, as seen on examination with a speculum. A tumor metastatic to the vagina may present with a firm, discolored mass. Occasionally, the patient presents with an **acute abdomen because of rupture of the uterus, liver, or theca lutein cyst. Neurologic signs,** such as partial weakness or paralysis, dysphasia, aphasia, or unreactive pupils, indicate probable central nervous system involvement.

DIAGNOSIS

Choriocarcinoma is a great imitator of other diseases, so unless it follows a molar pregnancy, it may not be suspected. **In females of reproductive age, a β-hCG measurement to screen for choriocarcinoma should be performed when any unusual symptoms or signs develop.**

INVESTIGATIONS

If the β-hCG level is elevated, the workup of a patient with choriocarcinoma is the same as that for patients with hydatidiform mole, but it should also include a computed tomographic scan of the abdomen, pelvis, and head. In addition, a lumbar puncture should be performed if the computed tomographic scan of the brain is normal, because simultaneous evaluation of the β-hCG level in the cerebrospinal fluid and serum may allow detection of early cerebral metastases. **Because the β-subunit does not readily cross the blood–brain barrier, a ratio of serum to cerebrospinal fluid β-hCG levels of less than 40:1 suggests central nervous system involvement,** with secretion of the β-hCG directly into the cerebrospinal fluid.

Treatment of Gestational Trophoblastic Neoplasia

An approach to treatment of GTN with nonmetastatic (good prognosis) and metastatic (poor prognosis) disease follows.

NONMETASTATIC AND METASTATIC GESTATIONAL TROPHOBLASTIC NEOPLASIA WITH A GOOD PROGNOSIS

The chemotherapy most often employed is either methotrexate or actinomycin D (Box 42-4). Methotrexate is usually given as a daily dose for 5 consecutive days or every other day for 8 days, alternating with folinic acid (leucovorin). This folinic acid "rescue" regimen is associated with significantly less bone marrow, gastrointestinal, and liver toxicity. Actinomycin D is given for 5 consecutive days intravenously or every other week as a single dose.

In appropriately selected patients, hysterectomy may be the primary therapy for hydatidiform mole. Women older than 40 years of age have an increased incidence of choriocarcinoma after molar pregnancy. These patients may decrease their risk of malignant sequelae by undergoing a hysterectomy.

BOX 42-4

SINGLE-AGENT CHEMOTHERAPY FOR MOLAR PREGNANCY

Actinomycin D Treatment

5-Day Actinomycin D

Actinomycin D 12 µg/kg IV daily for 5 days
CBC, platelet count, SGOT determination daily

Pulse Actinomycin D

Actinomycin D 1.25 mg/m^2 every 2 wk

Methotrexate Treatment

5-Day Methotrexate

Methotrexate 0.4 mg/kg IV or IM daily for 5 days
CBC, platelet count daily

Pulse Methotrexate

Methotrexate 40 mg/m^2 IM weekly

Protocol for Methotrexate with Folinic Acid "Rescue"

Methotrexate 1 mg/kg/day IM or IV on days 1, 3, 5, and 7, followed 24 hr later by 0.1 mg/kg/day of folinic acid "rescue" on days 2, 4, 6, and 8

CBC, Complete blood count; *IM,* intramuscularly; *IV,* intravenously; *SGOT,* serum glutamic oxaloacetic transaminase.

METASTATIC GESTATIONAL TROPHOBLASTIC NEOPLASIA WITH A POOR PROGNOSIS

For patients with disease having a poor prognosis, combination chemotherapy is always used. A regimen that has been successfully employed is the **modified "Bagshawe" regimen,** which is a six-drug chemotherapy regimen. The drugs used include etoposide, actinomycin D, vincristine, cyclophosphamide, methotrexate, and folinic acid. For patients whose disease fails to improve with these agents, combinations of cisplatin and etoposide or vinblastine, with or without bleomycin, have been used.

In patients with disease metastatic to the brain or liver, radiation is often employed to these areas in conjunction with chemotherapy. The whole brain tolerates an initial dose of 2000 to 3000 centigray (cGy), with fractions of approximately 200 cGy per day. Together with systemic chemotherapy, a 50% cure rate can be expected. Liver metastases are usually treated with about 2000 cGy.

Surgery plays a role in selected cases, especially hysterectomy and pulmonary resection for chemotherapy-resistant disease.

FOLLOW-UP STUDIES

All patients should have weekly β-hCG level measurements until three normal levels have been measured.

Patients with a hydatidiform mole should then have monthly level measurements until six normal levels have been measured.

For patients with GTN who have a good prognosis, monthly measurements should be done until 12 normal levels have been recorded.

Patients with GTN who have a poor prognosis should have monthly levels until 24 normal measurements have been recorded.

Patients should use effective contraception during follow-up, following which they may attempt pregnancy.

If a patient's levels become normal and later are found to be rising, a second metastatic workup must be undertaken before the initiation of secondary therapy.

PROGNOSIS

About 95-100% of patients with GTN who have a good prognosis are cured of their disease. Patients with poor prognostic features can be expected to be cured in only 50-70% of cases. **The majority of the patients who die have brain or liver metastases.**

Index

Note: Page numbers followed by "*f*" refer to illustrations; page numbers followed by "*t*" refer to tables; page numbers followed by "*b*" refer to boxes.

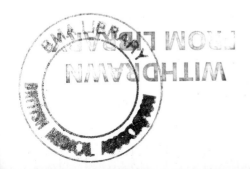